LEGAL & ETHICAL ISSUES IN NURSING

Fifth Edition

Legal & Ethical Issues in Nursing

Ginny Wacker Guido, JD, MSN, RN, FAAN
Regional Director—Nursing and Assistant Dean,
College of Nursing
Washington State University Vancouver
Vancouver, Washington

Pearson
Boston Columbus Indianapolis New York San Francisco Upper Saddle River
Amsterdam Cape Town Dubai London Madrid Milan Munich Paris Montreal Toronto
Delhi Mexico City Sao Paulo Sydney Hong Kong Seoul Singapore Taipei Tokyo

Library of Congress Cataloging-in-Publication Data

Guido, Ginny Wacker.
    Legal and ethical issues in nursing/Ginny Wacker Guido.—5th ed.
        p. cm.
    Includes bibliographical references and index.
    ISBN-13: 978-0-13-507998-0
    ISBN-10: 0-13-507998-5
    1. Nursing—Law and legislation—United States.   2. Nursing ethics—United States.   I. Title.
    [DNLM: 1. Legislation, Nursing—United States.   2. Ethics, Nursing—United States.   3. Jurisprudence—United States.
    4. Nursing—standards—United States. WY 33 AA1 G9L 2009]
    KF2915.N8G85 2009
    344.7304′14—dc22

2009018100

Publisher: Julie Levin Alexander
Publisher's Assistant: Regina Bruno
Editor-in-Chief: Maura Connor
Executive Acquisitions Editor: Pamela Fuller
Development Editor: Patricia Gillivan
Editorial Assistant: Jennifer Aranda
Managing Production Editor: Patrick Walsh
Production Liaison: Cathy O'Connell
Production Editor: Erin Melloy, S4Carlisle Publishing Services
Manufacturing Manager: Ilene Sanford
Art Director Cover: Jayne Conte
Cover Designer: Bruce Kenselaar
Director of Marketing: Karen Allman
Marketing Specialist: Michael Sirinides
Marketing Assistant: Crystal Gonzalez
Media Project Manager: Rachel Collett
Composition: S4Carlisle Publishing Services
Printer/Binder: STP Courier
Cover Printer: STP Courier
Cover Photos: Getty Images, Inc.

Notice: Care has been taken to confirm the accuracy of information presented in this book. The authors, editors, and the publisher, however, cannot accept any responsibility for errors or omissions or for consequences from application of the information in this book and make no warranty, express or implied, with respect to its contents.

The authors and publisher have exerted every effort to ensure that drug selections and dosages set forth in this text are in accord with current recommendations and practice at time of publication. However, in view of ongoing research, changes in government regulations, and the constant flow of information relating to drug therapy and drug reactions, the reader is urged to check the package inserts of all drugs for any change in indications of dosage and for added warnings and precautions. This is particularly important when the recommended agent is a new and/or infrequently employed drug.

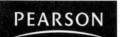

www.pearsonhighered.com

10 9 8 7 6 5 4 3 2
ISBN-10:   0-13-507998-5
ISBN-13: 978-0-13-507998-0

ABOUT THE AUTHOR

Ginny Wacker Guido has been active in legal and ethical issues in nursing for the past 30 years. She developed an interest in this area of nursing when she was teaching undergraduate nursing students in Texas, and her excitement for further knowledge and understanding of this content area encouraged her to pursue a doctorate of jurisprudence degree. She is active in nursing education and is currently employed as the Regional Director for Nursing and Assistant Dean, College of Nursing, Washington State University Vancouver. Over the years, she has authored numerous publications and presentations on legal and ethical issues, with special emphasis on a variety of clinical practice settings. She is also the editor of a newly published textbook on nursing care at the end of life.

As always, this book is lovingly dedicated to my family:

Ed, Jenny, and Joey Guido
and
Cecelia G. Wacker

REVIEWERS

We extend sincere thanks to our colleagues from schools of nursing throughout the country who gave their time generously to help create this textbook.

DeAnn Ambroson, MSN, MA, RN, LMSW, COI, CNE, PhD
Allen College
Waterloo, IA

Glenda Avery, APRN-BC, PhD
Troy University
Phenix City, AL

Debra Bacharz, RN, PhD
University of Saint Francis
Joliet, IL

Sarah Breier, RN, PhD
University of Missouri
Columbia, MO

Diane C. Bridge, BSN, MSN
Liberty University
Lynchburg, VA

Peggy N. Flannigan, RN, PhD
Bradley University
Peoria, IL

Joan Garity, RN, EdD
University of Massachusetts at Boston
Boston, MA

Karen Kovach, BSN, RN, PhD(c)
University of Pittsburgh
Pittsburgh, PA

Colleen M. Quinn, RN, MSN
Broward College
Pembroke Pines, FL

Penny Royal, RN-BC, DNP
Purdue University
West Lafayette, IN

Angela Stone Schmidt, MNSc, RNP, RN, PhD(c)
Arkansas State University
Jonesboro, AR

Kristi A. Wilkerson, RN, MSN
Southeastern Community College
West Burlington, IA

Mary Ellen Wurzbach, RN, MSN, FNP, PhD
University of Wisconsin
Oshkosh, WI

PREFACE

As with previous editions of the text, the fifth edition of *Legal & Ethical Issues in Nursing* reflects the continuing influence that the law, legal issues, and ethical issues have on the professional practice of the discipline of nursing. This influence indicates the expanding autonomous roles of nurses, whether in the public and community health arena, in acute care settings, or in long-term and hospice settings. It also reflects changes in the health care delivery structure, including mandatory nurse-patient ratios, the downsizing or closing of hospitals and other health care delivery agencies, and the continued shortage of professional nurses. These trends are occurring at the same time that professional accountability and responsibility are being enhanced as nurses complete newer degree programs in nursing, including the doctorate of nursing practice and the clinical nurse leader educational programs.

This edition of the text is, once again, written for practicing nurses as well as individuals studying in programs of nursing. The majority of the text addresses legal concepts and their application and is appropriate for nurses working in any clinical practice site. It is hoped that the text will continue to serve as a resource for practicing nurses and assist nurses in providing the most competent nursing care possible for the greatest number of patients. Nurses are again reminded that this text is not intended to take the place of procuring advice and counsel from practicing attorneys and agency legal services as needed; the book is meant to augment the role of legal counsel and assist nurses in understanding the legal process, potential liability as it relates to ethical nursing practice, and preventing possible lawsuits or other legal actions.

With each edition, some of the features are altered and others are retained. Popular features that were retained include the chapter previews, objectives, key terms, application exercises, guidelines, summaries, and the "You Be the Judge" feature at the conclusion of the chapter.

New to this edition is the inclusion of an ethical issues section toward the end of each chapter, highlighting some of the more frequently encountered ethical issues within an area of the law or clinical practice site. The chapter summary has also been reformatted so that key concepts in each of the chapters can readily be reviewed. As before, some of the content was placed in chapters where it was deemed most relevant and most natural, with the reader referred to these chapters for a review of content as appropriate. Finally, all of the content was updated, revised, and new content added so that this edition is as accurate and up-to-date as possible.

This edition of the text, recognizing that ethical issues often confront nurses in practice settings with the same frequency and depth as legal issues, begins with two chapters dedicated to ethical content. The first chapter provides a comprehensive review of ethical theories and principles and fully describes ethical committees as they exist within health care facilities. The second chapter applies this ethical content in nursing settings, addressing such issues as moral distress, the role of advocacy within nursing, and the application of therapeutic jurisprudence.

Part II of the text introduces the reader to the law and the judicial process, addressing sources and types of laws, the role of the court system in legal matters, and the importance of case law in determining standards of nursing care. This section of the text emphasizes the role of the nurse as an expert witness in defining professional standards of care and major legal doctrines and rules that underlie the practice of professional nursing.

Part III presents liability issues that can and do occur in all clinical practice areas, concluding with a chapter on professional liability insurance. Part IV contains multiple chapters that further explain how the law impacts professional nursing practice, beginning with a discussion of nurse practice acts and the scope of nursing practice. This chapter is followed by a chapter that describes the role of advanced nursing practice, including the newer nursing roles of the doctorate of nursing practice nurse and the clinical nurse leader. The remaining chapters in this section incorporate the multiple employment and federal laws that confront nursing, the role of the nurse manager, and laws as they pertain to delegation and supervision. The final chapters of the text, Part V, apply the impact of the law to individual clinical practice settings, including acute care settings, ambulatory and managed health care settings, public and community health settings, and long-term and home health care settings.

I am always amazed at how much I learn as I research and update new editions of this text. It is my hope that you will learn as much in reading and applying these materials.

Ginny Wacker Guido,
JD, MSN, RN, FAAN

CONTENTS

PART ONE

ETHICS

CHAPTER 1

Introduction to Ethics

PREVIEW

Nurses, in all practice arenas, continue to be confronted with the interplay between ethical and legal concepts, often asking themselves if the legal rights of the patients have been fully protected while also being sensitive to the individual's ethical rights. Though it may seem that these are two wholly separate issues, in reality, legal and ethical issues often intertwine and affect professional practice, and nurses must be knowledgeable about both concepts so that the legal and the ethical rights of patients are protected. For nurses, ethical issues may be encountered first, and thus they are presented first in this text.

Nurses continue to struggle with complex ethical concerns, including how to best ensure that the ethical issues of all involved persons are considered and evaluated. Though some of these decisions may seem more clear cut and easily made, all ethical situations demand considerable reflection and evaluation. Nurses often find themselves trapped in the midst of ethical dilemmas among physicians, patients, family members, and even their own peer groups. This chapter explores the distinction between law and ethics, describes the various ethical theories and principles employed in health care settings, and highlights the importance of institutional ethics committees.

LEARNING OUTCOMES
After completing this chapter, you should be able to:

1.1 Distinguish law from ethics.

1.2 Compare and contrast the different ethical theories that underlie ethical nursing practice.

1.3 Define and apply to nursing practice the ethical principles of autonomy, beneficence, nonmaleficence, veracity, fidelity, justice, paternalism, and respect for others.

1.4 Discuss the importance and role of hospital ethics committees and ethics grand rounds.

KEY TERMS

act deontology

act utilitarianism

applied ethics

autonomy

autonomy model

beneficence

compensatory justice

concept of double effect

deontological theories

detriment-benefit analysis

distributive (social) justice

duty ethics

ethical committees

ethics

fidelity

justice

metaethics

nonmaleficence

normative theories

paternalism (parentialism)

patient benefit model

principalism

relational ethics

respect for others

retributive or correctional justice

rule deontology

rule utilitarianism

situation ethics

social justice model

teleological theories

utilitarianism

veracity

virtue ethics

DEFINITIONS OF ETHICS AND VALUES

Ethics is the branch of philosophy concerned with evaluating human action. Derived from the Greek word "ethos," meaning character, customs, or habitual uses, ethics encompasses a process of determining right conduct from wrong. A broader conceptual definition is that ethics involves the principles or assumptions underpinning the way individuals or groups ought to conduct themselves; ethics is concerned with motives and attitudes and the relationship of these attitudes to the individual. Many people envision ethics as dealing solely with principles of morality, defining ethics in terms of what is good or desirable as opposed to that which is bad or undesirable. In such a context, morals and ethics might be viewed as interchangeable.

A more deliberate way of viewing morals encompasses the idea that morals are personal principles that are acquired from life experiences, family and peer relationships, religion, culture, and the law. Morals are generally seen as appropriate for routine decisions, but inadequate for resolving the more complex issues arising in clinical practice settings (Phillips, 2006). Ethics, what is right or wrong based on reason, can be distinguished from morals, what is considered right or wrong based on social custom. Thus ethics is a "system or philosophy of conduct and principles, whereas morals give the boundaries for acceptable behavior" (Barrocas, Yarbrough, Becnel, & Nelson, 2003, p. 37). In this context, ethics provides structure for placing conduct into action. As Levine (1977) noted over 30 years ago, ethical behavior is "the day-to-day expression of one's commitment to other persons and the ways in which human beings relate to one another in their daily interactions" (p. 846).

Using the broader conceptual definition interweaves values with ethics. Values are personal beliefs about the truths and worth of thoughts, objects, or behavior. Videbeck (2004) describes values as "abstract standards that give a person a sense of what is right and wrong and establish a code of conduct for living" (p. 4). Such abstract standards may include honesty, hard work, truthfulness, and sincerity. Values are usually derived from societal norms, family orientation, and religion; as one matures, values may change. Values may be subdivided into personal, professional, and societal value systems. Ultimately, one's values help determine the actions that one takes in his or her everyday life. To more fully understand one's own values, value clarification, a process aimed at understanding the nature of one's own value system and its vast impact on the individual, should take place.

Ethics, like values, is individualistic. One's values and ethics are fashioned by previous experiences, education, and the environment. It is essential to remember that nurses' ethics and values are just as individualistic as patients' ethics and values. How one views ethics may also change as the individual ages and matures or encounters new environments and cultures. Understanding one's ethics and values is the first step in understanding the ethics and values of others and in assuring the delivery of appropriate nursing care.

Similarly, health care values may change over time. For example, during the late 1960s the concept of resuscitation for all hospitalized individuals became a standard. The slogan, "A heart too good to die," was often cited as the reason that all hospitalized individuals, should they suffer a cardiac or respiratory arrest, had resuscitation efforts initiated rather then allowing the person to die without such heroics. As societal values changed, including allowing individuals to determine their own end-of-life decisions, the approach to resuscitation began to more accurately reflect the individual's value system as well as the value systems of individual practitioners.

DISTINCTION BETWEEN ETHICS AND THE LAW

The legal system is founded on rules and regulations that guide society in a formal and binding manner. Although made by individuals and capable of being changed, the legal system is a general foundation that gives continuing guidance to health care providers, regardless of their personal views and value system. For example, the law recognizes the competent patient's right to refuse therapy. The patient retains this right whether health care deliverers agree or disagree with the person's choice.

This right, however, is not absolute. If there are overriding state interests, treatment may be mandated against a patient's or parent's wishes. Cases concerning Jehovah's Witnesses, mandatory immunization statutes, and fluoridation of water enactments are three examples of overriding state interests.

Ethical values are subject to philosophical, moral, and individual interpretations. Both the health care provider and the health care recipient have a system of rights and values. Can one justify allowing competent adult patients to refuse therapy if the cost is their lives? Does ethics allow the refusal of health care therapies and treatments based on one's religious convictions that all medications and therapies are against God's law?

Most health care providers have difficulty in areas that transect both law and ethics, such as the issues of death and dying, genetics, abuse of others, and futility of health care. Table 1.1

TABLE 1.1 Distinction Between Law and Ethics

Concepts	Law	Ethics
Source	External to oneself; rules and regulations of society	Internal to oneself; values, beliefs, and individual interpretations
Concerns	Conduct and actions; what a person did or failed to do	Motives, attitudes, and culture; why one acted as one did
Interests	Society as a whole as opposed to the individual within society	Good of the individual within society as opposed to all of society
Enforcement	Courts, statutes, and boards of nursing	Ethics committees and professional organizations

Source: Adapted from *Legal Issues in Nursing: A Sourcebook for Practice,* by G. W. Guido, 1988, Norwalk, CT: Appleton and Lange.

distinguishes these two opposing concepts. To fully appreciate the interaction between these two areas, once must first understand ethics and ethical decision making.

ETHICAL THEORIES

Ethics involves systematizing, defending, and recommending concepts of appropriate and acceptable behaviors. A variety of different ethical theories have evolved over the course of history. The most basic distinction in ethics concerns non-normative and normative ethics. Non-normative ethics, often called **metaethics,** is the study of the kinds of things that exist in the universe. Metaethics attempts to analyze the meaning, justification, and inferences of moral concepts and statements, investigating where ethical principles originate and what they mean. The metaethical component of this type of ethical theory involves exploring whether moral values are external truths that exist in an "other-worldly" realm or merely aspects of human conventions. Said another way, metaethicists attempt to determine what is good or why one should act in a moralistic manner.

Normative theories of ethics concern norms or standards of behavior and values and the ultimate application of these norms or standards to everyday life, thus taking a more practical view to arrive at standards that regulate right and wrong conduct. Normative theories are universally applicable, involve questions and dilemmas requiring a choice of action, and entail a conflict of rights and obligations on the part of the decision makers. The key assumption in such ethical thought is that there is but one ultimate criterion of moral conduct.

Normative ethics may be subdivided into two overarching theories. **Deontological** (from the Greek *deon*, or "duty") **theories** derive norms and rules from the duties human beings owe one another by virtue of commitments that are made and roles that are assumed. Generally, deontologists hold that a sense of duty consists of rational respect for the fulfilling of one's obligations to other human beings. The greatest strength of this theory is its emphasis on the dignity of human beings.

Some ethicists further divide the deontological theory into virtue and duty theories. Essentially, **virtue ethics** places less emphasis on learning rules and regulations and more emphasis on the development of good character and habitually performing in this quality-character mode. For example, because a person has mastered the concept of benevolence, he or she will continue to act in a benevolent manner toward other persons. Virtues that are frequently listed by virtue ethicists include wisdom, courage, temperance, justice, fortitude, generosity, self-respect, good temper, and sincerity. The first four of these virtues were emphasized by Plato and dubbed *cardinal virtues* (Cooper, 1997). Virtue ethicists additionally denounce the acquisition of bad character traits, such as cowardice, insensibility, injustice, and vanity.

The second subdivision of the deontological theory is **duty ethics.** This subdivision is based on the premise that there are some obvious obligations that one has as a human being, such as the duty to not commit murder and to tell the truth. First advocated in the 17th century, these duties were classified as duties to God, duties to oneself, and duties to others (Frankena & Granrose, 1974). Duties to self include avoiding wronging others, treating people as equals, and promoting the good of others. More recently, W. D. Ross emphasized what he termed *prima facie duties*, which include:

- Fidelity, or the duty to keep promises
- Reparation, or the duty to compensate others when we harm them

- Gratitude, or the duty to thank those who help us
- Justice, or the duty to recognize merit
- Beneficence, or the duty to improve the conditions of others
- Self-improvement, or the duty to improve our virtue and intelligence
- Nonmaleficence, or the duty not to injure others (1930/2002, p. 6)

Deontological ethics look not to the consequences of an action, but to the intention of the action. It is one's good intentions that ultimately determine the praiseworthiness of the action. A branch of deontological ethics is commonly referred to as **situation ethics,** wherein the decision maker takes into account the unique characteristics of each individual, the caring relationship between the person and the caregiver, and the most humanistic course of action given the circumstances. Situation ethics are frequently relied on when the nurse has cared for a particular patient over a long time frame. Sometimes situation ethics are referred to as love ethics, conveying the deep respect for the human person.

Deontological theories can be subdivided into act and rule deontology. **Act deontology** is based on the personal moral values of the person making the ethical decision, whereas **rule deontology** is based on the belief that certain standards for ethical decisions transcend the individual's moral values. Example of such a universal rule could be "all human life has value" and "one should always tell the truth."

A second major division, **teleological** (from the Greek *telos*, or "end") **theories** derive norms or rules for conduct from the consequences of actions. Teleological theories became popular in the 18th century among philosophers who desired a means to quickly assess an action by appealing to experience rather than to a long list of questionable duties. Perhaps the most attractive feature of these theories was that one could quickly determine observable consequences of actions, with "right" consisting of actions that have good consequences and "wrong" consisting of actions that have bad consequences. Teleologists disagree, though, about how to determine the rightness or wrongness of an action.

This theory is often referred to as **utilitarianism**—what makes an action right or wrong is its utility, with useful actions bringing about the greatest good for the greatest number of people. An alternate way of viewing this theory is that the usefulness of an action is determined by the amount of happiness it brings.

Utilitarian ethics can be further subdivided into rule and act utilitarianism. **Rule utilitarianism** seeks the greatest happiness for all. It appeals to public agreement as a basis for objective judgment about the nature of happiness. **Act utilitarianism** attempts to determine, in a given situation, which course of action will bring about the greatest happiness, or the least harm and suffering, to a single individual. As such, utilitarianism makes happiness subjective.

A final way of viewing normative ethics is through applied ethics. **Applied ethics** is the branch of ethics that concerns the analysis of specific, controversial moral issues such as abortion, euthanasia, genetic manipulation of fetuses, and the status of unused frozen embryos. To be considered an applied ethical issue, two key characteristics are important. First, the issue needs to be controversial, with significant numbers of persons both for and against the issue. Second, the issue must concern a distinctly moral issue. Because of the controversial nature of the issues, resolution of these types of ethical issues is most often approached via the use of ethical principles, rather than through the application of ethical theories.

A theory that has emerged over the latter half of the 20th century is **principalism,** which incorporates various existing ethical principles and attempts to resolve conflicts by applying one or more of these principles. Ethical principles actually control professional decision making much more than do ethical theories, for a variety of reasons. McCarthy (2006) notes that the incorporation of principalism in nursing may emphasize the various ethical principles and create more "deliberate weighting of arguments" in a positive light (p. 163). Principles encompass basic premises from which rules are developed. Principles are the moral norms that nurses both demand and strive to implement daily in clinical practice settings. Each of the principles can be used solely, although it is much more common to see the principles used in combination.

Today, though, a newer framework appears to be evolving in assisting health care deliverers to apply ethical principles in clinical situations. Termed **relational ethics,** this concept redirects the issue of rights and responsibilities of the autonomous individual to view the relational commitments that individuals have to each other, thus moving the decisions into the context of the environment in which these decisions are made and creating a more "practical, action-oriented" ethics (Bergum & Dossetor, 2005). These authors note that there are four components of relational ethics: engagement, mutual respect, embodiment, and environment. Engagement requires that communications be expressed and considered that allow both the rational and emotional aspects of individuals' lives be included in ethical decision making. This component denotes a shared relationship with obligations and responsibilities to other persons. Mutual respect acknowledges differences and individuality, incorporating a broad understanding of culture and language as they affect ethical principles and issues. Embodiment reflects the connection needed between persons so that interactions between them are meaningful and fully acknowledged. Environment includes the breadth of the relationship, moving beyond individual personalities so that a broader relationship can be established and appreciated (Bergum & Dossetor, 2005). Relational ethics has been described in nursing using the terms *mutuality* and *caring* (Gadow, 1999).

Relational ethics is not meant to eliminate other ethical theories and guidelines, but to add a further method of understanding and applying a practical means of addressing the ethical issues that arise in everyday practice settings. Relational ethics, by engaging all parties to a potential dilemma, creates continued dialogue and consideration of all possible and realistic outcomes (Bergum & Dossetor, 2005).

ETHICAL PRINCIPLES

Nurses apply a variety of ethical principles in everyday clinical practice, some to a greater degree than others. Each principle is discussed separately in this chapter.

EXERCISE 1.1

In 1982, a woman in the United States gave birth to an infant who was severely retarded and who had multiple birth defects, including a separation of the esophagus from the stomach, resulting in the inability of the infant to receive oral nourishment. Although surgery could correct this deformity, the parents did not want to raise a severely retarded child and chose to deny consent for the surgery, food, and water. This decision was supported by the local court system and the infant died six days later. Using the ethical theories previously presented, conclude whether these theories assist in determining the ethics of allowing this infant to die. Do these theories support the refusal for surgical intervention? Does the fact that the infant was also severely retarded alter how the theories are applied? Could you argue, citing ethical grounds, that this child should have had the necessary surgery to correct this birth defect?

Autonomy addresses personal freedom and self-determination—the right to choose what will happen to one's own person. The legal doctrine of informed consent is a direct reflection of this principle. Autonomy involves health care deliverers' respect for patients' rights to make decisions affecting care and treatment, even if the health care deliverers do not agree with the decisions made. Because autonomy is not an absolute right, restrictions may be placed on a person's right to endanger others, as in the case of communicable diseases.

Beneficence states that the actions one takes should promote good. In caring for patients, *good* can be defined in a variety of ways, including allowing a patient to die without advanced life support. Conversely, *good* can also prompt nurses to encourage the patient to undergo extensive, painful treatment procedures if these procedures will increase both the quality and quantity of the patient's life. Nurses frequently consider this principle when viewing the long-term outcomes of invasive and noninvasive procedures. The difficulty with this principle is in defining *good*.

The corollary of beneficence, **nonmaleficence** states that one should do no harm, including the inflicting of pain and suffering on others. But not all actions bring intentional pain and suffering; often this aspect of harm is different for individual patients. Health care providers may employ the concept of a **detriment-benefit analysis** when the issue of nonmalificence is raised. Using such an analysis, the focus of the projected treatment or procedure is on the consequences of the benefits to the patient and not on the harm that occurs at the time of the intervention. An example is when a nurse gives a patient an injection for the relief of post-operative pain. Even though the injection imposes some degree of discomfort and suffering at the moment the injection is administered, the overall benefit is less suffering from the operative pain.

A second way to support interventions that may have harmful effects is through application of the **concept of double effect.** Four conditions must be present for this concept to be used. One, the action itself must be "good" or at least morally indifferent. Two, the practitioner must intend only a good effect. Three, the undesired effect must not be the means of attaining the good effect. Four, there is a proportional or favorable balance between the desirable and the undesirable effects of the action. Using this concept, one could be justified in administering a morphine drip in a terminally ill patient with pulmonary edema, as the desired effect is the relief of pain and suffering and not the further respiratory depression, which the medication will effect.

A means of distinguishing these two seemingly contradictory principles is that nonmaleficence is required, where beneficence is more a matter of individual choice. Ethicists often reserve the principle of nonmaleficence for issues of major impact, such as "Can one preserve the life of anencephalic infants merely as a source for organ transplantation?" Today, ethicists are concerning themselves with the issue of cloning, particularly cloning of human beings, and the negative effects that the Human Genome Project may have.

Veracity concerns truth telling and incorporates the concept that individuals should always tell the truth. This principle also compels that the whole truth be told. This principle is followed when one completely answers patients' questions, giving as much information as the patient and/or family can understand, and telling the patient when information is not available or known. An example of the difficulty in applying this principle occurs when nurses desire to convey knowledge that would enable the patient's autonomy in making a knowledgeable decision in an environment where family members are demanding that information be withheld from the patient. Often, the arguments that family members verbalize against giving the patient additional information center on their perceptions that the patient would forgo medical care if he or she knew the entire truth.

Fidelity is keeping one's promises or commitments. Staff members know not to promise patients what they cannot deliver or what they do not control, such as when the patient asks that nothing be done should he or she stop breathing, before consulting the patient's physician for such an order. Keeping one's promises may become an issue when a patient's family members are assured that they will be fully informed about their loved one's condition, yet emergencies occur and procedures must be implemented rapidly in order to prevent further complications.

Using the strictest definition, **paternalism** (also known as **parentialism**) involves making the final decisions for others and is often seen as an undesirable principle. Paternalism allows no collaboration in the decision-making process, but totally removes the decision from the patient or patient's family members. This principle, when used to assist in decision making with competent patients who lack the expertise or ability to fully comprehend data needed to make decisions, is generally seen as appropriate and acceptable. For example, when faced with a difficult decision, a patient may inquire what the nurse or physician would do in a similar case, allowing the health care deliverer to help in the decision-making process and further encouraging communication. When the entire decision is taken from the patient, the principle is to be avoided.

Justice states that people should be treated fairly and equally. Ideally, justice means giving to each person what he or she deserves, following a standard of rightness. Fairness often refers to the ability to judge without reference to one's feelings or interests, allowing each person to be treated equally. Generally, where people may differ is when decisions must be made about how benefits and burdens will be distributed among individuals. This principle frequently arises in times of short supplies or when there is competition for resources or benefits, such as when two equally deserving patients are awaiting a kidney transplant, when there is only one intensive care bed available and more than one individual requires intensive care monitoring, or when additional resources become available.

Justice may be subdivided into distributive justice, retributive or corrective justice, and compensatory justice. **Distributive justice** (also termed **social justice**) refers to the extent to which society ensures that benefits and burdens are distributed among society's members in ways that are fair and just. Disparities in health care delivery among various members of American society are frequently cited as not meeting distributive justice principles. **Retributive or correctional justice** refers to the extent to which punishments are fair and just, often cited when disciplinary outcomes appear to be very different for similar infractions of rules. **Compensatory justice** refers to the extent that people are fairly compensated for their injuries by those who have injured them, with just compensation proportional to the loss that has been inflicted on an individual. This latter type of justice forms the final issues in most medical malpractice suits and determines, once liability is shown, what fair and just compensation entails.

Respect for others, seen by many ethicists as the highest principle, incorporates all other principles. Respect for others acknowledges the right of individuals to make decisions and to live or die based on those decisions. Respect for others transcends cultural differences, gender issues, religious differences, and racial concerns. This principle is a core value underlying the Americans with Disabilities Act and several discrimination statutes. It is also the first principle enumerated in the American Nurses Association's *Code of Ethics for Nurses* (2001). Nurses positively reinforce this principle daily in actions with peers, interdisciplinary health team members, patients, and family members.

HOSPITAL ETHICS COMMITTEES

With the increasing numbers of legal and ethical dilemmas in patient situations today, health care providers often seek guidance with decision making. Perhaps one of the best solutions for both long-term and short-term ethical issues is the creation of an institutional ethics committee. **Ethical committees** can (1) provide structure and guidelines for potential problems, (2) serve as

GUIDELINES

Ethics

1. Recognize the difference between legal and ethical rights of individuals. While both concepts are important, if conflicts arise, legal rights must be afforded the patient.
2. Nurses understand and appreciate that their ethical views and values often differ greatly from those of the patient's culture and value system. Such an understanding allows nurses to remain objective when caring for patients and advocating for patients' decisions and desires.
3. When legal issues have not been addressed, nurses are guided by the ethics of the profession and personal values. There is never a time that ethics and values are not important considerations.
4. If the values of patients and nurses interfere with competent, quality nursing care, it is recommended that nurses remove themselves from those particular patients' care, if possible.
5. Ethical dilemmas have no perfect answers, just better answers. Legal questions have right and wrong answers. When in conflict, follow the established legal principles.
6. Know and follow the American Nurses Association's *Code of Ethics for Nurses* (2001).

EXERCISE 1.2

In the following examples, identify the ethical principles that would be appropriate for the nursing staff to employ.

1. Jody, an 8-year-old, has been admitted to an acute care hospital for an emergency appendectomy. Her parents have been given information about the surgery and what to expect in the immediate post-operative period. Three members of the nursing staff have also assured these anxious parents that they will be notified as soon as Jody is admitted to the post-anesthesia area or sooner if there are complications with the procedure.
2. Mrs. Hernandez, who speaks English as a second language, appears to be having difficulty understanding the discharge instructions that she was given prior to leaving her family doctor's office. The community health care nurse caring for Mrs. Hernandez has finally secured an interpreter to ensure that Mrs. Hernandez fully understands the instructions. The nurse also has the interpreter read the discharge instructions to the patient and the nurse answers all questions that Mrs. Hernandez asks.
3. Mr. Cho, a 72-year-old man, is admitted for acute lymphocytic leukemia. The hematologist caring for this patient has explained reasonable treatment options for an individual of Mr. Cho's age and general medical condition. His daughter, who is obviously distraught and unable to fully comprehend all that is happening, tearfully asks the nurse, "If it were your father, what would you do?" The nurse helps the daughter understand what the diagnosis means, the treatment options, and what would be a reasonable treatment option for Mr. Cho.
4. Jane is the nurse manager for a busy ICU. There are two patients awaiting admission to the ICU: one is a 42-year-old bank president admitted through the emergency center with a diagnosis of an acute myocardial infarction, and the second patient is an elderly woman who experienced a cardiac arrest in the general medical unit. Jane surveys all the patients already in the ICU and elects to contact Dr. Emerson about discharging Mr. Houseman so that there will be two beds available for the two patients awaiting admission.

an open forum for discussion, and (3) function as a true patient advocate by placing the patient at the core of the committee discussions.

To form such a group, if one does not already exist, the proposed committee should first begin as a bioethical study group so that ethical principles and theories as well as current issues can be explored by members of the group. The committee should be composed of nurses, physicians, clergy, clinical social workers, nutritional experts, pharmacists, administrative personnel, and legal experts. Adding this multidisciplinary aspect to the committee allows for varied perspectives from which to understand and broaden all members' understanding of ethics and their applications, as well as expanding possible committee outcomes (May, 2001). Once the committee has become active, individual patients or patients' family members may also be invited to the committee deliberations.

Ethics committees generally follow one of three distinct structures, though some institutional ethics committees blend the three structures, and others differ in their approach depending on the individual case:

1. The **autonomy model** facilitates decision making for the competent patient.
2. The **patient benefit model** uses substituted judgment and facilitates decision making for the incompetent patient.
3. The **social justice model** considers broad social issues and is accountable to the institution.

In most settings, ethics committees are a reality, in part because of the complex issues in health care. In 1992, the Joint Commission for the Accreditation of Healthcare Organizations (JCAHO) first mandated ethics committees or, in the alternative, other vehicles for addressing ethical concerns. Included in that JCAHO manual was a chapter on patient rights, further clarifying the important role of ethics committees.

These standards continue today. Standards that address the issues of a patient's participation in health care decisions, the creation of advanced directives, and the enactment of do-not-resuscitate orders and policies are included in the most current edition of the Joint Commission (JC, formerly the JCAHO) 2008 manual. The chapter's premise is that the hospital supports the rights of each patient and that the hospital's policies and procedures describe the means by which those rights are protected and exercised. The policies must also include a means for resolving conflicts in decision making and a description of the respective roles of physicians, nurses, and family members in decisions involving do-not-resuscitate orders or the withholding of treatment.

In many medical centers, ethical rounds, which are conducted on a weekly or monthly schedule, allow staff members who may be involved in later ethical dilemmas to begin viewing all the issues and become more comfortable with ethical issues and their resolutions. These ethical rounds serve as an alternative to ethics committees. Other institutions, to meet the requirements of the JC employ a bioethics consultant or pastoral staff care member rather than having the more traditional ethics committee.

Perhaps the more relevant ethical questions are yet to be addressed, though at some point they must be addressed, and nursing must be among those addressing the issues. Health care providers continue to debate the ethics of individual patients, but reject the need to look at the ethics of the social system itself. Untold amounts of time and resources are spent on debating informed consent, autonomy, and discontinuance of life support systems, while seemingly nothing is done about debating the ethics of the entire system, including the over- or undersupply of acute care beds in various geographical settings, continual duplication of revenue-generating procedures, and overproduction of medical specialists, to name but a few of the more pressing issues. As Richard Lamm so aptly stated, "The sum total of much of our ethical thinking about individuals has given us an unethical health care system" (1999, p. 14).

EXERCISE 1.3

If your health care institution has an ethics committee, attend one of its sessions. Who is on the committee? Were family members or patients allowed to attend? Which structural model was used in the deliberations? Was their final recommendation consistent with your expectations?

SUMMARY

- Ethics involves the principles or assumptions underpinning the way individuals or groups should conduct themselves and is concerned with motives and attitudes and the relationship of these attitudes to the individual.
- Values are personal beliefs about the truths and worth of thoughts, objects, or behavior.
- Ethical theories that pertain to clinical practice settings are generally divided into two overarching theories: deontological and teleological theories.
- Deontological theories derive norms and rules from the duties that human beings owe one another by virtue of commitments that are made or roles that are assumed.
- Teleological theories derive norms or rules for conduct from the consequences of actions.
- Ethical principles that are applicable in clinical settings include:
  - Autonomy, addressing personal freedom and self-determination
  - Beneficence, supporting actions that promote good

- Nonmaleficence, the concept that one should do no harm
- Veracity, concerning truth telling
- Fidelity, concerning keeping one's promises
- Paternalism, used to assist individuals in decision making
- Justice, the concept that all people should be treated fairly and equally
- Respect for others, which incorporates all other principles and transcends cultural differences, gender issues, religious differences, and racial concerns.
- Institutional ethics committees provide structure and guidelines for potential issues, serve as an open forum for discussion, and function as true patient advocates by placing the patient at the core of the committee discussions.
- Models for institutional ethics committees include the autonomy, patient benefit, and social justice models.

APPLY YOUR ETHICAL KNOWLEDGE

1. How can the professional nurse begin to ensure that ethical concepts will be applied in clinical practice settings?
2. Do professional nurses use ethical theories or ethical principles in clinical practice settings?

3. What types of ethical dilemmas do professional nurses face on a daily basis? How are these resolved so that it becomes a "win-win" situation for all involved parties?

YOU BE THE JUDGE

Until recently, Tyrell Dueck was a normal eighth grader in Canada, hoping that his favorite team would win the Stanley Cup for the third time. Then, early in the school year, he slipped climbing out of the shower and discovered a lump on his leg. He was then diagnosed with bone cancer.

After receiving two rounds of chemotherapy and being told that further therapy would mean the amputation of his leg, he announced that he wanted therapy stopped. He and his parents, devout fundamentalist Christians, decided to leave his health in God's hands and seek alternative therapy. The decision sparked a court battle between his parents, who supported Tyrell's decision, and the health care team, who sought to compel continued medical treatment and the planned amputation. The battle ultimately ended when doctors said that his cancer had spread to his lungs and that there was little more that could be done for Tyrell.

QUESTIONS

1. What are the compelling rights that this case addresses?
2. Whose rights should take precedence?
3. Does a child (specifically, this competent 14-year-old) have the right to determine what will happen to him? Should he ethically have this right?
4. How would you have decided the outcome if Tyrell's disease state had not intervened?

REFERFNCES

American Nurses Association. (2001). *Code of ethics for nurses with interpretive statements.* Washington, DC: Author.

Barrocas, A., Yarbrough, G., Becnel, P., & Nelson, J. E. (2003). Ethical and legal issues in nutrition support of the geriatric patient: The can, should, and must of nutrition Support. *Nutrition in Clinical Practice, 18*(1), 37–47.

Bergum, V., & Dossetor, J. (2005). *Relational ethics: The full meaning of respect.* Hagerstown, MD: University Publishing Group.

Cooper, J. M. (Ed.). (1997). *Plato: Complete works.* Indianapolis, ID: Hackett Publishing Company.

Frankena, W. K., & Granrose, J. T. (Eds.). (1974). *Introductory reading in ethics.* Englewood Cliffs, NJ: Prentice Hall.

Gadow, S. (1999). Relational narratives: The postmodern turn in nursing ethics. *Scholarly Inquiry for Nursing Practice, 13*, 57–70.

Joint Commission for Accreditation of Healthcare Organizations (JCAHO). (1992). *Accreditation manual for hospitals.* Oakbrook Terrace, IL: Author.

Lamm, R. (1999). The ethics of excess. *Hastings Center Report, 24*(6), 14.

Levine, M. (1977). Ethics: Nursing ethics and the ethical nurse. *American Journal of Nursing, 77,* 845–849.

May, T. (2001). The breath of bioethics: Core areas of bioethics education for hospital ethics committees. *Journal of Medicine and Philosophy, 26*(1), 101–118.

McCarthy, J. (2006). A pluralist view of nursing ethics. *Nursing Philosophy, 7,* 157–164.

Phillips, S. (2006). Ethical decision-making when caring for the noncompliant patient. *Journal of Infusion Nursing, 29*(5), 266–271.

Ross, W. D. (1930/2002). *The right and the good.* Oxford: Oxford University Press.

Videbeck, S. L. (2004). *Psychiatric mental health nursing* (2nd ed.). Philadelphia: Lippincott, Williams and Wilkins.

CHAPTER 2

Application of Ethics in Nursing Practice Settings

PREVIEW

Understanding ethical theories and principles is a first step in applying these concepts in nursing practice settings. As previously noted, the more familiar one is with ethical theories and principles, the more confident and prepared the individual becomes in applying these concepts. An appreciation of one's values and professional codes of ethics are equally essential in appropriately applying ethics in clinical settings. Additionally, knowledge of decision-making models to assist in resolving complex ethical dilemmas, how the nurse can employ the advocacy role, situations when moral distress may occur, and how therapeutic jurisprudence may begin to lessen the impact of future dilemmas is important in resolving ethical dilemmas. This chapter explores these concepts and concludes with a section outlining how implementing health policy complements nurses' ability to resolve ethical issues in everyday clinical practice settings.

LEARNING OUTCOMES
After completing this chapter, you should be able to:

2.1 Examine professional codes of ethics.

2.2 Analyze and apply decision-making models in resolving ethical dilemmas, with specific application of the MORAL model.

2.3 Evaluate slippery slope arguments in the application of ethical decision-making models.

2.4 Analyze the role of advocacy from an ethical perspective.

2.5 Describe moral distress, its affect on nurses in practice settings, and ways of coping with moral distress.

2.6 Discuss therapeutic jurisprudence and its place in ethical decision making.

2.7 Examine the role of health policy as it relates to resolving ethical dilemmas in nursing practice.

KEY TERMS

advocacy

health policy

moral dilemma

moral distress

MORAL model

moral stress

moral uncertainty

professional codes of ethics

respect for persons model

rights protection model

(autonomy model)

slippery slope argument

therapeutic jurisprudence

values-based decision model

PROFESSIONAL CODES OF ETHICS

Professional codes of ethics are formal statements that serve to articulate the values and beliefs of a given discipline, serving as a standard for professional actions and reflecting the ethical principles shared by its members. Professional codes of ethics generally serve the following purposes:

- Inform the public of the minimum standards acceptable for conduct by members of the discipline and assist the public in understanding a discipline's professional responsibilities.
- Outline the major ethical considerations of the profession.
- Provide to its members guidelines for professional practice.
- Serve as a guide for the discipline's self-regulation.

Codes of ethics have been established for nurses at the international, national, and state levels by professional nursing organizations. The International Council of Nurses (ICN), headquartered in Geneva, Switzerland, first established an international code of ethics in 1953. The code was most recently revised in 2006. The *ICN Code of Ethics for Nurses* (2006) has four basic elements that outline nurses' standards of ethical conduct, including nurses and people, nurses and practice, nurses and the profession, and nurses and co-workers. Each of these four basic elements has statements that assist the nurse in understanding his or her ethical responsibilities (ICN, 2006). Currently, the ICN code is available in 12 different languages.

On the national level, the American Nurses Association (ANA) first published a code for nurses in 1950, most recently revised in 2001. The *Code of Ethics for Nurses with Interpretive Statements* (ANA, 2001) has nine provisions regarding the professional practice of nursing and serves the following purposes:

- It is a succinct statement of the ethical obligations and duties of every individual who enters the nursing profession.
- It is the profession's nonnegotiable ethical standard.
- It is an expression of nursing's own understanding of its commitment to society. (p. 5)

The first three provisions of the code address fundamental values and commitments, the next three provisions address loyalty and one's duties, and the final three provisions address obligations and duties beyond individual nurse–patient encounters.

Along with establishing the ethical standard for the disciplines, the nursing codes of ethics provide a basis for ethical analysis and decision making in clinical situations. When making ethical decisions, consideration of the codes' mandates along with an understanding of ethical theories and principles, values, and decision-making models are essential.

ETHICAL DECISION-MAKING FRAMEWORK

In clinical practice, nurses seldom rely on a single ethical principle when caring for patients. Often, the ethical principles that nurses employ every day in practice settings come into conflict with each other. For example, envision the scenario of an elderly but independent patient who cherishes his independence. As a caregiver, one must balance the need to preserve this independence (autonomy) while discussing with his family alternative living situations (beneficence).

For most nurses, formal ethical decision-making models are only considered when complex ethical dilemmas present in clinical settings. In truth, though, nurses use ethical decision-making models each time an ethical situation arises, though the decision-making model may not be acknowledged or fully appreciated. Ethical dilemmas involve situations where a choice must be made between alternatives that an individual perceives he or she can accept and reasonably justify on a moral plane or where there is not a more favorable or appropriate choice that dominates the situation (Beauchamp & Childress, 2001). One's ability to respond to ethical dilemmas may be influenced by four factors:

- the nurse's perception of his or her level of influence within the health care setting
- level of clinical expertise and competence
- degree of ethical concern
- past experience with ethics education (Hamric, 1999)

One way to begin resolving such dilemmas is through ethical decision-making frameworks. Ethical decision making involves reflection on the following questions:

- Who should make the choice?
- What are the possible options or courses of action?
- What are the available options or alternatives?
- What are the consequences, both good and bad, of all possible options?
- Which rules, obligations, and values should direct choices?
- What are the desired goals and outcomes? (Guido, 2006, p. 8)

When making ethical decisions, nurses need to combine all the elements using an orderly, systematic, and objective method. Ethical decision-making models assist in this process.

The various models for ethical decision making typically have 5 to 14 ordered steps that begin with fully comprehending the ethical dilemma and conclude with the evaluation of the implemented decision. Perhaps the easiest model to use at the bedside remains the **MORAL model.** The MORAL model was first published by Thiroux (1977) and later refined by Halloran (1982) for use in nursing practice settings. Many nurses prefer this model, as the letters of the acronym remind nurses of the subsequent steps of the model, and thus the model can easily be used in all patient care settings.

The model includes the following steps:

- M—Massage the dilemma. Identify and define issues in the dilemma. Consider the opinions of the major players—patients, family members, nurses, physicians, clergy, and other interdisciplinary health care members—as well as their value systems.
- O—Outline the options. Examine all options fully, including the less realistic and conflicting ones. Make two lists, identifying the pros and cons of all the options identified. This stage is designed to fully comprehend the options and alternatives available, not to make a final decision.

EXERCISE 2.1

Jody Smith, a retired nurse with three adult children and numerous adult grandchildren, lives alone in a small rural area. Her income is limited. Two months ago, she fell and broke her left hip. After surgery for an artificial hip replacement, she was transferred to a rehabilitation center, where she had a left-sided cerebrovascular accident (CVA). She was then readmitted to the acute care facility, where she has received aggressive therapy for the CVA.

Completely paralyzed on her left side, Mrs. Smith has decided that she no longer desires aggressive therapy and frequently asks the staff why she cannot die in peace. "The rehabilitation is so painful and I'll never walk again. What's the use?"

Both the doctors and her family are much more optimistic. The orthopedic surgeon is convinced that she will walk again, and the neurologist believes that she will make a full recovery and be able to return home and care for herself. Both doctors have excluded Mrs. Smith from their conversations, assuring her children that she will be "as good as new" and ignoring her requests to discontinue anticoagulant and rehabilitative therapy.

While not in a life-threatening condition, Mrs. Smith refuses to cooperate with the physical and occupational therapists and to take her medications. She also refuses to perform simple tasks, relying on staff to meet her activities of daily living.

Using the MORAL model, how would you begin to resolve this dilemma? Does the *Code of Ethics* assist in resolving this dilemma: If so, which provisions are the most helpful?

- R—Resolve the dilemma. Review the issues and options, applying basic ethical principles to each option. Decide the best option based on the views of all those concerned in the dilemma.
- A—Act by applying the chosen option. This step is usually the most difficult because it requires actual implementation, whereas the previous steps had allowed for only dialogue and discussion.
- L—Look back and evaluate the entire process, including the implementation. No process is complete without a thorough evaluation. Ensure that all those involved are able to follow through on the final option. If not, a second decision may be required and the process must start again at the initial step.

Ethical decision making is always a process. To facilitate the process, use all available resources, including the ethics committee if the institution has one, and communicate with and support everyone involved in the process. Some decisions are easier to reach and support. It is important to allow sufficient time for the process so that a supportable option can be reached.

Varcoe et al. (2004) studied the meaning of ethics with particular focus on how ethics were enacted in nursing practice. They noted that nurses employed several different techniques in addressing ethical issues in clinical settings. Techniques that assisted the nurses in addressing ethical issues included more in-depth awareness of their own ethical values, in-depth understanding of their organizations' ethical values, working in between their own values and those of the organization, and working in between competing values and interests.

Nurses acknowledged that they experienced tension and conflict as they worked with patients, family members, and other health care providers, especially if the values of others contradicted their own values. Resources that these nurses sought included supportive colleagues, educators, and nursing managers. These same issues and resources are encountered as nurses confront ethical decision making in their practice settings. Decision-making models assist in providing guidance in reaching acceptable decisions for nurses involved in this process.

SLIPPERY SLOPE ARGUMENTS

When involved in ethical decision making, some nurses are reluctant to address issues for fear that what is an acceptable conclusion at the present time could later "slide" and become an unacceptable situation. Known to ethicists as a **slippery slope argument,** it suggests that an action will initiate a chain of events culminating in an undesirable event later in time without establishing or quantifying the relevant contingencies. Often, the basis for the slippery slope argument has little justification, but tends to be more speculative and presumes that there are no gray areas, but merely a definite transition from a certain point to an obvious conclusion. Examples of slippery slope arguments in bioethics include the debate over research using stem cells, the initiation of the Human Genome Project, the appropriateness of embryo cloning and in vitro fertilization, and allowing voluntary euthanasia.

For example, individuals argue that allowing voluntary euthanasia will lead to active euthanasia of patients who do not want to voluntarily end their lives or that it will actually lead to euthanasia without a patient's knowledge that such an intervention is being considered. Using a decision-making model to arrive at acceptable ethical solutions assists the nurse in avoiding being caught in a slippery slope argument.

ADVOCACY AS A NURSING ROLE

Advocacy concerns the active support of a cause or issue that has importance. Advocates are those who defend and speak for such a cause or issue. In nursing, one frequently addresses the role of the nurse in advocating for the legal rights of patients; equally important, though, is that nurses advocate for the ethical concerns of patients and peers.

Fowler and Levine-Ariff (1987) identified three models of advocacy that are still employed in clinical practice settings. The **rights protection model** is perhaps the best known model of advocacy. In this model, nurses advocate for the legal and ethical rights of the patient. Often seen as an **autonomy model,** nurses assist patients in asserting their autonomy rights, for example, in assisting an individual patient to successfully help health care providers understand why he or she does not want surgical intervention for coronary artery disease, but will accept medical management for the disease. Inherent in this model is the concept that actions taken promote the patient's best interest, coinciding with the interests expressed by the patient himself or herself. The third principle in the American Nurses Association's *Code of Ethics* (2001) reinforces this mandate: "The nurse promotes, advocates for, and strives to protect the health, safety, and rights of the patient" (p. 12).

A second approach to advocacy is the **values-based decision model.** Using this approach, the nurse assists the patient by discussing his or her needs and desires and helps the patient make choices that are most consistent with the patient's values, lifestyle, and desires. This model is predicated on the sharing of information and assisting the individual to become empowered to speak on his or her own behalf rather than relying on the nurse to speak or defend these rights. Thus, the patient is assisted to exert his or her right to autonomy and self-determination. Expressed differently, the model allows nurses to speak for patients in a manner in which the patient would speak for himself or herself if he or she could.

The third model is the **respect for persons model,** sometimes known as the patient-advocate model. Though not as fully developed as the two previous models, this model centers on inherent human dignity and the respect that is owed all persons. In this model, the nurse, valuing the human person who is involved, acts to protect the rights, dignity, and choices of the patient. If the patient is not able to assist in making decisions about his or her care and treatments, the nurse advocates for the best interests of the patient. The ultimate goal of this model is to promote the autonomy and individual uniqueness of the patient.

The American jurisprudence system has continually enforced the role of nurses as patient advocates through multiple court decisions, thus creating both the ethical and legal obligation of nurses to serve in this role. Recent court decisions include *Baby Doe v. (Confidential) Hospital* (2007); *Confidential v. Confidential* (2007); *Confidential v. Confidential* (2008); *Jaynes v. Centura Health Corporation* (2006); *Martin v. Abilene Regional Medical Center* (2006); and *Rettger v. UPMC* (2008). In *Baby Doe*, the court noted that the experienced labor and delivery nurses could plainly see that the first-year medical resident was not competently directing the mother's late-stage delivery and failed to alert more experienced physicians, who were literally a few steps away from the patient in another part of the labor and delivery suite. The court noted that when the fetal monitor tracing indicated no fetal heart rate, the first-year resident did not appreciate the extreme emergency nor was the resident able to respond appropriately when it became apparent that the umbilical cord was completely wrapped around the neck of the infant. At that point, the nurses had an obligation to serve as the patient's advocate and summon expert assistance.

In *Martin*, a patient who had been hospitalized for a coronary artery stent was discharged with information about how to begin Plavix therapy. There was, though, no prescription for Plavix in the discharge orders. The court noted that general principles of nursing practice require the nurse, as a patient advocate, to question any obvious inconsistencies in a physician's orders and to clarify any order or treatment regimen that the nurse has reason to believe is inaccurate. In this case, the medication error was not detected until after the patient was rehospitalized for an occluded coronary artery stent.

In *Confidential* (2008), the attending physician's assistant failed to diagnose a staphylococcal infection in a 4-year-old girl who presented with a fever of 103.1°F, petechial rash, diminished capillary refill, elevated heart rate, low oxygen saturation, and lethargy. The child had been seen in the emergency department by a physician's assistant, who sent the child home with instructions for the parents to take her to a children's clinic. Though the nurse triaged the patient as urgent, nursing personnel did not advocate for a further evaluation of the child by an attending physician before the child was discharged. The court held that the nursing personnel were negligent in not advocating that the emergency department physician see the child and that appropriate laboratory work was done before the child was allowed to leave the emergency center.

The *Rettger* case noted that despite the fact that an acute care hospital did not have a chain-of-command procedure detailing how a nurse was to communicate in emergency situations, the nurse should have known that there was a need to advocate for a 24-year-old-patient with a left-sided occipital brain tumor who suddenly developed a high fever, was short of breath, and had a blood pressure of 190/90. When the attending physician merely ordered Dilaudid and refused to see the patient, the nurse should have taken aggressive action to see that immediate action was taken.

In *Confidential* (2007), the court applauded the nurse for acting as the patient's advocate and continually alerting physicians and nursing supervisory personnel of the critical nature of a pediatric patient. Finally, in *Jaynes*, the court acknowledged that the nurse did have a duty to advocate for a patient, consistent with professional standards as outlined in the American Nurses Association *Code of Ethics* and the American Association of Critical-Care Nurses' *Role of the Critical Care Nurse*.

GUIDELINES

Acting as a Patient Advocate

1. Nurses should be aware of hospital policies and protocols, as well as acceptable standards of care. Question physicians when orders are contrary to the accepted standard of care or you believe following the order could harm the patient. Do not be intimidated into following orders, but use your professional and independent judgment. If physicians persist or refuse to change the order, consult nursing supervisory personnel.

2. In emergency situations in which the nurse believes that following the physician's order could result in harm to the patient, the nurse should refuse to follow the order, ensure patient safety and appropriate nursing care, then notify nursing supervisors and administrative supervisors.

3. If the patient is discharged early and such early discharge could cause direct harm to the patient, voice your concern to the attending physician and nursing supervisor. Remember, you have a duty to attempt to prevent early discharges if the patient's safety and well-being will be compromised.

4. Discharge planning and instruction must begin early, starting when the patient is first admitted and be completed before the patient's discharge. Include in your teaching potential complications for which the patient/family member must be alert and what to do if signs and symptoms of complications arise. Give the patient written instructions, if available, and carefully document your instructions in the patient's medical record.

5. The patient is your priority concern, and nurses have an affirmative duty to serve as patient advocates.

EXERCISE 2.2

In your clinical setting, consider how many times and ways in which you acted as a patient or family advocate. Which model did you follow in advocating for the patient: rights protection model, values-based model, or respect for persons model? Would having used a different model have changed the outcome? Were there also instances when you chose not to be an advocate for a particular patient? What circumstances or events prevented you from serving in this role?

MORAL DISTRESS

Nurses experience stress in clinical practice settings as they are confronted with situations involving ethical dilemmas. **Moral stress** most often occurs when faced with situations in which two ethical principles compete, such as when the nurse is balancing the patient's autonomy issues with attempting to do what the nurse knows is in the patient's best interest. Though the dilemmas are stressful, nurses can and do make decisions and appropriately implement those decisions.

Moral distress, first described within the discipline of nursing by Jameton (1984), is a painful state of imbalance seen when nurses make a moral decision, but are unable to implement the decision because of real or perceived institutional constraints. Jameton acknowledged that there are three categories in this phenomenon: moral uncertainty, moral dilemma, and moral distress. **Moral uncertainty** is characterized by an uneasy feeling wherein the individual questions the right course of action. Generally, this uncertainty is short lived. **Moral dilemma,** according to Jameton (1984), is characterized by conflicting but morally justifiable courses of action. In such a dilemma, the individual is uncertain about which course of action should be enacted. Moral distress involves the individual knowing the ethical course of action to take, but the individual cannot implement the action because of institutional obstacles.

Seen as a major issue in nursing today, moral distress is experienced when nurses are unable to provide what they perceive to be best for a given patient. Examples of moral distress include constraints caused by financial pressures, limited patient care resources, disagreements among family members regarding patient interventions, and/or limitations imposed by primary health care providers. Moral distress may also be experienced when actions nurses perform violate their personal beliefs. Corley (2002) further noted that lack of adequate education in nursing ethics, specifically in being able to apply ethical decision-making models, may also account for some of the moral distress experienced by nurses in clinical settings.

Moral distress may be further subdivided into initial moral distress and reactive moral distress (Jameton, 1993). Nurses who are experiencing initial moral distress generally experience frustration, anger, and anxiety when confronted with value conflicts and institutional obstacles. This frustration, anger, and anxiety results from being prevented from doing what the nurse sees as the correct course of action. Reactive moral distress incorporates negative feelings when the nurse is unable to act on his or her initial distress. Reactive moral distress involves the inability to identify the ethical issues involved or may result from a lack of knowledge regarding possible alternative actions. Signs and symptoms of reactive moral distress include powerlessness, guilt, loss of self-worth, self-criticism, and low self-esteem and physiologic responses evidenced by crying, depression, loss of sleep, nightmares, and loss of appetite. In extreme cases, moral distress may culminate in moral outrage, causing burnout and inability to effectively care for patients.

The impact of moral distress among nurses can be quite serious. The American Nurses Association (2008):

> attributes moral distress as a significant cause of emotional suffering, possibly causing nurses to give poor nursing care, change positions frequently or leave the profession entirely . . . It may be a significant contributing factor to nurses' feelings of loss of integrity and dissatisfaction with their work. It may also contribute to problems with nurses' relationships with patient and others and may affect the quality, quantity, and cost of nursing care. (paragraph 9)

There are several strategies for beginning to address moral distress in clinical practice settings. Nurses who feel empowered to voice their ethical concerns within their institutions may experience less moral distress. Storch, Rodney, Brown, and Starzomski (2002) concluded that nurses will continue to feel moral distress in clinical settings. This conclusion was based on the participant nurses' ongoing concerns about the ethical nature of the institution, appropriate resource utilization, and lack of time for working directly with patients. However, these researchers noted that there is an important relationship between ethics and power. When nurses have the ability to raise legitimate ethical concerns, power is manifested in ways that affect quality practice environments and allow the nurses to better cope with moral distress.

Additional aspects that may assist in reducing moral distress among nurses in nursing care settings include educating nurses about the concept and offering opportunities to discuss moral distress in neutral settings. Information about moral distress should be part of orientation programs for new

EXERCISE 2.3

Mrs. R., an 87-year-old patient, has a past history that includes coronary artery disease, a previous stroke, and advanced Alzheimer's disease. Ten days ago, Mrs. R. was hospitalized for aspiration pneumonia and has been ventilator dependent since being admitted to the intensive care unit in a small rural hospital. Family members visit daily and have repeatedly voiced their concern to the nursing staff about the continued ventilator support that Mrs. R. is receiving, most notably the fact that Mrs. R. would never have wanted such care. They also note that Mrs. R. has not recognized them in past months and that they plan to visit less in future days, but can be contacted should any change in Mrs. R.'s condition occur.

Her primary physician has practiced in this community for multiple years; he is well known for his reluctance to discontinue any type of life support for any patient. When questioned, Dr. G.'s consistent response is, if this were his frail 92-year-old mother, he would prescribe the very same treatment for her. Dr. G. has now requested that the nurses talk to the family about moving Mrs. R. to a major medical center, where she can receive more advanced care, including vigorous rehabilitation and physical therapy, so that she may eventually return to a long-term nursing care facility.

How might the nurses in this scenario respond to the physician's request? How would this scenario begin to cause moral distress among the nursing staff, and what are the positive actions that the nurses might begin to take to prevent moral distress?

---

employees. Other means of reducing moral distress include identifying and addressing impediments to delivery of quality nursing care, incorporating conflict resolution and mediation techniques so that nurses can work through their concerns and bring them to closure, and allowing nurses to serve on the institution ethics committees. This latter means of working with moral distress encourages nurses not only to identify and understand resources that are available to them, but to also use these valuable resources. Finally, open communications, establishing systems that value the active participation of nurses in clinical and ethical decision making, and encouraging and rewarding collaborative teamwork assist nurses in appropriately dealing with moral distress.

Individual nurses have learned to employ additional strategies in preserving their dignity and in compensating patients for perceived wrongdoings (McCarthy & Deady, 2008). These strategies include self-care, including working on a part-time basis and accepting personal limitations, assertiveness, collective action, and reexamining basic nursing ethical values. Lutzen, Cronqvist, Magusson, and Andersson (2003) noted that moral distress can also be an energizing factor that results in the person having an enhanced feeling of accomplishment of professional goals. They concluded that moral distress may begin to make individuals more aware of their own beliefs and strive to handle ethical issues more effectively in future encounters.

THERAPEUTIC JURISPRUDENCE

Though not often discussed in relation to ethical perspectives, the concept of **therapeutic jurisprudence** serves to ensure that the rights of patients are met in a humane and just manner. Therapeutic jurisprudence, which has as its premise that the law and legal processes have physical and psychological effects on the people who are involved, focuses on the positive aspects that legal outcomes may have. Therapeutic jurisprudence is the interdisciplinary study of law as a social force—understanding law's impact on an individual's emotional life and psychological well-being. First coined as a phrase in the early 1990s by law professors Bruce Winick and David Wexler (Wexler & Winick, 1991), therapeutic jurisprudence begins to describe the extent to which law and ethics affect the way in which health care is delivered. Primarily, therapeutic jurisprudence acknowledges the fact that "well-being" is one of the many goals of the legal system and begins to ensure that this goal is integrated when one applies legal remedies and processes.

Therapeutic jurisprudence, similar to applying ethical behavior in clinical settings, challenges nurses to always consider the outcome of one's actions. Perhaps the one case study that best depicts the effect that therapeutic jurisprudence might have involves the case of Theresa (Terri) M. Schiavo. Ms. Schiavo suffered a cardiac arrest in February of 1990. She was without oxygen for approximately 11 minutes, or 5 to 7 minutes longer than most medical experts believe is possible to sustain without suffering severe and permanent brain damage. She was resuscitated and, at the insistence of her husband, was intubated, placed on a ventilator, and eventually received a tracheotomy. The cause of her cardiac arrest was later determined to be a severe electrolyte imbalance caused by an eating disorder, as Ms. Schiavo had lost approximately 140 pounds, going from 250 to 110 pounds, in the months prior to her cardiac arrest.

Ms. Schiavo was in a coma for the first 2 months after her cardiac arrest. She then regained some wakefulness and was eventually diagnosed as being in a persistent vegetative state (PVS). She was successfully weaned from the ventilator and was able to swallow her saliva, both reflexive behaviors. Characteristic of PVS, Ms. Schiavo was not able to eat food or drink liquids, and a permanent feeding tube was placed so that she could receive nutrition and hydration.

For the next few years, there was no challenge to the PVS diagnosis or to the appointment of her husband as her legal guardian. In 1995, a successful lawsuit was filed by her husband, Michael Schiavo, against the fertility physician who failed to detect her electrolyte imbalance. A judgment of $300,000 was awarded to Michael Schiavo for loss of companionship, and $700,000 was placed in a court-managed trust fund to maintain and provide for the future care of Ms. Schiavo. Also during this time frame, Ms. Schiavo continued with extensive rehabilitation, including aggressive physical, occupational, and speech therapies. She also underwent multiple medical tests, primarily to determine the extent of her brain damage. The tests and the specialists who were consulted determined that she had no recognition of those around her and that there was no hope for improvement in her overall condition, though she could be sustained on artificial nutrition and hydration for multiple years.

Sometime after this successful lawsuit, the close family relationship between Michael Schiavo and Terri's parents had begun to erode, and the public first became aware of Ms. Schiavo's plight. Challenges to the husband's appointment as guardian and her future care were at the heart of their dispute. As her court-appointed guardian noted:

> Thereafter, what is for millions of Americans a profoundly private matter catapulted a close, loving family into an internationally watched blood feud. The end product was a most public death for a very private individual. . . . Theresa was by all accounts a very shy, fun loving, and sweet woman who loved her husband and her parents very much. The family breach and public circus would have been anathema to her. (Wolfson, 2005, p. 17)

Once the media became aware of Ms. Schiavo's condition, court battles regarding the removal or retention of her feeding tube were initiated. During these hearings and trials, sufficient medical and legal evidence to show that Ms. Schiavo had been correctly diagnosed and that she would not have wanted to be kept alive by artificial means was introduced. Laws in the state of Florida, where Ms. Schiavo resided, allowed the removal of tubal nutrition and hydration in patients with PVS. The feeding tube was removed, but was later reinstated following a court order.

In 2003, there was a second removal of the feeding tube after a higher court overturned the lower-court decision that had caused the feeding tube to be reinserted. With this second removal, the Florida legislature passed what has become to be known as Terri's Law. This law gave the Florida governor the right to demand that the feeding tube be reinserted and also to appoint a special guardian to review the entire case. The special guardian ad litem was appointed in October, 2003, specifically to serve as an objective individual in preserving the rights and dignity of Ms. Schiavo. Terri's Law was later declared unconstitutional by the Florida Supreme Court, and the U.S. Supreme Court refused to overrule that decision. In early 2005, during the last weeks of Ms. Schiavo's life, the U.S. Congress attempted to move the issue to the federal rather than the Florida state court system. The federal district court in Florida and the 11th Circuit Court of Appeals ruled that there was insufficient evidence to create a new trial, and the U.S. Supreme Court refused to review the findings of these two lower courts (Wolfson, 2005). Ms. Schiavo died on March 31, 2005, at the age of 41.

Ethical issues confronting the nurses in this case centered on preserving the dignity and rights of Ms. Schiavo, who was during the entire time unable to express her wishes and desires. At odds were her husband, who continually asserted that Ms. Schiavo had always stated she did not want to live in such a state of existence, and her parents, who exerted the need to continue her nutrition and hydration. Perhaps what should have been more evident was the ethical issue of respect for autonomy in the person of Ms. Schiavo and the right of patients to autonomy and respect for their wishes, even beyond their loss of competence.

Because of the national media attention and high profile of this particular case, the Terri Schiavo outcome will most likely remain controversial for some period of time. For a variety of reasons, including the facts that the case employed medical consensus to arrive at a correct diagnosis, withstood multiple legal challenges to the constitutionality of the law, and sought to preserve the right of the individual to her autonomy, the "case is an example of good standards and processes in medicine, law, and ethics" (Perry, Churchill, & Kirshner, 2005, p. 747). The question that remains concerns whether understanding and applying therapeutic jurisprudence could have made the outcome more acceptable to the multiple individuals involved in the case and to the millions of individuals who followed the case on a daily basis. Perhaps one means of applying the principle of therapeutic jurisprudence would have been in reinforcing one of the basic principles of American law and ethical thought: self-determination and the right of autonomy for the individual involved is paramount and takes precedent over what others may have wanted (Perry et al., 2005).

The Schiavo case has also resulted in an increase in the numbers of individuals who are seeking additional information about durable powers of attorney for health care, living wills, and other legislative documents that will preserve their autonomy rights should a similar catastrophe befall them. Perhaps, as Kollas and Boyer-Kollas (2006) concluded, this is the "lasting legacy of the Schiavo case" (p. 1159).

HEALTH POLICY

Policy "encompasses the choices that a society, segment of society, or an organization makes regarding goals and priorities and the ways it will allocate resources" (Mason, Leavitt, & Chaffee, 2002, p. 8). Policy is shaped by politics and is defined as the principles that govern actions directed toward specific aims and outcomes, reflecting the values of those who set the policy. **Health policy** concerns the choices that a society or a part of that society makes in regard to the health and welfare of its citizens.

Policy, including health policy, is a process that views issues and possible solutions to those issues. Consistent in all policies are a number of aspects. Policy has generality in that it addresses more than one person and more than one set of circumstances. Policy has normativity in that it formalizes judgments about what course of action is better among alternatives and the rules under which those alternatives will be determined. Policy has scale in that policies apply at different levels of an organization or society, and policies at one level can supersede policies at lesser levels. Policy is always decided by someone, though it is sometimes difficult to determine by whom a policy was made.

Policy may be generated in a number of ways. Often, policy is generated by the workplace and revolves around relevant issues in the workplace, such as the designation of nonsmoking areas, need for family leave, or patient–nurse ratios. Policy may also be generated by governmental agencies on a local, regional, state, or federal level and may also include the designation of nonsmoking areas or family leave. Community groups, whether a neighborhood group or a more regional group, may generate policies that are critical to the welfare of the given community. Finally, policy may be generated through the efforts of professional organizations at local or national levels. Nurses have been and continue to be an integral part of policy development and implementation in all of these spheres.

A framework for beginning to address policy and the need for new or additional policy in a clinical setting begins by addressing a series of questions, including:

- What is the problem?
- Where is the process?
- How many are affected?
- What possible solutions could be proposed?
- What are the ethical arguments involved?
- At what level is the problem most effectively addressed?
- Who is in a position to make policy decisions?
- What are the obstacles to policy interventions?
- What resources are available?
- How can I get involved? (Malone, 2005, p. 138)

Nurses are patient advocates, and extending one's advocacy skills to the policy arena is the beginning of making a greater impact on patient outcomes (Williamson & Drummond, 2000). The framework as proposed by Malone assists nurses individually and collectively to better educate and empower their patients and themselves and address health care issues in a more effective manner (Malone, 2005).

EXERCISE 2.4

You are one of the staff registered nurses in a busy emergency department in a large metropolitan area. Several of the patients have existing chronic health care problems and frequently return to the emergency center for reevaluation and follow-up treatment. As a means of working with these patients, you and some of your co-workers have increased the amount of time spent in discussing discharge orders and the need for compliancy with discharge orders, prescriptions, and treatment plans. This has resulted in longer "wait times" for incoming patients, and the nurse manager has dictated that nurses are to limit their discharge instructions to essential facts, informing patients that they need to read the written materials and call their family health care providers if further problems arise.

Examine the preceding scenario from the perspective of health care policy. How would you begin to evaluate the need for the policy and the possible support or lack of support for the policy from your peers, nursing management, and others who might be affected by the policy? Do the 10 questions outlined by Malone (2005) assist in this process? Draft a proposed policy to address the issues you have identified.

SUMMARY

- Understanding ethical theories and principles is a first step in applying relevant concepts.
- Nurses use ethical decision-making models each time there is an ethical situation or dilemma, and the MORAL model is perhaps the easiest model to use in everyday clinical practice sites.
- Consisting of constructs similar to the nursing process, the MORAL model has five steps:
  - Massage the dilemma.
  - Outline the options.
  - Resolve the dilemma.
  - Act by applying the chosen option.
  - Look back and evaluate.
- The use of a decision-making model assists nurses in avoiding slippery slope arguments, the concept that an acceptable solution could later "slide" and become an unacceptable solution.
- Advocacy concerns the active support of a cause or issue and is both an ethical and a legal responsibility for nurses.

- There are three models of advocacy:
  - rights protection (autonomy) model
  - values-based decision model
  - respect for persons model
- Moral distress, defined as a painful state of imbalance seen when nurses make a moral decision but are unable to implement the decision because of real or perceived institutional constraints, can be positively addressed in the workplace.
- Therapeutic jurisprudence, which serves to ensure that the rights of patients are met in a humane and just manner, focuses on the positive aspects that legal outcomes may have in clinical settings and challenges nurses to find appropriate ethical applications when dealing with clinical issues that overlap ethics and law.
- Health policy concerns the choices that a society or a part of society makes in regard to the health and welfare of its citizens.
- Nurses are frequently involved in health policy issues in everyday clinical settings.

APPLY YOUR ETHICAL KNOWLEDGE

1. Describe an ethical dilemma in which you used the MORAL model, including how you resolved the issue.
2. How can nurses begin to prevent moral distress from occurring in clinical situations?
3. Which of the advocacy models is most often employed by nurses, and why? Do different models for

advocacy depend on the type of patient population with which one works?

4. What are the more effective means of implementing new health policies within acute care institutions?

YOU BE THE JUDGE

A 53-year-old man, experiencing chest pains, was admitted to an acute care facility for a diagnostic cardiac catheterization following the determination that he had experienced a mild heart attack. During the catheterization, a cardiac stent was deemed necessary and the patient was started on Plavix and IV heparin at 1,000 units per hour. A partial thromboplastin time (PTT), done 6 hours into the therapy, indicated a prolonged

clotting time and the heparin was reduced to 900 units per hour. No further PTT tests were ordered or done. At trial, the nurse noted that a repeat PPT could have been done without a direct physician's order.

Eleven hours after the heparin dose was reduced to 900 units per hour, the patient experienced a severe headache, profuse sweating, nausea, vomiting, and a markedly increased blood pressure. Though the cardiologist was promptly notified, he did not immediately see that patient, did not order new laboratory tests nor further decrease the dosage of the heparin drip, and waited several hours for a neurology consultation. The patient subsequently had a fatal intracranial bleed, which occurred as he was being transported for an emergency CT scan.

The patient's family named in the subsequent lawsuit the cardiologist, the cardiac care nurse, and the hospital.

Questions

1. Did the nurse act appropriately in notifying the cardiologist of the patient's initial distress when he experienced the severe headache, nausea, vomiting, and increased blood pressure?
2. Did the nurse fully appreciate the gravity of the situation, including possible complications when a patient is receiving an IV heparin drip?
3. Did the nurse, in this case, act as a patient advocate?
4. Who should be found to have liability in this case?

REFERENCES

American Nurses Association. (2001). *Code of ethics with interpretive statements.* Washington, DC: Author.

American Nurses Association. (2008). Moral distress among nurses. Available online at http://nursingworld .org/MainMenuCategories/ThePracticeofProfessional Nursing

Baby Doe v. (Confidential) Hospital, 2007 WL 1576360 (Sup. Ct. King Co., Washington, January 30, 2007).

Beauchamp, T. L., & Childress, J. E. (2001). *Principles of biomedical ethics* (5th ed.). New York: Oxford University Press.

Confidential v. Confidential, 2007 WL 2389560 (Sup. Ct. Los Angeles Co, California, July 26, 2007).

Confidential v. Confidential, 2008 WL 3166820 (Sup. Ct. Orange Co., California, January, 2008).

Corley, M. (2002). Nurse moral distress: A proposed theory and research agenda. *Nursing Ethics, 9,* 636–650.

Fowler, M. D. M., & Levine-Ariff, J. (1987). *Ethics at the bedside: A source book for the critical care nurse.* Philadelphia: J. B. Lippincott Company.

Guido, G. W. (2006). *Legal and ethical issues in nursing.* (4th ed.). Upper Saddle River, NJ: Pearson Prentice Hall.

Halloran, M. C. (1982). Rational ethical judgments utilizing a decision-making tool. *Heart and Lung, 11*(6), 566–570.

Hamric, A. B. (1999). The nurse as a moral agent in modern health care. *Nursing Outlook, 47,* 106.

International Council of Nurses. (2006). *The ICN code of ethics for nurses.* Geneva, Switzerland: Imprimerie Fornara.

Jameton, A. (1984). *Nursing practice: The ethical issues.* Englewood Cliffs, NJ: Prentice Hall.

Jameton, A. (1993). Dilemmas of moral distress: Moral responsibility and nursing practice. *American Association of Women's Health, Obstetric and Neonatal Nurse's Clinical Issues in Perinatal Women's Health Nursing, 4,* 542–551.

Jaynes v. Centura Health Corporation, 2006 WL 1171858 (Colo. App., May 4, 2006).

Kollas, C. D., & Boyer-Kollas, B. (2006). Closing the Schiavo case: An analysis of legal reasoning. *Journal of Palliative Medicine, 9*(5), 1145–1163.

Lutzen, K., Cronqvist, A., Magusson, A., & Andersson, L. (2003). Moral stress: Synthesis of a concept. *Nursing Ethics, 10,* 312–322.

Malone, R. E. (2005). Assessing the policy environment. *Policy, Politics, and Nursing Practice, 6*(2), 135–143.

Martin v. Abilene Regional Medical Center, 2006 WL 241509 (Tex. App., February 2, 2006).

Mason, D. J., Leavitt, J. K., & Chaffee, M. W. (2002). Policy and politics: A framework for action. In D. J. Mason, J. K. Leavitt, & M. W. Chaffee (Eds.), *Policy and politics in nursing and health care* (4th ed., pp. 1–18). St. Louis; MO: Saunders.

McCarthy, J., & Deady, R. (2008). Moral distress reconsidered. *Nursing Ethics, 15*(2), 254–262.

Perry, J. E., Churchill, L. R., & Kirshner, H. S. (2005). The Terri Schiavo case: Legal, ethical, and medical perspectives. *Annals of Internal Medicine, 143,* 744–748.

Rettger v. UPMC, 2008 WL 2663155 (Ct. Comm. Pl., Allegheny Co., Pennsylvania, May 23, 2008).

Storch, J. L., Rodney, P., Brown, H., & Starzomski, R. (2002). Listening to nurses' moral voices: Building a quality health care environment. *Canadian Journal of Nursing Leadership, 15*(4), 7–16.

Thiroux, J. (1977). *Ethics: Theory and practice.* Philadelphia: Macmillan.

Varcoe, C., Doane, G., Pauly, B., Rodney, P., Storch, J. L., Mahoney, K., McPherson, G., Brown, H., & Starzomski, R. (2004). Ethical practice in nursing: Working the in-betweens. *Journal of Advanced Nursing, 45*(3), 316–325.

Wexler, D. B., & Winick, B. J. (1991). *Essays in therapeutic jurisprudence.* Durham, NC: Carolina Academic Press.

Williamson, D., & Drummond, J. (2000). Enhancing low-income patients' capacities to promote their children's health: Education is not enough. *Public Health Nursing, 17*(2), 121–131.

Wolfson, J. (2005). Erring on the side of Theresa Schiavo: Reflections of the special guardian ad litem. *The Hastings Center Report, 35*(3), 16–19.

PART TWO

INTRODUCTION TO THE LAW AND THE JUDICIAL PROCESS

CHAPTER 3

Legal Concepts and the Judicial Process

PREVIEW

The disciplines of law and professional nursing have been officially integrated since the first mandatory nurse practice act was passed by the New York legislature in 1938. The nursing profession has continuously relied on statutory law for its right to exist on a licensure basis and on court decisions for interpretation of these statutes. The civil rights movement of the 1960s and the malpractice crisis of the 1970s led to a heightened legal-mindedness of the 1980s and 1990s, which continues to escalate in practice settings today. Professional practitioners must know, understand, and apply legal decisions and doctrines in their everyday nursing practice. Part of this understanding comes from an appreciation of the court system. This chapter presents an overview of the legal system, sources and types of laws, and the role of the American court system.

LEARNING OUTCOMES

After completing this chapter, you should be able to:

3.1 Define the term *law* and describe four sources from which law is derived, including constitutional, statutory, administrative, and judicial (decisional) law.

3.2 Compare and contrast the doctrines of precedent (stare decisis) and res judicata.

3.3 Define and give an application of jurisdiction, as well as a landmark decision.

3.4 List four ways in which laws can be changed.

3.5 Define classifications of law, including common, civil, criminal, public, and private law.

3.6 Distinguish between substantive and procedural law, and state why each is important to professional nursing practice.

3.7 Discuss due process and equal protection of the law.

3.8 Differentiate between questions of law and questions of fact in trial settings, and give an example of both.

3.9 List two types of jurisdictions, giving the definition and an example of each.

3.10 Explain the functions of the trial courts, appellate courts, and supreme courts at both the state and federal levels.

3.11 Describe statutes of limitation, their significance, and their purpose in law.

KEY TERMS

administrative laws
attorney general's opinion
civil law
common law
constitutional law
criminal law
discovery rule
due process of law
equal protection of the law
fact-finder
felonies
judicial (decisional) laws
jurisdiction
landmark decision

law
misdemeanors
personal jurisdiction
procedural law
public law
questions of fact
questions of law
rational basis test
res judicata
specific performance
stare decisis (precedent)
state appellate courts
    (courts of intermediate
    appeals)

state supreme court
statutes of limitations
statutory laws
subject-matter jurisdiction
substantive law
territorial jurisdiction
tort law
trial court
U.S. district courts
U.S. Supreme Court
writ of certiorari

DEFINITION OF LAW

Law has been defined in a variety of ways, using simple to complex terms. The word *law* is derived from the Anglo-Saxon term *lagu*, meaning that which is fixed or laid down. *Black's Law Dictionary* defines law as "a set of rules or principles" (Garner, 2004, p. 900) and subdivides law into constitutional, judicial, and legislative law. **Law,** though, may be more completely defined as the sum total of rules and regulations by which a society is governed. Law includes the rules and regulations established and enforced by custom within a given community, state, or nation. As such, law is created by people and exists to regulate all persons.

The actual definition of law is not as important as the impact of law on society. Law is made by individuals, whether as legislative bodies or by justices of the court. Law reflects the ever-changing needs and expectations of a given society and is therefore dynamic and fluid. Law is not an exact science, but rather an ongoing and organized system of change in response to current conditions and public expectations.

SOURCES OF LAW

Understanding the various sources of law assists in determining their impact on the nursing profession. Each of the three branches of the government has the authority and right to create laws, and these laws form the basis of the judicial system. Table 3.1 gives an overview of the various sources of law with examples.

TABLE 3.1 Sources of Law with Examples

Constitutional Law	Statutory Law		Administrative Law	Judicial Law
	Civil Law	Criminal Law		
Bill of Rights	Tort law	Penal codes	Boards of nursing	Courts of law
Amendments to	Contract law		Regulatory boards	Trial level
the Constitution	Patent law		City ordinances	Appellate level
	Oil and			Supreme
	gas law			Court level

Source: Legal and Ethical Issues in Nursing (3rd ed.), by G. W. Guido, 2001, Upper Saddle River, NJ: Prentice Hall.

Constitutional Law

Constitutional law is a system of fundamental laws or principles for the governance of a nation, society, corporation, or other aggregate of individuals. The purpose of a constitution is to establish the basis of a governing system. The Constitution of the United States establishes the general organization of the federal government, grants specific power to the federal government, and places limitations on the federal government's powers.

The U.S. Constitution establishes, through the first three articles, the three branches of the federal government and enumerates their powers. Article I establishes the House of Representatives and the Senate. Congress has the power to regulate commerce with foreign nations and among selected states and to enact broad and powerful legislation throughout the nation. Article II establishes the presidency and the executive branch of government. While the powers of the president are not as clearly enumerated as those of Congress, the president has "executive" power, is the "commander and chief," and has power to grant pardons (except in cases of impeachment) for offenses against the United States. Article III establishes the role and duties of the Supreme Court and the judicial branch.

The general organization of the U.S. Constitution is, in reality, a grant of power from the states to the federal government, and the federal government has only the power granted to it by the Constitution (Article X). The federal government can collect taxes, declare war, and enact laws that are "necessary and proper" for exercising its powers. Federal constitutional law is the supreme law of the land, as federal law takes precedence over state and local law. Ideally, state and federal powers should be exercised so as not to interfere with each other, but if there is a conflict, federal laws prevail over state and local laws.

The U.S. Constitution also places limitations on the federal government. Such limitations have been enacted through the Bill of Rights (the first 10 amendments of the Constitution), which protects one's right to freedom of speech, trial by jury, free exercise of religious preference, and freedom from unreasonable search and seizure (United States Constitution, Amendments 1–10, 1787). Table 3.2 enumerates these rights and freedoms.

Constitutional law is the highest form of statutory law (defined in the next section). Statutory laws govern and meet existing conditions; constitutional laws govern for the future as well as the present in that the stability of constitutional law protects from frequent and violent fluctuations in public opinion (16 *American Jurisprudence*, 1995).

TABLE 3.2 United States Constitution, Amendments 1–10 and 14

1. Congress shall make no law respecting an establishment of religion, or prohibiting the free exercise thereof; of abridging the freedom of speech, or of the press; or the right of the people peaceably to assemble, and to petition the Government for a redress of grievances.

2. A well-regulated Militia, being necessary to the security of a free State, the right of the people to keep and bear Arms, shall not be infringed.

3. No Soldier shall, in time of peace, be quartered in any house, without the consent of the Owner, nor in time of war, but in a manner to be prescribed by law.

4. The right of the people to be secure in their persons, houses, papers, and effects, against unreasonable searches and seizures, shall not be violated, and no Warrants shall issue, but upon probable cause, supported by Oath or affirmation, and particularly describing the place to be searched, and the persons or things to be seized.

5. No persons shall be held to answer for a capital, or otherwise infamous crime, unless a presentment or indictment of a Grand Jury, except in cases arising in the land or naval forces, or in the Militia, when in actual service in time of War or public danger; nor shall any person be subject for the same offense twice put in jeopardy of life or limb; nor shall be compelled in any criminal case to be a witness against himself, nor be deprived of life, liberty, or property, without due process of law; nor shall private property be taken for public use, without just compensation.

6. In all criminal prosecutions, the accused shall enjoy the right to a speedy and public trial by an impartial jury of the State and district wherein the crime shall have been committed, which district shall have been previously ascertained by law, and to be informed of the nature and cause of the accusation; to be confronted with the witnesses against him; to have compulsory process for obtaining witnesses in his favor, and to have the Assistance of counsel for his defense.

7. In Suits at common law, where the value in controversy shall exceed twenty dollars, the right of trial by jury shall be preserved, and no fact tried by a jury, shall be otherwise reexamined in any Court of the United States than according to the rules of the common law.

8. Excessive bail shall not be required, nor excessive fines imposed, nor cruel and unusual punishments inflicted.

9. The enumeration in the Constitution, of certain rights, shall not be construed to deny or disparage others retained by the people.

10. The powers not delegated to the United States by the Constitution, nor prohibited by it to the States, are reserved to the States respectively, or to the people.

14. Section 1. All persons born or naturalized in the United States, and subject to the jurisdiction thereof, are citizens of the United States and the State wherein they reside. No State shall make or enforce any law which shall abridge the privileges or immunities of citizens of the United States; nor shall any State deprive any person of life, liberty, or property, without due process of law; nor deny to any person within its jurisdiction the equal protection of the laws.

Each state has its own constitution, establishing the organization of the state government, giving the state certain powers, and placing limits on the state's power. An important difference between federal and state constitutional law is that the federal government derives positive grants of power from the U.S. Constitution, while states enjoy plenary powers subject only to limitations by their individual state constitution, the U.S. Constitution, and any limitations necessary for the successful operation of the federal system.

Statutory Laws

Statutory laws are those made by the legislative branch of government. Statutory laws are designed to declare, command, or prohibit. Generally referred to as *statutes*, these laws are created by the U.S. Congress, state legislative bodies, city councils, or other elected bodies. Statutes are officially enacted (voted on and passed) by legislative bodies and are compiled into codes, collections of statutes, or city ordinances. Examples include the United States Code and Black's Statutes.

The federal and state governments have broad powers to legislate for the general welfare of the public. The U.S. Constitution grants the federal government's power, while the states have inherent power to act except where the Constitution restricts the power to the federal government. The states' power to legislate and govern is often referred to as *police power.* This term is generally seen as allowing the states to make laws necessary to maintain public order, health, safety, and welfare.

An example of statutory law is nursing licensure laws, which regulate health care providers within individual states. Licensure laws are designed to protect the general public from incompetent health care providers. Known as *nurse practice acts* or *nursing practice acts* depending on the individual state, these statutory laws give authority to qualified and licensed practitioners to practice nursing within a given state, the District of Columbia, and/or U.S. territories. Other statutory laws that affect the practice of professional nursing include statutes of limitations, protective and reporting laws, natural death acts, and informed consent laws. See Chapter 11 for a more complete discussion of nurse practice acts.

Administrative Laws

Administrative laws are enacted by means of decisions and rules of administrative agencies, which are specific governing bodies charged with implementing particular legislation. When statutes are enacted, administrative agencies are given the authority to carry out the specific intentions of the statutes, by creating rules and regulations that enforce the statutory laws. For example, legislative bodies pass the individual nurse practice acts (statutory laws) and create state boards of nursing or state boards of nurse examiners (state administrative agencies). These state boards implement and enforce the state nurse practice act by writing rules and regulations for the enforcement of the statutory law and by conducting investigations and hearings to ensure the law's continual enforcement.

Such authority is given to administrative agencies by the state legislature, since the elected legislative body has neither the resources nor the needed expertise to ensure that statutory laws are properly enforced. Administrative agencies are normally composed of persons with specific qualifications and experience and are given the single charge to implement and regulate the enforcement of a given statutory law. State boards of nursing are usually composed of predominantly registered nurse members, who are actively employed in educational or practice settings within nursing. Their charge is the enforcement of the state nurse practice act.

Administrative rules and regulations have validity only to the extent that they are within the scope of the authority granted by the legislative body. Legislative bodies have some limitations placed on them by state constitutional law. There must be specificity in the charge as given

EXERCISE 3.1

Read the table of contents of your state nurse practice act. Can you distinguish the state administrative body (board of nursing) that is created by the legislature? Which sections of your nurse practice act create the administrative body, and which sections serve to distinguish legislative intent?

to the administrative agency, and the legislative body remains ultimately responsible for the rules and regulations the administrative body passes.

Some procedural acts may also govern administrative bodies. Such procedural acts delineate how the agency promulgates rules and regulations and provides for comments from the public before the rules and regulations are enforceable. The procedural acts may also provide for publication in a state register prior to the enforcement of the new rules and regulations.

The administrative agency has the initial authority to decide how its rules and regulations are enforced, and the decisions of the administrative agency may be appealed through the state court system. If appealed, courts have limited their review of the agency's actions to one of the following five areas:

1. Was the delegation of power to the specific administrative agency constitutional and proper?
2. Did the specific administrative agency follow proper procedures in enforcing the statutory law?
3. Is there a substantial basis for the decision?
4. Did the administrative agency act in a nondiscriminatory and nonarbitrary manner?
5. Was the issue under review included in the delegation to the agency?

Attorney General's Opinions

A second example of administrative law is the **attorney general's opinion.** The national or state attorney general may be requested to give an opinion regarding a specific interpretation of a law. Individuals or agencies may request such an opinion, and the opinion is binding until a subsequent statute, regulation, or court order amends the attorney general's opinion.

The attorney general's opinions provide guidelines based on both statutory and common law principles. Sometimes statutes are written in such vague terms that nurses seek opinions concerning the interpretation of the statute. For example, a board of nursing may request a state attorney general's opinion regarding enforcement of the nurse practice act in agencies that fail to comply with the provision of the act. Such a request would seek guidance on how the board of nursing should proceed to ensure compliance with the nurse practice act.

Opinions can also be formal or informal. The greater the liability risks, the more likely it is that a formal opinion will be issued. If legal issues then arise and the nurse has a formal attorney general's opinion, the court is more likely to rule that the nurse acted in a reasonable and responsible manner in seeking clarification on the matter.

Judicial Laws

Judicial (or decisional) laws are made by the courts and interpret legal issues that are in dispute. Depending on the type of court involved, the judicial or decisional law may be made by a single justice, with or without the assistance of a jury, or by a panel of justices. As a rule of thumb, the initial trial courts have a single justice or magistrate, intermediary appeal courts have three justices, and the highest appeal courts have a panel of nine justices.

All courts serve to rule on issues in dispute. In deciding cases, the courts interpret statutes and regulations or may decide which of two conflicting statutes or regulations apply to a given fact situation. Courts may also decide if the statute or regulation violates a constitution (federal or state), because all statutes and regulations must be in harmony with the governing constitution. The landmark case of *Marbury v. Madison* (1803) established the power of the judiciary in interpreting constitutional law. For example, a nurse who questions the authority of the state board of nursing may file a court action if the nurse has cause to believe that there has been a legal or procedural error on the part of the board's action against him or her.

Two important legal doctrines, which are directly derived from the U.S. Constitution, guide courts in their decision-making role:

1. The doctrine of **precedent** or **stare decisis** literally means to "let the decision stand." This doctrine is applied by courts of law in cases with similar fact patterns that have been previously decided by the court system. The court looks at the facts of the current case before it reviews previous decisions that applied the same rules and principles with the similar fact situation and then arrives at a similar decision in the case currently before the court. This doctrine has great implications for nurses, because it gives nurses insight into ways in which the court has previously fixed liability in given fact situations. Nurses are cautioned to avoid two important pitfalls before deciding if the doctrine of precedent should apply to a given fact situation:

   a. The previous case must be within the jurisdiction of the court hearing the current case. For example, a previous New York case decided by an appellate court within New York does not set precedent for a California state court, although the California court may model its decision after the New York case. It is not compelled to do so because two separate jurisdictions are involved. Within the same jurisdiction, the case would set precedent. A New York appellate decision would be relied on by the lower courts in New York State.

   b. The court hearing the current case may depart from precedent and set a **landmark decision,** which signifies that precedent is changed by the current court decision. Such a landmark decision is usually arrived at for one of several reasons. Societal needs may have changed, or technology may have become more advanced. In addition, a court may find that to follow the previous decision would further harm an already injured person. A well-known example of a landmark decision was the U.S. Supreme Court holding in *Roe v. Wade* (1973). That court, for the first time in American history, recognized the right of a woman to seek and receive a legal abortion during the first two trimesters of pregnancy.

2. A second doctrine that courts employ in duplication of litigation and seemingly apparent contradiction in decisions is termed **res judicata,** which means literally "a thing or matter settled by judgment." Res judicata applies only when a legal dispute has been decided by a competent court of jurisdiction, and no further appeals are possible. This doctrine then prevents the same parties in the original lawsuit from retrying the same issues involved in the first lawsuit. Thus, res judicata prevents multiple litigation by parties who have lost in the original suit, in that those parties are prevented from taking the same issues to another court in hopes of persuading a second trial court in their favor.

   Res judicata does not apply to competent appeals to an appellate court, nor does it apply to parties who were not named in the original lawsuit. Res judicata likewise does not apply to issues that were not decided by the original trial court so that a second lawsuit could be filed by the same parties on different specific issues.

All laws, regardless of origin, are fluid and subject to change. Constitutional laws may be amended. Statutory laws may be amended, repealed, or expanded by future legislative action. Administrative bodies may be dissolved, expanded, or redefined. Judicial or decisional laws may be modified or completely altered by new court decisions.

CLASSIFICATIONS (TYPES) OF LAW

Laws may be further classified into several different types. Many nurses may have wondered about classifications such as (1) common law, (2) civil law, (3) public law, (4) criminal law, (5) private law, (6) substantive law, and (7) procedural law.

Common Law

Law may be classified according to the court in which it was first instituted. The federal courts and 49 state courts follow the common law of England. **Common law** is defined as law derived from principles rather than rules and regulations. It is based on justice, reason, and common sense. During the colonial period, the English common law was uniformly applied in the 13 original colonies. After the American Revolution, individual states adopted various parts of the common law, and differences in interpretation and enforcement began that still exist to this day. Individual state statutory and judicial findings also account for the variation of common law principles from state to state.

Civil Law

Louisiana elected to adopt civil or Napoleonic laws, because the origins of that state were of a predominantly French influence. Derived from the civil laws of the French, Romans, and Spaniards, Napoleonic or **civil law** may be said to be based on rules and regulations.

Civil law may also be used to distinguish that area of the law concerned with the rights and duties of private persons and citizens. Civil law is administered between citizens (private persons) and is enforced through the courts as damages or money compensation. No fine or imprisonment is assessed in civil law, and injured parties usually collect money damages from individuals who have harmed them.

The court, however, may also decide that an action, known as **specific performance,** be performed rather than allow money damages, if the court deems that specific performance best aids the injured party. For example, in a contract dispute, the court may force an employer to reinstate a previously discharged worker and to pay the worker compensation for the time he or she was without employment rather than merely paying the worker for the time spent without work.

Civil law may be further divided into a variety of legal specialties: contract law, labor law, patent law, and tort law, among others. Perhaps the most important area of law to the professional nurse, **tort law** involves compensation to those wrongfully injured by others' actions. This area of law is normally involved in medical malpractice claims. Tort law is covered in depth in Part III of this book.

Public Law

Public law is the branch of law concerned with the state in its political capacity. The relationship of a person to the state is at the crux of public law. Perhaps the best example of public law is the entire field of criminal law.

Criminal Law

Criminal law refers to conduct that is offensive or harmful to society as a whole. If an act is expressly forbidden or prohibited by statute or by common law principles, it is referred to as a *crime.* Most often, crimes are viewed as offenses against the state rather than against individuals, and the state, city, or administrative body brings the legal action against the offender. Examples of crimes include minor traffic violations, theft, arson, and unlawfully taking another's life. Punishment for the commission of crimes ranges from simple fines to imprisonment to execution.

Crimes can be classified as either misdemeanors or felonies. **Misdemeanors** are lesser criminal actions and are generally enforced through monetary fines rather than actual jail time. Fines that are imposed for misdemeanors are less than $1,000 or imprisonment, if it occurs, is for time periods of less than one year. **Felonies** are more serious criminal actions, most often involving fines of greater than $1,000, and punishment by prison terms of greater than one year or by death.

The same action by a given individual may be the basis for both a civil lawsuit and a criminal wrong. For example, if a nurse removes a ventilator-dependent patient from a ventilator and the patient subsequently dies, the state board of nursing may revoke the nurse's license to practice nursing (a criminal action), and the family may file a wrongful death suit (a civil suit) against the nurse. In the criminal case, the court would consider the intent of the defendant as well as the actual action. In the civil case filed out of the same action, the court only considers the action performed, and the standard of evidence is less stringent. Standards of evidence are more thoroughly discussed in the next chapter.

There are situations within nursing in which the nurse may be said to have violated criminal laws, and the number of criminal cases against nurses appears to be increasing. Examples include backdating of records (*Nevada State Board of Nursing v. Merkley*, 1997), mistreatment of patients (*Mississippi Board of Nursing v. Hanson*, 1997; *State v. Murphy*, 2004), substandard nursing care (*Leahy v. North Carolina Board of Nursing*, 1997), practicing without a license (*People v. Odom*, 1999), giving of a false nursing license to an employer (*People v. Cassadine*, 2003), chemically burning a disabled person with disinfectant bleach (*Kennerly v. State of Texas*, 2001), and the administration of drugs that cause or hasten a patient's death (*Jones v. State of Texas*, 1986). A more recent case in this area is *United States v. Occident* (2007), where a nurse's aide used her employment position to obtain confidential information from hospital patients' charts and co-workers' pay stubs. She subsequently sold the information to an accomplice who used the information to fraudulently apply for credit cards and purchase approximately $250,000 in merchandise. The nurse's aide was convicted for violation of the U.S. federal identity-theft statute. Additionally, in the "angel of mercy" line of cases, in which nurses administer fatal doses of lidocaine, insulin, or potassium chloride to elderly and/or terminally ill patients, nurses have been charged with criminal violations (*The People v. Diaz*, 1992; *Rachals v. State of Georgia*, 1987).

A recent case, *Shipman v. Hamilton* (2008), began as a criminal suit against a nurse for obstruction of a peace officer. Two officers came to the intensive care unit at midnight to deliver in person an emergency protective order to a 60-year-old male patient. The officers announced their purpose and requested to speak to the patient's nurse. The nurse readily pointed out the patient's room and, when asked about the patient's condition, the nurse said it would be better for the officers to speak with the patient's doctor before seeing the patient. The nurse at this point was worried that the patient could experience serious complications if confronted by a stressful stimulus.

The officers then requested that the nurse call her supervisor. After phoning the on-call physician, the nurse notified the police officers that the patient would be in the unit overnight and to come back in the morning. The on-call physician also advised the nurse to contact the supervisor, which she did. While the nurse was speaking with the supervisor, one of the officers became agitated and took the telephone from the nurse's hand. He then spoke with the nursing supervisor, who requested he return in the morning to deliver the protective order.

During the time that the officer was speaking with the nursing supervisor, the nurse caring for the patient returned to the nursing station. The officer went into the nursing station, arrested the nurse for obstructing service of process and obstructing a police officer, and had her taken from the hospital in handcuffs.

In the subsequent trial, the court noted that an arrest requires a warrant or probable cause. There was no way, the court ruled, that the officer could have thought the nurse's actions amounted to either of the offenses for which she was arrested. The nurse told the officer where the patient was located and did nothing to prevent him from contacting the patient. When the nurse advised the officer that it was not advisable for him to contact the patient, she had two responsible staff members collaborate that fact, leaving the officer to either leave or serve the patient with the emergency order. The court in finding for the nurse noted that obstruction of a peace officer, by definition, requires physical resistance intended to obstruct the officer in the execution of his lawful duties. While the nurse refused to give the officer permission to enter the patient's room, permission was not hers to give or withhold. Thus she did not obstruct the officer.

Other, less common, instances of criminal charges against professional nurses include the rape of patients (*State of North Carolina v. Raines*, 1987), manslaughter (*People of the State of New York v. Simon*, 1990), and attempted murder (*Caretenders v. Commonwealth of Kentucky*, 1991).

Private Law

Private law is synonymous with civil or common law, which has been discussed earlier in this chapter.

Substantive Law

Substantive law, which defines the substance of the law, may be further classified into civil, administrative, and criminal law. Thus, substantive law concerns the specific wrong, harm, or duty that caused the lawsuit or an action to be brought against an individual. Lawsuits brought to remedy violations of these laws must eventually prove the existence of the elements that comprise the actual claims.

EXERCISE 3.2

Describe instances in which the conduct of the professional nurse (with regard to the treatment of patients) might be cause for possible criminal charges. For example, the administration of toxic chemotherapeutic agents may place a patient in a more life-threatening condition than the disease process does. How might a court of law distinguish such a case? Which of the ethical principles is the nurse following when administering such therapies?

Procedural Law

Procedural law, which governs the procedure or rules to create, implement, or enforce substantive law, may vary according to the type of substantive law involved and the jurisdiction in which the lawsuit is brought. Procedural law concerns the process and rights of the individual charged with violating substantive law. Procedural issues that may be contested include admissibility of evidence, the time frame for initiating lawsuits, and the qualifications of expert witnesses.

DUE PROCESS OF LAW AND EQUAL PROTECTION OF THE LAW

Due process of law, a phrase often misquoted, applies only to state actions and not to actions of private citizens. Basically, the due process clause of the U.S. Constitution is intended to prevent a person from being deprived of "life, liberty, or property" by actions of state or local governments (Amendment 14, Section 1, 1787). Although difficult to define, the due process clause is founded on the fundamental principle of justice rather than a rule of law, and ensures that the government will respect all of a person's legal rights, not just some or part of those legal rights, when it deprives a person of life, liberty, or property.

Due process protects the public from arbitrary actions. Laws must operate equally among all persons, and laws must be definite, not vague. Due process is violated if a particular person of a class or community is singled out by the law. A "person of ordinary intelligence who would be law abiding can tell what conduct must be to conform to (the law's) regulation, and the law is susceptible to uniform interpretation and application by those charged with enforcing it" (*State v. Schuster's Express, Inc.*, 1969, at 792).

The two primary elements of due process are (1) the rule as applied must be reasonable and definite, and (2) fair procedures must be followed in enforcing the rule. This latter provision ensures that adequate notice be given before the rule is enforced so that persons who will be affected by it will have time to explain why the rule should or should not be enforced. Nurses become involved in the application of due process when requested to appear before state boards of nursing, in that they must be given proper notice of the upcoming hearing and of the charges that the board will be evaluating during the hearing. In the hospital setting, the concept of due process has been interpreted to include a hospital's right to licensure by the state and the right of qualified medical personnel to staff appointments in public hospitals.

A recent case example concerning due process of the law affecting boards of nursing is *Slagle v. Wyoming State Board of Nursing* (1998). In that case, an inmate in the Wyoming correctional system filed a complaint with the Wyoming Board of Nursing, claiming an advanced geriatric nurse practitioner was practicing illegally as an advanced practitioner in adult nursing. The board of nursing sent notice to the nurse, requesting that she substantiate her qualifications in adult advanced practice nursing. The nurse sent back numerous materials, including a letter of recommendation from the head of the University of Utah nursing program.

The nurse thought that the board was in the process of updating her qualifications and would be enlarging the scope of her license to include adult advanced practice. In fact, the board of nursing was conducting a disciplinary investigation to see whether the nurse had practiced beyond the scope of her geriatric advanced nurse practitioner standing.

In the subsequent lawsuit, the Supreme Court of Wyoming dismissed the board of nursing sanctions against the nurse, because the notice the board of nursing had sent was so misleading that it violated the nurse's constitutional right to due process of law. The final conclusion was that the board of nursing gave this nurse adult advanced nurse practitioner standing.

Note, however, that minor errors will not be seen as failing to give proper notice. In *Colorado State Board of Nursing v. Geary* (1997), the notice from the board of nursing was mailed to the nurse at an incorrect address. In Colorado, notice had to be sent to the nurse at the last known address and to the attorney, if any, who had notified the board that he or she was representing the nurse. In this case, the attorney received the notice, corrected the incorrect address, and sent the notice to the nurse at her correct address. The nurse received this latter notice from her attorney, but she decided not to appear at her disciplinary hearing. Because she was not at the hearing, the board placed a 2-year probation on the nurse's license.

In the subsequent lawsuit, the nurse argued that she had not received notice, as the original notice was misaddressed. The court ruled that when an agency mails out an administrative notice, the law presumes the notice was properly addressed and the person to whom it was addressed received it. The board does not have to prove the nurse received its notice. The nurse must prove she did not receive the notice and, because her attorney had been sent the notice, she had been "duly served." Thus, the court upheld the 2-year probation for the underlying charges of professional misconduct. A similar finding was upheld in *Beverly Enterprises v. Jarrett* (2007).

Like due process, the equal protection clause of the Fourteenth Amendment also restricts state actions and has no reference to private actions. The concept of **equal protection of the law** has become the source of many civil rights (Abboud, 2006). More than an abstract right, the equal protection clause guarantees that all similarly situated persons will be affected similarly. Laws need not affect every man, woman, and child alike, but reasonable classifications of persons must be treated similarly (*Dorsey v. Solomon*, 1984). Thus, states may not enforce rules and regulations based solely on classifications as determined by race, religion, and/or gender. The due process clause does not preclude states from resorting to classifications of persons for the purpose of litigation, but "the classification must be reasonable and not arbitrary and must rest upon some ground of difference having a fair and substantial relationship to the object of legislation so that all persons similarly circumstanced shall be treated alike" (*Ex Parte Tigner*, 1964, at 894–895).

In determining whether equal protection of the law has been achieved, courts use the **rational basis test,** which essentially states that persons in the same classes must be treated alike. In addition, this test states that reasonable grounds that further legitimate governmental interests exist in making distinction between those persons who fall within the class and those persons who fall outside the class (*Ohio University Faculty Association v. Ohio University*, 1984).

A case decided under the equal protection clause of both the U.S. and Arizona Constitutions held that it was unreasonable to allocate treatment within a service category solely on the criterion of age (*Salgado v. Kirschner*, 1994). In that case, a middle-aged Medicaid recipient was denied a lifesaving liver transplant based on an Arizona statue that limits Medicaid coverage for medically necessary transplants to persons under the age of 21. The court found that age was the only criterion used and that age was medically irrelevant to liver transplant outcomes, in that no evidence linking age to a greater survival rate was shown. This case is significant in that age, if used to set restrictions on care, cannot be the sole factor considered nor can it be medically irrelevant.

The distinction between due process and equal protection was perhaps best summarized in a 1983 case in which the court stated that "the difference between due process and equal protection of the law is that due process emphasizes fairness between state and individual regardless of how other individuals in the same situation are treated while equal protection emphasizes disparity in treatment by a state between classes of individuals whose situations arguably are indistinguishable" (*Peterson v. Garvey Elevators, Inc.*, 1983, at 897).

THE JUDICIAL PROCESS

To fully appreciate the various types and classifications of laws, substantive and procedural law, and the application of these specific procedures, an understanding of the court system is helpful. The next section addresses the judicial process in the United States.

Questions of Law or Fact

Facts are determined by evidence presented by both sides in a legal controversy. **Questions of fact** present the dispute that the jury answers. Facts are not necessarily what actually happened, because persons on both sides will have perceived a given incident through their own eyes. Each party to the controversy brings unique perceptions to the trial setting. The **fact-finder** has the responsibility to weigh admissible evidence as presented and to decide where the facts of the case really lie. For example, a question of fact could concern such issues as admission to a hospital. Was the patient formally admitted to a hospital so that a patient–hospital relationship was established? Questions of fact could also include the cost of an operation, the cost of a particular hospital service, or the people involved in a particular incident. Typically, questions of fact have concerned professional practice standards and whether these practice standards have set the standard of care for individual patients.

Sometimes both sides in a controversy agree to certain facts prior to the trial. In these cases, the only questions to be resolved concern **questions of law,** which involve the application or interpretation of laws and are determined by the judge in the court. For example, the judge may rule that a particular provision in a nurse's contract was against public policy and is therefore nonenforceable. Or the judge may rule that a particular provision in the contract is reasonable and thus enforceable. Federal and state statutes, rules and regulations, prior court decisions, new technology, and societal needs may all play a part in determining the law as it applies to a specific trial.

Fact-finders, usually the jurors at trial, determine the facts that are admissible. These selected people are charged with weighing the admitted evidence, while the judge or magistrate determines questions of law. If there is a trial without a jury, then the judge serves as both the fact-finder and the determiner of questions of law.

A case example may help illustrate this distinction. In *Hansen v. Universal Health Services of Nevada, Inc.* (1999), the facts of the case were fairly simple. The patient had surgery to implant a steel spinal fixation device in his back. After the surgery, the wound became severely infected and the patient incurred a series of additional operations on his back, costing more than $700,000. There was a serious dispute as to the medical cause of the infection.

In court, the patient's expert witness noted the patient was having episodes of bowel incontinence, which must have resulted in fecal matter being introduced into the wound. The hospital's expert witness related the infection to necrosis of muscle tissue near the surgical site.

The Supreme Court of Nevada agreed that fecal contamination of the surgical wound would be grounds for a negligent lawsuit against the hospital. However, in this case, the jury returned a verdict in favor of the hospital, apparently believing the hospital's expert witness's testimony about muscle necrosis. The court let the jury's verdict stand, as there were two fully plausible competing explanations for the events in question from which the jury made its own choice. Additionally, the court ruled that it was proper for the judge to exclude from the jury's attention hospital infection control reports not connected to this incident as potentially conflicting and prejudicial to the jury.

JURISDICTION OF THE COURTS

Jurisdiction, the authority by which courts and judicial officers accept and decide cases, is the power and authority of a court to hear and determine a judicial proceeding (Garner, 2004).

Jurisdiction determines the courts' ability to hear and rule on a given lawsuit. Jurisdiction may be divided into three categories.

Subject-matter jurisdiction, sometimes called *res jurisdiction*, refers to the court's competency to hear and to determine a given case within a particular class of cases. For example, a court may have jurisdiction only in cases that involve probate matters (wills and estates), family matters (adoptions, divorces, and child custody), or criminal matters. Subject-matter jurisdiction, along with the nature of the cause of action, may be determined by the amount or value of the claim as pled. For example, some courts have jurisdiction of a given case up to $1,000 or to cases that have a pled-damage figure of between $1,000 and $5,000.

Personal jurisdiction, sometimes referred to as *in personam jurisdiction*, refers to the power of a given court regarding a particular person. Personal jurisdiction is the legal power of a court to render a judgment against a party or parties to the action or proceeding. For example, personal jurisdiction often involves the county of the defendant. A court situated in the county of the defendant would have personal jurisdiction over the defendant. A court situated in the county of the plaintiff's residence can also have personal jurisdiction over the parties to the lawsuit.

The third jurisdictional issue concerns the court's ability to render the particular judgment sought. Any court possesses jurisdiction over matters only to the extent granted it by the constitution or legislation of the sovereignty on behalf of which it functions. **Territorial jurisdiction,** or the court's ability to bind the parties to the action, is a part of this third meaning of jurisdiction. Territorial jurisdiction determines the scope of federal and state court power. State court territorial power is determined by the U.S. Constitution's Fourteenth Amendment, and federal court jurisdiction is determined by the Fifth Amendment.

Courts may be either state or federal in origin. Federal courts seek to ensure that laws created through the U.S. Congress are enforced, and state courts have their sole jurisdiction within the given state. Overseeing the process is the U.S. Supreme Court, which has jurisdiction over all of the United States and its territories.

Overlapping or concurrent jurisdiction may occur when more than one court is qualified to hear a given dispute. In some areas of overlapping or concurrent jurisdiction and in some instances of specific subject-matter jurisdiction, the federal Constitution gives guidance. For example, the federal courts have original jurisdiction over admiralty cases, crimes involving federal laws, bankruptcy cases, and patent laws. The U.S. Constitution gives the U.S. Supreme Court original jurisdiction (that which is inherent or conferred to the court) over cases "involving ambassadors, other public ministers and consuls and those in which a state is a named party" (Article III, Section 2, 1787).

If there is no mandatory court of jurisdiction, the attorneys representing the party filing the lawsuit will advise their client of the optimal court in which to file the lawsuit. Concurrent jurisdiction frequently occurs in cases with multiple defendants and in cases that involve parties residing in different states. There are many reasons why one court may be more favorable to the party filing the lawsuit, including shorter length of time to trial, more favorable damage awards, and shorter distances for witnesses to travel.

STATE COURTS

Trial Courts

The court of original jurisdiction in most states is the **trial court,** and it is the first court to hear legal disputes. At this level, applicable law is determined, evidence is presented and evaluated to ascertain the facts, and either a judge or a jury functioning under the guidance of a judge applies the law to the admissible facts. As stated in the preceding sections, the judge determines questions of law and then guides the jury in applying this law to the questions of fact.

Even though the jury's tasks are to determine facts and, after proper instructions, to apply the law to the facts, the judge retains control over the entire trial process. The judge may find that the evidence is inadmissible or that the evidence as presented is insufficient to establish a factual issue for the jury to resolve. The judge may dismiss the case or may overrule a jury decision if he or she finds that justice has not been served.

Most state courts operate on a three-tier system. Sometimes called *inferior courts*, trial courts are the courts with original jurisdiction in most states with three-tier systems. Other names for this first court in which the lawsuit is filed include *circuit courts, superior courts, supreme courts* (New York), *courts of common pleas, chancery courts*, and *district courts*.

State Appellate Courts

The side that loses the case at trial level may decide to pursue the case at the appellate level if there are procedural or legal grounds on which to base an appeal. In a three-tier system, these **state appellate courts,** or **courts of intermediate appeals,** do not rehear the entire trial but base their decisions on evidence as presented in a record of the trial hearing. There are no witnesses, new evidence, or jurors. The intermediate court may concur (agree) with the previous decision, reverse the prior decision, or remand (send the case back to the trial level) and reorder a new trial.

Intermediate courts of appeal have different names throughout the states. They may be called *courts of appeal, intermediate appellate courts* (Hawaii), *appellate divisions of the supreme court* (New York), *superior courts, courts of special appeals* (Maryland), *courts of civil appeals*, and *courts of criminal appeals*. States that have a two-tier system, such as North Dakota, Rhode Island, and Maine, have no intermediate appellate courts.

State Supreme Courts

The ultimate court of appeal in the state is usually named the **state supreme court.** This court hears appeals from the intermediate appellate courts and also serves to adopt rules of procedure for the state and to license attorneys within the individual state. This court is the final authority for state issues, unless a federal issue or constitutional right is involved. The state supreme court may hear cases directly from the trial level. For example, if the trial-court case concerned the interpretation of the state constitution or a state statute, the case can be appealed directly to the state supreme court. An example of such a direct appeal involving the interpretation of the Missouri nurse practice act occurred in *Sermchief v. Gonzales* (1983).

Other names for this highest court of appeals within the state include *state court of last resort* (West Virginia), *supreme judicial court* (Maine and Massachusetts), and *court of appeals* (New York and Maryland). Some states may also have a separate supreme court of criminal appeals (Texas and Oklahoma).

EXERCISE 3.3

Explore your own state court system. What types of trial courts exist and what is their jurisdiction? Which court would most likely hear nursing malpractice cases? To which court would appeals be sent in your state system?

FEDERAL COURTS

The structure of the federal court system has varied a great deal throughout the history of the United States. The Constitution provides merely that the judicial power of the United States be "vested in one Supreme Court, and in inferior courts as Congress may from time to time ordain and establish" (Article III, Section 8, 1787). Thus, the only indispensable court is the Supreme Court. Congress has established and abolished other U.S. courts as national needs have changed over time.

Courts are presided over by judicial officers. In the Supreme Court, the judicial officers are called *justices.* In the courts of appeals, district courts, and specialty courts, most of the judicial officers are called *judges.* The authority, duties, and benefits assigned to judicial officers are enacted and amended by Congress.

District Courts

The federal court system mimics the majority of state court systems. The original trial courts in the federal three-tier system are the **U.S. district courts** and the specialty courts such as the U.S. court of claims, the U.S. bankruptcy courts, and the U.S. patent courts. There are currently 94 district courts, as well as specialized courts, including the Tax Court, Court of Federal Claims, Court of Veterans Appeals, and the Court of International Trade. The district courts normally hear cases in which a federal question (questioning a federal statute or violations of the rights and privileges granted by the U.S. Constitution) is involved or in which the parties to the suit have citizenship in different states (diversity of citizenship). In cases involving diverse citizenship, the federal court system applies rules of federal procedure in deciding applicable state law.

Courts of Appeal

The intermediary courts are the U.S. courts of appeal. These courts were known as the *circuit courts of appeal* prior to June 25, 1948. There are currently 13 courts of appeal, not including the U.S. Court of Appeals for the Armed Forces, and they are frequently called *U.S. circuit courts* even today. These courts are located in 13 areas (or circuits) of the country. The U.S. courts of appeal are numbered 1 through 12, with the District of Columbia Court of Appeals being the 13th court. Each of the first 12 courts of appeal consists of 1 to 9 state regions. These courts serve to correct potential errors that have been made in the decisions of the trial courts.

Supreme Court

The highest level of the federal court system is the **U.S. Supreme Court,** and its decisions are binding in all state and federal courts. This nine-justice court hears appeals from the U.S. courts of appeal and from the various state supreme courts when state court decisions involve federal laws or constitutional questions based on a **writ of certiorari,** or written petition to hear the case. The Supreme Court ensures the uniformity of decisions by reviewing cases in which constitutional issues have been decided or in which two or more lower courts have reached different conclusions.

Because most cases involving nursing practice concern tort law or state licensure issues, it is rare for lawsuits involving nurses as primary defendants to be heard in the federal court system. Exceptions to this rule are nurses working in the military and veterans' hospitals or other federally funded health care centers. Cases involving these nurses are frequently settled in federal courts.

EXERCISE 3.4

Find out which district court and federal court of appeals have jurisdiction over your city and state. What types of nursing malpractice cases have these courts heard in the past? How did the courts rule on those issues? How did their decisions affect the professional practice of nursing in your state?

STATUTES OF LIMITATIONS

Statutes of limitations, procedural law time frames, are essentially time intervals during which a case must be filed or the injured party is barred (prevented legally) from bringing the lawsuit. Statutes of limitation establish a time frame within which a suit must be brought. Set by the state legislature, most states allow 1 to 2 years for the filing of a personal injury lawsuit. The majority of the states do not begin measuring time until the injured party has actually discovered the injury that will become the basis of the ensuing lawsuit. According to the **discovery rule,** patients have 2 years from the time that they knew or should have known of the injury to file a personal injury lawsuit in the majority of states. These time frames vary according to state law. For example, California has amended its laws so that medical malpractice issues must be filed 3 years from the date of injury or 1 year from the date of discovery, whichever occurs first, except for foreign objects, where the statute of limitations runs from when the object is, or should have been, discovered. Texas allows 2 years in which to file a medical malpractice case, with a maximum of 10 total years. Washington state specifies 3 years with the discovery rule, but no more than 8 years from the wrongful act, unless there is an intentional concealment of a foreign object.

Some courts have distinguished between traumatic injury cases and disease cases. In traumatic injury cases, the injury is normally of the type that the patient knows or should have known of immediately. For example, the patient who has an operation on the opposite extremity or wrong area of the body will immediately know that an injury has occurred. In traumatic injury cases, the 1- or 2-year statute of limitations is strictly applied.

In disease cases, the statute of limitations may be less strictly applied, because it may be some time before the patient becomes aware of the possible malpractice event. The statute of limitations would begin to measure time when the patient became aware of the injury (event) or when the reasonable patient would have become aware of the injury. California's statute allows for this disease state, but further limits the actual time frame during which a successful lawsuit may be filed. For example, in *Melendez v. Beal* (1985), the patient had entered the hospital for gallbladder surgery in May 1968. She had no complications following the surgery and was discharged. Late in 1981, she began experiencing abdominal pain and entered the hospital for tests. The tests revealed an abscess under her liver caused by a surgical sponge that had been retained in the abdomen following the 1968 surgery. Additionally, the retained sponge had eroded into the small intestine at the time of surgery, thus necessitating extensive repair to the small intestine.

The patient filed a lawsuit for the retained sponge against the surgeon, nurses, and hospital. The trial court ruled in favor of the defendants because of the 14-year gap from the time of the original surgery to the time that the tests revealed the retained sponge.

The court of appeals reversed and remanded the case for a new trial. The court concluded that the "two-year limitation period could not be applied constitutionally to this patient, who had no way of discovering the negligent act within the two years from the date of the medical treatment. The filing of the action within two years after the patient's discovery of the negligence was, in fact, timely" (*Melendez v. Beal*, 1985, at 873). The court further concluded that a 2-year limitation may be appropriate, but that it should not be used when the results would be "unreasonable, absurd, or unjust" (at 877).

Similarly, in *Perkins v. HEA of Iowa, Inc.* (2002), a nurse was caring for a renal dialysis patient when the leg shunt portal disconnected and the patient, nurse, and dialysis center were covered in blood. The nurse was tested for hepatitis C for 1 year, during which the results were negative for hepatitis C. She tested positive for the disease at 6 years post-incident. Ruling in her favor that the statute of limitations did not bar her lawsuit, the court noted that the statute started to run when she discovered the infection, not at the date of the infecting episode.

Finally, in *Alcott Rehabilitation Hospital v. Superior Court* (2001), a California court allowed the 1-year statute of limitations for health care malpractice to be extended to 3 years, noting that the patient in this instance was incompetent to sue on her own behalf and that this was the type of case that was intended when the state legislature permitted cases to be filed beyond the 1-year limit. Her family could file on her behalf for acts of negligence that had occurred during her stay in the nursing home.

Note, though, that courts apply the statute of limitations and dismiss causes of action if the facts support such conclusions. For example, in *Blackburn v. Blue Mountain Women's Clinic* (1997), the patient was given negligent advice by the clinic nurse and, believing her child to be HIV positive and capable of passing the disease to the patient in utero, had an abortion. Complications followed the abortion, including a hospitalization for severe depression.

The patient filed a lawsuit against the clinic for negligence. She claimed damages for her own physical and mental suffering and for the wrongful death of her unborn child. The court, in dismissing the suit, relied on the Montana 5-year time limit for filing such a case, stating that a malpractice suit was not valid more than 5 years after the events in question.

The Ohio Appellate Court reached similar conclusions in *Scott v. Borelli* (1996) and in *Long v. Warren General Hospital* (1997). In the first case, the patient sued her psychotherapist for sexual assault and professional malpractice that had occurred during her therapy 25 years earlier. The court even said that the patient could rely on memories recovered during Eye Movement and Desensitization and Reprocessing Therapy in bringing such a suit. However, once the patient's memory of past abuse is recovered, the statute of limitations begins to run, and this case was filed after the applicable time limit.

In *Long*, the court ruled that when a patient falls, is seriously injured, and files a lawsuit, even the simplest aspects of the patient's care can come under scrutiny. The patient was taken into an examination room in preparation for a colonoscopy. Because it was cold, the nurse told the patient to keep his socks on, rather than getting for him the nonskid slippers that the hospital used for patients.

When the orderly came for the patient, he told the patient to walk to the gurney. Two feet from the gurney, the orderly told the patient to turn around and go back and get his pillow for the ride on the gurney. In turning around, the patient slipped, lost his balance, and fell, hitting his head on the wall and his elbow on the floor. He sustained a comminuted fracture of his elbow, requiring surgery and extensive physical therapy.

The patient filed suit against the hospital. The court was highly critical of the care this patient had received. However, because the lapses in judgment that led to this patient's injuries occurred in a health care setting, the court believed that the case should be considered under the rules for medical malpractice. In Ohio, there was a 1-year statute of limitations for such suits, and the case was dismissed.

Parties cannot be added to an already-filed lawsuit after the statute of limitations has expired. In *Reynolds v. Thomas Jefferson University Hospital* (1996), the patient reported hoarseness and a sore throat to her family practice physician almost immediately after her emergency cesarean section. The physician said he would wait 2 weeks to see what happened. Although there was some improvement in the patient's voice, her persistent hoarseness did not improve. After 4 months, he sent her to an eye, ear, nose, and throat specialist who diagnosed and repaired a dislocated right arythenoid cartilage. The surgical procedure was considered a success but left the patient, a semiprofessional singer, with a residual "airy" quality in her voice.

The patient first sued the anesthesiologist for faulty intubation and extubation. The anesthesiologist prevailed, because the court held that some cartilage damage can occur even with the best intubations. She then sued the family practice physician for his failure to refer her to a specialist more promptly. Although the allegations of malpractice against the family practice physician were valid, he was not added to the lawsuit until after the statute of limitations had run. Thus, the case was dismissed.

Some states have begun to use a continuous-treatment time frame doctrine, which states that the time limit for filing a medical malpractice case is calculated not from the date of the alleged malpractice but from the date that the patient was last treated for the condition. The treatment for the same condition must have been continuous, not sporadic, for this doctrine to apply.

In *Stilloe v. Contini* (1993), a New York appellate court unanimously ruled that if there was no personal contact between the patient and the physician, where the two parties intend for their professional relationship to continue and the patient continues to rely on the doctor for care and treatment, there is continuous care and treatment for the purpose of satisfying the statute of limitations. Under this doctrine, the time in which to file a medical malpractice suit is extended when the course of treatments that includes the alleged wrongful acts or omissions has run continuously and is related to the same original medical condition or complaint. Thus, patients have an extended time period during which they may file lawsuits for medical malpractice.

The rationale behind statutes of limitations is that potential defendants should have the opportunity to defend themselves within a reasonable time period. The purpose of statutes of limitations is to suppress fraudulent claims after the facts concerning them have become obscured from lapse of time, defective memory, or death or removal of witnesses (*Noll v. City of Bozeman*, 1975). If too much time has lapsed between the occurrence and the lawsuit, facts become stale and witnesses cannot be identified or found.

At one time, courts uniformly allowed one major exception, in the case of minors, to the prompt filing of a lawsuit for personal injury. Because parents may not always seek what is in the best interest of their child, the court allowed minors to reach their majority before the statute of limitations began to be measured. In most states, this means the statute begins to be counted when the child reaches his or her 18th birthday. The lawsuit must be filed by the time the injured minor reaches his or her 20th birthday or the suit is barred by law. Today, most states have become more restrictive and have opted to disallow the right of a minor to bring suit upon reaching adulthood. For example, in Montana, a child under 4 years of age has until his or her 8th birthday to file suit. For minors 4 or older, the state's general 3-year discovery rule to a maximum of 5 years for foreign objects and 10 years for legal cases applies. In New Mexico, if the child is under 6 years of age at the time of the injury, he or she must file by his or her 9th birthday. In at least one state, though, the statute of limitations has recently been increased for parents who sue on behalf of their minor child. In Ohio state, the time frame for filing a medical malpractice suit has been increased from 1 year up to the child's 19th birthday. Minors continue to have until their 19th birthday to file a medical malpractice suit.

EXERCISE 3.5

Decide the following fact scenario: A nursing home resident filed a lawsuit alleging that nurses caring for him were negligent in their care. Specifically, the nurses did not follow the care plan in that they failed to turn him every 2 hours, they frequently failed to get him out of bed so that he could sit in a wheelchair, and he remained in spoiled bedding for long periods of time. As a result, he had multiple open wounds on his buttocks, hips, and heels, which are slowly resolving. He filed this lawsuit 3 years after being removed from the nursing home. How would the statute of limitation affect this suit? Are there any circumstances he could plead that would allow this lawsuit to continue despite the 3-year interval?

SUMMARY

- Law may be defined as the sum total of rules and regulations by which a society is governed.
- The four sources of law are constitutional, statutory, administrative, and judicial law.
- Attorney general's opinions, requested at either the national or state level, provide guidelines based on both statutory and common law principles.
- Law may be classified into several different types, including common, civil, criminal, public, private, substantive, and procedural law.
- Due process of the law and equal protection of the law are special applications of the Fourteenth Amendment, and both pertain only to state actions.

- In courts of law, questions of law and fact are determined in reaching a conclusion to the lawsuit.
- Jurisdiction pertains to the power and authority of a court to hear and determine a judicial proceeding and can be subdivided into subject-matter, personal, and territorial jurisdiction.
- State and federal courts are generally dived into a three-tier system: trial courts, appellate courts, and supreme courts.
- Statutes of limitations are time intervals during which a case must be filed or the injured party is prevented from bringing the lawsuit.

APPLY YOUR LEGAL KNOWLEDGE

1. Which classifications of law are more commonly applied to professional nursing?
2. How do attorney generals' opinions protect the practice of professional nursing?
3. Do all four sources of law protect the practice of nursing? Why or why not?
4. Does the court in which a case is filed affect the ability of the injured party to have a more favorable or less favorable verdict?
5. How do statutes of limitations favor defendants in a lawsuit?

YOU BE THE JUDGE

Mrs. Casey was expecting her second child. Because she had atypical postpartum eclampsia during her first pregnancy, she chose to be cared for by a group of obstetricians who specialized in complicated obstetrical care. She delivered a healthy daughter during the 9th month of her pregnancy. Shortly after delivery, she reported swelling in her hands and face, headaches, and visual changes she associated with the postpartum symptoms she had experienced following the birth of her first child 2 years earlier. One of the physicians authorized her to stay an additional day in the acute care setting for further evaluation, but she was dismissed when the hospital nursing staff said her insurance would not approve the additional hospital day.

Three days later she presented to the emergency center with high blood pressure, severe headaches, and 4+ swelling in both of her lower extremities. She was admitted to the intensive care unit for treatment and was released 3 weeks after this second admission.

She later filed a lawsuit for the early dismissal and the subsequent readmission.

At trial level, the plaintiff's attorney argued that the case had been timely filed, as the patient filed this lawsuit within 2 years after she was discharged from the intensive care unit stay. The defendants' attorney countered that she had not timely filed the lawsuit, as it was filed more than 2 years after the initial discharge following the birth of her daughter.

QUESTIONS

1. How does the statute of limitations affect this case?
2. Is there evidence to support the claim that the statute of limitations barred Mrs. Casey's cause of action?
3. Is there evidence to support the plaintiff's claim that the statute of limitations should not bar this action?
4. How would you decide this case?

REFERENCES

Abboud, A. (2006, January 20). Equal protection essential component of rule of law. *The Washington File.* Washington, DC: U.S. Department of State.

Alcott Rehabilitation Hospital v. Superior Court, 112 Cal Rept.2d 807 (Cal. App., 2001).

Beverly Enterprises v. Jarrett, 2007 WL 466810 (Ark. App., February 14, 2007).

Blackburn v. Blue Mountain Women's Clinic, 951 P.2d 1 (Montana, 1997).

Caretenders v. Commonwealth of Kentucky, 821 S.W.2d 83 (Kentucky, 1991).

Colorado State Board of Nursing v. Geary, 954 P.2d 614 (Colo. App., 1997).

Dorsey v. Solomon, 435 F. Supp. 725 (DC Md., 1984).

Ex Parte Tigner, 132 S.W.2d 885, 139 Tx. Cr. Rept. 452 (Texas, 1964).

Garner, B. A. (Ed.). (2004). *Black's law dictionary* (8th ed.). St. Paul, MN: Thompson West Publishing.

Hansen v. Universal Health Services of Nevada, Inc., 947 P.2d 1158 (Nevada, 1999).

Jones v. State of Texas, 716 S.W.2d 142 (Texas, 1986).

Kennerly v. State of Texas, 40 S.W.3d 718 (Tex. App., 2001).

Leahy v. North Carolina Board of Nursing, 488 S.E.2d 245 (North Carolina, 1997).

Long v. Warren General Hospital, 700 N.E.2d 364 (Ohio App., 1997).

Marbury v. Madison, 5 U.S. (1 Cranch) 137 (1803).

Melendez v. Beal, 683 S.W.2d 869 (Texas, 1985).

Mississippi Board of Nursing v. Hanson, 703 So.2d 239 (Mississippi, 1997).

Nevada State Board of Nursing v. Merkley, 940 P.2d 144 (Nevada, 1997).

Noll v. City of Bozeman, 534 P.2d 880, 166 Mont. 504 (Montana, 1975).

Ohio University Faculty Association v. Ohio University, 449 N.E.2d 792, 5 Ohio App. 2d 130 (Ohio, 1984).

People v. Cassadine, N.W.2d (Mich App., 2003).

People v. Odom, 82 Cal. Rptr.2d 184 (Cal. App., 1999).

People of the State of New York v. Simon, 549 N.Y. Supp. 701 (New York, 1990).

Perkins v. HEA of Iowa, Inc., N.W.2d (Iowa, 2002).

Peterson v. Garvey Elevators, Inc., 850 P.2d 893, 252 Kan. 976 (Kansas, 1983).

Rachals v. State of Georgia, 361 S.E.2d 671 (Georgia, 1987).

Reynolds v. Thomas Jefferson University Hospital, 676 A.2d 1205 (Pa. Super., 1996).

Roe v. Wade, 410 U.S. 113 (1973).

Salgado v. Kirschner, 878 P.2d 659 (Arizona, 1994).

Scott v. Borelli, 666 N.E.2d 322 (Ohio App., 1996).

Sermchief v. Gonzales, 600 S.W.2d 683 (Mo. En Banc., 1983).

Shipman v. Hamilton, 2008 WL 8521444 (7th Cir., April 1, 2008).

16 *American Jurisprudence* (2nd ed.). Constitutional Law (1995).

Slagle v. Wyoming State Board of Nursing, 954 P.2d 979 (Wyoming, 1998).

State v. Murphy, 2004 Ohio 638, 2004 WL 254217 (Ohio App., 2004).

State of North Carolina v. Raines, 334 S.E.2d 138 (1987).

State v. Schuster's Express, Inc., 5 Conn. Cir. 472, 256 A.2d 792 (Connecticut, 1969).

Stilloe v. Contini, 1993 WL 233404 (N.Y.A.D. 3 Dept, 1993).

The People v. Diaz, 834 P.2d 1171 (California, 1992).

United States Constitution, Amendments 1–10, 14; Article III, Sections 2 and 8 (1787).

United States v. Occident, 2007 WL 1988454 (4th Cir., July 6, 2007).

CHAPTER 4

Anatomy of a Lawsuit

PREVIEW

The ultimate goal of any court system is to resolve, in an orderly and just process, controversies that exist between two or more parties. To reach this orderly and just conclusion, the trial process has evolved. This chapter presents all aspects of the trial process, from initiation of the complaint to appeals, and highlights nursing's role, with special emphasis on the role as an expert witness, in the process. Alternate means of resolving controversies and conflicts, including alternative dispute resolution, mediation, arbitration, and prelitigation panels are also discussed.

LEARNING OUTCOMES
After completing this chapter, you should be able to:

4.1 List and explain the purpose of the six procedural steps in the trial process.

4.2 Examine alternate means of resolving controversies, including alternative dispute resolution, mediation, arbitration, and prelitigation panels.

4.3 Distinguish between traditional depositions, court reporter–recorded depositions, and the more modern videotaped depositions, stating the pros and cons of each of these methods.

4.4 Distinguish between lay and expert witnesses and their roles in the trial process.

4.5 Examine levels of evidence and state which level is most appropriate in criminal and civil court cases.

4.6 Enumerate the trial process, including the purposes and steps of the various stages in the process.

4.7 Discuss some of the ethical issues facing the expert witness.

KEY TERMS

alternative dispute resolution (ADR)
arbitration
clear and convincing standard of proof
complaint
counterclaim
cross-examination
default judgment
defendant
deposition
expert witness

injunction
interrogatories
lay witness
legal consultant
level of evidence
mediation
motion to dismiss
motions
opening statements
plaintiff
pleadings
prelitigation panels

preponderance of the evidence standard of proof
pretrial conference (hearing)
proof beyond a reasonable doubt
right of discovery
settlement
trial
verdict (decision)
voir dire

THE TRIAL PROCESS

There are six procedural steps to any given lawsuit. (See Table 4.1.) Each step, with its special application to nursing, is discussed in the following sections.

Step One: Initiation of the Lawsuit

A party, the **plaintiff,** who believes he or she may have a valid cause of action against another individual initiates the lawsuit. The answering party or parties, the **defendant**(s) in the lawsuit, may then respond. (In reality, the attorneys execute the intentions of their clients, but the parties to the suit are always referenced as though they are the ones controlling and instigating the proper motions, claims, forms, and defenses.)

In most instances, it is rare to have a single plaintiff versus a single defendant. More commonly, there are multiple parties on either or both sides to the lawsuit. In medical malpractice suits, a single plaintiff typically sues multiple defendants, including physicians, the health care institution's board of directors, and various members of the nursing staff. Naming as defendants all possible persons or entities involved in the cause of action may be a wise strategy for the plaintiff, since the plaintiff could be barred by the statute of limitations from later adding defendants to the lawsuit. (Review Chapter 3 for a detailed discussion about statutes of limitations.) Should plaintiffs subsequently discover that a named defendant has been incorrectly named as a party to the suit, that defendant may be nonsuited (sometimes called *dismissed*) and removed from the case entirely.

When the plaintiff's cause of action is well identified, a **complaint** is filed in a court with competent jurisdiction to hear the case. Upon filing the complaint, the court serves the defendant(s) with a summons to appear before the court at a specified time. This process, known as *service* in both state and federal court systems, alerts the named defendants that a lawsuit is now pending against them. The complaint outlines the names of the parties to the suit, the allegations of the breaches of standards of care, injuries or damages, and the demand for an award. In some states, the demand for damages is a specified amount, whereas other states determine the amount of the award based on the evidence as presented at court.

Once served, the defendants must respond to the complaint within a specified period of time or forfeit their right to defend the suit. The time frame for answering is determined by state or federal law and varies according to the jurisdiction. When served, each defendant should promptly notify his or her liability insurance carrier for representation by one of the retained attorneys or

TABLE 4.1 Procedural Steps in the Trial Process

Initiation of the Lawsuit

1. Complaint or summons is initiated by the plaintiff.
2. Service of the complaint is made to the defendant.
3. Health care provider contacts insurance carrier for attorney, or provider obtains independent attorney.
4. Answer (response) is filed by the defendant.
5. If no answer (response) is made within the legal time frame, a default judgment is entered by the court against the defendant.
6. Alternate means of resolving the dispute, including a prelitigation panel, is held if state has such a pretrial review mechanism/requirement.

Pleadings and Pretrial Motions

1. Plaintiff makes initial complaint.
2. Defendant files original pleadings or answer.
3. Motion to dismiss is initiated by either plaintiff or defendant.
4. Counterclaims are filed with the court.
5. Amended and/or supplemental pleadings are entered.
6. Motion for judgment is based on the pleadings.

Discovery of Evidence

1. Interrogatories are served to both plaintiff and defendant.
2. Depositions of witness and named parties are taken.
3. Request to produce documents is made.
4. Requests for an independent medical examination of the plaintiff are made.
5. Subpoenas of witnesses are issued as needed.
6. Pretrial conference or hearing is held.
7. Settlements are initiated and may be accepted.

Trial Process

1. Jury is selected (voir dire).
2. Opening statements are made, first by plaintiff, then by defendant.
3. Plaintiff's case is presented, with cross-examination by defendant.
4. Defendant's case is presented, with cross-examination by plaintiff.
5. Motion is made by defendant for directed verdict against plaintiff.
6. Closing statements are made, first by defendant, then by plaintiff.
7. Jury instructions are given.
8. Jury deliberates.
9. Verdict is decided and announced.

Appeals

1. Appellate level or state intermediate level court.
2. State supreme court or highest state court.
3. Federal court.

Execution of Judgment

1. Payment of damages.
2. Specific performance or injunction.
3. Imprisonment or fine of defaulting party.

Source: From *Legal and Ethical Issues in Nursing* (4th ed.), by G. W. Guido, 2006, Upper Saddle River, NJ: Prentice Hall.

procure a personal attorney. Never ignore the complaint because complaints do not disappear when ignored. If not properly answered within the time period allotted by law, a default judgment will be entered in the court against the defendant. A **default judgment** means that the defendants automatically lose the lawsuit, whether they had any liability or not. Each defendant should act promptly, because each jurisdiction sets specific time periods for each phase of the pretrial procedures and motions. Additionally, defendant nurses should never assume that other defendants will respond on their behalf; the named defendant must respond within the set time frame.

Nurse-defendants should remember two points. First, after notifying their insurance carrier and arranging to be represented by an attorney in the impending suit, they should also notify the health care institution's administrative staff of the lawsuit (assuming that they are still employed at the institution named in the lawsuit). This notification allows the health care institution's attorney to better represent the institution's and the nurses' interests. Second, nurse-defendants should not discuss the impending suit with anyone except their attorney and the health care institution's attorney. The less said, the less likely the nurse-defendants will be misquoted, and the less likely that their comments will be introduced into evidence.

Mandated by law in some states, **alternative dispute resolution (ADR)** refers to any means of settling disputes outside of the courtroom setting. Typically, ADR includes arbitration, mediation, early neutral evaluation, and conciliation. Although all of these processes are somewhat different in application, all serve to provide ways for parties to legal disputes to avoid formal lawsuits and costly trials. Other advantages of ADR include time saved (most disputes take in excess of 6 years from actual cause to resolution through the nation's court systems) and privacy (the details of the disagreement and its resolution are confidential). Thus, institutions and health care providers can avoid public disclosure and adverse publicity. A major disadvantage to ADR is possible compromise of fairness and due process.

Two of the more common approaches to ADR include mediation and arbitration. **Mediation** involves one or more professional mediators, usually experts in the discipline, listening to both sides of the dispute and helping each side see the other side's position. Hopefully, the two sides to the dispute will be able to solve their differences. Although this approach frequently is helpful in contract disputes, it has rarely been effective in medical malpractice issues because emotions tend to dominate and health professionals have their careers at stake. Additionally, agreements reached through mediation are generally not enforceable unless both sides agree to a binding decision before initiating the process.

Arbitration is a more formal process and is often seen as a "mini-trial." Attorneys are present at arbitration, questioning the parties to the arbitration and witnesses. Testimony is given under oath, so that the process does look like a trial. The differences are that there are no rules of evidence, no court reporter, and no formal record made of the arbitration process. The arbitrator's judgments are legally binding, as agreed to before the process is initiated (*Ash v. Kaiser Foundation Health Plan, Inc.*, 2003; *McGuffey Health and Rehabilitation Center v. Gibson*, 2003).

For example, in *Unidad Laboral v. Hospital De Damas, Inc.* (2001), a hospital employee was terminated for excessive absenteeism and overall inferior work. Her union filed a grievance, requested arbitration, and asked that the nurse be reinstated. The arbitrator ruled for the hospital, stating that there was no basis to see that the dismissal was unfair or discriminatory. The union appealed by filing a lawsuit in federal court.

The court for the District of Puerto Rico upheld the arbitrator's decision. The court ruled that when both sides have bargained for arbitration to resolve disputes, the arbitrator's decision will be final. Arbitrators have "no duty to provide the reasons for their decisions, unlike judges in court, as their decisions are not meant to be appealed" (*Unidad Laboral v. Hospital De Damas, Inc.*, 2001, at 41). Similarly, in *Potts v. Baptist Health System, Inc.* (2002), the court upheld a hospital's right to compel arbitration and ruled that the nurse, who had filed this case in federal court, had no standing to bring such a lawsuit.

Recent lawsuits in this area of the law have concerned residents in nursing homes (*Broughsville v. OHECC, LLC,* 2005; *Bland v. Health Care and Retirement Corporation,* 2006; *Consolidated Resources Healthcare Fund I, Ltd. v. Fenelus,* 2003; *Flaum v. Superior Court,* 2002; *Northport Health Services v. Estate of Raidoja,* 2003). In each of these cases, the court upheld the arbitration clause, following the emerging trend toward arbitration as a viable alternative to jury trial in nursing home liability cases.

Note, though, that the court will reject arbitration agreements if the parties were not fully informed of the significance of the agreement or if the agreement takes away legal rights mandated to a person by state law. In *Romano v. Manor Care, Inc.* (2003), the court set aside an arbitration agreement and allowed the case to be filed in court. The facts of the case were fairly straightforward. An elderly woman had fallen in her home, sustaining a nonoperable hip fracture, and sought immediate admission to a nursing home because her elderly husband could not care for her in their home. The paperwork, concerning her rights and mandate for arbitration rather than filing lawsuits directly in court, was presented after she had already been admitted. No explanation of the six-page document was given, and no meaningful choice was offered as to whether or not to sign the arbitration agreement. The agreement specifically disallowed the resident's right to punitive damages and reimbursement of the resident's legal fees, both allowed under the state's Nursing Home Resident's Bill of Rights. Thus, the court invalidated the arbitration agreement in favor of a court trial before a judge and jury.

In *Prieto v. Healthcare and Retirement Corporation of America* (2005), an elderly nursing home patient contracted a urinary tract infection that lead to his death. Though the nursing home insisted that the subsequent lawsuit could not be validly filed because of an existing arbitration agreement, the court looked at the language of the agreement and allowed the lawsuit to proceed. Not only was the agreement not fully explained, but the family member signing the agreement was instructed that, if she did not sign the agreement, her father could not receive care. The court further noted that nursing home residents' rights laws amount to a legislative statement of public policy against abuse and neglect of vulnerable adults residing in the nursing home, and the nursing home cannot limit those rights through arbitration agreements. *SA-PG-Ocala, LLC v. Stokes* (2006) reached similar conclusions.

Recent lawsuits have also centered around whose signature is required for binding arbitration as a means of resolving conflicts (*Ashburn Health Care Center, Inc. v. Poole,* 2007; *Buie v. Mariner Health Care, Inc.,* 2006; *Compere's Nursing Home, Inc. v. Estate of Farish,* 2008; *Covenant Health and Rehabilitation v. Estate of Lambert,* 2006; *Covenant Health v. Moulds,* 2008; *Del Prado v. THC Orange County, Inc.,* 2006; *Gulledge v. Trinity Mission Health and Rehabilitation,* 2007; *Jones v. Kindred Healthcare,* 2008; *Ricketts v. Christian Care Center,* 2008; *Waverly-Arkansas, Inc. v. Keener,* 2008). Generally, these cases held that a family member (husband, daughter, son, or nephew) could not legally serve as the signer on arbitration agreements for a competent adult. Fundamental to arbitration, said the court in *Ashburn,* is the requirement that the patient knowingly and voluntarily agreed to arbitration. The authority of an agent to act on behalf of the principal must be made apparent by the statements or conduct of the principal, not the agent. For the arbitration agreement to be valid, the court concluded, there must be some means of showing that the competent patient had given her right of consent to her husband. In *Gulledge,* the arbitration agreement was upheld because the daughter was the appropriate surrogate for her incompetent and legally incapacitated mother.

Arbitration in malpractice cases becomes problematic because neither party typically wants to give up the ability to be heard in court. Also, because no rules of evidence apply, testimony that is inadmissible in courts of law may be freely offered in arbitration sessions. For example, a health care provider may be asked about substance abuse if that issue is relevant to the case.

Finally, there is no appeal process with arbitration, unless one can show that the arbitrator was biased in favor of or against one of the parties.

A separate mechanism for ensuring the appropriateness of causes of actions is the prelitigation panel. **Prelitigation panels** ensure that there is an actual controversy or fact question before the case is presented at court. At prelitigation hearings, a panel of medical and legal experts reviews evidence concerning the injury, its cause, and the extent of the injury. Evidence presented may include medical records, expert reports, photographs, x-rays, authoritarian texts, medical journal articles, and medical or legal memoranda.

Not all states employ prelitigation panels because arguments abound as to whether they should exist. In some states, the prelitigation panel is mandatory (for example, Idaho, Maine, and Utah), while in others it is voluntary (for example, Connecticut, Indiana, and Kansas). Defendants' attorneys argue that such panels reduce frivolous lawsuits and expedite the trial process, whereas plaintiffs' attorneys contend that they merely prolong the legal process and increase the overall expense of the trial. Most malpractice cases take 3 to 6 years from the time of injury to a decision, and in states with prelitigation panels, the time is increased by 6 to 12 months.

EXERCISE 4.1

List four reasons why nurse-defendants might not seek the hospital attorney as the attorney to represent their impending case, and list four reasons why they might desire the hospital attorney to be involved as their legal representative. What ethical issues might arise in determining whether to seek assistance from a hospital attorney rather than an attorney not associated with the institution? How would the nurse involved resolve such ethical issues?

Step Two: Pleadings and Pretrial Motions

Pleadings, written documents setting forth the contentions of the parties, are statements of facts as perceived by the opposing sides to the lawsuit. Pleadings give the basis of the legal claim to opposing parties and prevent unfair surprise to either side. In actuality, the initial complaint or petition is also a pleading to the court setting out the plaintiff's facts and declaring that an injustice or wrong has been done. Each defendant responds with a pleading, giving his or her version of the facts to the court. In the defendants' original pleadings, the defendants set forth objections to the plaintiff's complaint. These objections cite possible errors in the plaintiff's case. Possible errors may be procedural (e.g., the process of service was incorrectly performed or the lawsuit is filed in a court that lacks personal jurisdiction over the defendant). Possible errors may also be factual (e.g., the defendant named in the suit was in reality on vacation or scheduled off at the time of the occurrence and thus has no liability in the matter before the court).

The defendant may also file a **motion to dismiss,** stating that there is no valid cause of action on which a claim may be made. The judge may either dismiss the suit upon such a filing or decline to dismiss. If the case is dismissed, the plaintiff may appeal the dismissal. If the motion to dismiss is declined, the defendant must answer the complaint.

A third alternative for the defendant is to file a counterclaim. A **counterclaim** states a cause of action the defendant has against the plaintiff, such as failure to timely pay a hospital bill or comparative negligence on the part of the injured party. For example, if the plaintiff is suing for the improper casting of a broken arm, but failed to keep scheduled appointments to check the alignment of the fracture, the plaintiff could have contributed to the purported negligence.

Either side may then file amended or supplemental pleadings as needed. Amended pleadings correct or add new material to the original pleadings before the court; supplemental pleadings add to the statement of facts already before the court. For example, an amended pleading would be filed to correct a deficiency in the original pleading. Instead of stating that one injection had been negligently given to the plaintiff by the nurse-defendant, the amended pleading might state that two injections, at two separate times, were administered by the nurse-defendant and that both injections resulted in injury to the plaintiff. A supplemental pleading allows the original pleading to stand while supplying additional facts. For example, a supplemental pleading might be filed to bring a third party into the lawsuit.

Pleadings may raise questions of fact or law. If there are no questions of fact, the case may be decided by the judge merely upon the pleadings. Usually, there are a variety of questions of fact and law, necessitating a full trial with or without a jury.

Once the pleadings have been completed, either or both parties may move for a judgment based on the pleadings. Some state courts allow the party seeking a judgment based on the pleadings to introduce sworn statements as evidence showing that the claim or defense is false. Normally, a substantial controversy is involved, and the motion for a judgment based on the pleadings is denied.

Motions, formal requests by one of the parties asking the court to grant its request, may also be filed. Motions may include the need for a speedy trial date owing to the elderly status of the plaintiff or a major witness, the need for a later trial date owing to the length of time needed to obtain necessary documents, or the need for additional documents. Motions are supported with a written narrative, known as a *brief,* that sets out legal arguments for granting the motion. Motions are then argued before the judge, who issues a ruling regarding the motion.

Step Three: Pretrial Discovery of Evidence

Many state courts and federal courts allow parties the **right of discovery,** which permits:

1. witnesses to be questioned by the opposing side prior to the trial.
2. the finding of relevant written materials.
3. possible additional examinations of the plaintiff.

Because of the right of discovery, this step of the trial process may take up to 2 or 3 years to complete.

There are several methods of allowable pretrial questioning of witnesses. **Interrogatories** are written questionnaires mailed to opposing parties that ask specific questions concerning the facts of the case. Most states limit the number of questions on the questionnaire that a given party may be required to complete. Interrogatories must be answered under oath and returned within a time period that is set by state law.

Parties should not attempt to answer interrogatories on their own. Most attorneys instruct their clients to answer the questions as completely as possible on a separate sheet of paper. The attorneys then complete the interrogatory with their clients, appropriately objecting to objectionable questions, and wording answers so as not to suggest or admit liability. Clients should read the answers as completed carefully before signing and, because they are given under oath, make sure that the answers are true as stated.

A second means of obtaining witness testimony is through **deposition,** which is a witness's sworn statement made outside the court that is admissible as evidence in a court of law. Depositions are taken of a witness, who is questioned by the attorney representing the opposing side of the controversy. The deposition's purpose is to assist opposing counsel in preparing for the court case by revealing potential testimony from witnesses before the trial.

One must not be fooled by the fact that a deposition is taken at an attorney's office with few persons present. A deposition is a crucial part of the discovery phase, and one must be alert to the questions being asked and their answers. The deposing witness is under oath during the entire deposition. The attorney representing the person deposed normally does not ask any questions during the deposition or take an active part in the deposition. The attorney for the deposing party already knows the extent of the testimony and does not need to reveal strategy to the opposing side.

Also present at the deposition is a court reporter, who records all questions and answers exactly as they are stated. The deposing party will be allowed to see and read the final written document before signing it, and the deposition becomes sworn testimony. When reviewing the final copy, the deposing witness may correct typographical errors, such as the misspelling of a name, but may make no substantive change to the record, such as changing a previous "yes" answer to a "no" answer.

Deposing witnesses should give their attorneys sufficient time to object to the various questions, and time should be taken when answering each question. The witness may bring medical records, notes, and literature sources to the deposition, and may refer to them as needed during the deposition. Information should not be guessed, but the witness should ensure its accuracy before responding. This same information will be given in court.

An error that physicians and nurses frequently make during depositions is in giving too much information. Often, such information is given because the health care provider knows the right questions to ask and the essential information to elicit. Opposing counsel may not be as well versed and may have ignored an entire area of pertinent information during questioning. Do not assist opposing counsel by giving them the answers needed to pursue the case. That is the domain of attorneys, who have the ultimate responsibility to their clients.

A newer concept in taking depositions is to videotape the witness during the entire deposition rather than to record the deposition through a court reporter. If the witness giving the deposition has a pleasing personality and appears to be caring and compassionate on tape, playing of this type of deposition in court mimics the personal effect of a live appearance. It is the option of deposing parties (and their counsel) to choose this type of deposition.

A fairly recent case, however, illustrates the danger of videotaped depositions. In *Parkway Hospital, Inc. v. Lee* (1997), the hospital's attorneys objected vigorously during the trial, asserting that the plaintiff's attorneys were trying to embarrass the hospital and prejudice the jury against the hospital by playing back pretrial videotaped depositions of the nurses who had cared for the injured patient.

In that case, a nurse had administered Pitocin to a patient in labor, causing the uterus to quickly rupture, and the infant was born with severe neurological injuries. The obstetrician claimed he had never ordered Pitocin. One nurse gave a videotaped deposition saying that there had been no order for Pitocin, but that the physician's routine orders were to be followed. This same nurse testified that she told the oncoming nurse at the change of shift that the physician's routine orders were to be followed. She also testified that she had never said anything about Pitocin or that it had been ordered.

The second nurse testified in her taped deposition that the first nurse told her to administer Pitocin, so she proceeded with the administration. These two depositions were played back to back at trial. The depositions were dramatic proof that the nurses were confused about the physician's orders and the ultimate care of this patient. The jury was led to conclude that negligence by the hospital's nursing staff caused a nurse to give Pitocin to a patient in the labor and delivery unit, especially since the medication had not been ordered by the patient's physician. The jury found that the physician had no liability in the case, but found liability against both the hospital and its nursing staff.

The court ruled it was a perfectly acceptable trial tactic to place into evidence the conflicting testimony of two different agents of the same defendant. The court also upheld the showing to the jury of an 11-minute videotape that showed the child attempting to walk forward and backward, draw on a piece of paper, and talk, to demonstrate graphically the profound limitation in the child's motor control and functional abilities.

Taped depositions are frequently reserved for witnesses who will not be present for the actual trial. For example, witnesses who are outside the jurisdiction of the court or who may be unavailable during the time of the trial hearing may choose to have their depositions videotaped. Although the same evidence could be read at trial from a traditional deposition, the impact of having the witness in the courtroom setting via a taped deposition carries much more weight with the jury.

Depositions serve to uncover facts for the opposing side and to perpetuate the testimony of witnesses. Elderly witnesses or very ill witnesses may actually have their testimony preserved for trial through pretrial depositions.

Either side in the controversy may also obtain and examine copies of the medical records, business records, x-ray films, and the like through a request to produce documents. The court may also require a physical or mental examination of a party through a request for an independent medical examination of the plaintiff, if the medical information so obtained is pertinent to the case. Either party may object to these requests based on grounds that they are unduly burdensome, seek confidential or privileged information, or are protected as part of the attorney's work product. Generally, the scope of discovery is large, and parties are allowed to discover all relevant materials that would be admissible in the subsequent trial.

During the discovery phase, both sides decide on their strategy for the subsequent trial and interview the witnesses they need to testify in court. Both sides also obtain evidence to submit at trial in the form of x-ray films, medical records, consultation reports, and other tangible items that affect the case.

The final phase of the pretrial discovery of evidence is a **pretrial conference,** or **pretrial hearing**. This is a fairly informal session during which the judge and the representing attorneys agree on the issues to be decided and settle procedural matters. The pretrial conference may result in a finalization of a **settlement,** which is favored by the judicial system because it allows for a quick resolution. A settlement is not synonymous with the admission of guilt or liability, but is a means of allowing the parties to forgo the trial process and settle for an agreed-upon dollar figure. Included among the many reasons for settling a case prior to trial are the expense of the trial process, lengthy delays in reaching a trial date, emotional and physical drain on an already injured plaintiff, uncertainty of the jury trial process, and the nature of the harm complained of and its potential ability to shock a jury. As the following case illustrates, a final reason for a settlement may be because there is no adequate means of defending prior actions.

An example of a case that was settled prior to a court determination was *Ballard v. Henry* (2007). In that case, the patient presented to the hospital in active labor, 2 weeks before she was scheduled for her third cesarean section. She had a fever of 101.3°F, which did not abate despite active Tylenol therapy. A fetal monitor was placed, showing that the fetal heart rate was 170. During the next 4 hours, the fetal heart rate was recorded as 170 to 180. The neonate, who was diagnosed with moderate right-sided hemiparesis and cognitive impairment from cerebral infarctions and is today developmentally delayed, was finally delivered approximately 7 hours after the patient was admitted. The main issue for the court concerned why an immediate cesarean section was not done, given the mother's presenting symptoms and the fetal heart rate. The defendants elected to settle the case before the trial was initiated.

Similarly, in *Weatherspoon v. San Francisco General* (2008), a 40-year-old patient was over-sedated with Versed and sent to the radiology department for an abdominal scan. The nurse who was with him during the scan noted nothing abnormal until he arrested. A code was called and the patient has severe residual hypoxic brain damage. The patient's filed lawsuit was settled during the pretrial discovery phase for $6,000,000.

Step Four: The Trial

At the **trial,** the evidence is presented, facts are determined by the jury, principles of law are applied to determined facts, and a solution is formally reached. Evidence is usually presented through various witnesses' answers to specific questions. The jury relies on the testimony and credibility of the witnesses in determining the facts of the case.

If a jury trial has been requested, the trial begins with the selection of the jury, or **voir dire.** Attorneys representing both sides to the controversy question a panel of qualified persons and a 4-, 6-, or 12-person jury is selected and sworn in by the judge. In some jurisdictions, parties to the lawsuit may be allowed to stipulate a jury of 6 rather than the more traditional jury of 12. If no jury is requested or mandated by law, the judge serves as both judge and jury.

After jury selection, both sides make their opening statements. **Opening statements** generally indicate for the jury what each side intends to show by the evidence it presents. Because the plaintiff has the legal burden of proof to show not only that an incident occurred but also that the incident did in fact cause the plaintiff's injury, the plaintiff's attorney has the first opening statement.

Witnesses are then called, one by one, to answer specific questions. The witnesses are directly questioned first by the attorney calling the witness. The opposing side then has the opportunity for **cross-examination,** during which the questioning attorney attempts to discredit or negate the witness's testimony. The attorney originally calling the witness may then ask additional questions in an attempt to reestablish the credibility of the witness once the cross-examination is concluded.

The **level of evidence** or standard of proof that is presented at trial often depends upon the type of case being tried. The standard of proof required in a legal action depends upon "the degree of confidence society thinks should have in the correctness of factual conclusions for a particular type of adjudication" (*Addington v. Texas*, 1979, at 423). Another way of expressing the standard of proof is what is necessary to convince the judge and/or jury that a given proposition is true and to "minimize the risk of an erroneous decision" (*Addington v. Texas*, 1979, at 425).

In civil court cases, the standard of proof is **preponderance of the evidence.** Preponderance of the evidence is based on the probable truth or accuracy of the evidence presented, not on the amount of evidence. The judge or jury must be persuaded that the facts are more probable one way than another way. Thus, one clearly knowledgeable witness may provide the preponderance of the evidence over other witnesses who have merely a general idea of what occurred. Likewise, a signed agreement with definite terms and definitions will provide the preponderance of the evidence over witnesses' speculations of what may have been intended. Note that this level of evidence remains subjective, despite a witness's best efforts to be as objective as possible.

The intermediate standard of proof is **clear and convincing** evidence. Defined by one court as "proof beyond a reasonable doubt is proof that a fact is almost certainly true, while clear and convincing evidence means simply proof that a fact is highly probable (*Allen v. Bowen*, 1987, at 152). For most courts, this is the highest level of proof that can be applied in a civil case and is generally the standard of proof seen in cases involving withdrawal of life-sustaining treatment. *Cruzan v. Director, Missouri Department of Health* (1990) remains the classic case where this level of evidence was required. This level of evidence was supported, in the court's view, as the right to life is a fundamental interest, the person whose life was in question could not protect herself, and the extent of harm was irreversible. Chapter 8 presents more detailed information concerning this case and withdrawal of life-sustaining therapies.

The highest level of evidence is **proof beyond a reasonable doubt** and is generally the standard required in criminal cases. This means that the proposition presented by the government must be proven to the extent that there is no "reasonable doubt" in the mind of a reasonable person that the defendant is guilty of the crime with which he or she is charged. Doubts can linger, but only to the extent that these doubts do not affect a reasonable person's belief that the defendant is guilty as charged.

> The reasonable doubt standard plays a vital role in the American scheme of criminal procedure. It is a prime instrument for reducing the risk of convictions resting on factual error. The standard provides concrete substance for the presumption of innocence—that bedrock. . . . principle whose enforcement lies at the foundation of the administration of our criminal law." (*In re Winship*, 1970, at 358)

The plaintiff presents his or her side of the case through the oral testimony of his or her witnesses. The plaintiff's side then rests the case, meaning that it has attempted to meet the burden of proof and has legally established its cause of action. At that point, the defendants' attorneys may petition for a directed verdict, indicating from their perspective that the plaintiff has failed to present sufficient facts on which to decide the case in the plaintiff's favor. This motion for a directed verdict is typically overruled, and the defendants then call their witnesses one by one to present their case to the jury.

At the conclusion of the defendant's entire case, both sides or either side may again move for a directed verdict. If these attempts are overruled (and they traditionally are), the attorneys make their final arguments, and the judge instructs the jury as to their charge and the principles of law involved. This last step varies greatly from jurisdiction to jurisdiction. The jury retires to deliberate and to reach a **verdict** (decision).

If the verdict that the jury reaches is against the weight of the evidence, the judge may elect to disregard the verdict and determine the ultimate verdict. In *Boxie v. Lemoine* (2008), the jury returned a verdict of no negligence on the part of the defendants. The case involved a patient who had cervical surgery in the not-often-used seated position, where members of the surgical team needed to continuously evaluate the patient for chin-to-sternum clearance. During the surgical procedure, the patient suffered a stroke when his carotid artery blood flow became compromised. The judge found that there was negligence on the part of the surgical team and disregarded the jury's verdict.

Once the verdict is known, the losing side may move for a new trial. If the motion is granted, the entire trial is repeated before a new jury panel. If it is denied, the judgment becomes final, and the losing side may appeal to the proper appellate court if there are legal grounds for such an appeal.

A case example illustrating legal grounds for an appeal is *Pivar v. Baptist Hospital of Miami, Inc.* (1997). In that case, an elderly patient had been hospitalized for several days following hip replacement surgery. The patient was known by the nursing staff to waken several times during the night with the urgent need to arise and go to the bathroom. On the night of the patient's fall, she awoke, feeling the urgency to urinate, and rang her call bell. When no one responded to the call bell, the patient got out of bed by herself and used her walker to get to the bathroom. She placed the walker next to the toilet and transferred herself to the toilet. When she finished urinating, the patient rose, took a step toward the walker, and fell on the water that still remained in the bathroom from an earlier shower.

Detailed for the court was the institution's procedure for showering a patient who had a recent hip replacement. The last part of the procedure was that the nurse assisting the patient is to return to the bathroom once the patient is safely back in bed and clean up any water that may be on the floor from the shower.

In the patient's civil lawsuit against the hospital, the trial judge exercised his prerogative to dismiss the lawsuit without submitting the issues to the jury. The District Court of Appeals held that the trial judge was guilty of a legal error, because there were valid grounds for a civil negligence suit against the institution.

Specifically, the Court of Appeals held that a hospital is "legally bound to exercise such reasonable care as the patient's condition may require, the degree of care in proportion to the patient's known physical and mental impairments" (*Pivar v. Baptist Hospital of Miami, Inc.,* 1997, at 277). Applying this concept to the current case, the court held that it was the nurse's responsibility, given the patient's unsteadiness on her feet and her propensity to use the bathroom unaided when she felt an urgency to urinate, to ascertain that the water had been wiped up after the evening shower and to document that fact in the nursing notes.

EXERCISE 4.2

Jedidiah Monroe has sued Thomas Smith for malpractice, stating that he was given an oral medication by Nurse Smith and that he then suffered a severe allergic reaction to the medication. What additional information might cause the court to enter a directed verdict for the plaintiff?

Step Five: Appeals

The appropriate appellate court reviews the case based on (1) the trial record, (2) written summaries of the principles of law applied, and, in many states, (3) short oral arguments by the representing attorneys. Depending on the outcome at the intermediate appellate level, the case may be eventually appealed to the state supreme court. Once decided at this highest level, the judgment typically becomes final, and the matter is closed. A few cases may be appealed to the U.S. Supreme Court, but this is a rarity in medical malpractice cases.

Step Six: Execution of Judgment

Most lawsuits involving nurses result in one of two possible conclusions: the awarding of money damages against the nurse-defendant or the dismissal of all causes of action against the nurse-defendant. Nothing can return plaintiffs to their original, pretrial status, and the American judicial system attempts to compensate plaintiffs (if the evidence supports compensation) with money damages. Other forms of conclusion include an **injunction** requiring the nurse-defendant to either perform or refrain from performing a certain action and a restraining order.

Restraining orders may be granted when preventing an ongoing action is the only logical outcome to the facts as presented. A case example is the recent case of *Johnson v. Berg* (2008). In this case, the judge ordered the restraining order against the daughter of a nursing home resident, preventing her from any further communication or contact with the nursing home management and staff. The court's decision was based on a finding that the daughter's conduct met the legal definition of harassment.

A family member, noted the court, has the right to consult with caregivers, to voice his or her opinions, and to advocate for alternatives. However, the situation in this case went far beyond reasonable advocacy and became harassment. The resident's daughter repeatedly sent harassing letters of complaint to the nursing staff and followed up with harassing phone calls to staff members. She verbally accused the administrator face-to-face on at least six different occasions and personally interfered with the care of other residents. On one occasion, a security guard had to remove the daughter from the facility. While being bodily removed, she screamed at the nurse and waved some legal-appearing papers in the nurse's face, causing the nurse to fear for her personal safety. On another occasion, she phoned the nursing station and demanded that the nurse who took the phone call conduct an immediate review of her mother's care plan to determine if her mother had been assisted to the restroom no later than 7:00 that morning. That was but one of a long series of repeated, angry, demanding, and demeaning phone calls and letters, which finally forced management to file a lawsuit for the restraining order. The court concluded that the nursing home was entitled to a restraining order so that the daughter would cease and desist from harassing conduct.

After all appeals, the plaintiff will ask that the judgment as provided for by the court be executed. This procedure gives legal relief to the plaintiff if a losing defendant chooses to ignore a court order. If an injunction has been mandated by the court, the defendant may be fined or imprisoned if the injunction is not fulfilled.

A case example of the use of an injunction in a medical context is *Wyckoff Heights Medical Center v. Rodriquez* (2002). In that case, a patient with quadraparesis who had non-insulin-dependent diabetes had been admitted to an acute care facility after his home care was discontinued by the local visiting nurses association. The visiting nurses refused to provide further care because of his violent, threatening, and harassing behavior toward the home health aides who either treated him or attempted to treat him. Ten days after his admission, his medical evaluation indicated that he needed no further acute hospital care and he was discharged.

The hospital found him a placement in an adult home. The patient refused to enter the adult home, and the hospital filed suit seeking a mandatory injunction requiring him to leave the hospital voluntarily or, in the alternative, allow the hospital the legal authorization to have him transported to the adult home. The Supreme Court of New York issued the injunction, noting that the very purpose of an acute care hospital is in jeopardy when a patient who no longer requires acute care services refuses to leave, thereby preventing patients who do require the acute care from using the space to receive inpatient care. The court also noted that it would be pointless for the hospital to sue this patient for the money that his continued stay cost. The court concluded by noting, "To evict a person from the hospital who does require a certain level of professional care is a drastic step, but the patient's unreasonable conduct is equally drastic" (*Wyckoff Heights Medical Center v. Rodriquez*, 2002, at 404).

For a default judgment or money damages award, the defendant's wages may be garnished (i.e., a certain amount of money is taken from the defendant's earnings and given to the winning plaintiff on a weekly or monthly basis) or property may be confiscated and sold to pay the amount of the award. Not all states apply garnishment laws in the same manner, and some states have restrictions on the type of property that may be confiscated. As a result, the execution of judgment varies from state to state.

EXPERT AND LAY WITNESSES

Lay Witness

Most nurses are aware of the expert-witness status. Equally important in the judicial system is the **lay witness,** who establishes facts at the trial level, stating for the judge and jury exactly what transpired. The lay witness is allowed to testify only to facts and may not draw conclusions or form opinions. Lay witnesses define for the jury what actually happened. Both sides to the controversy will present lay witnesses who attempt to describe for the jury what, when, and how a particular event occurred. The lay witness thus has a direct connection with the case in controversy. Lay witnesses at trial include patients, patients' family members, nurses not named in the lawsuit, and other interdisciplinary staff members. In *LeBlanc v. Walsh* (2006), family members served as lay witnesses to testify that the patient's back and bed linens were completely soiled with blood immediately before the patient coded. The jury discounted the nursing personnel version that the only visible blood was the approximate 5 to 10 ccs of fluid in the drain reservoir immediately prior to the patient's code.

Nurses may be called to serve as lay witnesses. In *Hurd v. Windsor Garden Convalescent Hospital* (2002), the court refused a nurse's testimony, stating that a nurse could not testify as an expert in orthopedics, even if she had 20 years of work experience. But she could testify as a lay witness concerning the pain, suffering, and limitations of activities that would result from the fall that was at the heart of the resident's lawsuit.

Expert Witness

The second type of witness, the **expert witness,** explains highly specialized technology or skilled nursing care to the jurors, who typically have little or no exposure to medicine and nursing. Expert testimony is required when conclusions by a jury depend on facts and scientific information that is more than common knowledge. Three recent cases, holding that what is common knowledge requires no expert testimony, iterate this fact. In *Brown v. Tift County Hospital Authority* (2006), an occupational therapist required that a patient stand while showering. Twice the patient told the occupational therapist that she was slipping and needed help. Nevertheless, the patient was left standing in the shower while the occupational therapist went to get the patient's bathrobe. The patient fell while the occupational therapist was getting the bathrobe. The patient's fall risk had been well documented in the chart and her need for maximum assistance with activities of daily living was also well documented. The court concluded that no expert witness was needed in order for this lawsuit to proceed.

In *Rush v. Senior Citizen's Nursing Home District of Ray County* (2006), an elderly diabetic patient died following complications when his blood sugar level rose to 540. There were standing orders for sliding-scale insulin, though the nurse caring for the patient left phone messages for the physician and did not follow the sliding-scale orders. The court ruled in this case that expert witnesses were not needed for the jury to understand the importance of following standing orders when the patient had an ever-increasing blood glucose level. In *Willaby v. Bendersky* (2008), the court held that the patient who had surgery for the removal of a sponge following discharge from the hospital did not need an expert witness, as the negligence is obvious to the common knowledge of lay persons.

The use of nurses as expert witnesses has evolved since the late 1970s and early 1980s. Before then, physicians served as nursing's voice and testified at court regarding the role and accountability of professional nurses. Two precedent court cases in 1980, one in North

Carolina and one in Georgia, set the stage for acceptance by the court of nurses serving as expert witnesses in defining the role of nursing (*Maloney v. Wake Hospital Systems* and *Avet v. McCormick*). In *Maloney,* the court held that "the role of the nurse is critical to providing a high standard of health care in modern medicine. Her expertise is different from, but no less exalted than, that of the physician" (1980, at 683). The court in *Manor Care Health Services, Inc. v. Ragan* (2006) held that to testify as an expert in a health care malpractice lawsuit, a witness must be practicing health care in a field that involves the same type of care or treatment and must have knowledge of the accepted standards of care. A physician is not necessarily disqualified for testifying against nurses just because the physician is not a nurse, if the physician is familiar with nursing standards.

Other courts, though, have concluded that physicians may not establish the nursing standards of care. In *Young v. Board of Hospital Directors, Lee County* (1984), the court held that a psychiatrist was not familiar with the daily practices of psychiatric nursing and therefore could not testify to a deviation from nursing standards. In *Greenberg v. Empire Health Services, Inc.* (2006), the court held that nurses are the experts when testifying to nursing standards of care.

The courts have continued to define qualifications and expectations of nurse expert witnesses. In *Kent v. Pioneer Valley Hospital* (1997), the court allowed a nurse to testify about the legal standard of care for nursing, but ruled that the nurse was not qualified to state an opinion making a cause-and-effect connection between a departure from accepted nursing standards and the injury that the patient had incurred. In two cases, *Stryczek v. Methodist Hospital, Inc.* (1998) and *Taplin v. Lupin* (1997), the court ruled that a nurse is not legally qualified to render an opinion about a medical diagnosis. There is, in the words of the *Stryczek* court, "a significant difference in the scope of nurses' and physicians' legal authority with respect to diagnosis and treatment" (1998, at 697). A more recent case, *Gaines v. Comanche County Medical Hospital* (2006), concluded that courts are seeing a wider role for nurses in medical litigation and that nurses from various states have testified in cases as experts regarding:

- standards for assisting post-operative patients with ambulation (Delaware)
- standards for wound care for post-operative patients with a screw-pin head restraint (Minnesota)
- standards for maintaining the sterility of needles used to draw blood (Georgia)
- issues of a parent's parenting skills, or lack thereof, in child-custody cases (Colorado)
- standards for assessing a patient for signs of preeclampsia and for monitoring the patient for seizure (Ohio)
- the cause of a hospital patient's staph infection, if the nurse has a background in infection control (Kentucky)

The role of an expert witness in assisting the jury and judge to determine nursing interventions can be seen in *Taylor v. Cabell Huntington Hospital, Inc.* (2000). In *Taylor,* a female patient was seen in the emergency center for treatment of a bee sting. The physician ordered 125 mg of Solu-Medrol and 25 mg of Benadryl to be administered intramuscularly. The registered nurse in the emergency center used one syringe to administer the medications, charting that the medications were given by IM injection in the left upper outer quadrant of the patient's buttocks, using a 1½-inch needle.

The patient returned to the emergency center a few days later, complaining of pain in her right hip, which was diagnosed as piriformis muscle spasm. She subsequently sued the hospital, physician, and nurse, claiming that the nurse had in fact injected her in the right hip and had done so negligently. The jury exonerated all defendants.

At trial, a registered nurse testified to the compatibility of the two medications, noting that she herself had given these two medications in combination during her nursing career. "If two medications produce a cloudy solution they are not syringe-compatible" (*Taylor,* 2000, at 723). The expert nurse demonstrated this fact for the jury by mixing these two medications, which remained in a clear solution. Additionally, the nurse demonstrated the extent to which a 1½-inch needle would perforate the patient's muscle mass, concluding that this type of needle could not have reached as far as the patient's piriformis muscle. Thus, the nurse could not have caused this patient's injury. The court accepted the nurse's testimony as an expert witness, noting that it is within a nurse's scope of practice to determine syringe compatibility of medications and which needle size is indicated for IM injections.

Note, though, that the court will not allow a nurse to testify if it can be shown that the witness has no expertise in the specifics of the care in question. In *Tuck v. Healthcare Authority of the City of Huntsville* (2002), a nurse who was a faculty member at a local school of nursing testified about the use of restraints. On cross-examination, it was noted that she had not practiced in a clinical setting in 20 years, that she had never researched or written about restraints, and that she had never used the type of restraint at issue in this case. The court disallowed her testimony as an expert witness. Similar results occurred in *Doades v. Syed* (2002) and *Perdieu v. Blackstone Family Practice Center, Inc.* (2002). In *Perdieu,* the court specifically stated that extensive experience with geriatric patients in acute care settings did not make a nurse an expert on nursing home care.

The minimum credential for a nurse expert witness is current licensure to practice professional nursing within a state or territory. Other criteria for selection include total lack of involvement with the defendants either as an employee or consultant, clinical expertise in the area of nursing at issue, certification in the clinical area if possible, and recent continuing or formal education relevant to the specialty of nursing at issue. Ideally, the expert witness should also have earned graduate degrees and authored publications in nursing. Some attorneys will substitute status as a nurse manager, nurse educator, or preceptor for advanced degrees. It is ultimately the role of the trial judge to decide whether an expert witness possesses adequate skill, training, education, knowledge, and/or experience to serve as an expert witness in a specific lawsuit (*People v. Munroe,* 2003).

The purpose of these criteria for the nurse expert witness is to display for the jury that the nurse is well qualified to be an expert witness. Therefore, credentials that speak to the highest level of nursing expertise and knowledge of the appropriate standard of care weigh favorably with judges and jurors. Such criteria also further ensure the objectivity of the nurse expert. Expert witnesses who have either worked for the defendant institution or who are associated with defendant nurses on a personal level may be seen as giving subjective testimony. Such subjective testimony is most likely to result in a verdict for the plaintiff and against the defendants.

When nurses are first contacted about the possibility of serving as expert witnesses, they should consider some guidelines. First, is the case of interest to them and is it in their area of expertise? Second, all materials sent should be reviewed carefully and a determination made as to whether a standard of care has been upheld or breached. The nurse should not put thoughts and opinions in writing at this stage, because such writings may be viewed by both sides to the controversy. Formal writings can be done once the position of expert witness has been confirmed. Third, the nurse should decide on the fee schedule before proceeding. Acceptable fee schedules can be determined by the geographic area and whether the nurse will appear at trial. Finally, the nurse should know the time frames for discovery and the actual court trial, so that the expert witness can be available for an extended period of time, if that is foreseen.

An expert witness may also serve as a **legal consultant** whose name is not revealed to the opposing side and whose reports or comments are not disclosed. Nurses who are named as expert witnesses should understand that their reports and comments are discoverable by counsel on both sides of the controversy.

When the need for an expert witness arises, both sides in the controversy retain their own experts. Testimony is generally in the form of opinions and answers to hypothetical questions. This practice has evolved because expert witnesses have the ability to analyze facts presented and to draw inferences from those facts, something the lay witness is not allowed to do.

Once selected as an expert witness, the nurse is prepared for this role by the attorney. Legal doctrine or state procedural rules that pertain to the individual case are discussed. Each nursing expert witness should review the following:

1. The facility or area where the incident occurred, to identify special environmental factors and the location of the patient in relation to needed equipment, medications, and staff
2. The state nurse practice act and any relevant rules that the board of nursing may have promulgated
3. Relevant nursing literature to ensure the status of acceptable practice at the time of the occurrence
4. The applicable nursing process of the institution during the time of the occurrence
5. All written records pertaining to the incident or that may have implications for assessment, planned actions, implementation, and evaluation of the incident
6. Supportive management records and/or patient classification acuity records
7. Support functions provided by the institution for nursing

Each of these has implications for the applicable standard of care during the incident.

Unfortunately, the number of lawsuits naming nurses as defendants is currently on the rise (Domrose, 2007). The role of the expert nurse is therefore becoming more vital. The role of expert nurse witnesses is anticipated to continue to increase in importance as nurses testify not only in malpractice cases, but in custody and abuse cases.

Nurses are the only professionals with the competency, credentials, and right to define nursing or to judge whether the appropriate standard of care has been delivered. As nurses come forward to assume this role, the system will adjust to incorporate them and to actively solicit their professional testimonies.

GUIDELINES

For Testifying as an Expert Witness

1. Personal characteristics are important. Be attentive and alert. Look at the person asking the question, showing that you are giving great thought to what is being asked. Do not try to impress anyone. Use normal, conversational language, and refrain from using jargon or "hospital talk." The judge and jury must be able to understand your answers.
2. Time must be taken when considering the answer to each question. Once spoken, an answer cannot be retracted. Understand the question or ask that it be repeated or rephrased. Give your attorney time to object to the question. Objections after an answer is given serve little value in jurors' minds.

3. A favorite ploy of opposing counsel is to fluster, confuse, or anger an expert witness. Such ploys may prevent a clear and concise answer and may cause you to blurt out the first thought that enters your mind. All answers must be considered carefully, giving only the information that answers the questions. The battle being played out in court is about the facts of the case, not about people and personalities. Remain as objective as possible, take a deep breath if needed, and answer objectively, not defensively. Strive to portray yourself as an individual to whom the judge and jury will want to listen.

4. Remember that there are several ways to accomplish any given intervention. The selection of an alternative approach does not equate with substandard care. Do not allow yourself to be backed into a corner where only one means of implementing an intervention is correct. Keep your options open, and reiterate that any of these approaches could have been selected.

5. Ensure that interventions as presented were appropriate at the time of the occurrence, not at the time of the court case. The expert witness should not be manipulated into discussing current practice standards, because they are most likely not reflective of the standard at the time the incident occurred.

6. Testimony previously given during a deposition is sworn testimony and cannot be changed at trial. If you are unsure of your previous testimony, such as quoting the patient's blood pressure or pulmonary wedge pressure, verify the information before speaking. You may refer back to your deposition or to the patient record before responding. If the answers are different, the next question by opposing counsel will inevitably be, "Tell me, nurse, are you lying now or were you lying before?" Either answer destroys all credibility you may have had with the jury.

7. The expert witness should answer only what pertains to nursing, a nursing role, or standards of nursing care. If you cannot answer the attorney's questions without testifying to medical standards, then say it is outside the scope of nursing and you cannot answer. You may ask the attorney to rephrase the question so that it pertains to nursing standards of care.

8. Remember to dress appropriately, in a suit or more conservative dress, because appearance makes a valuable first impression with the jury. Look at the jury as you give your answers, thus showing your sincerity and knowledge.

9. Give only enough information to answer the question. If a simple yes or no will suffice, stop after stating yes or no. Frequently, nursing experts undermine their credibility by trying too hard to ensure that the jury is aware of their knowledge base. The jury will already know that you are a knowledgeable expert by the introduction of your credentials.

10. If opposing counsel asks if you are being paid to appear and testify, the answer is yes. However, stress that the payment is not for testimony, but for any provisions or inconveniences you had to make to be in court, such as travel to a distant court, lost work hours, child care, and review of pertinent facts and standards. The difference is subtle, but extremely important.

11. Expect opposing counsel to question your credentials. Remember, they are trying in every way possible to lessen the weight of your testimony in the eyes of jurors. Rather than credentials, it may be ethics that are attacked, such as a question asking if you had solicited the attorney of record for the opportunity to testify.

12. Be positive in your answers. Do not predicate your answers with "I believe," "I think," or "in my opinion." These are words of equivocation that impair your credibility as a witness.

13. Remember the three Cs of testifying: Be calm, courteous, and consistent in your demeanor.

EXERCISE 4.3

List three possible instances in which no expert witness testimony is needed to assist the jury in their deliberations. An example: Mr. Gonzales is an elderly man who was admitted to the general surgical unit from the post-anesthesia care unit. Earlier in the day, he had surgery to remove his gallbladder. After his admission, Mr. Gonzales fell out of bed, breaking his knee and right wrist. Judy, his primary care nurse, admitted leaving both siderails down and the bed in its highest position.

ETHICAL ISSUES AND THE EXPERT WITNESS

Perhaps the major ethical concern in the trial process concerns the expert witness and his or her testimony. The expert, who was not present at the occurrence or event that triggered the lawsuit, has the task of re-creating the events and testifying on what should have occurred or why what did occur was appropriate given the circumstances, the community standard, and the expertise and education of those involved at the time of the occurrence/event. Thus, the expert witness has the task of being objective and unbiased and conveying these qualities to the judge and jury so that they can come to a fair decision or, as a Federal Rule of Evidence states, that "the truth be ascertained and proceedings justly determined" (Superintendent of Documents, 2006, Rule 102).

The ethical dilemma of being an expert witness begins with the review of the patient records and other reports that comprise the written record of the occurrence or event. These materials are often all that the expert has upon which to base his or her conclusions, and they are predicated on the supposition that they are truthful and contain all the details of the events that occurred at the time of the incident. How does one proceed if the records and reports clearly show that the interventions were inappropriate or that the minimal standard of care was barely completed by those involved in the incident? What obligations does the expert witness have to disclose such findings to the attorney representing the defendants? The expert witness knows that nursing is not an exact science and that human factors often intervene. How does one begin to explain these unexpected outcomes in a way that does not create liability or prejudice a patient who should be compensated for untoward outcomes?

SUMMARY

- There are six procedural steps in any lawsuit:
  - the initiation of the lawsuit
  - pleadings and pretrial motions
  - discovery of evidence
  - trial process
  - appeals
  - execution of judgment
- Alternative dispute resolution, including mediation and arbitration, can be a means of settling a lawsuit outside of the courtroom.
- Pleadings are written documents setting forth the contentions of the parties to the lawsuit.
- Discovery of evidence includes interrogatories, written questionnaires mailed to opposing parties to a lawsuit, and depositions, which are witnesses' sworn statements made outside a courtroom that are admissible as evidence in a court of law.
- Depositions serve to uncover facts for the opposing sides of a lawsuit and also to preserve the testimony of witnesses.
- Settlements may occur during the third phase of the trial process, serving as a quick resolution to the dispute.
- During the trial process, evidence is presented, facts are determined, principles of law are applied to determine facts, and a solution is reached.

- The level or standard of evidence presented during the trial process includes:
  - Lay witnesses establish facts for the judge and jury, defining what actually happened.
  - Expert witnesses explain highly specialized technology and skilled nursing care for the judge and jury, so that they can reach a conclusion based on the evidence presented.
- The ethical issues of being an expert witness are multifaceted and complex.

APPLY YOUR LEGAL KNOWLEDGE

1. Does the trial process ensure that both plaintiffs and defendants have equal opportunity to present their case?
2. When is it advisable to settle a case rather than persist with a lengthy trial?
3. How does understanding the trial process aid the professional nurse?

YOU BE THE JUDGE

Mrs. M. was admitted to an acute care facility for removal of a noncancerous brain lesion. Following her surgical procedure, she had problems swallowing, but no difficulty with respirations and breathing. On x-ray, her lungs showed no signs of congestion or infiltration. She was receiving humidified oxygen via an oxygen mask.

During transport from her hospital room to x-ray for a repeat chest film, the humidifier attached to her oxygen line was allowed to lay on its side, allowing water to accumulate and enter the patient's lungs. The sole person who transported Mrs. M. to the x-ray department was an untrained patient transporter. The patient subsequently experienced aspiration pneumonia and was readmitted to the intensive care unit.

Following her recovery, the patient brought suit for the mishandling of the oxygen humidifier, subsequent aspiration pneumonia, and additional recovery time. At the trial, the patient transporter admitted that he had received no training regarding the transportation of patients receiving humidified oxygen and was not aware that there were any special precautions needed for transporting a patient who was receiving humidified oxygen. The plaintiff's attorney presented no expert witness testimony regarding professional standards for patient transport. The court ruled in favor of the medical center, noting that expert testimony was required, and the patient appealed.

QUESTIONS

1. Was an expert witness needed for the jury to understand the issues being tried?
2. Did the patient transporter's testimony negate the need for expert testimony regarding standards for patient transport when the patient was receiving humidified oxygen via an oxygen mask?
3. If it was determined that expert testimony was needed, what type of qualifications would you have chosen for the expert in this case?
4. How would you decide the appeal?

REFERENCES

Addington v. Texas, 441 U. S. 418 (1979).

Allen v. Bowen, 657 E. Supp. 148 (N. D. Ill., 1987).

Ash v. Kaiser Foundation Health Plan, Inc., 2003 WL 21751207 (Cal. App. July 30, 2003).

Ashburn Health Care Center, Inc. v. Poole, 2007 WL 1764217 (Ga. App., June 20, 2007).

Avet v. McCormick, 271 S.E.2d. 833 (Georgia, 1980).

Ballard v. Henry, 2007 WL 2491531 (Sup. Ct. Kings County, New York, April 19, 2007).

Bland v. Health Care and Retirement Corporation, 2006 WL 1235910 (Fla. App., May 10, 2006).

Boxie v. Lemoine, 2008WL 2744238 (La. App., July 16, 2008).

Broughsville v. OHECC, LLC, 2005 WL 3483777 (Ohio App., December 21, 2005).

Brown v. Tift County Hospital Authority, 2006 WL 1914585 (Ga. App., July 13, 2006).

Buie v. Mariner Health Care, Inc., 2006 WL 3858330 (S. D. Miss., December 29, 2006).

Compere's Nursing Home, Inc. v. Estate of Farish, 2008 WL 2139548 (Miss., May 22, 2008).

Consolidated Resources Healthcare Fund I, Ltd. v. Fenelus, 2003 WL 21750370 (Fla. App., July 30, 2003).

Covenant Health and Rehabilitation v. Estate of Lambert, 2006 WL 3593437 (Miss. App., December 12, 2006).

Covenant Health v. Moulds, 2008 WL 3843820 (Miss. App., August 19, 2008).

Cruzan v. Director, Missouri Department of Health, 110 S. Ct. 2841 (1990).

Del Prado v. THC Orange County, Inc., 2006 WL 3555563(Cal. App., December 11, 2006).

Doades v. Syed, 2002 WL 31249906 (Tex. App., October 9, 2002).

Domrose, C. (2007). Malpractice suits against nurses on the rise. *New Hampshire Nurse, 31*(4), 8–9.

Flaum v. Superior Court, 2002 WL 31852905 (Cal. App., December 20, 2002).

Gaines v. Comanche County Medical Hospital, 2006 WL 1628094 (Oklahoma, June 13, 2006).

Greenberg v. Empire Health Services, Inc., 2006 WL 1075574 (Wash. App., April 25, 2006).

Gulledge v. Trinity Mission Health and Rehabilitation, 2007 WL 3102141 (N. D. Miss., October 22, 2007).

Hurd v. Windsor Garden Convalescent Hospital, 2002 WL 1558600 (Cal App., July 16, 2002).

In re Winship, 397 U.S. 358 (1970).

Johnson v. Berg, 2008 WL 3897846 (Minn. App., August 26, 2008).

Jones v. Kindred Healthcare, 2008 WL 3861980 (Tenn. App., August 20, 2008).

Kent v. Pioneer Valley Hospital, 930 P.2d 904 (Utah App., 1997).

LeBlanc v. Walsh, 2006 WL 329839 (La. App., February 14, 2006).

Maloney v. Wake Hospital Systems, 262 S.E.2d. 680 (North Carolina, 1980).

Manor Care Health Services, Inc. v. Ragan, 2006 WL 57355 (Tex. App., January 12, 2006).

McGuffey Health and Rehabilitation Center v. Gibson, 2003 WL 21040590 (Alabama, May 9, 2003).

Northport Health Services v. Estate of Raidoja, 2003 WL 21713988 (Fla. App., July 25, 2003).

Parkway Hospital, Inc. v. Lee, 946 S.W.2d 580 (Tex. App., 1997).

People v. Munroe, 2003 N.Y. Slip Op. 16136, 2003 WL 21709674 (N.Y. App., July 24, 2003).

Perdieu v. Blackstone Family Practice Center, Inc., 2002 WL 31048324 (Virginia, September 13, 2002).

Pivar v. Baptist Hospital of Miami, Inc., 699 So.2d 273 (Fla. App., 1997).

Potts v. Baptist Hospital System, Inc., 2002 WL 31845929 (Alabama, December 20, 2002).

Prieto v. Healthcare and Retirement Corporation of America, 2005 WL 3479850 (Fla. App., December 21, 2005).

Ricketts v. Christian Care Center, 2008 WL 3833660 (Tenn., App., August 15, 2008).

Romano v. Manor Care, Inc., 2003 WL 22240322 (Fla. App., October 1, 2003).

Rush v. Senior Citizen's Nursing Home District of Ray County, 2006 WL 3361856 (Mo. App., November 21, 2006).

SA-PG-Ocala, LLC v. Stokes, 2006 WL 2347369 (Fla. App., August 11, 2006).

Stryczek v. Methodist Hospital, Inc., 694 N.E.2d 1186 (Ind. App., 1998).

Superintendent of Documents. (2006). *Federal rules of evidence.* Washington, DC: U.S. Government Printing Office.

Taplin v. Lupin, 700 So.2d 1160 (La. App., 1997).

Taylor v. Cabell Huntington Hospital, Inc., 538 S.E.2d 719 (West Virginia, 2000).

Tuck v. Healthcare Authority of the City of Huntsville, 2002 WL 31663594 (Alabama, November 27, 2002).

Unidad Laboral v. Hospital De Damas, Inc., 171 F. Supp.2d 38 (D. Puerto Rico, 2001).

Waverly-Arkansas, Inc. v. Keener, 2008 WL 316149 (Ark. App., February 6, 2008).

Weatherspoon v. San Francisco General, 2008 WL 2736708 (Sup. Ct. San Francisco Co., California, May 8, 2008).

Willaby v. Bendersky, 2008 WL 2550708 (Ill. App., June 25, 2008).

Wyckoff Heights Medical Center v. Rodriquez, 741 N.Y.S.2d 400 (N.Y. Super., 2002).

Young v. Board of Hospital Directors, Lee County, #82-429 (Florida, 1984).

LIABILITY ISSUES

CHAPTER 5

Standards of Care

PREVIEW

Standards of care are implemented daily in all aspects of health care delivery and in all practice settings, forming the basis for quality, competent health care. Standards of care are the criteria for determining if less-than-adequate care was delivered to health care consumers. This chapter explores the foundations of standards of care, describing how they are derived and defined within courts of law.

LEARNING OUTCOMES
After completing this chapter, you should be able to:

5.1 Define *standards of care* from a legal and a nursing perspective.

5.2 Compare and contrast internal versus external standards of care.

5.3 Discuss the concept of the reasonably prudent nurse in defining standards of care.

5.4 Differentiate national versus local standards of care.

5.5 Describe the importance of standards of care to the individual nurse.

5.6 Discuss some of the ethical issues that arise concerning standards of care.

KEY TERMS
error in judgment rule
external standards

internal standards
national standards

standards of care
two schools of thought
    doctrine

DEFINITION OF STANDARDS OF CARE

Standards of care are generally defined as the level or degree of quality considered adequate by a given profession. Standards of care are the skills and knowledge commonly possessed by members of a profession. Created by the duty undertaken, standards of care describe the minimal requirements that define an acceptable level of care, which is to exercise ordinary and reasonable care to see that no unnecessary harm comes to the patient. The court, in *King v. State of Louisiana* (1999), further defined standards of care: "legal duty of care or standards of care means a nurse must have and use the knowledge and skill ordinarily possessed and used by nurses actively practicing in the nurse's specialty area" (at 1029).

The basic purposes of standards of care are to protect and safeguard the public as a whole. Were there no standards of care, consumers would open themselves to varying levels of care and varying degrees of quality of care, and the consumers would eventually be the persons who suffered. Standards of care have evolved to help the health care recipient avoid substandard health care and to give guidance to health care providers.

Standards of care may easily be differentiated from objectives, philosophies, and guidelines. Objectives are goals that give direction to what must be accomplished. For example, a goal may be to ambulate the patient 20 steps. Philosophies state why an action is performed. Ambulation of the post-operative patient helps to prevent complications due to thrombus formation and orthostatic hypotension. Guidelines describe recommended courses of action. For example, patients should be ambulated more than once per day, preferably when they are most rested and steady on their feet.

Standards are authoritative statements promulgated by a profession by which the quality of practice, service, or education can be evaluated (American Nurses Association, 1998). A standard of care might be written as follows:

The early post-operative patient should be ambulated during the first 24 hours following surgery pursuant to a valid order and with two nurses or assistants in attendance. Vital signs will be taken and recorded both before and after ambulation.

EXERCISE 5.1

Review your institution's current policy and procedure manual. Randomly select a policy and procedure and show how the language used makes this a standard as opposed to an objective, philosophy, or guideline. Rewrite the policy so that it is an objective, a philosophy, and a guideline.

Why do standards give the most guidance to nurses for effective patient care? Do standards of care also give ethical guidance for the practicing nurse? Why or why not?

ESTABLISHMENT OF NURSING STANDARDS OF CARE

Nursing standards of care may be established in a variety of ways and often are classified into two broad categories: internal and external standards.

Internal Standards

Internal standards are those set by the role and education of the nurse or by individual institutions. These include the professional nurse's job description, education, and expertise as well as an institution's policies and procedures. An illustration of how a court of law judges the importance of one's expertise may be found in *Miller v. Jacoby* (2001). In that case, the patient had a Penrose drain placed to promote post-operative drainage following renal surgery. The physician ordered the drain removed on the third post-operative day. The nurse who removed the Penrose drain had more than 30 years of experience in post-operative care and had removed in excess of 100 Penrose drains during her nursing career. Resistance was met when the drain was removed;

the removed piece had a jagged edge, and it was discovered during imaging studies 3 months later that a 5.5 centimeter portion of the drain had been retained in the patient.

In finding for the patient, the court noted that when resistance is encountered during the removal of such a drain and there is a jagged edge at the end of the removed portion, the nurse should know that something is wrong. At that point, the nurse, especially one with vast experience in this field of nursing, has a legal duty to bring the matter to the physician's attention so that further evaluation and intervention can be made.

The institution's policies and procedures also set internal standards of care. The importance of following the institution's policies and procedures cannot be understated. In court cases, the institution's policies and procedures are presented and evaluated to determine if a nurse defendant has met the standards of care. For example, *Weiner v. Kwait* (2003) illustrates the importance of adhering to written policies and procedures in avoiding potential liability. In that case, a patient's next of kin sued the physician and a skilled nursing home for a patient's untimely death due to sepsis. An 86-year-old man, whose medical diagnosis included hypothyroidism, depression, and prostate cancer, was admitted to a skilled nursing facility. The standard of care as dictated in the institution's policy and procedure manual was for vital signs to be taken and recorded twice per day and for the patient to be seen by his or her physician at least every 30 days unless the nursing staff detected a problem that required the patient to be seen immediately.

The court noted in its finding that the nursing staff did take and record the patient's vital signs twice daily. When the nursing staff detected a low-grade fever and a drop in the patient's blood pressure, the physician was called and blood was drawn for a possible overdose of the thyroid medication. That evening, the patient's blood pressure was still low and his temperature was higher than earlier in the day, and the physician was again notified of the change in the patient's condition. Following the physician's order, the patient was transported to the emergency center, where he died the following day. In dismissing the case in favor of the defendants, the court noted that the institution's policies and procedures had been followed in the care of this patient.

Note how the *Weiner* case differs from the finding in *Beck v. Director, Arkansas Employment Security Department* (1999). In *Beck,* a clearly written policy existed for the dispensing and charting of medications. The nurse in this case said she made it a practice to wait until the end of her shift to chart all medications she had given during the shift. She admitted that at the end of the day in question she could not remember what she had given or to whom it was given. The nurse also admitted on one occasion that she had given Darvocet without looking at the patient's record and that the patient had received the medication earlier than it should have been administered. The court upheld the termination of this nurse because she was guilty of misconduct by intentionally violating a policy established for the patients' well-being and safety.

While nurses are required to follow institutional policies and procedures, *Smith v. Silver Cross Hospital* (2003) illustrates that they are not required to do more than the policy requires. In *Smith,* a patient was admitted to the emergency center with flulike symptoms, including nausea, cough, fever, and difficulty breathing. He was triaged, treated by the physician for bronchitis, and released. Later that day, his condition worsened, and he was admitted to a second hospital, where he subsequently died from meningococcemia.

Though the patient was discharged at 5:50 A.M., he did not get a ride home until 7:00 A.M. The nurse who discharged the patient testified that at 5:50 A.M., his condition had been stabilized and the patient did not have any obvious skin rash or petechial hemorrhages characteristic of meningococcemia. His brother testified that when the patient left the hospital at 7:00 A.M., he had difficulty walking, his speech was slurred, and he had red and purple discoloration on his face. The brother admitted that he did not inform anyone of the patient's condition, but merely took the brother home.

The court, in finding for the defendants, noted that there is generally no requirement for nurses to check on patients sitting in the waiting room following discharge. The court also noted that there was no institutional policy for the nurses to do so; thus the discharge nurse had not fallen below the standard of care. It is interesting to note that the hospital subsequently implemented a policy requiring a patient to be reevaluated when he or she actually left the hospital, but that was a later policy and not in effect at the time of the incident and thus had no bearing on this specific case.

Courts expect nurses and health care providers to use their professional judgment before blindly following written policy and procedures. In *Vede v. Delta Regional Medical Center* (2006), the patient sustained a severe inhalation injury and burns over 18% of his body in a motor vehicle accident. During the 2 months he was hospitalized at a regional burn center, he developed a decubitus ulcer on his coccyx. The subsequent lawsuit alleged that the nurses at the burn center were negligent for failing to follow the center's protocols and nationally accepted patient care standards for frequent patient turning to prevent skin breakdown.

Though the court acknowledged that the center's internal standards as well as the nationally accepted patient care standards do require in general terms that patients at risk for skin breakdown be turned every 2 hours, the court found substantial evidence that justified departures from these general standards of care. Specifically, the priority for a patient with severe inhalation and burn injuries is survival, and keeping to the center's standing protocols for frequent turning would have compromised the patient's ability to breathe. Documentation regarding his care noted that the patient's oxygen saturation fell to dangerously low levels when he was turned on his side and that the oxygen saturation level returned to normal values when he was lying on his back, the difference apparently caused by airway obstruction in the side-lying position. Documentation also supported that the nurses did note that an ulcer was forming on the patient's coccyx and that a special flotation mattress was used so that he could remain in a supine position and that the nurses carefully and frequently charted their observations regarding further skin breakdown.

In a case that had an opposite finding, the court ruled that nurses must use their professional judgment when following facility procedures and protocols (*Pages-Ramirez v. Hospital Espanol,* 2008). In that case, the nurses were faulted for continuing a Pitocin drip despite signs and symptoms that the fetus was in distress. Hospital policy also mandated that the nurses ensure that an internal monitor be initiated if none is present when the external monitor readings indicate fetal distress. In *Pages-Ramirez,* the nurses blindly followed the attending physician's orders rather than discontinuing the Pitocin, and they also failed to notify their nursing supervisor that the established standards of care were not being followed.

Sheridan v. St. Luke's Regional Medical Center (2001) and *Schultz v. Ingham Regional Medical Center* (2006) illustrate what can happen when no policy and procedure exists. In *Sheridan,* the nurses failed to report increasing jaundice in a newborn to the attending physician and did not instruct the mother at discharge about seeking further medical attention if the jaundice increased or failed to abate. The court said the hospital's neonatal nurses should have taken more seriously the threat posed by signs of jaundice in a newborn and should have advocated for early intervention. The court further stated that there should be a policy for nurses to take patient care issues to hospital administration, and it faulted the hospital for not having a policy for incompatible maternal and umbilical cord blood to be brought immediately to the pediatrician's attention.

In *Schultz,* a patient developed compartment syndrome in his right calf after a lengthy orthopedic procedure on his left knee. During the 6-hour procedure, the circulating nurse twice reached under the sterile drapes to exercise the non-operative leg. At trial, the expert witness related the patient's post-operative complications to the fact that the range-of-motion exercises did not fully exercise the non-operative leg and that they were not performed as frequently as they should have been. The judge dismissed the case, noting that there were no established standards of care setting the acceptable parameters for exercising and repositioning the non-operative leg during orthopedic cases. The court of appeals, though, overruled the trial court, noting that the jury should hear from both the plaintiff's and defendant's expert witnesses before rendering a verdict.

Santa Rosa Medical Center v. Robinson (1977), which remains the leading case in this area, extended internal standards to include hospital in-service films. In that case, the standard of care for closed-head injuries was reduced to an in-service film, and the viewing of the film was mandatory for all staff members. When members of the staff violated the standard of care as outlined in the film, the court allowed the jury to view the film to show what the hospital's standard of care should have been.

While courts have allowed policy and procedure manuals to be introduced as criteria for the acceptable standard of care, policies and procedures need not be in writing to be considered legally enforceable. Unwritten policies may actually potentiate liability because not all employees are aware of the policy's existence. In *Boring v. Conemaugh Memorial Hospital* (2000), a patient was admitted for surgery on his ear. During the operation, the surgeon encountered uncontrollable bleeding that made it necessary for the surgeon to stop the surgery. It was later determined that the patient had received Naprosyn less than 72 hours prior to the surgery and that the surgeon routinely contradicted Naprosyn for his presurgical patients due to the risk of excessive bleeding. There was no evidence that the nurses knew that the physician's standing preference for excluding this medication during the immediate presurgical care of patients.

The hospital did have a policy that surgeons' general preferences regarding presurgical care were to be brought to the attention of the nursing staff without any specific orders. What the hospital's policies and procedures lacked was a means of communicating this information to the nursing staff. There must be, said the court, "specific directions for recording surgeon's preferences ahead of time and for communicating these to the nursing staff" (*Boring v. Conemaugh Medical Hospital,* 2000, at 864).

External Standards

External standards are those set by the state boards of nursing, professional organizations, specialty nursing organizations, current nursing literature, federal organizations, and federal guidelines. These standards are seen as external because they transcend individual practitioners and single institutions. In many instances, external standards are synonymous with national standards.

State boards of nursing publish acceptable standards in the state nurse practice act or in rules and regulations promulgated to enforce the state nurse practice act. These rules and regulations have the force of law because they are created to carry out the law. Courts consider whether standards of care were met or violated based on the evidence presented. An example of a state's standards of nursing practice is presented in Figure 5.1.

(1) Standards Applicable to All Nurses. All vocational nurses, registered nurses and registered nurses with advanced practice authorization shall:

(A) Know and conform to the Texas Nursing Practice Act and the board's rules and regulations as well as all federal, state, or local laws, rules or regulations affecting the nurse's current area of nursing practice;

(B) Implement measures to promote a safe environment for clients and others;

(C) Know the rationale for and the effects of medications and treatments and shall correctly administer the same;

(D) Accurately and completely report and document:

   (i) the client's status including signs and symptoms;

   (ii) nursing care rendered;

   (iii) physician, dentist or podiatrist orders;

   (iv) administration of medications and treatments;

   (v) client response(s); and

   (vi) contacts with other health care team members concerning significant events regarding client's status;

(E) Respect the client's right to privacy by protecting confidential information unless required or allowed by law to disclose the information;

(F) Promote and participate in education and counseling to a client(s) and, where applicable, the family/significant other(s) based on health needs;

(G) Obtain instruction and supervision as necessary when implementing nursing procedures or practices;

(H) Make a reasonable effort to obtain orientation/training for competency when encountering new equipment and technology or unfamiliar care situations;

(I) Notify the appropriate supervisor when leaving a nursing assignment;

(J) Know, recognize, and maintain professional boundaries of the nurse-client relationship;

(K) Comply with mandatory reporting requirements of Texas Occupations Code Chapter 301 (Nursing Practice Act), Subchapter I, which include reporting a nurse:

   (i) who violates the Nursing Practice Act or a board rule and contributed to the death or serious injury of a patient;

   (ii) whose conduct causes a person to suspect that the nurse's practice is impaired by chemical dependency or drug or alcohol abuse;

   (iii) whose actions constitute abuse, exploitation, fraud, or a violation of professional boundaries; or

   (iv) whose actions indicate that the nurse lacks knowledge, skill, judgment, or conscientiousness to such an extent that the nurse's continued practice of nursing could reasonably be expected to pose a risk of harm to a patient or another person, regardless of whether the conduct consists of a single incident or a pattern of behavior.

   (v) except for minor incidents (Texas Occupations Code §§301.401(2), 301.419, 22 TAC §217.16), peer review (Texas Occupations Code §§301.403, 303.007, 22 TAC §217.19), or peer assistance if no practice violation (Texas Occupations Code §301.410) as stated in the Nursing Practice Act and Board rules (22 TAC Chapter 217).

(L) Provide, without discrimination, nursing services regardless of the age, disability, economic status, gender, national origin, race, religion, health problems, or sexual orientation of the client served;

(M) Institute appropriate nursing interventions that might be required to stabilize a client's condition and/or prevent complications;

(N) Clarify any order or treatment regimen that the nurse has reason to believe is inaccurate, non-efficacious or contraindicated by consulting with the appropriate licensed

FIGURE 5.1 Examples of a state's standards of nursing practice. (*continued*)

practitioner and notifying the ordering practitioner when the nurse makes the decision not to administer the medication or treatment;

(O) Implement measures to prevent exposure to infectious pathogens and communicable conditions;

(P) Collaborate with the client, members of the health care team and, when appropriate, the client's significant other(s) in the interest of the client's health care;

(Q) Consult with, utilize, and make referrals to appropriate community agencies and health care resources to provide continuity of care;

(R) Be responsible for one's own continuing competence in nursing practice and individual professional growth;

(S) Make assignments to others that take into consideration client safety and that are commensurate with the educational preparation, experience, knowledge, and physical and emotional ability of the person to whom the assignments are made;

(T) Accept only those nursing assignments that take into consideration client safety and that are commensurate with the nurse's educational preparation, experience, knowledge, and physical and emotional ability;

(U) Supervise nursing care provided by others for whom the nurse is professionally responsible; and

(V) Ensure the verification of current Texas licensure or other Compact State licensure privilege and credentials of personnel for whom the nurse is administratively responsible, when acting in the role of nurse administrator.

(2) Standards Specific to Vocational Nurses. The licensed vocational nurse practice is a directed scope of nursing practice under the supervision of a registered nurse, advanced practice registered nurse, physician's assistant, physician, podiatrist, or dentist. Supervision is the process of directing, guiding, and influencing the outcome of an individual's performance of an activity. The licensed vocational nurse shall assist in the determination of predictable healthcare needs of clients within healthcare settings and:

(A) Shall utilize a systematic approach to provide individualized, goal-directed nursing care by:
  (i) collecting data and performing focused nursing assessments;
  (ii) participating in the planning of nursing care needs for clients;
  (iii) participating in the development and modification of the comprehensive nursing care plan for assigned clients;
  (iv) implementing appropriate aspects of care within the LVN's scope of practice; and
  (v) assisting in the evaluation of the client's responses to nursing interventions and the identification of client needs;

(B) Shall assign specific tasks, activities and functions to unlicensed personnel commensurate with the educational preparation, experience, knowledge, and physical and emotional ability of the person to whom the assignments are made and shall maintain appropriate supervision of unlicensed personnel.

(C) May perform other acts that require education and training as prescribed by board rules and policies, commensurate with the licensed vocational nurse's experience, continuing education, and demonstrated licensed vocational nurse competencies.

(3) Standards Specific to Registered Nurses. The registered nurse shall assist in the determination of healthcare needs of clients and shall:

(A) Utilize a systematic approach to provide individualized, goal-directed, nursing care by:
  (i) performing comprehensive nursing assessments regarding the health status of the client;
  (ii) making nursing diagnoses that serve as the basis for the strategy of care;
  (iii) developing a plan of care based on the assessment and nursing diagnosis;
  (iv) implementing nursing care; and
  (v) evaluating the client's responses to nursing interventions;

FIGURE 5.1 Examples of a state's standards of nursing practice.   (*continued*)

(B) Delegate tasks to unlicensed personnel in compliance with Chapter 224 of this title, relating to clients with acute conditions or in acute are environments, and Chapter 225 of this title, relating to independent living environments for clients with stable and predictable conditions.

(4) Standards Specific to Registered Nurses with Advanced Practice Authorization. Standards for a specific role and specialty of advanced practice nurse supersede standards for registered nurses where conflict between the standards, if any, exist. In addition to paragraphs (1) and (3) of this subsection, a registered nurse who holds authorization to practice as an advanced practice nurse (APN) shall:

(A) Practice in an advanced nursing practice role and specialty in accordance with authorization granted under Board Rule Chapter 221 of this title (relating to practicing in an APN role; 22 TAC Chapter 221) and standards set out in that chapter.

(B) Prescribe medications in accordance with prescriptive authority granted under Board Rule Chapter 222 of this title (relating to APNs prescribing; 22 TAC Chapter 222) and standards set out in that chapter and in compliance with state and federal laws and regulations relating to prescription of dangerous drugs and controlled substances.

Source: Rule 217.11, effective November 15, 2007, 32 Texas Register, p. 8165

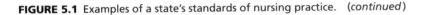

FIGURE 5.1 Examples of a state's standards of nursing practice. *(continued)*

Professional organizations add to the body of acceptable standards of care for professional nursing. The profession has the inherent right to direct and control its activities. The most active professional organization in this area is the American Nurses Association (ANA) and its state components. The ANA Congress for Nursing Practice set eight basic standards of care in 1973. Based on the nursing process, these eight standards are applicable to all nurses, regardless of clinical specialty. These standards of care for nursing practice represent the first step in unifying standards of care throughout all jurisdictions.

The ANA and the state nurses associations have lobbied to encourage enactment of these generic standards of care through state legislative processes. One of the basic arguments for such generalized standards of care is to upgrade the standards set by individual hospitals and institutions that were traditionally based on a local standard of acceptability.

In 1974, the ANA's publication of specialty standards of care was first published. These specialty standards of care were published for various clinical specialties, including (1) community health nursing, (2) geriatric nursing, (3) maternal–child health nursing, (4) mental health nursing, and (5) medical–surgical nursing. Standards published in the past few years have greatly expanded clinical applications to areas outside acute care settings, including standards for advanced nurse practitioners, standards of college health nursing practice, standards for hospice and palliative nursing practice, standards for pain management nursing practice, standards for corrections nursing practice, standards for plastic surgery nursing practice, standards of genetics/genomics nursing practice, and standards of faith community nursing. Today, ANA publishes multiple standards that pertain to specialty practice areas (ANA, 2008), including standards that pertain to holistic nursing, forensic nursing practice, and diabetes nursing.

Professional standards of care are also created by the National League for Nursing Accrediting Commission (NLNAC), an arm of the National League of Nursing (NLN).

The NLNAC evaluates the quality of nursing education and accredits schools of nursing, both at the undergraduate and graduate levels. Directly and indirectly, these standards of education influence the quality of acceptable nursing within a community.

A recent court case that illustrates the importance of adhering to professional standards is *MacTavish v. Rhode Island Hospital* (2002). In that case, the patient had a history of chest pains and shortness of breath. She was to have surgery to correct her spinal stenosis. Before the surgery, though, she was scheduled for an outpatient treadmill test to assess her cardiac status. The nurse competently assessed the patient, finding that the patient was fit for the cardiac assessment test. Because of a 3-hour span between this assessment and the scheduled treadmill test, the nurse suggested that the patient go to the cafeteria for lunch. The patient did not need or request assistance. She walked to the cafeteria and ate her lunch without incident. On the way back to the treadmill test, she fell and sued the hospital for negligence.

As there was no expressed hospital policy nor written physician order for this situation, it became a matter of nursing judgment. In finding for the nurse and against the hospital, the court noted that there was no evidence that the nurse's judgment had departed from professional nursing standards.

Individual nursing specialty practice organizations also publish standards of care to upgrade and generalize the standards for patients within a given clinical setting or within a given category. For example:

1. The American Association of Critical-Care Nurses (AACN) publishes standards of care for critically ill patients.
2. The Emergency Nurses Association (ENA) publishes standards of care for trauma and urgent care patients.
3. The Oncology Nursing Society (ONS) publishes standards for cancer patients.
4. The Association of Operating Room Nurses (AORN) publishes standards of care for patients in the perioperative setting.
5. On an international perspective, the International Council of Nursing (ICN) has published its standards through an ethical code (2006).

A case that illustrates how courts enforce specialty nursing practice guidelines is *Ledesma v. Shashoua* (2007). The patient sued the hospital for a radial nerve palsy caused by the failure to correctly position and pad the patient's arm during surgery. The court relied on the standards of care published by the American Association of Operating Room Nurses and the American Nurses Association in their holding that the circulating room nurse has responsibility for the IV, arm board placement, padding, and positioning of this patient as well as for intra-operative nursing documentation. Those organizations' publications are widely recognized by the court as authoritative references in the legal standard of care in various nursing settings.

Federal organizations and federal guidelines are other examples of external standards. The Joint Commission (JC) sets nursing standards by publishing the *Accreditation Manual for Hospitals* on a yearly basis (JC, 2008). JC's requirements for individualized nursing care plans set a standard of care. For example, one of its standards states that patients must be assessed and individualized care plans must be written. Such a requirement may actually assist nurses if a subsequent lawsuit is filed. The individualized care plan may indeed show that the nursing staff did meet the standard of care for safety by innovative measures aimed at preventing an individual patient's injury or further injury.

In *Pugh v. Mayeaux* (1998), a patient had intermittent labor contractions and was slightly dilated on admission to the acute care setting. Pancreatitis, not explained by her history, developed while she was in the hospital. The physicians determined that the pancreatitis did not threaten the fetus, but the patient was continuously assessed for signs of fetal distress. When signs of distress occurred, an emergency cesarean section was performed, but not quickly enough to prevent permanent damage due to hypoxia.

The court applauded the nurses for their individualization of this patient's care. When the patient was admitted, the nurses were alert to the possibility that another medical condition could manifest itself. In fact, it was the nursing staff who first assessed signs of pancreatitis and alerted the physicians. The patient was transferred to the intensive care unit after the nurse notified the physician of the patient's worsening condition and called to recommend such a transfer. In the intensive care unit, labor and delivery nurses were available to check the fetal monitor and assess the infant's condition.

Although there were catastrophic complications to the baby, the court indicated in its final summary the respect the justices had for the nurses and how competently they both cared for the patient and communicated all aspects of that care with the physicians.

A similar conclusion was reached in *Barnett v. University of Cincinnati Hospital* (1998). In that case, a home health care patient became increasingly more forgetful and irrational. The social worker who saw her determined that these were signs of her inability to live independently and arranged for admission to an acute care geriatric psychiatric unit of the hospital.

At the hospital, the patient was diagnosed with dementia and agitation, for which Ativan was prescribed. The nurses assisted the patient out of bed and into a "geri chair," where the patient slept for a few hours. They repositioned her in bed, where she slept for the majority of the morning. She was awakened for meals and medications, and the nurses assisted in feeding the patient.

She was assessed on a routine basis and was later found on the floor after she fell while trying to get out of bed. The Court of Claims of Ohio dismissed the resulting lawsuit. The justices ruled that close supervision of a dementia patient sedated with Ativan requires periodic checks to ensure the patient's safety. But close supervision does not mean one-to-one in-room supervision. The court praised the nurses for placing this patient in a room next to the nurses' station so that they could keep a closer watch on her, and in conducting and documenting frequent periodic checks. They also did not fault the nurses for not restraining the patient while she was asleep in her room.

Other federal agencies, such as the Social Security Administration (overseeing Medicare and Medicaid funding, nursing home qualifications, and maternal and child health programs), also are directly responsible for setting nursing standards of care. These agencies serve a vital role in setting standards of care as they periodically publish rules and regulations regarding the care of patients, and in setting minimum qualifications for those who care for patients receiving their support. For example, the requirement that registered nurses perform and record complete physical assessment data on hospitalized patients on a 24-hour basis was initially introduced by federal funding agencies as a Medicare and Medicaid requirement.

Current nursing literature, including journal articles and textbooks, also creates standards of care. An interesting case that illustrates this concept is *Wolff v. Washington Hospital Center* (2007). In *Wolff*, a patient filed a lawsuit alleging that the nurses' negligence caused him to develop pressure sores that progressed to decubitus ulcers. The patient had been hospitalized for open-heart surgery, which was complicated by additional surgeries to revise his surgical site. The patient's expert witness testified that nursing standards adamantly required that patients be turned every 2 hours, even if a special bed such as a Baribed was used. The hospital's expert witness testified that there are significant risks involved in moving some post-cardiac surgical patients and that it is more appropriate to use a special bed and mattress to change pressure points continuously, thus minimizing the risk of skin breakdown.

When reviewing the nursing literature, the court found that though nursing textbooks stress the importance of turning patients on a regular schedule, the current nursing literature does not support the conclusion that turning is required when a special bed, such as a Baribed, is in use or that turning plus special beds produce measurably better outcomes than a special bed alone. The literature also supports the fact that a patient with co-morbidity factors such as diabetes is at risk for loss of skin integrity and slow healing even with the most competent of nursing care. The court concluded that the nurses were not responsible for this patient's skin breakdown.

Finally, the court has also seemed to create a new source of external standards in *Hall v. Huff* (1997). In that case, a patient's care providers were having difficulty managing his end-stage renal disease. Peripheral venous access sites had been damaged by repeated dialysis, and a central venous catheter was inserted for medications. During insertion, the catheter was advanced too far, perforating the heart muscle, and the patient subsequently died. The family brought a lawsuit for the patient's wrongful death.

In holding both the physician and the nurses accountable for the death, the court noted that despite several warnings printed on the manufacturer's label insert for the central venous catheter, cautioning health care personnel to be alert for signs and symptoms of cardiac tamponade, neither the attending physician nor the nurses caring for this patient discovered the condition until after the patient died. The court noted that the nurses' notes, charted on the days following the insertion of the catheter, reflected that the nurses were seeing signs and symptoms of cardiac tamponade, though none of the nurses recognized the signs and symptoms for what they were. The court ruled that it was within the standard of care for the competent nurse to detect such a complication following the insertion of a central venous catheter.

EXERCISE 5.2

The patient was a quadriplegic following a motor vehicle accident. He filed a lawsuit claiming the skin lesions he contracted in the hospital were the result of negligent care on the part of his nurses. At trial, it was noted that the patient's sacral bedsores and decubitus ulcers did first appear while he was immobile in a Minerva brace and on a ventilator. The patient's expert witness noted that documentation by the nurses showed that he was turned every 2 to 3 hours, his tube feedings and supplements were correctly given, and he was continually assessed for additional skin breakdown. This expert also testified that the policy and procedures for turning a patient who was ventilator dependent and a high risk for skin breakdown was every 2 to 3 hours.

Was there a deviation from the standards of care in this instance? Review professional organizations' standards of care as you decide this case.

NATIONAL AND LOCAL STANDARDS OF CARE

Appropriate standards of care may be decided based on a national versus local standard. **National standards** are based on reasonableness and are the average degree of skill, care, and diligence exercised by members of the same profession. Such a national standard means that nurses in rural settings must meet the same standards as those members of the profession practicing in large urban areas.

In areas of specialty practice, courts are almost universally holding health care providers to a national standard of care. The precedent case in this area of the law is *Brune v. Belinkoff* (1968). In that case, the court ruled that a person holding himself out as a specialist should be held to the same standard of skill and care as the average member of that specialty, not merely the skill and ability of specialists practicing in a particular city.

There are two important reasons for national standards of care, and both are fairly obvious. With the advent of educational programs, educational videos, the ability to transport specialists across the nation, and the ability to perform patient assessment via electronic transmissions, all areas with health care delivery systems have access to the same information and educational opportunities. This is increasingly true today as advancing technology allows patient data and test results to be reviewed by consultants worldwide. A second—and perhaps more important—reason is that all patients have the right to quality health care, whether hospitalized in a small community or a large, university institution.

IMPORTANCE OF STANDARDS OF CARE TO THE INDIVIDUAL NURSE

Standards of care are referenced in malpractice cases against nurses to show that they breached the duty of care owed the patient. Duty of care has frequently been defined to mean the applicable standard of care. The test for the court to apply is what a reasonable, prudent nurse, with like experience and education, would do under similar conditions in the same community (*King v. State of Louisiana,* 1999).

A court case that distinguishes the acceptable standard of care for various services within a health care setting is *Sobol v. Richmond Heights General Hospital* (1996). In that case, the patient was admitted to the intensive care unit of a general acute care hospital following an attempt to commit suicide with a medication overdose. The attending physician wanted to stabilize the patient's condition while his family made arrangements for transfer to a psychiatric facility. There was a delay in obtaining the patient's transfer because of lack of insurance coverage.

At the time of admission, the institution agreed to the patient's hospitalization, even though the institution had no inpatient psychiatric unit. After admission, the patient became more paranoid and delusional. A nurse sat at his bedside and tried to calm him. The nursing staff deliberated whether to restrain the patient, but decided against it, fearing that it would only compound the situation by making him more agitated and increasing his level of paranoia. The patient got out of bed, knocked down the nurse in his room, fought his way past two other nurses who were trying to corral him, and ran off the unit. Once away from the unit, he kicked out a third-story window and jumped, fracturing his arm and sustaining other relatively minor injuries.

The Court of Appeals of Ohio ruled that the nurses were not negligent. The nurses realized that the patient was a danger to himself, and they acted reasonably under the circumstances. Their actions were fully consistent with basic professional standards of practice for medical–surgical nurses in an acute care facility. They did not have, nor were they expected to have, specialized psychiatric nursing education and would not be judged as though they did.

When deciding which standards of care apply, courts also consider the *error in judgment rule* and the *two schools of thought doctrine*. The honest **error in judgment rule** allows the court to evaluate the standards of care given a patient even if there was an honest error in judgment, including an error in the diagnosis. What the court evaluates is the care given and whether that care met the prevailing standards, not whether the judgment was correct. *Fraijo v. Hartland Hospital* (1979) stands as the landmark case in this matter. In that case, the court stated that a nurse is not bound to do exactly what another nurse would do, only to select one approach among several that exists at the time and is reasonable.

The second consideration by courts is the **two schools of thought doctrine,** which supports the nurse who chooses among alternative means of delivering quality health care. In this instance, the court evaluates the standards of care given when the nurse chooses among the alternative modes of treatment. Were standards of care met in the chosen mode of treatment? If the answer is yes, courts support the quality of care as delivered, even though other nurses would choose a different course of action. *Fury v. Thomas Jefferson University* (1984) remains the leading case illustrating this doctrine.

Standards of care can provide the criterion for determining if a nurse has violated the state nurse practice act. The court in *Botehlo v. Bycura* (1984) held that when patients choose a practitioner of a recognized branch of the health care professions, they elect to undergo the care and treatment common to that profession. Thus, nurses must meet the standards of care of the profession. Each state publishes acceptable standards of care as part of the nurse practice act or through the rules and regulations promulgated by the state board of nursing. Violations of those standards open the nurse to possible disciplinary action by the board. See Chapter 11 for a full explanation of nurse practice acts and the board of nursing.

GUIDELINES

Standards of Care

1. Recognize that all professions have standards of care. Standards are the minimal level of expertise that must be delivered to the patient. Standards of care are the starting point for acceptable nursing care.
2. Standards of care may be set externally or internally. Internal standards of care pertain to the individual practitioner or institution while external standards of care pertain to nurses in all states and territories.
3. Standards of care may be found in:
   a. The state nurse practice act
   b. Published standards of professional organizations and specialty practice groups such as the American Association of Critical-Care Nurses or the Association of Operating Room Nurses
   c. Federal agency guidelines and regulations
   d. Hospital policy and procedure manuals
   e. The individual nurse's job description
   f. Manufacturer's published materials
   g. In-service films and materials
4. Nurses are accountable for all standards of care as they pertain to their profession. To remain competent and skillful, the nurse is encouraged to read professional journals and to attend pertinent continuing education and in-service programs.
5. Standards of care are determined for the judicial system by expert witnesses. Such persons testify to the prevailing standards in the community—standards that all nurses are accountable for matching and exceeding. Adherence to such standards ensures that patients receive quality, competent nursing care.

Standards of care may be used to determine if nurses have violated criminal or civil codes. Two cases illustrate this point. In *Fairfax Nursing Home, Inc. v. U.S. Department of Health and Human Services* (2002), standards of care were examined to show that the nursing home staff had failed to follow policies and procedures related to comprehensive nursing assessment of ventilator-dependent patients following episodes of respiratory distress. One patient died before the policy was implemented and two patients died after the policy was implemented. An additional three patients, while not suffering irreversible harm, might also have been harmed by the immediate jeopardy to their health and safety caused by the nurses' failure to adhere to the newly written policy. In *United States v. Bell* (2006), a nursing home operator was convicted for violating the U.S. health care fraud statute. Evidence showed that there was more than a mere failure to provide the standard of care required by federal nursing home regulations. The nursing home operator falsified residents' treatment records to conceal the fact that required care was not furnished to the residents of the home.

Standards of care may also be used to determine if there has been a violation of a person's constitutional rights. In *Holloway v. Oguejiofor* (2006), a prisoner incarcerated in a state prison brought suit for a violation of his constitutional rights as outlined in the Eighth Amendment. Specifically, he argued that deliberate indifference to his health care needs constituted cruel and unusual punishment.

The patient had suffered a mild heart attack and was seen in the prison clinic. The nurse obtained three EKGs over a 2-hour period and did not release the patient until a normal EKG was obtained. When he returned to the clinic a second time, the prisoner complained of symptoms of indigestion, for which he was given antacids, and again a normal EKG was obtained.

His lawsuit alleged that the second nurse was negligent in her diagnosis and that the standards of care for a cardiac event should have been followed. The court used the patient's admitting symptoms and complaint as the basis for selecting the appropriate standards of care to be implemented by this second nurse and found that the patient was treated appropriately for the condition that the patient truly believed he had. The standards of care were completely followed by the first nurse. The court ultimately ruled that the lawsuit was frivolous.

Finally, standards of care provide the criterion for placing nursing practice on a professional level. Standards of care both increase the status of the nursing profession and, at the same time, set minimal standards for nursing practice. National standards of care have further increased this acceptance of professional status. National standards dictate that all patients receive the same expert nursing care, whether they are cared for in a major medical center or in a small community hospital. All professions have standards. The ANA, through its *Code of Ethics* (2001), has delineated standards promoting professionalism and quality nursing care.

EXERCISE 5.3

Before beginning surgery on a young boy, an order was written for the RN to insert a Foley catheter. The nurse first tried a #16 French latex rubber Foley catheter, but was unable to pass the catheter through the urethra. She then tried with a #12 French latex rubber Foley catheter and again met resistance. She then deferred to a surgical resident, who was equally unsuccessful. The surgical resident eventually inserted a supra-pubic catheter. Postoperatively, the patient developed a bladder fistula, and his parents brought suit alleging that standards of care were not met.

How would you show that this nurse had met the standards of care for this patient? Did she also meet the ethical obligations that were owed this patient? What arguments would you use to show that the nurse had met the legal standards of care?

EXPERT TESTIMONY

In courts of law, deviation from the standard of care is shown through the use of expert witnesses. See Chapter 4 for a review of this concept.

EXPANDED NURSING ROLES

With the advent of expanded roles in nursing and the rewriting of several state nurse practice acts to accommodate these expanded roles, the standard of care that is owed the patient by advanced nurse practitioners is frequently that of a medical (physician) standard of care or a nurse practitioner standard of care. Chapter 12 discusses the expanded nursing role and further clarifies this concept.

 EXERCISE 5.4

Read the "Example of a State's Standards of Nursing Practice" in this chapter. Compare these with the standards of nursing practice endorsed by your state board of nursing. Give examples from your clinical practice to show how these standards might be met.

ETHICAL ISSUES AND STANDARDS OF CARE

Average, prudent, cautious, and *reasonable* are words that are most often used to characterize standards of care. By using words such as average or reasonable, health care professionals imply that they are not perfect or all-knowing, but are acting in the manner in which the profession generally acts. What these words do not take into account is that standards of care are not "frozen in time," but are fluid and dynamic. What they also fail to take into account is how one proceeds if a patient presents with a complex of signs and symptoms that no one has ever seen before. In the age that evidence-based practice has become the gold standard, how do we begin to develop standards of care that consistently involve the best approach for the patient, and how does the profession tolerate health care professionals who are slow to adopt these new standards of care?

One way that the profession begins to assure that all of its practitioners meet current standards of care is by creating policy and procedure manuals that are updated and are not so overwhelming that it is possible for health care providers to readily implement the procedures. The ethical object of policy and procedure manuals is to protect patients and advance their welfare. Means to meet this ethical objective include remembering that one should avoid the temptation to deviate from standards of care and take a quicker route, albeit riskier route, of implementing interventions. Another means is to remember that standards of care should be based on national standards, such as those created and published by one's professional organization. Finally, professionals must be patient advocates, performing in a manner that places the patient's needs first and foremost.

SUMMARY

- Standards of care are the skills and knowledge commonly possessed by members of a profession.
- Standards of care describe the minimal requirements that define an acceptable level of care.
- Standards of care are classified in two broad categories: internal and external.
- Internal standards of care are established by the:
  - Nurse's job description
  - Nurse's education and expertise
  - Institution's policies and procedures
- External standards of care are established through:
  - State boards of nursing
  - Professional organizations
- Specialty nursing organizations
- Current nursing literature, including textbooks and journal articles
- Federal organizations
- Federal guidelines
- National standards ensure that all patients, regardless of location, receive the same quality of care.
- There are two concepts that assist in deciding which standard of care should apply:
  - Error in judgment rule
  - Two schools of thought doctrine
- Ethical issues that arise around standards of care generally concern how to continually develop standards that meet the ethical objective of safeguarding the patient.

APPLY YOUR LEGAL KNOWLEDGE

1. Does the fact that many institutional policy and procedure manuals have similar standards of care move these standards of care from an internal standard to an external standard? Why or why not?

2. Should standards of care be written at more than a minimal level of care? What might be the outcome if standards of care are written at this higher level?
3. What additional ethical issues may be involved in the area of standards of care?

YOU BE THE JUDGE

The patient, a very competent 77-year-old, was admitted to the acute care facility for treatment of a kidney stone. He was taking a variety of medications, including those for the primary diagnosis as well as medications for his renal failure, sepsis, and atrial fibrillation. His fall risk was classified as moderate to high.

The nurse had him get out of bed for his breakfast. After he finished the meal, he asked the nurse if he could use the restroom. Though the nurse tried to get him to use a bedpan, he insisted on using the bathroom and the nurse agreed. The nurse assisted him to the bathroom, showing the patient the safety rail and how to call for assistance. When he called for assistance, the nurse came and helped him stand, but the patient began to fall and, because of his weight, the nurse helped him

gently to the floor. In the course of being helped to the floor, the patient fractured his ankle and he brought a lawsuit against the hospital for nursing negligence.

The expert witness for the patient testified at trial that it is a breach of the legal standard of care for only one person to assist a patient in standing, walking, and using the bathroom when the patient has a high or moderate fall risk, weighs in excess of 250 pounds, and is dizzy or not alert. The defendant's expert witness countered that it is not necessarily a breach of a standard of care for one person to assist with transferring, standing, ambulating, or using the bathroom. The critical question is the patient's level of alertness and whether the patient has sufficiently stable alertness and safety awareness for one-person assistance.

The trial level dismissed the case and the appeal court remanded the case back to the trial level. How would you decide the case?

QUESTIONS

1. Had the nurse fully assessed the patient's level of alertness so that one-person assistance was sufficient?

2. Did the fact that the patient had been determined to be a moderate to high fall risk and that he weighed greater than 250 pounds alter the standard of care in his individual case?

3. How would one decide the standard of care for this patient?

4. How would you decide the outcome of this case?

REFERENCES

American Nurses Association. (1998). *Standards of clinical nursing practice* (2nd ed.). Washington, DC: Author.

American Nurses Association. (2001). *Code of ethics with interpretive statements.* Kansas City, MO: Author.

American Nurses Association. (2008). *Catalogue of publications.* Washington, DC: Author.

Barnett v. University of Cincinnati Hospital, 702 N.E.2d 979 (Ohio Ct. Cl., 1998).

Beck v. Director, Arkansas Employment Security Department, 987 S.W.2d 733 (Ark. App., 1999).

Boring v. Conemaugh Memorial Hospital, 760 A.2d 860 (Pa. Super., 2000).

Botehlo v. Bycura, 320 S.E.2d 59 (Pa. Super., 1984).

Brune v. Belinkoff, 354 Mass. 102, 235 N.E.2d 793 (1968).

Fairfax Nursing Home, Inc. v. U.S. Department of Health and Human Services, 2002 WL 1869592 (7th Cir., August 15, 2002).

Fraijo v. Hartland Hospital, 99 Cal. Rptr.3d 331, 160 Calif. Rptr. 848 (1979).

Fury v. Thomas Jefferson University, 472 A.2d 101 (Louisiana, 1984).

Hall v. Huff, 957 S.W.2d 90 (Tex. App., 1997).

Holloway v. Oguejiofor, 2006 WL 346304 (5th Cir., February 15, 2006).

International Council of Nursing. (2006). *Code of ethics for nurses.* Geneva, Switzerland: Author.

Joint Commission. (2008). *Accreditation manual for hospitals.* Oakbrook Terrace, IL: Author.

King v. State of Louisiana, 728 So.2d 1027 (La. App., 1999).

Ledesma v. Shashoua, 2007 WL 2214650 (Tex. App., August 3, 2007).

MacTavish v. Rhode Island Hospital, 795 A.2d 1119 (R.I., 2002).

Miller v. Jacoby, 33 P.3d 68 (Wash., 2001).

Pages-Ramirez v. Hospital Espanol, 2008 WL 1213051 (D. Puerto Rico, April 7, 2008).

Pugh v. Mayeaux, 702 So.2d 988 (La. App., 1998).

Santa Rosa Medical Center v. Robinson, 560 S.W.2d 751 (Tex. Civ. App., San Antonio, 1977).

Schultz v. Ingham Regional Medical Center, 2006 WL 1451557 (Mich. App., May 25, 2006).

Sheridan v. St. Luke's Regional Medical Center, 25 P.3d 88 (Idaho, 2001).

Smith v. Silver Cross Hospital, 2003 WL 21107135 (Ill. App., May 15, 2003).

Sobol v. Richmond Heights General Hospital, 676 N.E.2d 958 (Ohio App., 1996).

32 Texas Register. Licensure and practice. Rule 211.17. (2007).

United States v. Bell, 2006 WL 052214 (W. D. Pa., April 12, 2006).

Vede v. Delta Regional Medical Center, 2006 WL 1737631 (Miss. App., June 27, 2006).

Weiner v. Kwait, 2003 Ohio 3409, 2003 WL 21487995 (Ohio App., June 27, 2003).

Wolff v. Washington Hospital Center, 2007 WL 4438935 (D.C., December 20, 2007).

CHAPTER 6

Tort Law

PREVIEW

Health care providers are acutely aware of potential legal claims that may be filed against them. Much of this concern involves unknowns about the legal process and civil liability. Although most cases filed against nurse-defendants concern negligence and malpractice, nurses may be held equally accountable for intentional and quasi-intentional actions. Health care providers and the general public frequently interchange the terms *malpractice* and *negligence.* While the distinction is technical, nurses should be able to distinguish between the two terms and apply both in the provision of quality nursing care. This chapter discusses the elements of negligence and malpractice, intentional torts and quasi-intentional torts, and presents guidelines for nurses practicing in all settings for preventing potential lawsuits in this area of the law.

LEARNING OUTCOMES
After completing this chapter, you should be able to:

6.1 Distinguish negligence from malpractice.

6.2 List the six elements of malpractice and give examples of each element in professional nursing practice.

6.3 Define the three tests currently used by courts in establishing cause-in-fact.

6.4 Analyze the doctrine of res ipsa loquitor and give an example of when the doctrine would apply to professional nursing practice.

6.5 Compare and contrast the locality rule to a national standard.

6.6 List ways to avoid or lessen the potential of future malpractice cases.

6.7 Define and differentiate between intentional and quasi-intentional torts.

6.8 List the more commonly occurring intentional torts in health care settings and give an example of each.

6.9 List the more commonly occurring quasi-intentional torts in health care settings and give an example of each.

6.10 Discuss some of the ethical issues involved in nursing and tort law.

KEY TERMS

alternate causes	defamation	malpractice
assault	duty of care	negligence
battery	false imprisonment	professional negligence
breach of duty	foreseeability	proximate cause
"but for" test	injury or harm	quasi-intentional torts
causation	intentional infliction of	res ipsa loquitor
cause-in-fact	emotional distress	substantial factor test
compensatory damages	intentional torts	tort
conversion of property	invasion of privacy	tortfeasor
damages	locality rule	trespass to land

DEFINITION OF TORTS

A **tort** is a civil wrong committed against a person or the person's property. Torts, a term derived from the French, include personal injuries that one person inflicts upon another, whether through actions performed or actions omitted. Tort law is based on fault. The accountable person either failed to meet his or her responsibility or performed an action below the allowable standard of care. Torts are civil wrongs, not based on contracts, but on personal transgressions in that the responsible person performed an action incorrectly or omitted a necessary action. Tort law is the most commonly seen classification of law in health care settings.

NEGLIGENCE VERSUS MALPRACTICE

Of primary importance to health care providers is the area of negligence and malpractice. Though most often used interchangeably, there is a fine distinction between the two terms.

Negligence is a general term that denotes conduct lacking in due care. Thus, negligence equates with carelessness, a deviation from the standard of care that a reasonable person would use in a particular set of circumstances. Negligence may also include doing something that the reasonable and prudent person would not do. As such, anyone, including nonmedical persons, can be liable for negligence. An example is a fall by an elderly person who is being cared for by a sitter. The reasonable person in the place of the sitter has a standard of care to prevent such a fall.

A case that illustrates the concept of negligence is *Dent v. Memorial Hospital of Adel* (1998). In this case, a child had an episode of apnea and was brought to the facility's emergency center by her parents. The emergency center physician admitted the child for observation and ordered a pediatric apnea monitor.

After admission to the pediatric unit, the child again suffered an apneic episode, which was not discovered for several minutes, despite the fact that the apnea monitor had been placed on the child by the nursing staff. The reason for the delay was that the monitor was never turned to its "on" position. A code was called, but it too was delayed because the items appropriate for pediatric patients (airways, endotracheal tubes, and laryngoscope blades) were not on the unit's crash cart and had to be retrieved from other areas of the facility.

Simple acts, the court held, are not exercises in professional judgment. "It is ordinary negligence for nurses not to check that the on/off switch on a pediatric apnea monitor is on. . . . It is ordinary negligence for nurses not to make sure that a crash cart is stocked with items for pediatric patients" (*Dent,* 1998, at 514). Interestingly, the court held that the selection of items appropriate for placement on a crash cart involves professional judgment, but the restocking or validation of whether those items are on the cart does not involve professional judgment.

A more recent example of how negligence can occur in health care settings by other than hospital personnel is *Thomas v. Sheridan* (2008). In this case, a reserve sheriff's deputy without training in handling prisoners was assigned to guard a recently arrested criminal suspect who was in the institution's intensive care unit recovering from an overdose of Oxycontin. The inexperienced officer did not have the patient shackled to the bed nor had he reapplied the patient's handcuffs after the patient finished eating. The patient was able to grab the officer's gun, fire a shot into the ceiling, and take a nurse hostage. The patient was eventually restrained and the nurse was freed unharmed. The court found that the sheriff's department was liable to the nurse for negligence.

Malpractice, sometimes referred to as **professional negligence,** is a more specific term that addresses a professional standard of care as well as the professional status of the caregiver. To be liable for malpractice, the **tortfeasor** (person committing the civil wrong) must be a professional, such as a physician, nurse, accountant, or lawyer. Courts have continually defined malpractice as any professional misconduct, unreasonable lack of skill, or fidelity in professional or judiciary duties. Moreover, this wrong or injudicious treatment results in injury, unnecessary suffering, or death to the injured party, and proceeds from ignorance, carelessness, want of proper professional skill, disregard of established rules and principles, neglect, or a malicious or criminal intent. In a more modern definition, malpractice is the failure of a professional person to act in accordance with the prevailing professional standards or failure to foresee consequences that a professional person, having the necessary skills and education, should foresee.

The same types of acts may form the basis for negligence or malpractice. If the action is performed by a nonprofessional person, the result is negligence. When the same action is performed by a professional person, the acts form the basis for a malpractice lawsuit. The court in *Pender v. Natchitoches Parish Hospital* (2003) outlined six elements that assist in determining whether an action is negligence or malpractice. In *Pender,* an elderly resident was allowed to fall from a wheelchair. The six elements outlined were:

1. The injury is treatment-related or caused by a dereliction of professional skill.
2. Expert evidence is required to determine whether the appropriate standard of care was breached.
3. The act or omission involved an assessment of the patient's condition.
4. The incident occurred in the context of the health care provider–patient relationship or was within the scope of activities a hospital or other care facility is licensed to perform.
5. The injury occurred because the patient sought treatment.
6. The act of omission was unintentional. (*Pender,* 2003, at 21017352)

Quintanilla v. Coral Gables Hospital, Inc. (2006) concerned the definition of professional negligence. In that case, the nurse spilled hot tea on a patient, causing a burn on his skin. The legal issue was whether this was a case of ordinary negligence or professional negligence, and the court concluded that the nurse was guilty only of ordinary negligence.

Some actions will almost always constitute malpractice because only a professional person would be performing the actions. These include the drawing of arterial blood gases via a direct arterial stick or the initiation of blood transfusions. According to Croke (2003), the most common categories of malpractice and negligence among nurses are the failure to follow standards of care, use equipment in a responsible manner, communicate, document, assess and monitor, and act as a patient advocate.

Is the distinction important? Many authorities have concluded that the general public has a right to expect and receive a higher standard of care from a professional person than from a nonprofessional worker. Courts have likewise concluded that this increased expectation of duty exists, and, as a result, substantially higher awards have been given to injured parties in malpractice cases.

EXERCISE 6.1

List the types of nursing actions you perform on a daily basis in your clinical setting. Could all types of the nursing actions you listed be the basis for both negligence and malpractice? Why or why not?

ELEMENTS OF MALPRACTICE OR NEGLIGENCE

To be successful in either a malpractice or negligence cause of action in court in most jurisdictions, the plaintiff (injured party) must prove the following elements to establish liability on the part of the defendant(s):

1. Duty owed the patient
2. Breach of the duty owed the patient
3. Foreseeability
4. Causation
5. Injury
6. Damages

Remember, malpractice is negligence as it pertains to a professional person. Therefore, the elements are the same. The only difference is the status of the person committing the action or failing to act when legally required to act. (See Table 6.1.)

Duty Owed the Patient

Duty of care is owed to others and involves how one conducts oneself. When engaging in an activity, an individual is under a legal duty to act as an ordinary, prudent, reasonable person would act. The ordinary, prudent, reasonable person will take precautions against creating unreasonable risks of injury to other persons. The duty of care that is owed has two distinct

TABLE 6.1 Negligent Torts

Elements	Examples of Nursing Actions
Duty owed	Failing to monitor the patient
Breach of the duty owed the patient	Failing to report a change in patient status
Foreseeability	Failing to report another health care provider's incompetence
Causation	Failing to provide for the patient's safety
Cause-in-fact	Restraining a patient improperly
Proximate cause	Improper medication administration
Injury	Allowing a patient to be burned
Damages	Failing to question an inappropriate medical order
General	Using equipment incorrectly
Special	Failing to follow ordered treatments
Emotional	Failing to provide patient education and discharge instructions
Punitive/exemplary	Acting in a manner that wholly disregards the patient's safety

aspects: (1) it must first be shown that a duty was indeed owed the patient, and (2) the scope of that duty must be proven. The first aspect may be the easier to prove.

The duty of care owed to a given patient may be fairly easily established, especially if the nurse is employed by a hospital or clinic. This duty of care is more difficult to establish when the professional nurse is not the individual directly caring for the patient. Shorter hospital stays and use of unlicensed assistive personnel have served to distance the patient from the professional nurse. The importance of the nurse–patient relationship, though, cannot be overemphasized, as the patient is relying on the professional nurse to provide the necessary competent, quality nursing care. Means of establishing this relationship could be as simple as taking a moment or two to meet with the patient and establish his or her care needs. The nurse–patient relationship may also be established by working with unlicensed assistive personnel as they care for a selected patient. Once the nurse–employer and patient–hospital contractual entities are established, the doctrine of duty arises. The patient has a right to rely on the fact that the nursing staff has a clear-cut duty to act in the patient's best interest.

Duty, however, is created by a relationship and not merely by an employment status. More important than employment is the concept of a nurse–patient relationship or a patient–provider relationship. This reliance relationship—of one person depending on another for quality, competent care—actually forms the basis of the duty-owed concept.

Today's primary nursing easily creates a concept of reliance in that the nurse is assigned the entire nursing care of a given patient. Thus, the duty of care and the establishment of a nurse–patient relationship are readily seen. But even the more traditional, team nursing approach creates such a duty of care. In that functional mode, several nurses were assigned a particular group of patients, and both reliance and a nurse–patient relationship existed.

Even if the nurse is not assigned to a particular patient, a general duty of care arises if the patient presents with an emergency or is in need of instant help. For example, a general duty of care would exist if the nurse was on the way to another part of the hospital and happened to pass the open door of a patient about to fall out of bed. Although not assigned to that given patient or even to the nursing unit, the nurse has a limited duty to assist patients in times of crisis and imminent harm.

Most cases have not concerned themselves with this portion of the nursing duty element because a showing of hospital employment usually is considered sufficient in proving that a duty is owed to the patient. An exception to this rule is *Lunsford v. Board of Nurse Examiners* (1983), a landmark decision concerning when the nurse–patient relationship arises. There the nurse attempted to show that, because the patient was never formally admitted to the hospital and there was no physician–patient relationship, a nurse–patient relationship had never been formed. Thus, according to her argument, there was no duty owed the patient. The court refused this argument, stating that by virtue of licensure, a nurse–patient relationship automatically existed when the patient presented at the hospital's admitting office for emergency care and was met by the nurse.

The second aspect of duty is the scope of care that must be delivered. The standard of care owed is that of the reasonably prudent nurse under similar circumstances as determined by expert testimony, published standards, and common sense. The test for the court to apply is what a reasonable, prudent nurse, with like experience and education, would do under similar conditions in the same community (*Fraijo v. Hartland Hospital*, 1979). See Chapter 5 for a more extensive discussion of the standards of care that must be delivered to a particular patient.

Breach of Duty Owed the Patient

Breach of duty owed naturally follows as the second element of malpractice and negligence. This element involves showing a deviation from the standard of care owed the patient; that is, something was done that should not have been done or nothing was done when it should have been done. For example, an incorrect medication was administered to a patient or a scheduled medication was omitted. Omissions entail as much potential liability as commissions.

A case illustrating this breach of duty owed the patient is *Patel v. Williams* (2007). The patient, who had been treated for a hip fracture and had a gastrostomy tube, was transferred to a nursing care facility. When the patient became agitated and removed the gastrostomy tube, the nurses reinserted the tube incorrectly, without medical supervision, and with no follow-up. This allowed the nutrient supplement to infuse into the patient's peritoneum. Multiple surgeries were performed to remove the abscesses that resulted, and the patient ultimately died from complications associated with the surgeries and the incorrect placement of the gastrostomy tube.

The court noted that, in this case, there were several instances where standards of care were not followed, including failure to have the gastrostomy tube reinserted by trained personnel, failure to verify the placement of the tube prior to restarting nutrient supplements, and the primary failure to adequately address the patient's agitation that caused the gastrostomy tube to be removed by the patient.

Foreseeability

Foreseeability involves the concept that certain events may reasonably be expected to cause specific results. For example, the omission of an ordered insulin injection to a known diabetic patient will foreseeably result in an abnormally high serum glucose level. The challenge is to show in a court of law that one could reasonably foresee a certain result based on the facts as they existed at the time of the occurrence rather than what could be said based on retrospective thinking and results. In the preceding example, could one foresee, at the time of omission of the ordered insulin, that the patient would lapse into a diabetic coma and suffer a cardiopulmonary arrest?

A case example illustrating foreseeability is *Palafox v. Silvey* (2007). In that case, an elderly nursing home resident was found nonresponsive and not breathing in her room at the hospital where she had been admitted for minor elective surgery. She was resuscitated, intubated, and admitted to the intensive care unit. A large volume of stomach contents was suctioned from her lungs when she was intubated. Her death was linked to failure by the hospital staff to check to see if she had any specific dietary needs. In the nursing home, the resident had been on a mechanical soft diet, due to her poor dentition and difficulty with chewing and swallowing. In the nursing home, all of her solid food was pureed. The court noted, in finding liability against the hospital and its staff, that this patient should have been adequately assessed before advancing her from a liquid to a regular diet.

The fact that nurses may not be aware of potential complications does not overshadow the concept of foreseeability. In *Christus Spohn v. De La Fuente* (2007), a patient in labor ruptured her uterus when nursing staff failed to appreciate the fact that Pitocin can cause uterine hyperstimulation and the nurses failed to monitor the patient, induced for a vaginal delivery after a prior cesarean section, for such hyper-stimulation.

The issue of foreseeability was the main issue in three recent cases involving patient assault by other patients. *Casas v. Paradez* (2008) concerned a patient who was accepted from a locked psychiatric ward of a Veteran's Administration hospital to a nursing home. The new resident immediately began assaulting other patients in the nursing home and the nurses insisted that he be moved to a facility that could securely handle him, but the nursing home administrator refused to have him moved. The resident was placed with a new roommate who was unable to protect himself; when this new roommate was attacked and badly injured, he sued. Based on the new resident's violent history at the time he was admitted and subsequent to his admission, the court held it was foreseeable that he would act as he did.

Estate of Thurston v. Southwood Nursing Center (2007) concerned a lawsuit filed by the deceased's family after she was sexually assaulted by an 83-year-old Alzheimer's resident. Though the victim died of unrelated causes, the court held that the assaulting resident had an extensive history of striking the nursing staff of the facility and threatening to stab them. Expert witnesses testified that once the resident displayed such violent behavior, he should have been discharged and moved to a more secure facility.

In *Glanda v. Twenty Pack Manufacturing Corporation* (2008), an aide walked into a resident's room and discovered a dementia patient about to have sexual intercourse with her, as the dementia patient thought the resident was his wife. When the female resident's family sued the long-term care facility, the court held that the facility could be held liable if it could be shown that they had reason to foresee that the demented resident would act as he did. In this case, the facility prevailed as the resident had never before wandered from his room at night nor had he shown any violent actions aimed at others.

Some of the more common cases concerning foreseeability include those involving medication errors and patient falls. The questions of when and how to provide siderails, restraints, and other protections have been addressed by most jurisdictions in the United States (*Crane v. Lakewood Hospital,* 1995; *Delaune v. Medical Center of Baton Rouge, Inc.,* 1996; *Dickerson v. Fatehi,* 1997; *Hardman v. Long Island Urological Associates, P.C.,* 1998; *Lane v. Tift County Hospital Authority,* 1997; *McGraw v. St. Joseph's Hospital,* 1997; *Young v. University of Mississippi Medical Center,* 2005). In *Delaune,* the hospital had equipped a bathroom with a wheelchair ramp, and the patient, who was using a walker rather than a wheelchair, fell when she exited the shower unassisted. In *Hardman,* the patient was allowed to fall from an examining table, and in *Crane,* a visitor to the hospital fell from a chair that was lightweight and unstable. *Dickerson* concerned an operating room case in which the final needle count was incorrect because a marker needle was not included in the final count. In *Lane,* an elderly patient, confused from medications, was allowed to fall while in the radiology department for x-rays, and in *McGraw,* a patient was dropped during transfer from a wheelchair to his bed. In *Young,* the patient died from a pulmonary embolus following the failure to apply anti-embolic stockings as ordered.

Note that in none of these cases was there any high technology involved or what could be considered advanced nursing skills. These cases represent the most commonly occurring injuries to patients—injuries that occur because of lack of foresight, common sense, and/or adherence to standards of care.

For example, in *Siegel v. Long Island Jewish Medical Center* (2003), a hospital staff nurse and two private-duty nurses were sued for administering a fatal 3% saline solution instead of a 0.3% saline solution to a 33-year-old patient. The staff nurse handed the 3% solution to the private-duty nurse, who started the solution and then was relieved by the second private-duty nurse, who then completed the infusion of the 3% solution. In *Sisters of St. Joseph of Texas, Inc. v. Cheek* (2001), a post-operative patient was allowed to remain immobile despite orders for early ambulation. The patient subsequently died from a pulmonary embolus.

Note, however, that foreseeability is equally important in imputing liability. A case that illustrates this fact is *Mitchell v. University Hospital and Clinic-Holmes County* (2006). The patient, who was diagnosed with acute renal failure, congestive heart failure, and diabetes, was also a paraplegic, having sustained a gunshot injury 16 years earlier. Though he had supplemental oxygen at home, he had not used it for some time.

En route to the hospital, he was started on 15 liters of supplemental oxygen, which was reduced to 2 liters in the emergency center. After being observed for 2 hours, he was to be admitted to the medical-surgical unit. During the transfers from the emergency center to the medical-surgical unit, his oxygen was discontinued. He coded as he was wheeled into the elevator, revived, transferred to the intensive care unit, and subsequently discharged back to his home a week after this intensive care unit admission. He sued for the failure to provide oxygen during the hospital transfer.

The court held that there was no proof that this short interval while he was not receiving supplemental oxygen had any bearing on the subsequent code. The complex medical problems that caused him to be admitted in the first place were the reason for the code and subsequent admission to the intensive care unit.

Causation

Somewhat more difficult to prove is **causation,** which means that the injury must have been incurred directly as a result of the breach of duty owed the patient. Causation is frequently subdivided into the concepts of (1) cause-in-fact and (2) proximate cause.

Cause-in-fact denotes that the breach of duty owed caused the injury. If it were not for the breach of duty, no injury would have resulted. For example, a medication is incorrectly administered in the wrong dosage, and the patient subsequently suffers direct consequences due to the medication. In *Brown v. Southern Baptist Hospital* (1998), a patient received Bunnell's irrigation solution following surgery for a severely infected finger. The irrigating solution was to be dripped on the patient's surgical wound for 24 hours. A pharmacy student extern mixed the solution at about 100 times the ordered strength, creating a 47% glacial acetic acid solution rather than the ordered 0.49% solution. The patient suffered serious complications to the surgical site, had to have numerous follow-up surgeries, and ultimately lost the finger.

In assessing blame, the court concluded that the majority of the liability fell on the nursing staff. Even though they did not know of the pharmacy error, the nurses did know that the patient repeatedly complained of the burning pain in his arm, and they should have known that Bunnell's solution is supposed to have a soothing effect and should not cause pain and burning. Thus, they were negligent for not listening to the patient's repeated complaints of pain and for not discontinuing the solution and notifying the patient's physician.

Medication errors remain the most common type of errors where there is a direct connection between a breach of duty owed the patient and the actual injury caused by that breach of duty (e.g., *Hatton v. Interim Healthcare,* 2007; *Kunz v. Little County of Mary Hospital,* 2007; *Lakos v. Kaiser Permanente,* 2008; *Moc v. Children's Hospital,* 2007; *Morrison v. Mann,* 2007; *People v. Gutierrez,* 2006; *Schroeder v. Northwest Community Hospital,* 2006; *Turner v. United States,* 2008; *Weeks v. Eastern Idaho Health Services,* 2007). In all of these cases, if the nursing staff had followed the five rights of medication administration (right patient, right medication, right dose, right route, and right time), the errors could have been avoided.

Courts have continually held it is not sufficient that the standard of care has been breached, but that the breach of the standard of care must be the direct cause of the patient's injury (*Henderson v. Homer Memorial Hospital,* 2006; *Long v. Wade,* 2007; *Nayman v. Huntsville Hospital,* 2007; *O'Shea v. State of New York,* 2007; *Piro v. Chandler,* 2001; *Radish v. De Graff Memorial Hospital,* 2002; *Skikiewicz v. Mount Clemens General Hospital,* 2007). In *Henderson,* the patient, assessed as a low-fall risk, was found lying on the floor. In ruling for the hospital and the defendant nurses, the court ruled that the patient's nursing care plan was adequate and that hindsight was not sufficient to find liability. Merely because a tragic accident occurs does not equate with liability. In *Long,* one twin was delivered without complications and the second twin died due to water filling both brain hemispheres. The court held that the "patient must prove the link between negligence and the harm caused the patient and that it was inconclusive that the care-givers negligence damaged the baby's brain" (*Long v. Wade*, 2007, at 2459976). *O'Shea* concerned a patient who sustained an accident in which two fingers were severed while using a power saw. The patient permanently lost the two fingers when the nursing staff failed to follow the order for an immediate orthopedist consultation. *Radish* concerned a patient's friend who brought suit alleging that the nurse's failure to assist a falling patient caused the friend to intervene, and the fall herniated a disc in the friend's neck. The court, based on witnesses' testimony, found that the injury sustained was due to degenerative arthritis and not a herniated disc; thus, cause and effect was lacking. In *Skikiewicz*, a special speaking device was negligently inserted by a nurse and the patient suffocated. Unknown to the nurse were the facts that the speaking valve must be inserted by a person specially trained in its use and that the patient must be closely monitored while the valve is in place.

Perhaps the most interesting of these cases, from a nursing perspective, is *Piro*. In that case, the court found that the nursing staff of a Louisiana hospital was not liable for the death of a patient admitted with hypertension who subsequently died of a stroke. Admitting orders for the patient included that vital signs were to be taken and recorded every 4 hours and that the patient was to receive Procardia for blood pressure readings above 160/95. At 4:00 P.M. his blood pressure was recorded as 170/100 and he was not given the Procardia. At 7:30 P.M. his blood pressure was 173/100 and the Procardia was given as ordered. The patient became unresponsive at midnight, and he was diagnosed as having experienced a stroke.

At trial, considerable deliberation was given to the fact that the Procardia was to be given without unreasonable delay when the patient's blood pressure exceeded 160/95. One of the defenses offered by the nursing staff was that they had faxed the order for the medication to the pharmacy and that they were waiting for the pharmacy to bring the Procardia to the nursing unit. All the experts who testified at trial agreed that a 4-hour delay was unreasonable and that how quickly a pharmacy fills an order has no bearing on how quickly nurses must give something the patient urgently needs. But, said the court, "even if a caregiver's professional conduct is negligent, there must be cause and effect linking the negligence with harm to the patient or no judgment to pay damages will be entered" (*Piro v. Chandler*, 2001, at 398). In this case, medical expert witnesses testified that the patient had died due to a thrombolytic stroke, not a stroke, and whether the nurses' actions fell below the standard of care or not, there was no direct link to the failure to give the Procardia and the patient's ultimate death.

Two recent cases reinforce the concept that the patient's injury must be directly related to the substandard care (*Estate of Garrison v. Dailey*, 2006; *Houston v. Baptist Medical Center*, 2007). In the first case, the patient had a myocardial infarction, incurred a cardiac arrest, and suffered permanent brain damage due to anoxia during the arrest. He was discharged to a nursing home with a gastrostomy tube in place. The gastrostomy tube was dislodged while at the nursing home. The aide promptly informed the nurse, who requested the nurse practitioner to replace the tube. The tube was reinserted, the tube placement was verified, and the nursing staff resumed his feedings. Later in the day, about 90 minutes after his last tube feeding, the nurse noted that the patient was shaking and making facial grimaces. She called 911 and the patient was transported to the hospital. An x-ray revealed that the gastrostomy tube was not in the patient's stomach and he died 9 days later from peritonitis.

The court ruled that the evidence was inconclusive regarding nursing liability. In health care negligence, the court noted that "the patient must be able to prove by a preponderance of the evidence that negligence occurred and caused harm" (*Estate of Garrison v. Dailey*, 2006, at

1547759). The expert witnesses in this case testified that the tube might not have been correctly positioned or may have been correctly positioned and then repositioned to an incorrect position at some time prior to the x-rays being taken.

In the second case, a newborn was given an injection of vitamin K shortly after birth. Several months later, the infant developed a blood clot in the leg, which was later amputated. The court found no liability in this case, noting that a bad result does not show that the nurse who administered the vitamin K had used an improper technique.

Tests for Causation

Several tests have been established to determine cause-in-fact. The **"but for" test** answers the question of whether the act or omission is a direct cause of the injury or harm sustained. Would the injury have occurred but for the act or omission by the defendant? Would the patient have developed complications, such as an abscess, but for the sponge that was inadvertently left in the abdomen during surgery?

The **substantial factor test** has been developed to aid in pinpointing liability when several causes occur to bring about a given injury. With several possible causes, the but for test is inadequate, because the answer to each defendant's liability would be that no one defendant caused the entire set of circumstances, and therefore the entire result could not have been foreseen. Rather than allow such a result, the substantial factor test is used, not to determine certainty but to establish a causal link between actions and injury. This test asks if the defendant's act or omission was a substantial factor in causing the ultimate harm or injury. If the answer is yes, there is cause-in-fact. For example, in *Brown v. Southern Baptist Hospital (1998)*, the court had to determine which of the multiple defendants was most responsible for the patient's ultimate loss of his finger—the student pharmacist, her university, her pharmacy preceptor at the hospital, the hospital, the physician, or the nursing staff.

An equally complex example of substantial factor is *Depesa v. Westchester Square Medical Center* (1997). In this case, a 49-year-old patient entered the emergency center with severe abdominal pain. Physicians prescribed Mylanta and sent her home, advising her to contact her personal physician if her condition worsened.

She took the medication but continued to experience increasing abdominal pain. After 20 days, the patient visited a different hospital's emergency center. Tests revealed a perforated bowel and peritonitis. Following surgery, the personnel at this second hospital administered almost double the prescribed amount of IV fluids, and the patient died of acute heart failure. The court was left to determine the exact cause of the patient's death—the initial failure to diagnose the perforated bowel or the substandard care at the second hospital. In addition, the court had to decide to what degree each of the defendants shared responsibility—the physicians, nurses, and individual institutions. Ultimately, the court apportioned liability between the two hospitals and their employees.

The **alternate causes** approach also addresses the problem in which two or more persons have been accused of negligence. Under this test, the plaintiff must show that the harm or injury was caused by one of the multiple defendants, and the burden of proof then shifts to the defendants to show who actually caused the harm or injury at issue. In *Donahue v. Port (1994)*, a 32-year-old male lost his leg due to failure to diagnose vascular problems associated with a dislocated knee. At trial, the defendant orthopedic surgeon claimed that the nurses were negligent in not reporting vascular problems until it was too late to save the leg. An expert witness for the nurses testified that, if there was an initial popliteal artery injury, there was only a 12-hour window in which to successfully repair the artery and that the 12-hour window had expired before the patient was treated. The patient has the burden of proof to show that the harm was caused by one of the defendants, and the defendants have to show which one of them did (or did not) cause the harm. If neither defendant can establish his or her own innocence or the other's negligence, they may both be liable. The alternate causes approach is frequently seen in a negative light by judges and juries.

Proximate Cause

Proximate cause attempts to determine how far the liability of the defendant extends for consequences following negligent activity. Thus, proximate cause builds on foreseeability. Could one foresee the extent to which consequences will follow a negligent action? Several cases in this aspect of the law involve subsequent automobile accidents that occurred after medicated patients were released from acute care settings (*Cheeks v. Dorsey,* 2003; *Robinson v. Health Midwest Development Group,* 2001; *Shortnancy v. North Atlanta Internal Medicine, P.C.,* 2001). As a general rule, courts have held no liability against health care providers when patients operate motor vehicles after taking medications that may cause drowsiness. The rationale for this decision is that the health care providers have no control over the patient who elects to take the medication and then drive a motor vehicle. The exception to this rule exists for patients committed involuntarily for psychiatric treatment on the grounds that they may pose a threat of harm to others. Their caregivers do have legal obligations to control this classification of patients to prevent their harming others.

To win at trial, the injured party must show that the health care providers were negligent in their legal responsibilities to adequately inform, assess, monitor, and supervise the patient (*Robinson*), or the injured party must show that the medication was administered to a patient who should not have received it (*Cheeks*). In this latter case, the patient, who was visibly intoxicated, was medicated with methadone and then released from the outpatient clinic. In *Shortnancy,* the patient received medications 2 months following surgery for a herniated disc. These were the same medications he had received on an outpatient basis in the preceding weeks. The patient was given clear instructions that he should not drink, drive an automobile, or operate machinery for at least a 12-hour period. He was given the medications at 11:30 A.M. and left the physician's office at 12:30 P.M. At 6:45 P.M., he was involved in an automobile accident. Blood and urine samples taken at the time of the accident were positive for marijuana. The court noted that the legal obligations of the health care providers had been met.

Another case example that illustrates proximate cause is *Silves v. King* (1999). Donald Silves presented to the hospital, complaining of a sore and swollen toe. Because of a history of blood clots, Silves feared he might be experiencing another one. Dr. King, the emergency center physician, took his medical history, performed a physical examination, diagnosed gouty arthritis, and prescribed indomethacin. She instructed Silves to follow up with his regular physician within 5 days. She testified she knew that Silves was currently taking heparin for his history of blood clots.

The emergency center nurse gave Silves two pages of discharge instructions. The list of warnings concerning indomethacin included a caution not to take the medication if the patient has problems with blood clotting or bleeding. Silves signed the discharge instruction sheet, which contained a statement that he had received and could read the instructions. At trial, he testified that he did not read the discharge instructions prior to taking the indomethacin. Approximately 2 weeks after he started the indomethacin, he suffered a pulmonary hemorrhage that left him permanently disabled.

Silves sued the physician, her employer, the hospital, and its staff. The trial court entered summary judgment in favor of the hospital and its staff and found that Dr. King had not violated the standard of care, but did fail to obtain Silves's informed consent prior to the use of the indomethacin. However, the jury found that the failure to obtain informed consent was not a proximate cause of Silves's injury.

In the finding against liability on the part of the nursing staff, the court rejected Silves's claim that the discharge nurse had a duty to inform him of possible drug interactions. The nurse does not need to review the medication discharge instructions with the patient if the patient has read and signed the form. Assuming the patient can read and understand the medication instructions, there is no reason to require nurses to read these same instructions to the patient. This, too, said the court, was not a proximate cause of his injury.

Proximate cause is fairly clear as long as the result is directly related. Proximate cause becomes less clear when intervening variables are present. Intervening forces may combine with the original negligent action to cause injury to the patient. As a rule of thumb, in medical malpractice cases, the health care provider is frequently liable for intervening forces when they are foreseeable.

Often, though, intervening factors are not foreseeable. In *Van Horn v. Chambers* (1998), a patient admitted for seizures and alcohol withdrawal was sedated, given antiseizure medications, and restrained. He was admitted to the neurological intensive care unit. The following day, the attending neurologist determined that the restraints were no longer indicated and transferred the patient to a private room on a medical-surgical unit.

The patient decided to leave against medical advice. Three individuals, a patient care technician, a medical student, and a food service worker, attempted to prevent his leaving. In the subsequent fight that occurred, two of the hospital personnel were injured and one was killed. The Supreme Court of Texas ruled that each had acted at his or her own risk and could not sue the neurologist for malpractice. The neurologist did not misdiagnose the patient and had no duty to control the patient. Thus, proximate cause did not exist.

Injury

The fifth element that must be shown is an actual **injury or harm.** The plaintiff must demonstrate that some type of physical, financial, or emotional injury resulted from the breach of duty owed the patient. Generally speaking, courts do not allow lawsuits based solely on negligently inflicted emotional injuries. Such emotional injuries are actionable only when they accompany physical injuries.

Pain and suffering are allowed if they accompany a physical injury but not by themselves (*Jones v. Department of Health,* 1995; *Majca v. Beekil,* 1998). *Jones* involved the potential damages for pain and suffering, loss of capacity for the enjoyment of life, and the reasonable expectation for life following a false-positive test result for human immunodeficiency virus (HIV). *Majca* concerned the fear of contracting acquired immune deficiency syndrome (AIDS) without evidence of exposure to HIV. This contrasts with intentional infliction of emotional harm, an intentional tort, which is covered later in this chapter.

Note, however, that negligent actions coupled with pain and suffering may provoke the court to find that psychological harm is sufficient to sustain a cause of action against defendants. The court in *Curtis v. MRI Imaging Services II* (1998) acknowledged that, as a general rule, the law does not allow lawsuits for damages for emotional distress in negligence cases unless the victim had sustained some type of physical harm. Having noted such, the court identified a major exception to the rule—the relationship between patients and their health care providers. Health care professionals, said the court, are held to a legal standard of care that includes the specific duty to be aware of and guard against particular adverse psychological reactions or consequences of medical procedures.

Certain specific interventions carry with them known foreseeable risks of adverse psychological reactions. Steps must be taken to assess the particular patient's susceptibility to foreseeable adverse reactions and to minimize or avoid them. In this case, the patient had a magnetic resonance imaging (MRI) scan, but no explanation of the potential for claustrophobic effects was provided to the patient before the examination. No adequate history was taken, which would have made known the patient's preexisting asthmatic condition and his propensity to panic reactions and breathing difficulties. During the MRI, the patient was not closely monitored, and the caregivers could not terminate the procedure quickly and extract the patient from the MRI device once he began having difficulty breathing and respiratory distress.

A second exception to the nonrecovery for emotional harm concerns instances related to parents and their offspring, such as when a parent views an injury to his or her child. In these types of cases, the courts have frequently allowed damages for a purely emotional injury. In *Gooch v. North Country Regional Hospital* (2006), delivery was induced after a fetus had died in utero. Hospital staff wrapped the fetus in a blanket, placed him in a basket, and encouraged the parents to hold him if they so desired. The parents were given three options: cremation, a private funeral, or the fetus could be kept in the hospital morgue until the spring when it would be possible for a local funeral home to bury the fetus in a shared casket with other fetal remains. The parents chose the shared-casket option.

In the spring when the parents asked the funeral home about the shared-casket burial observance, the funeral home said that it had never received the remains. Eventually the hospital chaplain determined that the remains were most likely transported from the pathology laboratory and incinerated with medical wastes and surgical byproducts. The court ruled that the parents had a right to sue for emotional damages.

Rayford v. Willow Ridge (2008) presents another exception to recovery for emotional damages. The court ruled that a nursing home was liable for making no effort to contact the next of kin before allowing the burial of a long-term resident who died at the age of 93. The nursing home administrator knew who the family members were and where they lived. In fact, they lived in the same small town where the nursing home was located. The final settlement to the family was $5,000 for the family's mental anguish and emotional distress and the cost of disinterment and reburial of the resident in a manner more consistent with the resident's wishes.

Damages

Unlike intentional torts, damages are not presumed. Nominal (e.g., a $1 or $2 award) damages do not exist for negligent torts. The basic purpose of awarding damages is compensatory, with the law attempting to restore the injured party to his or her original position so far as is financially possible. The goal of awarding damages is not to punish the defendants but to assist the injured party.

Essentially four types of **damages** may be compensated:

1. General damages are inherent to the injury itself. Included in general damages are pain and suffering (past, present, and future) and any permanent disability or disfigurement because of the injury. In *Synder v. Arrowhead Community Hospital* (2007), a newborn infant was scalded when a nurse spilled hot coffee on him. The jury awarded damages only to compensate the baby for the injury, which amounted to $7,000.
2. Special damages account for all losses and expenses incurred as a result of the injury. These include medical bills, lost wages (past, present, and future), cost of future medical care, and cost of converting current living areas to more easily accommodate the injured party.
3. Emotional damages may be compensated if there is apparent physical harm as well. A limited number of cases, such as the *Curtis v. MRI Imaging Services II* (1998) case cited previously, do allow for such emotional damages without evidence of physical injury. Repeatedly, courts have rejected fear of contracting HIV or AIDS cases (*Brooker v. Galen of Kentucky, Inc.,* 2003; *Rustvold v. Taylor,* 2000). Note, though, that the court will allow damages for pain and suffering

even if the patient may appear to be unable to feel pain. In *Keel v. West Louisiana Health Services* (2001), the court allowed a quadriplegic patient who was scalded and burned to be compensated for his pain and suffering. This was appropriate, said the court, because the patient "had to sleep in an unaccustomed and awkward position while his injuries healed" (*Keel v. West Louisiana Health Services*, 2001, at 383).

4. Punitive or exemplary damages may be awarded if there is malicious, willful, or wanton misconduct. The plaintiff must show that the defendant acted with conscious disregard for his or her safety. *Luby v. St. John's Episcopal Hospital* (1995) expanded this definition to include "conduct which is wanton, malicious, or activated by evil or reprehensible motives" (at 776). Punitive damages are usually considerable and are awarded to deter similar conduct in the future. A nursing malpractice case illustrating punitive damages is *Mobile Infirmary Medical Center v. Hodgen* (2003).

A 58-year-old patient, following coronary artery bypass surgery, developed a cardiac arrhythmia while in the intensive care unit (ICU). The graduate nurse caring for the patient phoned the cardiologist, who ordered 0.25 mg of digoxin. The graduate nurse told her supervising nurse that the cardiologist had ordered 1.25 mg of digoxin, which the supervising nurse relayed to the pharmacy. Before the pharmacy could deliver the dosage of digoxin, the supervising nurse told the graduate nurse not to wait, but to use digoxin from the medication cabinet that stocked emergency drugs for the ICU. The graduate nurse, acting without supervision, opened three 0.5-mg digoxin vials and pushed 1.25 mg of the medication into the patient's intravenous line. Shortly after the administration of the medication, the pharmacist called to question the amount of medication ordered. Only then did the supervising nurse realize that she had allowed the graduate nurse to give five times the amount of medication that was actually ordered.

The following evening, the patient began to experience complications from the digoxin toxicity. He was given Digibind, the digoxin-specific antidote, and arrested shortly after the administration of the Digibind. He was revived, but suffered permanent organ damage, including brain injury.

The Supreme Court of Alabama found that the nurses' actions had gone beyond professional negligence and that they had acted wantonly and callously. Punitive damages amounting to $1.5 million were assessed against the defendants. The court faulted the graduate nurse for giving a medication with which she obviously was unfamiliar, the supervising nurse for her failure to safeguard the patient, and the institution's system for assigning patients, tasking, and supervising nurses. At trial, the graduate nurse testified that she had never administered digoxin to a patient before this event and that she made no effort to obtain more information about the medication prior to its administration. The supervising nurse testified that she had only been licensed herself for about 7 months. She further testified that she had her own patients and that she understood she was only available if the graduate nurse had questions. The supervising nurse did not believe she was responsible for directly overseeing the graduate nurse and thus did not assist the graduate nurse in administering the medication. Further, she had never worked with this graduate nurse before and knew nothing of the graduate nurse's experience or skill level.

Similarly, in *Miller v. Levering Regional Healthcare Center* (2006), a 92-year-old resident of a nursing home, who had difficulty ambulating and for whom there was a specific order that she was not to be left unattended while using her walker, fell and hit her head while unattended in the facility's dining room at 6:30 P.M. The facility's policy mandated neurological assessments immediately after a fall involving an apparent head injury and every 4 hours until the patient was medically stable. A neurological assessment was performed immediately after the fall and once at midnight. At 5:30 the next morning she was found unresponsive. She had vomited sometime during the time interval between midnight and 5:30. She was transferred to an acute care facility, where she died of an epidural hemorrhage.

The court noted that though the actual damages in the case were relatively small, punitive damages were not. Punitive damages, held the court, "are not meant to compensate the family for their loss but are intended to punish the civil wrongdoer for reprehensible conduct" (*Miller v. Levering Regional Healthcare Center,* 2006, at 1889883).

Sometimes general and special damages are grouped into one category called **compensatory damages.** The last two classifications are retained, and thus there are three categories for damage awards.

GUIDELINES

Avoiding Negligent Torts

1. Treat patients and their families with respect and honesty. Communicating in a truthful, open, and professional manner may well prevent a negligence cause of action.
2. Use your nursing knowledge to make appropriate nursing diagnoses and to implement necessary nursing interventions. You have an affirmative duty not only to make correct nursing diagnoses, but to take the actions required to implement your diagnoses.
3. Remember that the first line of duty is to the patient. If the physician is hesitant to order necessary therapy or to respond to a change in the patient condition, call your supervisor or another physician. Question orders if they are (a) ambiguous or unclear, (b) questioned or refused by the patient, (c) telephone orders, or (d) inappropriate, such as when a major change occurs in the patient's status and the orders remain unchanged. For telephone orders, reread the orders to the physician and clarify them prior to hanging up the phone.
4. Remain current and up to date in your skills and education. Take advantage of continuing education programs and in-service programs on a regular basis. Read professional journals. Refuse to perform skills and procedures if you are unfamiliar with them, have never performed them before, or lack the necessary materials and equipment to perform them safely.
5. Base your nursing care on the nursing process model. Using all five steps of the model prevents the inadvertent overlooking of a vital part(s) of required nursing care for a given patient.
6. Document completely every step of the nursing care plan and the patient's responses to interventions. Express yourself clearly and completely. Chart all entries as soon as possible while the facts and observations are still clear in your mind.
7. Respect the patient's right to education about his or her illness, and ensure that the patient and family are taught about the disease entity, therapy, and possible complications prior to discharge. Chart any discharge instructions in the medical record.
8. Delegate patient care wisely, and know the scope of practice for yourself and those whom you supervise. Never accept or allow others to accept more responsibility than they can handle or than they are allowed to accept by law.
9. Know and adhere to your hospital's policies and procedures. Help to update those that are outdated, and ensure that the personnel you supervise are also aware of hospital policies and procedures. All personnel should reread the manual periodically.
10. Keep your malpractice liability insurance policy current, and know the limits of coverage. This may not help you to give better care, but it will help you if a patient should name you in a malpractice cause of action.

With multiple defendants, courts apportion the harm caused the plaintiff according to each defendant's portion or percentage of actual harm. Harm is seen as a total percentage of 100% and each defendant's part in the harm is calculated, with all the defendants' portions, to equal 100%. Then the court multiplies the total damage award by each defendant's percentage. *Estate of Chin v. St. Barnabas Medical Center et al.* (1998) illustrates the concept. In that case, the patient died following a hysteroscopy. The total damages awarded by the jury were $200,000. Five defendants were involved:

1. The circulating nurse was 20% at fault and was assessed $40,000.
2. One scrub nurse was 25% at fault and was assessed $50,000.
3. Another scrub nurse was 0% at fault and was assessed no dollar amount.
4. The hospital was 35% at fault and was assessed $70,000.
5. The physician was 20% at fault and was assessed $40,000.

In *Quesenberry v. Beebe Medical Center, Inc.* (2006), the nursing staff members were apportioned 40% of a $570,000 verdict for their part in the patient's injury, and the physician who had misdiagnosed the patient's condition was apportioned 60% of the verdict. Similarly, in *Jacobs v. Leesburg Regional Medical Center* (2007), the hospital was apportioned 55% and the physician apportioned 45% at fault for rupture of an artificial urinary sphincter in a 70-year-old patient.

EXERCISE 6.2

A patient's family sued a nursing home, alleging that the patient died due to neglect by the nursing staff. Specifically, the family alleged that the 86-year-old had been left lying for hours in her bed, without being bathed or turned for prolonged periods of time, and she had dried feces under her fingernails at the time of her death. Unhealed bedsores were present on her heels, coccyx, and both hipbones. She was contractured and had lost 15 pounds in the preceding 2 months. Listed on her death certificate was the entry that she died from dehydration and malnutrition.

What types of damages could be assessed against the defendant nursing home and nursing staff in such a case? How would you apportion the damages? What types of legal and ethical responsibilities did the nurses have to this patient? Can you devise a scenario in which nursing staff members would not be held liable in such a case?

DOCTRINE OF RES IPSA LOQUITOR

The doctrine of **res ipsa loquitor** allows a negligence cause of action without requiring that all six elements of malpractice or negligence be proven. Essentially, res ipsa loquitor allows the jury to find the defendant negligent without any showing of expert testimony on the plaintiff's part.

Res ipsa loquitor—"the thing speaks for itself"—is a rule of evidence that emerges when plaintiffs are injured in such a way that they cannot prove how the injury occurred or who was responsible for its occurrence. The negligence of the alleged wrongdoer may be inferred from the mere fact that an accident or incident happened. The proviso is that the nature of the incident and the circumstances surrounding the incident lead reasonably to the belief that, in the absence of negligence, it would not have occurred. The instrument that caused the injury must be shown to have been under the management and control of the alleged wrongdoer, not the injured party.

This doctrine is used by the courts in cases in which the person injured has an insurmountable burden in proving the facts of the case. For example, the landmark case for this doctrine is a California case in which the injured party underwent a routine appendectomy and suffered a permanent loss of neuromuscular control of the right shoulder and arm as a result of the surgery (*Ybarra v. Spangard,* 1944). The injured party had no means of accurately showing how or when this permanent injury occurred. All the patient could show was that this was not the type of complication normally incurred with an appendectomy and that he had full range and movement of the affected arm prior to the surgical procedure.

To prevent injured parties from an unfair disadvantage and to prevent wrongdoers from benefiting by their silence, the court enacted the doctrine of res ipsa loquitor. The injured party must prove three elements for this doctrine to apply:

1. The accident must be the kind that ordinarily does not occur in the absence of someone's negligence.
2. The accident must be caused by an agency or instrumentality within exclusive control of the defendant.
3. The accident must not have been due to any voluntary action or contribution on the part of the plaintiff (*Ybarra v. Spangard,* 1944, at 687).

Once these three elements are shown, the defendant must disprove them. The courts view the defendants as being in a better position to actually explain what happened, because they had exclusive control during the time the incident occurred.

The doctrine of res ipsa loquitor is normally applied in medical malpractice cases in which the injured party is unconscious, was in surgery, or was an infant. Typical examples of cases for which the courts have allowed the doctrine of res ipsa loquitor to be applied include those in which a foreign object has been left in the patient during surgery, infection was caused by unsterile instruments, neuromuscular injury occurred due to the improper positioning of an unconscious patient, burns occurred during surgery, or a surgical procedure was performed on the wrong limb or part of the body.

Recognized by a majority of the states, not all states apply the doctrine of res ipsa loquitor in the same manner. Some states have actually expanded the doctrine through recent court cases. Other states have tended to limit the application of the doctrine, especially in areas where more than common knowledge is needed to ensure the jury's understanding of the facts, such as in the area of secondary infections. A third group of states has rejected application of the doctrine, noting that malpractice must be shown and not presumed (e.g., *Boling v. Stegemann,* 2007).

Several cases illustrate the application of res ipsa loquitor. *Babits v. Vassar Brothers Hospital* (2001), *Cleary v. Manning* (2008), *Pillers v. The Finley Hospital* (2003), and *Rosales-Rosario v. Brookdale University Hospital and Medical Center* (2003) all concerned patients who had been burned during surgical procedures. *Thomas v. New York University Medical Center* (2001) and *Schallert v. Mercy Hospital of Buffalo* (2001) concerned unconscious patients who had fallen from operating room tables during positioning for the surgical procedure. *Quinby v. Plumsteadville Family Practice, Inc.* (2006) involved a quadriplegic patient who fell in a doctor's office following an outpatient procedure. In *Collins v. Superior Air-Ground Ambulance Service, Inc.* (2003), the court allowed a case to proceed under res ipsa loquitor even though there were two distinct defendants in the case. An 83-year-old diabetic patient who was totally bedridden, unable to speak because of a stroke, and fed via a gastrostomy tube was transported to the hospital by a local ambulance service. The same ambulance service transported the patient to her home 5 days later. Upon return to her home, the daughter noted that her mother winced in pain when her right leg was moved and that the leg was extremely swollen. A second ambulance service subsequently transported the patient to a second hospital where a fractured right distal tibia and fibula and dehydration were diagnosed. The court noted that this was the type of injury that supported a ruling of res ipsa loquitor and that, while the case was somewhat different than the traditional res ipsa loquitor case as there were two totally separate defendants, the two defendants had the burden of proof to show which one of them was or was not at fault.

Courts struggle under this doctrine to ensure that all elements of res ipsa loquitor are met before deciding the case. For example, in *Garcia v. Bronx Lebanon Hospital* (2001), a patient woke with bruises over his entire body. He testified that he had been drinking and went to the emergency center when he experienced chest pains. Once at the emergency center, the patient went to the restroom, sat down, and later woke to find himself bruised. Two hospital security guards testified that the patient had come in extremely intoxicated and picked up and swung a chair, breaking a window. The patient had to be physically restrained for the safety of the staff and other patients. The court ruled that res ipsa loquitor did not apply in this case. The security guards may or may not have used excessive force in this case. Under the circumstances, the court ruled that the injury, in and of itself, did not prove the hospital was negligent.

Similarly, in *Maquette v. Goodman* (2001), a patient arrested after an emergency cesarean section at the end of the surgical procedure. The courts refused to apply the doctrine of res ipsa loquitor because patients can arrest during anesthesia in the absence of negligence. The anesthetist did not have the burden of showing there was no negligence, but rather the widower had the duty of showing that negligence occurred.

A third case in which the court refused to apply this doctrine is *Walston v. Lakeview Regional Medical Center* (2000). In this case, a patient had emergency surgery to repair an aortic aneurysm. The sponge counts during the procedure showed that all of the health care providers could account for all of the sponges used during the case. Shortly after the patient was admitted to the post-operative recovery unit, the patient's blood pressure fell and the patient encountered a second operation. At the end of the second procedure, the surgeon was notified that one of the sponges used in the case could not be found. The surgeon, because of the patient's hemodynamic instability, elected to leave the sponge rather than spend additional time locating the sponge. The patient died 2 weeks later, and a suit was brought alleging malpractice on the part of the physician and nurses. A medical panel that reviewed the case prior to its being filed with the courts concluded that there had been no negligence, noting that the retained sponge had not been a factor in the patient's subsequent demise. This court concurred, noting that there had been a correct sponge count and a conscious decision made to leave the sponge in the patient. Thus, the elements of res ipsa loquitor had not been met.

Res ipsa loquitor may be invoked on behalf of the nursing staff and health care facility. In *Slease v. Hughbanks* (1997), a patient was admitted following an industrial mishap for orthopedic ankle surgery. One or two days after the surgery, he noticed a burn on his thigh and filed a malpractice suit. In court, the plaintiff's attorney did not produce expert witnesses to show that the burn was the type consistent with an electrical burn from a bovie pad, but rested the case solely on the doctrine of res ipsa loquitor.

In finding for the hospital and against the plaintiff, the court relied on the admission note as charted when the patient first came to the hospital. The admission nurse had noted that there was a burn on the patient's thigh as one of the multiple traumas he had incurred in the industrial accident. Thus, res ipsa loquitor did not apply.

Two recent cases appear to signal a newer application of the res ipsa loquitor application. *Flowers v. HCA Health Services of Tennessee* (2006) and *Tucker v. University Specialty Hospital* (2005) both concern patients who died of drug overdoses while hospitalized. In *Flowers*, the patient was receiving morphine, intramuscularly and via a patient-controlled analgesia (PCA) pump, following removal of a kidney stone. Early the morning of her second day post-operatively, she was found unresponsive with no pulse and could not be resuscitated. She was found to have a lethal level of morphine in her blood post mortem. An investigation into her death revealed that the PCA pump was not defective and had been functioning normally during the time it was in use with this patient.

The court held that the doctrine of res ipsa loquitor was appropriate in this case, as a patient dying of an overdose of morphine could not have happened in the absence of negligence on the part of the health care providers. The patient's family members were not required to explain further how the deceased's health care providers were negligent.

In *Tucker*, the coroner's report established that the hospitalized patient died from a lethal dose of Oxycontin, ingested within an hour of the patient's death. Though there was no direct proof of how the patient received the overdose, the patient was in the exclusive control of hospital employees at the time of the events in question. The court concluded that the "element of exclusive control leads to a logical inference that some act of negligence must have been committed by the hospital" (*Tucker v. University Specialty Hospital*, 2005, at 3213897).

LOCALITY RULE

Whenever the legal system refers to the reasonable, prudent practitioner, there is a statement to the effect that the professional is viewed by a prevailing community standard, "in a similar community" or "under the same circumstances." Known as the **locality rule,** such a statement attempts to hold the standard of the professional to that of other professionals practicing in the same geographic area of the country.

The locality rule arose because of wide variations that once existed in patient care, depending if the hospital was in an urban or rural setting. Rural hospitals and health care providers did not have the same sophistication and means of technology available within large medical centers.

In 29 states, the locality rule has been abolished either by statute or by judicial rulings. Today, a national standard continues to emerge that offers to all persons an acceptable minimal standard of care, though there appears to be some resurgence of the locality rule as a tort reform measure and because of the issue of access to health care in rural areas.

Several factors arose to help abolish the locality rule. First, because of mass media, national conferences, and improved transportation, health care providers were no longer able to defend the acceptance of a lower standard of care for rural areas. The practitioner has available all the teaching aids and continuing education programs needed to stay informed about new and innovative therapeutic approaches and to understand technological advances. The rule does not require that rural settings have the same medical facilities available, but that practitioners in that setting have the same education and exercise the same level of judgment and diligence of an urban health care provider.

Second, professional organizations (e.g., the Joint Commission or the American Association of Critical-Care Nurses) have moved toward the creation of an acceptable standard for given patients by publishing national standards of care. Additionally, state nurse practice acts have enacted standards of nursing practice for all nurses within the jurisdiction, not just for nurses within large medical centers.

Third, standards for accreditation of health care facilities should be the same no matter where the hospital is located geographically.

AVOIDING MALPRACTICE CLAIMS

Nurses frequently inquire about the impact that the medical malpractice crisis will have on the professional practice of nursing. This is especially true as more and more nurses are being sued along with physicians or hospitals. The National Practitioner Data Bank (2008) reports that approximately 4,418 malpractice reports were filed against registered nurses—1,276 against nurse anesthetists, 701 against nurse midwives, 802 against nurse practitioners, and 12 against clinical nurse specialists—for the period September 1, 1990 through September 4, 2008. The number of reports filed against clinical nurse specialists is for the period 2002–2008, as that classification was added at a later date.

Can anything be done to stop the increased litigation? What should nurses do to protect themselves? From a legal perspective, nurses may be able to limit their potential liability in several ways. Possibly the first and most important concept to remember is that patients and their families who are treated honestly, openly, and respectfully and who are apprised of all facets of treatment and prognosis are not likely to sue. Communicating in a caring and professional manner has been shown time and time again to be a major reason why more people do not sue, despite adequate grounds for a successful lawsuit. Even given untoward results and a major setback, the patient is less likely to file suit if there has been an open and trusting nurse–patient relationship or physician–patient relationship. Remember, people sue, not the action or event that triggered a bad outcome.

Second, nurses should know relevant law and legal doctrines and combine these concepts with the biological, psychological, and social sciences that form part of the basis of all rational nursing decisions. The law can and should be incorporated into everyday practice as a safeguard for the health care provider as well as the health care recipient.

Third, nurses should stay well within their areas of individual competence and become lifelong learners. To remain competent, nurses should upgrade technical skills consistently, attend pertinent continuing education and in-service programs on a regular basis, and undertake only those actual skills they can perform competently.

Fourth, joining and actively supporting professional organizations will allow nurses to take advantage of excellent educational programs and to become active in organizations' lobbying efforts, which might be focused on a stronger nurse practice act or the creation or expansion of advanced nursing roles. Far too many nurses are afraid to become politically involved; yet, as a unified profession, nursing could have a strong voice, particularly in upgrading and strengthening nurse practice acts.

Fifth, nurses should recognize the concept of the suit-prone patient. This type of patient is more likely than other patients to initiate a malpractice action in the event that something untoward happens during the treatment process. Because the psychological makeup of these persons breeds resentment and dissatisfaction in all phases of their lives, they are much more apt to initiate a lawsuit.

Suit-prone patients tend to be immature, overly dependent, hostile, and uncooperative, often failing to follow a designated plan of care. They are unable to be self-critical and shift blame to others as a way of coping with their own inadequacies. Suit-prone patients actually project their fear, insecurity, and anxiety to health care providers, overreacting to any perceived slight in an exaggerated manner.

Recognizing such patients is the first step in avoiding potential lawsuits. The nurse should then attempt to react on a more human or personal basis, such as expressing satisfaction with the patients' cooperation, showing empathy and concern with their suffering and setbacks, and repeating needed information to keep patients less fearful of unknown treatments and procedures. An atmosphere of attentiveness, caring, and patience may help prevent the suit-prone patient from filing future lawsuits.

Sixth, recognize that nurses' personality traits and behaviors may also trigger lawsuits. Suit-prone nurses are those who (1) have difficulty establishing close relationships with others, (2) are insecure and shift blame to others, (3) tend to be insensitive to patients' complaints or fail to take the complaints seriously, (4) have a tendency to be aloof and more concerned with the mechanics of nursing than establishing meaningful human interactions with patients, and (5) inappropriately delegate responsibilities to peers to avoid personal contact with patients. These nurses need counseling and education to change these behaviors into more positive attitudes and behaviors toward patients and staff. Such positive changes have the ability to lessen future potential lawsuits.

A case example of suit-prone activity is *Jackson v. Waquespack* (2002). In that case, an African American sued a dialysis clinic because she was placed on a machine in the fourth row; Caucasian patients occupied the machines in the first three rows. This particular patient had called the dialysis clinic at 6:30 A.M. Saturday, informing the nurse that she could not keep her scheduled appointment. The nurse with whom the patient spoke told the patient to come in anytime during the evening shift (4:00 P.M. to 8:00 P.M.), as those were the only appointments available later in the day. The patient came at 3:45 P.M. and was allowed to begin her 4-hour treatment at that time.

The patient became upset when she was escorted to a machine in the fourth row, noting that in the first three rows there were only Caucasian patients. The nurse escorting the patient was adamant that the machine in the fourth row was where the patient would have to sit for her treatment. The patient sued for racial discrimination.

In the subsequent lawsuit, testimony was presented to show that the patients seated in the first three rows were "regulars" on the evening shift and were accustomed to using the machines where they were sitting. The only unused machines in the first three rows at 3:45 P.M. that Saturday were on "heat-clean" mode and were unavailable for use by any person. The court noted that the nurse sued for discrimination was also the charge nurse and was busy with administrative duties as well as caring for her assigned patients. That, said the court, could have explained her undiplomatic attitude toward this one particular patient. The case does reinforce the need for nurses to be reasonable and diplomatic at all times, especially as the patient was herself suit prone.

Seventh, while it may not prevent lawsuits, nurses are encouraged to investigate having professional liability insurance. This will better protect them should a lawsuit be filed. Chapter 10 presents more detail about this subject.

Eighth, it seems inevitable that at some point the consumer of health care must begin to accept some responsibility for risks along with the health care providers. One of the reasons cited for high medical malpractice claims against obstetricians is that consumers want total assurance they will have only healthy, perfectly formed children. Perhaps one of nursing's most important tasks is in helping to educate consumers. All health care entails some risks, no matter how remote or far-fetched.

While patients must begin to take this responsibility for their own health care, nurses have a responsibility to be patient advocates. The court in *Coleman v. Christian Home Health Care* (2001) reiterated this aspect for the nurses and patients. The patient in this case was a paraplegic who was being seen in his home by health care aides because of severe bedsores. During one of the home health care aide's visits, she noted that the patient's penis and scrotum were red and swollen and that there was blood in his urine. The aide reported this finding to the LPN, and the LPN went to see the patient. The LPN contacted the patient's nephew, who had the patient seen at the local hospital. At the hospital, the patient was given antibiotics and told to return in 10 days.

Two days after being seen at the hospital, the LPN returned to the patient's home and found that the patient's penis and scrotum were more swollen and discolored than before. The LPN told the patient to return to the hospital; the LPN made no effort to see that the patient was transported to the hospital. Three days later, the LPN returned to the patient's home and again told the patient that he should go to the hospital for care as the condition was continuing to worsen. Two days after this second visit by the LPN, the nephew took his uncle to the hospital, where the patient had surgery for a debridement of necrotic tissue from his penis.

The patient sued for the necrosis and the surgery, which he claimed would not have been necessary if there had been more prompt medical intervention. The court found both parties to the suit, the patient and the home health care agency (the LPN's employer) to be equally responsible for the outcomes in this case. Specifically, the court found that the nurse has a responsibility to be a patient advocate and should have intervened when it was apparent that the patient was not abiding by the professional advice given him by the LPN. The nurse's responsibility, said the court, was more acute as the patient was disabled and lived alone. The patient, though, also had some responsibility for his own care. He was a paraplegic, but not totally helpless. He had no cognitive impairment to prevent him from understanding the LPN's instructions and he had previously contacted his nephew to secure a ride to the hospital. Thus, both parties were equally responsible for the outcomes that occurred.

Finally, remember that many malpractice claims that arise today involve patient education and discharge planning issues. All patients and/or significant others must be taught before discharge from any health care setting, acute care and community-based, and this education may include both formal and informal education. Instructions that are given and information that is learned must become part of the patient record.

EXERCISE 6.3

Review all of the patient encounters that have occurred in the past 7 to 10 days. Were any or all of the patients classifiable as suit-prone patients? Did you observe nurses who could meet the definition of a suit-prone nurse? Do the nurses' ethical principles affect such patients? Which ethical principles should the nurse consider when caring for these suit-prone patients or in assisting suit-prone nurses?

PATIENT EDUCATION AND TORT LAW

Patient education, especially through discharge planning and instruction information, is one of the more visible ways of preventing malpractice claims. As health care providers have become more aware of standards of care and are delivering quality, competent care in the acute care setting, fewer malpractice cases are being filed against nurses. But the same is not true of the outpatient setting and the home setting. Patients are now returning to their homes, failing to follow instructions or claiming that no instructions were given, and filing suits for injuries that arose in the home setting. For example, the newly diagnosed diabetic patient can properly do a blood test for his blood sugar content, give himself the necessary dose of insulin, and correctly select the foods necessary to prepare healthy meals. But what happens when he decides to replant his flowerbed and sustains an open foot injury? Unfortunately, that is the exact scenario being played out across the nation. The patient received excellent acute care, but is unable to follow the medication regime or does not know when to seek emergency medical care after returning to the community.

A recent case that illustrates the importance of discharge planning is *Lewis v. State* (2008). The patient had been admitted to an acute care facility for surgery to correct a misalignment of his jaw. In the post-surgical area, the patient required two doses of Apresoline, a short-acting antihypertensive agent, with a 2-hour interval between doses. He required no additional antihypertensive medication while in the hospital setting, though he had a history of hypertension.

He was discharged at 5:30 P.M., but did not actually leave the setting until 6:30 P.M. Ten minutes after leaving the hospital, he began bleeding profusely from his mouth. His wife drove him back to an office building on the hospital grounds, paramedics were called, but the patient could not be saved. An autopsy established the cause of death as asphyxia from hemorrhage into his airway. At trial, the verdict for the widow and his children was $1,834,914.

The nurse had taken his blood pressure at 5:00 P.M. in anticipation of his discharge; it was 179/88. According to testimony at trial, the nurse did not convey any information about the patient's blood pressure to the surgeon who signed the patient's discharge orders. The court found that the nurse had breached the standard of care by failing to identify a potentially danger-ous situation, failing to communicate the patient's blood pressure to the physician, and failing to take the patient's blood pressure immediately before discharge. The jury concluded that the patient should have been kept in the hospital for observation and treatment of his hypertension and would have been, but for the nurse's errors and omissions in his discharge process.

The court in *C. W. v. The Cooper Health System* (2006) extended the responsibility that health care providers have toward patients who are tested for HIV and the result is not known before the patient is discharged: health care providers must ensure that the patient is aware of the necessity of finding out the result of the test. If the patient does not recontact the health care providers, they must make every attempt to contact the patient.

Because of such instances, acute care settings and outpatient settings are developing more formalized discharge instructions. These instructions may be in English or other languages, they are usually one to two pages and printed in larger fonts, and they are geared toward an eighth-grade educational level. When using these discharge instruction forms, remember to evaluate the patients' and families' understanding of the content. Did they ask pertinent questions? Were they able to perform a repeat demonstration of the skill? Were they able to answer simple questions about the skill? Did they know possible side effects and what to do if such side effects occurred? Retain a copy of the discharge instruction form for the medical record and carefully chart what was taught, how it was evaluated, and what printed information the patient and family were given. More information on legally defensive charting is discussed in Chapter 9.

DEFINITION OF INTENTIONAL TORTS

Intentional torts share three common elements:

1. There must be a volitional or willful act by the defendant.
2. The person so acting must intend to bring about the consequences or appear to have in-tended to bring about the consequences.
3. There must be causation. The act must be a substantial factor in bringing about the injury or consequences.

Intentional torts may be differentiated from negligence in the following manner:

1. Intent is necessary in proving intentional torts. The nurse must have intended an action. For example, the nurse must have intended to hold the patient so that an injection might be given to the patient or so that a nasogastric tube might be inserted into the patient's stomach.
2. There must be a volitional or willful action against the injured person. In intentional torts, there cannot be the omission of a duty owed as with negligence. In the preceding

example, the nurse held the patient so that the injection could be given or the nasogastric tube inserted.

3. Damages are not an issue with intentional torts. The injured party need not show that damages were incurred. Whether the patient encounters out-of-pocket expenses or not, the patient could still show that an intentional tort had occurred.

INTENTIONAL TORTS

The more commonly seen intentional torts within the health care arena are assault, battery, false imprisonment, conversion of property, trespass to land, and intentional infliction of emotional distress (see Table 6.2). Defamation and invasion of privacy are usually discussed with intentional torts, although these two wrongs are more correctly classified as **quasi-intentional torts.**

Assault

An **assault** is any action that places another person in apprehension of being touched in a manner that is offensive, insulting, or physically injurious without consent or authority. No actual touching of the person is required. The action or motion must create a reasonable apprehension in another person of immediate harmful or offensive contact.

Usually thought of as a violent, angry, or unwarranted contact with the patient, assault requires the patient's knowledge. For example, the nurse cannot assault a patient who is sleeping or

TABLE 6.2 Intentional Torts

Tort	Elements	Examples of Nursing Actions
Assault	Shared elements, plus places another in apprehension of being touched in an offensive, insulting, or physically injurious manner	Threatening patients with an injection or with starting an intravenous line
Battery	Shared elements, plus the actual contact with another person or the person's clothing without valid consent	Forcing patients to ambulate against their will; holding a patient so that a nasogastric tube can be inserted
False imprisonment	Shared elements, plus unjustified detention of a person without legal warrant to so confine the person	Refusing to allow patients to leave against medical advice; restraining competent patients against their wishes
Conversion of property	Shared elements, plus interference with the patient's right of possession in his or her property	Searching patients' belongings and taking medications or removing patients' clothing
Trespass to land	Shared elements, plus unlawful interference with another's possession of land	Patient refusing to leave the hospital after being discharged; visitor's refusal to leave the hospital when so requested
Intentional infliction of emotional distress	Shared elements, plus conduct that goes beyond that allowed by society; conduct that is calculated and causes mental distress	Handing a mother her stillborn child in a gallon jar of formaldehyde

unconscious because, no matter how angry or violent the nurse might be or how irrational his or her actions, the patient has no knowledge of the potential contact and is therefore not apprehensive of the potential contact. In *Baca v. Velez* (1992), an operating room nurse sued for assault and battery when an orthopedic surgeon struck her on the back with a bone chisel. In finding that there was no assault (although a battery had occurred), the court concluded that since she was struck in the back, there was "no act, threat or menacing conduct that causes another person to reasonably believe that he is in danger of receiving an immediate battery" (at 1197).

Words alone are not enough for assault to occur, although the addition of words may accompany the overt act. For example, the nurse moves toward the patient with a syringe in one hand while telling the patient why the injection is necessary or while telling the patient to "lie still or this will really hurt!" Either example is an assault if the patient is apprehensive of an offensive touching of his or her body.

Assault also requires a present ability to commit harm. For example, if someone is threatened over a telephone, there is no present ability to commit a harm, and thus no tort has been committed.

Two important reminders: (1) The actual touching of the person (battery) does not have to follow an assault, and (2) either the nurse or the patient may be the tortfeasor (person committing the tort). Assault is apprehension of an unwarranted touching, and the apprehension is all that is needed to prove a tort has occurred. The nurse may approach the patient or the patient may approach the nurse.

Battery

A **battery,** the most common intentional tort within the practice of nursing and medicine, involves a harmful or unwarranted contact with the patient-plaintiff. Liability for such an unwarranted contact is based on the individual's right to be free from unconsented invasions of the person.

The legal system recognizes several factors regarding battery:

1. A single touch, however fleeting and faint, is sufficient for the tort to have occurred. Everyday examples include brushing against another person in a crowded elevator or auditorium or placing one's hand on the patient's shoulder for reassurance. It is the touching, not the manner of the touch, that creates the tort.
2. No harm, injury, or pain need befall the patient. The unwarranted contact frequently will not harm or physically hurt the patient.
3. The patient need not be aware of the battery for the tort to have occurred. Unlike assault, in which knowledge is a key factor, taking a pulse of a sleeping patient could be considered a battery at law.
4. Causation is an important factor, and the nurse may be liable for direct as well as indirect contact. For example, the nurse, intending to restrain a patient for the purpose of starting an intravenous infusion, accidentally drops the intravenous tray on the patient. Even though the nurse has not directly touched the patient, a battery has occurred because the nurse put the scenario into motion.
5. The nurse may also commit a battery by the unwarranted touching of the patient's clothes or of an article held by the patient, such as a purse or a suitcase. For purposes of a battery, anything that is connected with the patient's person is viewed as part of the person.

Most health-care-related lawsuits in this area have focused on consent for medical or surgical procedures. Lack of consent always sets the stage for a potential assault and battery lawsuit. The classic and landmark case of *Schloendorff v. Society of New York Hospitals* (1914) held that the medical practitioner had committed a battery when he removed a tumor from a patient who had authorized merely an examination. *Mohr v. Williams* (1905) had reached a similar previous conclusion when that court found the practitioner liable for performing surgery without prior consent. That court also limited damages because of the good faith of the practitioner and the beneficial results of the surgery to the patient.

More recent examples of such unwarranted treatment are *Loungbury v. Capel* (1992), *Foflygen v. R. Zemel* (1992), and *Anderson v. St. Francis-St. George Hospital* (1992). Each of these cases held that treatment without prior consent by the patient resulted in a battery.

Nurses may also be the plaintiffs in assault and battery cases, rather than the patient, because the rules of law apply to all persons. In *Creasy v. Rusk* (1998), a certified nursing assistant filed a civil personal injury case against a patient who had hurt him. The Court of Appeals of Indiana acknowledged that health care workers can sue patients for personal injuries if the worker is harmed by the patient. But *Berberian v. Lynn* (2002) illustrates the difficulty health care providers encounter when filing such lawsuits. In *Berberian,* an elderly patient suffering from Alzheimer's disease pushed the nurse and caused the nurse's injury. At trial, the patient's diminished mental capacity became the turning point, and the court noted that these patients require special care and that allowing such lawsuits would jeopardize the care for such patients. Second, the courts noted that health care providers who work with such patients recognize and voluntarily accept special risks, for which they should have specialized training.

False Imprisonment

False imprisonment is the unjustifiable detention of a person without legal warrant to confine the person. Nurses falsely imprison the patient when they confine the patient or restrain the patient in a bounded area with the intent to prevent the patient from freedom and nonrestraint. The confined area may be the patient's room or bed. False imprisonment may also occur if the act is directed at the patient's family or possessions. For example, one has effectively been confined if the nurse refuses to give the patient her purse, car keys, or clothing, or refuses to allow the patient to see his family members unless the patient stays in bed.

There must be knowledge of the restraint for false imprisonment to occur. Sedated patients who are incapable of realizing their confinement do not have a suit for false imprisonment. Likewise, future threats are not enough to sustain the tort of false imprisonment. Threatening a patient who is about to leave against medical advice with "if you leave now, no physician will ever take your case in the future" does not constitute false imprisonment, though it may be inadvisable from a nursing perspective. Detaining the patient who wishes to leave against medical advice until the supervisor can be located or until the patient's physician can be contacted to come and see the patient is false imprisonment.

Some of the more recent cases involving false imprisonment in the health care setting concern the area of mental health. In *Arthur v. Lutheran General Hospital, Inc.* (1998), the patient prevailed when he was held against his will after refusing voluntary admission to an inpatient psychiatric facility. The court noted that the patient could be held if there had been a physician's certification to show why the patient was a grave danger to others. State law must be followed, the court held, "to the letter when a citizen's liberty is at stake, and if not, the citizen can sue for false imprisonment" (at 1242).

A second case, *Wingate v. Ridgeview Institute, Inc.* (1998), involved a patient who was held against his will in an alcohol rehabilitation program. The patient had voluntarily admitted himself and then changed his mind and desired to leave. Again, the court held that the legal standard for involuntary mental health treatment is grave danger of serious harm or death of the person or another.

Williams v. Fairlane Memorial Convalescent Home (2007) ruled that a nursing home cannot rely solely on statements of other persons about a resident's mental capacity in deciding to hold a resident against his will, or the resident can file a lawsuit for false imprisonment. Nursing home staff have a legal duty to make and act upon their own independent evaluation of a resident's mental status.

Note that the patient must be aware of the detention for a successful false imprisonment lawsuit. *Remmers v. DeBuono* (1997) was decided as a case of mistreatment of a patient rather than false imprisonment of the patient, because of the patient's inability to understand he had been imprisoned. Here, a nurse's aide was assigned to a patient in a nursing home setting. The patient was confined to a wheelchair but was highly mobile, and he could wheel himself about easily. He was labeled a "wanderer" by the staff, because he frequently roamed away from the nursing unit and could be found in other patients' rooms.

One evening, he wheeled himself off the unit and into other patients' rooms four times. After the fourth time, the aide requested permission to put the patient to bed early. The charge nurse said no, but to keep the patient under watch and go get him when he wandered off the unit. The aide then wheeled the patient into his room, slammed the door closed, and moved the bed into such a position that the door barely opened. There was no way that the patient could exit the room in his wheelchair. The court found the aide had mistreated the patient by barricading him in his room and fined her $1,500.

Some circumstances, however, justify detainment. Hospitals have a common law duty to detain persons who are confused or disoriented. Most states have laws authorizing the detainment of mentally ill persons or persons with a contagious disease who would be a threat to society. In *Blackman for Blackman v. Rifkin* (1988), the hospital was allowed to detain a highly intoxicated, head trauma patient in the emergency center despite her insistence that she be allowed to leave.

As a rule of thumb, mentally ill persons may be detained only if they are a grave threat to themselves or are capable of jeopardizing others. The only force that may be used to detain such persons is that necessary under the circumstances; otherwise, the patient may be able to show battery and false imprisonment.

Restraints are an interference with the patient's liberty, but relatively few cases exist in which a patient has filed for false imprisonment due to use of restraints. Care, caution, and reasonableness are the prerequisites to use of restraints. See Chapter 17 for a more thorough discussion concerning the use of restraints.

Conversion of Property

The tort of **conversion of property** arises when the health care practitioner interferes with the right to possession of the patient's property, either by intermeddling or by dispossessing the person of the property. Examples include searching a patient's suitcase and removing prescription drugs from the patient's possession or taking the patient's car keys or clothing without just cause. This tort is often seen in combination with other torts. Taking a patient's car keys to prevent the patient from leaving the hospital could also be termed false imprisonment. As with the other intentional torts, however, the practitioner may be free from liability if there is adequate justification for the action. For example, taking the car keys to prevent the confused, disoriented person from driving is permissible.

A case that illustrates this concept is *New Jersey Department of Health v. Robert* (2008). Residents in the long-term care facility had the option of paying extra for a phone in the resident's room and receiving an itemized statement for outgoing calls, local or long distance. Though this particular resident could not herself make outgoing calls, the family had a phone installed so that they could call the resident. When they received a bill for outgoing calls, it was discovered that an aide at the facility made a total of nine calls, over a 3-day period, to her next-door neighbor. Though the aide testified that the resident had given her permission to use the phone, the court dismissed this claim because the resident was incapable of making any knowing decision. The court also dismissed the fact that the bill for the nine phone calls came to $1.73, stating that it was not the size of the bill that was relevant, but the fact that the aide had taken what was not hers to take.

Trespass to Land

Trespass to land, the tort of unlawful interference with another's possession of land, may occur either intentionally or as the result of a negligent action. This tort occurs when a person (1) intrudes onto another's property, (2) fails to leave the property when so requested, (3) throws or places something on the property, or (4) causes a third person to enter the property.

Institutions and health care facilities, including their respective parking areas, are private property and people do not have an absolute right to remain on the property. Trespass to land thus occurs when a patient refuses to leave the institution after having been properly discharged or when visitors refuse to leave the area. Trespass may also occur when protestors enter the health care facility as part of a dispute.

Saucier v. Biloxi Regional Medical Center (1998) raised the issue of trespass to land. A group of teenage boys broke into an abandoned hospital to hide and smoke marijuana and to see if ghosts really inhabited morgues as rumored. They found that the pharmacy in the abandoned hospital still had medications on several of the shelves. They returned the next night and looted pills from the pharmacy shelves. They then went to one of the boys' homes to look in a copy of the *Physician's Desk Reference* to identify the pills before consuming them. One of the boys overdosed on amphetamines and barbiturates. The boy's mother sued the hospital on her son's behalf.

The Supreme Court of Mississippi ruled that the boys who had broken into the hospital were trespassers. They knew the hospital was not open for business, that they were not entering the building for a purpose associated with the owner's business, and that they had no permission to be there. Thus, the court ruled that there were no grounds for a civil lawsuit against the owner for injuries associated with a trespasser's unlawful entry on the premises.

Intentional Infliction of Emotional Distress

Sometimes called *extreme and outrageous conduct,* the tort of **intentional infliction of emotional distress** includes several types of outrageous conduct that cause severe emotional distress. Three conditions must be met to prove this tort:

1. The practitioner's conduct goes beyond behavior that is usually tolerated by society.
2. The conduct is calculated to cause mental distress.
3. The conduct actually causes the mental distress.

Rude and insulting behavior is not sufficient to recover under this tort; the behavior must be beyond all realms of decency. Depending on state law, patients' families who witness the conduct may also recover damages. A case that illustrates these points is *Roddy v. Tanner Medical Center, Inc.* (2003).

In that case, a patient, 10 weeks pregnant, experienced severe abdominal cramps, and was driven to the hospital by her husband. En route to the hospital, she bled heavily, even soaking her shoes. At the hospital, nurses removed her blood-soaked clothing, and the patient told the nurses that she felt as if she had passed "something big" on the way to the hospital. She passed several large blood clots at the hospital and she was discharged following a dilatation and curettage (D&C).

At the time of discharge, the nursing staff inquired of the patient if she wanted her clothing returned to her. She said she did, so the nurses placed her soiled clothing in a large plastic bag and gave the bag to her. When the patient returned home, she removed the clothing from the bag so that she could wash the clothes. In her laundry room, the patient found the remains of her stillborn fetus in her blood-soaked trousers. She then filed a lawsuit for intentional infliction of emotional distress.

The court noted in its findings that the individual had indeed suffered severe shock and emotional distress, and that the nurses could be said to be negligent for not inspecting the clothing before returning the clothes to the patient. But, said the court, there was no intent on the part of the nurses to cause her such shock and distress. And, lacking intent, there was no basis for such a lawsuit. Thus, there were no grounds to sue the hospital for intentional infliction of emotional distress.

A similar finding occurred in *Goode v. Bayhealth Medical Center* (2007). Though a close family member was allowed to inadvertently see the deceased relative who had not yet been prepared for viewing on an autopsy table, the court held that there was no intent on the part of health care facility to cause the plaintiff any distress.

Unless the conduct goes outside the reasonable bounds of decency, courts are reluctant to allow plaintiff recovery for this tort. This tort can be easily avoided by treating patients and their families in the same civil, reasonable manner that one would want for oneself or loved ones.

EXERCISE 6.4

A deaf patient, admitted to the emergency center in acute respiratory failure, died within 90 minutes of her admission to the emergency center. The cause of death was listed as suffocation. Following the patient's death, her mother sued the hospital for intentional infliction of emotional distress for the hospital's failure to supply an interpreter for the patient, despite the mother's numerous requests for an interpreter and the fact that impaired communication was noted on the patient's care plan as critical for her care.

How might the court rule in such a case? Does the failure to communicate and understand what is happening to the patient meet the requirements for intentional infliction of emotional distress? Does the fact that the patient failed to survive strengthen the case? Are there other causes of action the mother might have asserted? What are the nurses' ethical responsibilities for such a patient?

QUASI-INTENTIONAL TORTS

The law also recognizes quasi-intentional torts. A tort becomes quasi-intentional when intent is lacking but there is a volitional action and direct causation. In other words, more than mere negligence is involved, but the intent that is necessary for an intentional tort is missing in quasi-intentional torts. As with intentional torts, quasi-intentional torts have no use to society and damages are not an issue. Table 6.3 outlines these torts.

Invasion of Privacy

The right to protection against unreasonable and unwarranted interferences with the individual's solitude is well recognized. The tort of **invasion of privacy** includes the protection of personality as well as the protection against interference with one's right to be left alone. This right to privacy

TABLE 6.3 Quasi-Intentional Torts

Tort	Elements	Examples of Nursing Actions
Invasion of privacy	Act must intrude or pry into person's seclusion; intrusion must be objectionable to a reasonable person; intrusion must concern private facts or published facts and pictures of a private nature; must be public disclosure of private information	Using patients' pictures without their consent or in a manner that was not authorized by them; releasing confidential information to others without the person's consent; giving status reports about a patient to someone not authorized to receive such information
Defamation	Defamatory language about a living person that would adversely affect his or her reputation, published to a third person; damage to reputation	Making false chart entries about a patient's lifestyle or diagnoses; falsely accusing staff members in front of visitors or other staff members

concerns one's peace of mind in that he or she is to be free from unwarranted publicity. Within a medical context, the law recognizes the patient's right against:

1. Appropriation or usage of the plaintiff's name or picture for defendant's sole advantage
2. Intrusion by the defendant on the patient's seclusion or affairs
3. Publication by the defendant of facts that place the patient in a false light
4. Public disclosure of private facts about the patient by hospital staff or medical personnel

Elements of invasion of privacy include:

1. An act that must intrude or pry into the seclusion of the patient
2. Intrusion that is objectionable to the reasonable person
3. An act or intrusion that intrudes or pries into private facts or publishes facts and pictures of a private nature
4. Public disclosure of private information

Information concerning the patient is confidential and may not be disclosed without authorization. Authorization may be either by patient waiver or pursuant to a valid reporting statute. Most hospitals and institutions have policies regarding who and under what circumstances information may be released. Liability could exist if nurses and hospital personnel fail to follow their published policies and procedures.

Nurses are cautioned about releasing information concerning current patients over the telephone. Remember, even family members may not be privileged to patient information. The patient may elect not to disclose information concerning diagnosis and treatments to family members. Short of a valid reporting statute, the nurse may not violate this privacy right.

Frequently, relatives and friends call to inquire about the patient's status, diagnosis, or prognosis. Before releasing any information, the patient must authorize such release, and the nurse should verify who the inquirer is, as most patients allow release of information only to family and close friends. For callers who are not allowable recipients of patient knowledge, an appropriate response is to ask the caller to contact the family or relatives directly.

Patients have a right to their names as well as to their pictures. Pictures or photos may not be used, even for medical journals or technical publications, without proper authorization (*Vessiliades v.*

Garfinckel's, Brooks Brothers, 1985). In that case, the court held that a plastic surgeon had violated the privacy of a patient when he allowed, without her consent or prior knowledge, "before" and "after" pictures of her to be used for a department store presentation and by a television station.

Nor is it important if the patient is the subject of the picture in the foreground or part of the background or if the photograph was taken with no intent to infringe on the patient's rights. Photographing a patient without the patient's consent is a violation of the patient's right to medical confidentiality (*Strango v. Hammond*, 2008).

A case that illustrates the court's reluctance to expand privacy rights is *Rothstein v. Montefiore Home* (1996). In this case, the deceased's wife had filed the original application for his admission to a nursing home. Included in the application packet were financial records and tax returns. The deceased died before the application could be processed, and the application packet was returned to the deceased's daughter, not his widow.

According to the court, the daughter carefully examined the financial papers and, based on what she learned, filed a suit to contest her father's will in probate court. The will contest threatened the widow's position as beneficiary under the will, and the widow sued the nursing home for releasing the financial records to the daughter. The widow's case listed the cause of action as invasion of privacy.

In dismissing the invasion of privacy lawsuit, the court noted that such a lawsuit is meant to compensate a person for mental anguish when a private facet of a person's life is exposed to the public. The deceased, ruled the court, suffered no mental anguish. Additionally, the records were released in privacy to another member of the family, so no invasion of the widow's privacy occurred.

In limited circumstances, the newsworthiness of the event makes disclosure acceptable. The public's right to know can exceed the patient's right to privacy, as seen in the 1981 attempt on President Reagan's life or in the implantation of innovative life-support systems. Dr. Barney Clark (1982), the first man to have an implanted artificial heart would be an example of such a newsworthy event (Lerner, 2007), although his name might have been protected, as was done in the 1993 case of Baby K in which a Virginia hospital was ordered to provide treatment for an anencephalic infant (*Matter of Baby K*, 1994).

Even though there may be a right to public knowledge, courts have not allowed public disclosure to undermine a patient's dignity. Two landmark cases, *Barber v. Time, Inc.* (1942) and *Doe v. Roe* (1978), both stand for the need to protect the patient's privacy rights. One cannot divulge so much information about the patient that the patient's identity becomes readily obvious.

Valid reporting statutes may allow disclosure of limited patient data. Nurses must protect the patient's privacy over and above what is required by disclosure statutes (*Prince v. St. Francis-St. George Hospital*, 1985). Chapter 8 discusses reporting statutes, including the newer Health Insurance Portability and Accountability Act (HIPAA) of 1996 regulations, in more detail.

Defamation

Defamation, comprised of the torts of slander and libel, concerns wrongful injury to another's reputation (his or her good name, respect, and esteem). It involves written or oral communication to someone other than the person defamed of matters concerning a living person's reputation. A claim of defamation may arise from inaccurate or inappropriate release of medical information or from untruthful statements about other staff members.

Five elements are necessary to prove the quasi-intentional tort of defamation:

1. Defamatory language that would adversely affect one's reputation
2. Defamatory language about or concerning a living person

3. Publication to a third party or to several persons but not necessarily the world at large
4. Damage to the person's reputation as seen by adverse, derogatory, or unpleasant opinions against the person defamed
5. Fault on the part of the defendant in writing or telling another the defamatory language

The tort may be harder to prove if the person affected is a public figure. The law recognizes that such public figures would have a greater possibility of publicly defending themselves than the private person and could more easily explain or counteract the potentially defamatory statement. For example, politicians could call a press conference or request that the local newspaper write their version. A private housewife or health care provider could not command such actions and thus has greater protection for this quasi-intentional tort at law.

Generally, no actual damages need to exist for slander (oral communications), but must exist for libel (written defamation). Exceptions include slanderous statements that concern contagious or venereal diseases, crimes involving moral turpitude, or comments that prejudice persons in their chosen profession, trade, or business. Two older but still applicable cases illustrate this point. *Schessler v. Keck* (1954) concerned a case wherein a nurse told a second person that a particular caterer was currently being treated for syphilis, and the false statement destroyed the catering business. *Farrell v. Kramer* (1963) concerned a similar defamatory statement.

A case that points out the idea that the statements as communicated must be false is *Columbia Valley Regional Medical Center v. Bannert* (2003). In that case, an operating room scheduler discovered a memo on the hospital's shared computer memory drive in which the chief nursing officer made accusations of unprofessionalism about a nursing manager. The memo also noted that the chief nursing officer was not recommending this individual for promotion. The scheduler copied the file to a disc, and the memo was then widely circulated among hospital personnel.

The court denied the nursing manager's suit for defamation, noting that to be defamation, "a statement must be false and must subject a person to public hatred, contempt, or ridicule or impeach the person's honesty, integrity, or virtue" (*Columbia Valley Regional Medical Center v. Bannert*, 2003, at 200). In this case, the court ruled, based on the wording and tone of the memo, that what had been circulated was an opinion, perhaps issued by the chief nursing officer, and that opinions are not defamatory. There was no proof, said the court, that the chief nursing officer had indeed issued the memo, as the authorship of the computer file was not proven. Additionally, there is a legal privilege for supervisors to share opinions with others concerning individuals they supervise.

Nurses are cautioned against defamatory statements in chart references about patients. For example, charting that a patient is a prostitute or acts "crazy" may raise potential liability issues. When a person exhibits unusual behavior, chart exactly the behavior as perceived rather than conclusory statements.

EXERCISE 6.5

Imagine that you are required to design a 1-hour continuing education offering for nurses to learn more about intentional torts. What content would you include in the presentation? How should you present the information to the audience? How should you evaluate the effectiveness of your continuing education offering?

DEFENSES

In some instances, a health care provider may commit an intentional tort and incur no legal liability. Called *defenses,* these specific instances and circumstances are the subject of the next chapter.

ETHICAL ISSUES AND TORT LAWS

One of the premises upon which tort law is based concerns the duty owed to the patient. Inherent in this duty is the common law interpretation that no duty was owed a stranger, but once the duty was undertaken, then one could be found liable for failure to care for the patient. There are some exceptions to this rule, including the right to refuse care based on religious beliefs, such as when a nurse refuses to care for a patient seeking an abortion. Concern over one's own health issues was raised when the first cases of HIV and AIDS were detected, and the concern seems to have resurfaced with each advent of a newly confirmed infectious disease, such as severe acute respiratory syndrome (SARS), avian influenza (bird flu), and now the swine flu pandemic. These concerns continue to be discussed and debated from an ethical perspective, particularly as the duty to provide care is rooted in several longstanding ethical principles. Clark (2005) notes that health care providers have greater ethical standards in such outbreaks for the following reasons:

1. The ability of the health care professionals to provide care is greater than that of the public, thus increasing the obligation to provide care.
2. Health care professionals have assumed the risk of care for these individuals based on their choice of a profession dedicated to the care of the sick.
3. Members of the profession should be available in times of emergency, as the profession is part of a social contract with the public. This latter reason is also consistent with the ANA's *Code of Ethics for Nurses* (2001), point 8.

A second ethical issue concerns the number of medication errors that occur within health care facilities and in the home. Issues arise concerning the amount of disclosure that is made available to the patient and family, fairness in the manner in which all medication errors are investigated by management, and how to ensure future trust and confidence in all staff members regarding patient safety. Nurses must be held accountable for their own errors, but they also need to be treated in a respectful and assistive manner. Nurses may need assistance in understanding that some harm occurs with every medication error, even the smallest errors, such as when a medication dose is missed. In a survey by Cohen, Robinson, and Mandrack (2003), the authors discovered that only 18% of the nurses surveyed would fully disclose an error to the patient or a family member when a medication error occurred. Many of the nurses explained that they would not fully disclose the error as they did not wish to frighten the person or persons involved. Ethically, though, the disclosure of errors is the correct approach, as another cannot make health care decisions unless he or she has full knowledge upon which to base a decision.

A final area of ethics in this area of the law involves the locality rule, discussed earlier, which seems to be making a resurgence in some areas of the country. The central idea of the locality rule is that some patients, usually those in more rural settings and potentially the most deserving of care, may not receive the same type of care that they would receive in more urban settings or in different locations.

SUMMARY

- A tort is a civil wrong committed against a person or a person's property.
- Negligence equates with carelessness, can be either a commission or an omission, and is performed by a nonlicensed person.
- Malpractice, sometimes termed *professional negligence*, is the failure of a professional person to act in accordance with the prevailing standard of care or the failure of the professional person to foresee consequences that a professional person would foresee.
- Six elements must be shown in malpractice lawsuits:
  - Duty owed the patient
  - Breach of duty owed the patient
  - Foreseeability
  - Causation
  - Injury
  - Damages
- Duty owed the patient incorporates both the obligation as well as the level of the obligation.
- Breach of duty owed the patient involves showing a deviation from the standard of care owed to the patient.
- Foreseeability is the concept that certain events may reasonably be expected to cause specific outcomes.
- Causation means that the injury caused to the patient must be a direct result of the breach of duty owed to the patient and may be subdivided into cause-in-fact and proximate cause.
- The tests for causation include the "but for" and substantial factor tests.
- Injury involves some type of physical, financial, or emotional harm that occurred as a result of the breach of duty owed the patient.
- Damages can be subdivided into four categories:
  - General damages
  - Special damages
  - Emotional damages
  - Punitive or exemplary damages
- The doctrine of res ipsa loquitor ("the thing speaks for itself") allows a negligence cause of action without requiring that all of the six elements of negligence or malpractice be proven.
- The locality rule has been abolished in the majority of states and a national standard of care has emerged.
- Patient education and discharge planning are two of the more visible means of preventing future malpractice claims.
- Intentional torts include:
  - Assault: an action that places another person in apprehension of being touched in a manner that is offensive, insulting, or physically injurious without consent or authority.
  - Battery: involves a harmful or unwarranted contact with another person.
  - False imprisonment: the unjustifiable detention of another person without legal warrant to confine the person.
  - Conversion of property: involves the interference with the right of possession of another person's property.
  - Trespass to land: the unlawful interference with another's possession of land.
  - Intentional infliction of emotional distress: sometimes called extreme and outrageous conduct, this involves conduct that causes another person severe emotional distress.
- Quasi-intentional torts include:
  - Invasion of privacy, or the right to protection against unreasonable and unwarranted interferences with the individual's solitude.
  - Defamation, including libel and slander, concerns the wrongful injury to another's reputation.
- Ethical issues that can arise include the obligation to provide competent care to all patients, including those who may place the health care provider at risk, disclosure concerning actions that place patients at risk, and the ethics involved with the locality rule.

GUIDELINES

Intentional Torts and Quasi-Intentional Torts

1. Recognize that the patient has several rights at law for freedom from intentional torts and quasi-intentional torts and that the nurse must act to ensure these rights.
2. Know the elements of each of the intentional and quasi-intentional torts so that you will not violate the rights of patients for whom you care. Some torts are more common than others. The nurse should know that the tort of battery is the most common one seen within the health care arena and possibly the easiest one to commit. Stop and think before making unwarranted contacts with patients.
3. Know that there are limited circumstances in which the absolute rights of the patient may be transgressed. Understand the full impact of the law in these limited areas, and seek legal guidance before transgressing the patient's rights.
4. Treat all patients with the same competent, courteous care that you would want for yourself and your loved ones.
5. Be particularly selective when answering questions about patients over the telephone. Recognize that patients have the right to refuse, unless there exists a state reporting statute to the contrary, to allow disclosure of details about their illness and prognosis to others, including close family members.
6. Be cautious of the patient who is also a public figure. Public figures, whether voluntarily placed before the public eye or not, are owed the same privacy and reputation rights as the private patient.

APPLY YOUR LEGAL KNOWLEDGE

- What types of patients are more likely to bring nursing malpractice suits?
- When a patient injury occurs, is the nurse or another staff member always legally responsible?
- What are the more common types of nursing malpractice today?
- Is the distinction between malpractice and negligence important? Why or why not?
- How do intentional torts differ from negligence and malpractice?

- If a teaching session were to be given on intentional torts seen in clinical settings, which torts would be included? Would you answer differently if time was limited and you could include additional materials?
- What can staff nurses do to protect patients from quasi-intentional torts? Does this differ from the nurse manager's role in preventing quasi-intentional torts?

YOU BE THE JUDGE

The nurse was counseled for improperly documenting wastage of a controlled substance. She had signed for three 100-mg doses of fentanyl, but had only documented giving doses of 25 mg to each of three patients. The counseling session was attended by the nurse in question and her immediate supervisor.

Following this initial session, a second meeting was convened with the nurse, two nurse managers, and a representative from the hospital's employee assistance program. The nurse was told that she was suspected of narcotics conversion and on-the-job drug abuse.

The nurse was assured that she was free to leave, but was not allowed to drive her car parked on the street two blocks away, based on the suspicion that she was under the influence of drugs. A female police officer drove the nurse and her supervisor to the nurse's car to get some personal items, then back to the hospital. The nurse's boyfriend came to take her out to dinner and then returned to get her car.

Drug tests were negative, but the nurse was subsequently fired for substandard performance related to the medication documentation errors. She sued the hospital for false imprisonment based on the way she had been confined.

QUESTIONS

1. Did the manner in which the nurse was treated conform to the definition of false imprisonment?
2. Were the hospital supervisor and nurse manager justified in not allowing the nurse to drive her car until the results of the drug test were returned?
3. Did the fact that the nurse was faced with disciplinary action that was extremely prejudicial to her continued employment cause the nurse to fail to stand up for her rights and leave of her own accord rather than follow the dictates of her supervisor and nurse managers?
4. How would you decide this case?

REFERENCES

American Nurses Association. (2001). *Code of ethics for nurses with interpretive statements.* Washington, DC: Author.

Anderson v. St. Francis-St. George Hospital, 614 N.E.2d 841 (Ohio, 1992).

Arthur v. Lutheran General Hospital, Inc., 692 N.E.2d 1238 (Ill. App., 1998).

Babits v. Vassar Brothers Hospital, 732 N.Y.S.2d 46 (N.Y. App., 2001).

Baca v. Velez, 833 P.2d 1194 (N.M. App., 1992).

Barber v. Time, Inc., 348 Missouri 1199, 159 S.W.2d 291 (1942).

Berberian v. Lynn, 355 N.J. Super. 210, 2002 WL 31557027 (N.J. App., November 20, 2002).

Blackman for Blackman v. Rifkin, 759 P.2d 54 (Colo. App., 1988), cert. denied (1988).

Boling v. Stegemann, 2007 WL 778621 (N.Y. App., March 16, 2007).

Brooker v. Galen of Kentucky, Inc., 2003 WL 21828795 (Ky. App., 2003).

Brown v. Southern Baptist Hospital, 715 So.2d 423 (La. App., 1998).

C. W. v. The Cooper Health System, 2006 WL 2590107 (A. J. App., August 10, 2006).

Casas v. Paradez, 2008 WL 2517135 (Tex. App., June 25, 2008).

Cheeks v. Dorsey, 2003 WL 21014391 (Fla. App., May 7, 2003).

Christus Spohn v. De La Fuente, 2007 WL 2323989 (Tex. App., August 16, 2007).

Clark, C. C. (2005). In harm's way: AMA physicians and the duty to treat. *Journal of Medical Philosophy, 30,* 65–87.

Cleary v. Manning, 2008 WL 1701176 (Ind. App., April 14, 2008).

Cohen, H., Robinson, E. S., & Mandrack, M. (2003). Getting to the roots of medication errors: Survey results. *Nursing 2003, 33*(9), 36–45.

Coleman v. Christian Home Health Care, 786 So.2d 819 (La. App., 2001).

Collins v. Superior Air-Ground Ambulance Service, Inc., 2003 WL 1971813 (Ill. App., April 29, 2003).

Columbia Valley Regional Medical Center v. Bannert, 112 S.W.3d 193 (Tex. App., Corpus Christi, 2003).

Crane v. Lakewood Hospital, 658 N.E.2d 1088 (Ohio App., 1995).

Creasy v. Rusk, 696 N.E.2d 442 (Ind. App., 1998).

Croke, E. M. (2003). Nurses, negligence, and malpractice. *American Journal of Nursing, 103*(9), 54–63.

Curtis v. MRI Imaging Services II, 956 P.2d 960 (Oregon, 1998).

Delaune v. Medical Center of Baton Rouge, Inc., 683 So.2d 859 (La. App., 1996).

Dent v. Memorial Hospital of Adel, 509 S.E.2d 908 (Georgia, 1998).

Depesa v. Westchester Square Medical Center, 657 N.Y.S.2d 419 (A.D. 1 Dept. 1997).

Dickerson v. Fatehi, 484 S.E.2d 880 (Virginia, 1997).

Doe v. Roe, 93 Misc.2d.201, 400 N.Y.S.2d. 958 (1978).

Donahue v. Port, Case #92-CIV-4477 (Pennsylvania, 1994).

Estate of Chin v. St. Barnabas Medical Center et al., 711 A.2d 352 (N.J. Super., 1998).

Estate of Garrison v. Dailey, 2006 WL 1547759 (Tex. App., June 7, 2006).

Estate of Thurston v. Southwood Nursing Center, 2007 WL 866450 (Fla. Cir. Ct., February 22, 2007).

Farrell v. Kramer, 193 A.2d 560 (Maine, 1963).

Flowers v. HCA Health Services of Tennessee, 2006 WL 627183 (Tenn. App., March 14, 2006).

Foflygen v. R. Zemel, 615 A.2d 1345 (Pennsylvania, 1992).

Fraijo v. Hartland Hospital, 99 Cal. Rptr.3d 331, 160 Calif. Rptr. 848 (1979).

Garcia v. Bronx Lebanon Hospital, 713 N.Y.S.2d 702 (N.Y. App., 2001).

Glanda v. Twenty Pack Manufacturing Company, 2008 WL 4058590 (E. D. Mich., August 28, 2008).

Gooch v. North Country Regional Hospital, 2006 WL 771384 (Minn. App., March 28, 2006).

Goode v. Bayhealth Medical Center, 2007 WL 2050761 (Delaware, July 18, 2007).

Hardman v. Long Island Urological Associates, P.C., 678 N.Y.S.2d 365 (N.Y. App., 1998).

Hatton v. Interim Healthcare, 2007 WL 902176 (Ohio App., March 27, 2007).

Henderson v. Homer Memorial Hospital, 2006 WL 217933 (La. App., January 27, 2006).

Houston v. Baptist Medical Center, 2007 WL 4522998 (Cir. Ct., Duval Co., Florida, April 19, 2007).

Jackson v. Waquespack, 2002 WL 31427316 (E.D. La., October 25, 2002).

Jacobs v. Leesburg Regional Medical Center, 2007 WL 1976951 (Cir. Ct. Lake Co., Florida, March 30, 2007).

Jones v. Department of Health, 661 So.2d 1291 (Fla. App., 1995).

Keel v. West Louisiana Health Services, 803 So.2d 382 (La. App., 2001).

Kunz v. Little County of Mary Hospital, 2007 WL 1309558 (Ill. App., May 4, 2007).

Lakos v. Kaiser Permanente, 2008 WL 3822331 (Med. Mal. Arbitration, Los Angeles, California, February 5, 2008).

Lane v. Tift County Hospital Authority, 492 S.E.2d 317 (Ga. App., 1997).

Lerner, B. H. (2007). Hero or victim? The 25th anniversary of Barney Clark's artificial heart. Available online at http://hnn.us/articles/44902.html

Lewis v. State, 2008 WL 1777227 (La. App., April 16, 2008).

Long v. Wade, 2007 WL 2459976 (Alabama, August 31, 2007).

Loungbury v. Capel, 836 P.2d 188 (Utah, 1992).

Luby v. St. John's Episcopal Hospital, 631 N.Y.S.2d 773 (N.Y. App. Div., 1995).

Lunsford v. Board of Nurse Examiners, 648 S.W.2d 391 (Tex. Civ. App., Austin, 1983).

Maquette v. Goodman, 771 A.2d 775 (Pa. Super., 2001).

Majca v. Beekil, Nos. 83677, 83886 (Illinois, 1998).

Matter of Baby K, 16 F. 3rd 590 (4th Cir., 1994).

McGraw v. St. Joseph's Hospital, 488 S.E.2d 389 (West Virginia, 1997).

Miller v. Levering Regional Healthcare Center, 2006 WL 1889883 (Mo. App., July 11, 2006).

Mitchell v. University Hospital and Clinics-Holmes County, 2006 WL 3290844 (Miss. App., November 14, 2006).

Mobile Infirmary Medical Center v. Hodgen, 2003 WL 22463340 (Alabama, October 31, 2003).

Moc v. Children's Hospital, 2007 WL 5624414 (March 23, 2007).

Mohr v. Williams, 95 Minn. 261, 104 N.W. 12 (1905).

Morrison v. Mann, 2007 WL 655578 (N.D. Georgia, February 27, 2007).

National Practitioner Data Bank Healthcare Integrity and Protection Data Bank. (2008). *NPDP summary report*. Available online at http://www.npdb-hipdb .hrsa.gov/summaryrpt.html

Nayman v. Huntsville Hospital, 2007 WL 2988258 (Cir. Ct. Madison Co., Alabama, February 23, 2007).

New Jersey Department of Health v. Roberts, 2008 WL 4066426 (N.J. App., September 4, 2008).

O'Shea v. State of New York, 2007 WL 1516492 (N.Y. Ct. Cl., January 22, 2007).

Palafox v. Silvey, 2007 WL 3225512 (Tex. App., November 1, 2007).

Patel v. Williams, 2007 WL 3286800 (Tex. App., November 6, 2007).

Pender v. Natchitoches Parish Hospital, 2003 WL 21017325 (La. App., May 7, 2003).

People v. Gutierrez, 2006 WL 2875504 (Ca. App., October 11, 2006).

Pillers v. The Finley Hospital, 2003 WL 22087488 (Iowa App., September 10, 2003).

Piro v. Chandler, 780 So.2d 394 (La. App., 2001).

Prince v. St. Francis-St. George Hospital, 484 N.E.2d 265 (Ohio App., 1985).

Quesenberry v. Beebe Medical Center, Inc., 2006 WL 515455 (Del. Super., February 28, 2006).

Quinby v. Plumsteadville Family Practice, Inc., 2006 WL (Pennsylvania, October 18, 2006).

Quintanilla v. Coral Gables Hospital, Inc., 2006 WL 3078909 (Fla. App., November 1, 2006).

Radish v. De Graff Memorial Hospital, 738 N.Y.S.2d 780 (N.Y. Super., 2002).

Rayford v. Willow Ridge, 2008 WL 3394662 (La. App., August 13, 2008).

Remmers v. DeBuono, 660 N.Y.S.2d 159 (N.Y. App., 1997).

Robinson v. Health Midwest Development Group, 58 S.W.3d 519 (Missouri, 2001).

Roddy v. Tanner Medical Center, Inc., 2003 WL 21525268 (Ga. App., July 8, 2003).

Rosales-Rosario v. Brookdale University Hospital and Medical Center, 2003 N.Y. Slip Op. 18447, 2003 WL 22717881 (N.Y. App., November 17, 2003).

Rothstein v. Montefiore Home, 689 N.E.2d 108 (Ohio App., 1996).

Rustvold v. Taylor, 14 P.3d 675 (Or. App., 2000).

Saucier v. Biloxi Regional Medical Center, 708 So.2d 1351 (Mississippi, 1998).

Schallert v. Mercy Hospital of Buffalo, 722 N.Y.S.2d 668 (N.Y. App., 2001).

Schessler v. Keck, 271 P.2d 588 (California, 1954).

Schloendorff v. Society of New York Hospitals, 211 N.Y. 125, 105 N.E. 92 (1914).

Schroeder v. Northwest Community Hospital, 2006 WL 3615559 (Ill. App., December 12, 2006).

Shortnancy v. North Atlanta Internal Medicine, P.C., 556 S.E.2d 209 (Ga. App. 2001).

Siegel v. Long Island Jewish Medical Center, 2003 N.Y. Slip Op. 17790, 2003 WL 22439814 (N.Y. App., October 27, 2003).

Silves v. King, 970 P.2d 790 (Wash. App. 1999).

Sisters of St. Joseph of Texas, Inc. v. Cheek, 61 S.W.3d 32 (Tex. App., 2001).

Skikiewicz v. Mount Clemens General Hospital, 2007 WL 5157903 (Cir. Ct. Macomb Co., Michigan, November 6, 2007).

Slease v. Hughbanks, 684 N.E.2d 496 (Ind. App., 1997).

Strango v. Hammond, 2008 WL 501322 (S. D. Tex., February 21, 2008).

Synder v. Arrowhead Community Hospital, 2007 WL 2592401 (Sip. Ct. Maricopa Co., Arizona, January 16, 2007).

Thomas v. New York University Medical Center, 725 N.Y.S.2d 35 (N.Y. Super., 2001).

Thomas v. Sheridan, 2008 WL 426289 (La. App., February 8, 2008).

Tucker v. University Specialty Hospital, 2005 WL 3213897 (Md. App., December 1, 2005).

Turner v. United States, 2008 WL 2726508 (M. D. Fla., July 1, 2008).

Van Horn v. Chambers, 970 S.W.2d 542 (Texas, 1998).

Vessiliades v. Garfinkel's, Brooks Brothers, 492 A.2d 580 (D.C. App., 1985).

Walston v. Lakeview Regional Medical Center, 768 So.2d 238 (LA. App., 2000).

Weeks v. Eastern Idaho Health Services, 2007 WL 600830 (Idaho, February 28, 2007).

Williams v. Fairlane Memorial Convalescent Home, 2007 WL 750387 (Mich. App., March 13, 2007).

Wingate v. Ridgeview Institute, Inc., 504 S.E.2d 714 (Ga. App., 1998).

Ybarra v. Spangard, 154 P.2d 687 (California, 1944).

Young v. University of Mississippi Medical Center, 2005 WL 3112420 (Miss. App., November 22, 2005).

CHAPTER 7

Nursing Liability: Defenses

PREVIEW

Health care providers are acutely aware of potential legal claims that may be filed against them. Much of this concern involves unknowns about the legal process and the extent of one's civil liability. Concern may also surface about possible defenses to lawsuits that are filed. This chapter explores possible legal defenses to nursing liability and how such defenses may lessen the individual practitioner's potential legal liability. The chapter concludes with a discussion of products liability and collective and alternative liability.

LEARNING OUTCOMES

After completing this chapter, you should be able to:

7.1 Define the term *defense* and give examples of defenses that may be used against intentional, quasi-intentional, and negligence torts.

7.2 Review the concept of statute of limitations, including the importance this statute has in the health care field.

7.3 Examine the Good Samaritan laws and their relevance for health care deliverers.

7.4 Define and explain products liability and collective and alternative liability defenses.

KEY TERMS

abuse
access
alternative liability
assumption of the risk
collective liability
consent
contributory and comparative negligence
contributory negligence rule

defense of others
defenses
disclosure statutes
exculpatory agreements
exculpatory contracts
Good Samaritan laws
immunity
modified comparative negligence

necessity
privilege
products liability
pure comparative negligence
qualified privilege
release
self-defense
statutes of limitations
truth

DEFENSES AGAINST LIABILITY

Several defenses are available to the health care practitioner in the event that a legal claim or lawsuit is filed. **Defenses** are "arguments in support of or used for justification" (Merriam-Webster, 2008, paragraph 1). These defenses may be based on statutory law, common law, or the doctrine of precedent. These defenses may also be classified according to the cause of action filed against them.

DEFENSES AGAINST INTENTIONAL TORTS

As much as is practical, defenses used in relation to intentional, nonintentional, and quasi-intentional torts are divided according to those broad categories. Some of the defenses overlap and are discussed in the most appropriate category. Defenses against intentional torts generally include (1) consent, (2) self-defense, (3) defense of others, and (4) necessity (see Table 7.1).

Consent

Consent may be oral, implied by law, or apparent. There can be no lawsuit for battery if the patient approved of the touching. For example, the nurse enters the patient's room with a syringe in one hand and an alcohol wipe in the other hand. As she enters the room, she states, "Mr. Jones, I have your vitamin injection. In which arm would you prefer that I give it?" The patient extends his left arm and helps the nurse roll up his left sleeve with his right hand. Apparent consent has been given, because the reasonable person would infer from the patient's conduct that he both understood what was said to him and that he consented to the action of giving the injection.

Consent may also be implied by law. Many examples of implied consent occur in emergency settings. When the person is not capable of either giving or denying consent, the law adopts the granting of consent if the following four elements are met:

1. An immediate decision is required to prevent loss of life or limb.
2. The person is incapable of giving or denying consent.
3. There is no reason to believe that consent would not be given if the patient were capable of such.
4. A reasonable person in the same or similar circumstances would give consent.

A complete discussion of consent may be found in Chapter 8.

TABLE 7.1 Defenses to Torts

Intentional Torts	Quasi-Intentional Torts	Nonintentional Torts
Consent	Consent	Release
Self-defense	Truth	Contributory negligence
Defense of others	Privilege	Comparative negligence
Necessity	Disclosure statutes	Assumption of the risk
Access laws	Immunity statutes	Statute of limitations
Duty to disclose laws		
Qualified privilege		

Self-Defense and Defense of Others

Self-defense and **defense of others** may be justifiable to protect oneself and others in the area from harm. For example, a patient suddenly becomes combative, and there is imminent danger to the nursing staff, other patients, and visitors. The nurses would be justified in forcibly restraining the patient, even though no order for restraints had been obtained. In such an example, defense of others could be extended to include the defense of the patient as well. The caveat is that one can use only reasonable force—that which is necessary to prevent injury to oneself or to defend others in the situation.

In *Mattocks v. Bell* (1963), one of the landmark cases in this area, a male medical student was allowed to strike a 23-month-old child on the cheek to free his finger from the child's mouth. In finding that no battery or assault occurred, the court concluded that no unnecessary force was used nor was the force applied inappropriately. The court did say, however, that it was not condoning the striking of the child.

A more recent example of an acceptable use of defense of others is *Wyatt v. Department of Human Services* (2008). In that case, the Supreme Court of Iowa overturned the initial ruling in which the court had found liability. The certified nursing assistant (CNA) in question had used a pillow to stifle the cries of a patient who had severe dementia and was diagnosed with a brain tumor. The reason the nurse used a pillow to stifle the patient's constant cries was to avoid unnecessary alarm to a second neurological patient, who was recovering from a subarachnoid hemorrhage and who was resting quietly in a nearby, darkened room. A co-worker reported the nurse to the state department of human services and, at trial, the CNA was found to be liable for abuse of a dependent adult. The Supreme Court overturned the original verdict, noting that to commit abuse an individual must possess the mental state of intent to harm a patient or dependent person. The CNA in this instance had no intent to harm anyone and was actually motivated by concern for the safety and welfare of another very fragile individual in her care. In both of these cases, *Mattocks* and *Wyatt*, remember that the actions in question concerned an intentional tort, where intent is critical to the commission of the tort.

A more common example of self-defense and defense of others may be seen in the following example. A nurse is employed in a medical-surgical unit of a large, urban, acute care institution. A male patient, newly post-operative from an appendectomy, approaches the nurse and demands "more pain medication now!" After being told that his next scheduled medication is not for over an hour, he grabs the nurse, saying, "I want my medicine now!" Since the nurse is alone and no one is available to assist her, she jabs her elbow into his sternum. Once freed, she returns to the central nurse's area and immediately calls security. Has the nurse acted prudently, using only "reasonable" force given the circumstances?

Many legal experts would agree with the nurse's action, given the specifics of this scenario. At court, a jury would be asked to determine if force was necessary and if the amount of force used was "reasonable." In the preceding scenario, because the patient was capable of using force and did so, added to the fact that he was angry, most experts would concur that some degree of force was appropriate. The nurse struck only one blow, one that was sufficient for the patient to move away from the nurse and allow her to run for assistance. Again, striking a patient should not be one's first line of defense, but it may well be the most appropriate course of action given the circumstances. Remember to accurately document the incident and complete an unusual occurrence report; information on these issues is described in detail in Chapter 9.

A recent case that supports the conclusions of the preceding scenario is *Estate of Klein v. North Shore University Hospital* (2007). A 79-year-old patient was admitted to the institution's intensive care unit for diabetic ketoacidosis. The next evening, she removed the monitor leads, rose, and announced that she was leaving the facility. Three nurses put her back to bed and reattached the monitor leads. Within hours, the patient's behavior became combative. Multiple staff members intervened, and during the ensuing struggle the patient's arm and both legs were broken. She required surgery for the multiple broken limbs, developed complications following the surgery, and died a week later. The family brought a lawsuit, naming all involved in the incident as well as the hospital.

At trial, the attorney for the family argued that sedatives, specifically Haldol, should have been given when the patient first became confused. The jury, though, accepted the fact that no chemical restraint was required at the time of the first episode of confusion. Nothing in that initial episode indicated that a full-blown combative episode would follow or that the patient, who had advanced osteoporosis, would be so injured. The jury further found that there was no liability on the part of the staff members or the hospital.

Necessity

Necessity, which is similar to self-defense, allows the nurse to interfere with the patient's property rights to avoid threatened injury. For example, suppose the suddenly combative patient approaches the staff with a knife or attempts to use a belt to strangle the nurse. This defense allows the nurse to take the knife or belt away from the patient. Thus, self-defense allows reasonable force against a person, while necessity allows the person's property to be confiscated. Two caveats to remember are:

1. A defense of necessity does not allow the nurse the right to search the patient's property.
2. The defense of necessity mandates that the patient's property must be the threatening factor.

DEFENSES AGAINST QUASI-INTENTIONAL TORTS

Consent

Consent may be a defense against the quasi-intentional torts of defamation and invasion of privacy as well as against the intentional torts. The nurse cannot be charged in a lawsuit with invasion of privacy if the patient allowed the nurse right of access to personal property. Consent does not need to be formal or well thought out. Allowing a nurse to remove a nightgown from a piece of luggage would also constitute consent to notice a stash of drugs packed alongside the nightgown.

Two cases illustrate this concept. In *State v. Welch* (2006), the patient was taken by ambulance to an acute care facility following an automobile accident. After his arrival, the nurse and another hospital staff member removed his clothing so that they could more accurately assess the patient's extent of injuries. A medication bottle fell out of his clothing. Wanting to know what medications the person was taking, the nurse opened the medication bottle and noted that the contents of the bottle contained a substance that the nurse thought might be illegal, such as cocaine or methamphetamines.

The nurse called hospital security, who called the police. The police officer who responded took the bottle and its contents, read the patient his Miranda rights, questioned him, and obtained permission for a blood test. The substance was analyzed as containing methamphetamines, and the patient's laboratory tests also showed the presence of methamphetamines. At trial, the patient was convicted of possession of methamphetamines. In striking down the patient's Fourth Amendment rights, the court ruled that all parties to the case (nurse, security guard, and police officer) acted lawfully. The bottle was discovered on the patient's person in the course of necessary, good-faith medical care, not in the course of a police search. It was in "plain sight." No search warrant was required to open the bottle and ascertain its contents.

Similarly, in *United States v. Clay* (2006), a nurse was following standard hospital practice for inventorying a patient's possessions when she found cocaine and ammunition in the patient's coat. The nurse in this case notified her supervisor, who alerted the police. The cocaine and ammunition were given to the police officer, who read the patient his Miranda rights and then questioned the patient. The patient admitted that the items were his and also gave the officer permission to search his car, where a firearm and digital scales were found. This court also found that there was no violation of the patient's constitutional rights. The court noted that the policy of the hospital was reasonable and that its purposes were to prevent injury to patients and personnel and to protect the institution from possible liability.

EXERCISE 7.1

The patient was involved in a motor vehicle accident while being chased by police. He was placed under arrest and taken to the emergency center of a local hospital. In the emergency room, with the arresting officers standing by, the patient told the nurse he had taken heroin an hour earlier. Charges of illicit drug possession were added to the other charges against the patient. At trial, the patient requested that the charges of illicit drug possession be dropped. How should the court rule in this instance? Were the patient's constitutional rights violated?

Truth

Truth is a valid defense against defamatory statements. Nurses should be aware that in using this defense, the entire statement must be true and not merely parts of the statement. Someone who states, "Many patients have perished for her want of skill" must be able to show that the entire statement is truthful or face a possible defamation suit.

Truth may be a defense against defamatory statements, but may also lead to other torts such as invasion of privacy. The nurse, in proving the truth of a defamatory statement, may unwillingly make public facts that concern the nature of the patient's hospitalization or the fact that the person was even a patient within a given setting. For example, for a nurse to prove that a specific patient was hospitalized for drug abuse, the nurse would need to divulge facts about the drug abuse that may invade the patient's privacy rights. As a practical matter, this usually does not occur, because the injured party or patient forfeits this privacy right when filing the lawsuit.

A case that illustrates this concept is *Board of Trustees v. Martin* (2003). The nurse's neighbor kept a large number of dogs that were raised as sled dogs. As there was an upcoming sled-dog race, local media interviewed neighbors of this individual to see if living next to such a large number of dogs was problematic. The nurse was interviewed and she acknowledged that it was problematic for her. The nurse also stated that the owner was a drunk who belonged in a detoxification unit.

Unknown to the nurse was the fact that the owner had been treated for drug and alcohol abuse at the same hospital that employed the nurse. The hospital board of directors fired the nurse for breach of confidentiality and the nurse appealed her dismissal. Should the dog owner later sue the nurse for defamation, the case does show that the nurse's sole means of proving such an allegation would be by breaching the patient's right to privacy and confidentiality.

Gunnells v. Marshburn (2003) concerned a nurse who had tried to fill a prescription ostensibly written by a retired physician. When the pharmacy called the physician who had been the retired physician's partner about the prescription, the practicing physician phoned the local police and personnel department at the hospital about this incident. The police reported it to the U.S. Drug Enforcement Agency, but they declined to prosecute the case. The local hospital required a drug test of the nurse, which was positive, and the hospital suspended her from employment.

The nurse subsequently sued the physician for defamation of character. The court found that his comments were completely accurate and truthful; he merely described what had occurred. The physician purported to have written the prescription had surrendered his license and thus was unable to write such a prescription. Truth, said the court, is a perfect defense to such a case. The court will look literally at what the defendant said. "Nuances and implications drawn by others are not important. If what was said was literally true, the lawsuit must be dismissed" (*Gunnells v. Marshburn,* 2003, at 274).

Privilege

Privilege, another defense against defamation, is a disclosure that might ordinarily be defamatory under different circumstances, but such disclosure may be allowable to protect or further public or private interests recognized by law. Examples of privilege include the mandate to report persons with certain diagnoses or diseases or those suspected of abusing others.

Disclosure Statutes

Both federal and state laws compel disclosure of health-related information to proper agencies to protect the public. The reporting laws require health care providers to be familiar not only with the types of information that must be disclosed, but also with the governmental agency requiring the information. The giving of required information is protected, and there may be liability for disclosure of such privileged information to the wrong governmental agency.

Disclosure statutes mandate the reporting of certain types of health-related information to protect the public at large. A judge may also mandate that certain information be disclosed by issuing a subpoena. These statutes mandate that the health care providers or those standing in the place of health care providers voluntarily give the required information to the proper agency. The most common example of reporting statutes is vital statistics. All states require births and deaths to be reported, and a majority of states require an accounting of neonatal deaths and abortions.

Public health agencies may require a variety of disease states to be reported. Communicable and venereal diseases must be reported to protect the public. Additionally, some states require that the names of patients suffering from any type of seizure activity be reported to the state drivers' licensing agency. Cancer and other related diseases are to be reported in a handful of states.

If practitioners disclose only the limited information they must disclose, there is no liability for the disclosure under either a defamation or invasion of privacy lawsuit. These statutes, therefore, serve as a defense against both defamation and invasion of privacy.

Communicable-disease-reporting laws, informing public health officials of infectious cases, are among the oldest compulsory reporting statutes in most states. The statutes or regulations usually list the diseases to be reported and mandate practitioners to give local public health officials the patient's name, gender, age, address, and other identifying information as well as details of the patient's illness. In the cases of sexually transmitted diseases, other identifying information would include the names of all sexual partners within a reasonable time frame. Under the Health Insurance Portability and Accountability Act of 1996 (HIPAA) statutes, patients have the right to know that such information, including which personal identifiers, are released to state public health officials or employees of the Centers for Disease Control in Atlanta, Georgia. A more comprehensive discussion of HIPAA may be found in Chapter 9.

Because of the sensitivity of human immunodeficiency virus (HIV) and acquired immune deficiency syndrome (AIDS) issues, many states have enacted legislation regarding the confidentiality of HIV test results. This concept is likewise more thoroughly explored in Chapter 9.

The National Childhood Vaccine Injury Act of 1986 mandates that all health care providers and institutions record each administration of any vaccine to a child and report any illness, disability, or death resulting from the administration of a vaccine to the U.S. Department of Health and Human Services. This act was passed following the national and international concern regarding the safety and efficacy of vaccines given to newborns and infants.

Child abuse is reportable to child welfare offices and/or other state-designated offices. Such statutes usually require that both suspected cases of child abuse and suspected neglect of a child be reported. **Abuse** encompasses physical, mental, and sexual assaults as well as physical, emotional, and medical neglect. Similar protection against abuse and neglect is currently being given to adults in some states, particularly residents in nursing and convalescent homes.

Generally, the nurse reports any suspected cases through the administration of the institution. In most institutions, nurses report the suspected abuse to their immediate supervisor and the treating physician. All information concerning the notification is then documented in the patient's chart. Both civil and criminal liability may flow from the nonreport of such suspected cases, especially if further abuse or neglect occurs because of nondisclosure.

The landmark case of *Landeros v. Flood* (1976) held that a physician who fails to report suspected child abuse can be exposed for liability on the theory of medical malpractice. In that case, an 11-month-old was brought to the emergency center with a leg fracture. The fracture was the type for which a reasonable and careful physician would have started an investigation of possible abuse. Instead, the child was treated and released to her parents. Shortly afterward, the child was admitted with severe and permanent injuries due to abuse. After being removed from her parents' care, this lawsuit was brought against the treating physician and health care institution.

In its findings, the court held that the hospital, through its agents or employees, either knew of or should have suspected that the child requiring care was a victim of abuse. Health care professionals who failed to report the case could be held liable for the subsequent injuries done to the child by her abusers. The decision makes it clear that liability for failure to report suspected child abuse is a greater risk than reporting suspected child abuse that, upon investigation, proves to be erroneous.

Nurses could easily have been part of the *Landeros* case. Reporting laws grant immunity from prosecution to those health care providers who report suspected abuse in good faith and who report such violations to the correct governmental agency. This means that nurses who report a battered child to their supervisor and to the treating physician, following institution policy, have not violated the patient's or the parents' right to privacy.

In fact, nurses are more open to liability if they fail to report the abuse. If the parents fail to assert the child's rights against the nurse for nondisclosure of abuse, the state child welfare agency could sue the nurse in a civil suit for the injuries inflicted on the child after the failure to disclose (*Kempster v. Child Protection Services of the Department of Social Services,* 1987).

Health care providers are protected when they in good faith report suspected child abuse, even if the subsequent investigation shows the report to be groundless. In *Heinrich v. Conemaugh Valley Memorial Hospital* (1994), a Pennsylvania Superior Court found that the hospital was immune from suit when a child abuse report, which later proved groundless, was filed.

Pennsylvania's Child Protective Services Law mandates that suspected child abuse must be reported and that a plaintiff seeking to prove that an injury resulted from a false report of abuse must show bad faith on the part of those reporting the suspected abuse. Courts presume good faith on the part of the health care providers unless shown to be incorrect.

A more recent case upholds this principle. In *Sager v. Rochester General Hospital* (1996), a 5-month-old child was taken to the emergency center with a fractured femur, an unusual injury for such a young child and one for which the parents had no explanation.

An orthopedist casted the leg and told the parents the child would be held for 24 hours for medical observation. The hospital social worker was notified of the child's admission, and after she consulted with her supervisor, she called the local protective services hotline. Child protective services posted a police officer at the child's hospital door to prevent the parents from removing the child. The child was subsequently placed in foster care and was then placed with a grandmother.

Criminal charges of abuse were never conclusively proven against the parents. The parents sued in civil court for intentional infliction of emotional distress, interference with the custodial relationship with their child, violation of their civil rights, and false imprisonment of their child.

The court dismissed the parents' causes of action. Hospital personnel stated the court must report evidence of apparent child abuse. They must hold the child pending completion of a child protective services investigation of possible abuse and the filing of legal procedures to remove the child into foster care. "When acting under a reasonable belief that their actions are warranted to prevent further imminent harm to an apparently abused child, hospital personnel are immune from liability in civil and criminal court for their actions" (*Sager v. Rochester General Hospital*, 1996, at 412).

Remember, though, that violations of the statutes, even in good faith, may not protect the nurse from liability. In *Perez v. Bay Area Hospital* (1992), a child was examined in the emergency room for genital irritation. Medication was prescribed, the child was instructed in proper hygiene, and a culture was obtained. The child was discharged, and the culture came back negative for sexually transmitted diseases.

Two days later, the Oregon Children Services Division (CSD) received a phone call from an unnamed nurse at the defendant hospital, stating that the child had tested positive for gonorrhea. Later that day, a CSD employee and a local police officer went to the child's school, told the school secretary that there was reason to believe the child had been infected with a sexually transmitted disease, and questioned the child. The child's mother was also questioned in her home by the CSD employee and the police officer. Later in the week, the mother was notified of the negative report by the defendant hospital.

The mother subsequently filed this cause of action, asserting that the CSD employee was "negligent in disclosing information and identifying misinformation" (*Perez v. Bay Area Hospital*, 1992, at 706). The court granted summary judgment for the defendants on the grounds that the CSD employee's disclosures were protected by the Oregon abuse-reporting statutes. On appeal, the mother argued that the CSD employee should have contacted the hospital independently to verify the report, and that failure to do so constituted negligence. The defendants countered that the Oregon law requires that the CSD immediately investigate reported abuse after receiving a report of suspected child abuse.

The trial court agreed with the plaintiffs. Had the case against the hospital been filed within the required statute of limitations, both the CSD employee and the defendant hospital would have been charged with negligence. Thus, careful reporting of suspected abuse, according to the strict requirements of local and state law, is encouraged to prevent possible liability.

Though it does not fall within the traditional definition of disclosure, the law also recognizes that physicians and nurses have a duty to protect the public at large. In *State v. Cummings* (2008), a patient was discharged following an outpatient medical procedure after having received four (4.0) mg of Dilaudid. The patient was instructed not to drive; he was seen immediately after his release driving a semi tractor-trailer truck from the hospital parking lot. The nurse who had cared for the patient and seen him drive away called the police to report that he was driving under the influence of a powerful narcotic. The patient was quickly stopped by the police and a standard roadside horizontal-gaze nystagmus test gave the officers grounds to take the driver to the police station to obtain a urine sample. Evidence from the urine test was later used to show that the driver was driving illegally.

The court upheld the patient's detention and arrest. Based on the nurse's conversation with the police dispatcher, the patrol officers had reasonable suspicion to stop the driver, administer the field sobriety tests that showed he had signs of intoxication, and take him to the police station for further testing.

GUIDELINES

Disclosure Statutes

1. Know both federal and individual state laws concerning the duty to report versus privileges to access laws.
2. Report only the information that is required to the proper governmental agency, and ensure that others who have a duty to disclose health-related information do so promptly.
3. Comply with reporting laws (such as abuse statutes) in good faith; civil and criminal liability may be incurred for failure to report under a statutory duty to disclose.
4. With access laws, follow hospital policy carefully, and ensure that those persons requesting access to medical records are allowed such access by law. Ask for proper identification as needed and consult the institution's legal department or risk manager when in doubt.
5. Remember, if you work in home health care or community settings, you may be the only person with the firsthand information needed to file reports to the appropriate governmental agency. Review the agency's rules and regulations regarding how to correctly file such reports and consult with supervisors when in doubt.
6. Avoid any breach of confidentiality, which is often considered unprofessional conduct and grounds for disciplinary action by the state board of nurse examiners. Report only the information that is required; no freedom from liability exists for information that was not required or for information that is given to other than the proper governmental agency.

Access Laws

This group of statutory disclosure laws permits access to patient records and information without securing permission of the individual patient. The caveat is to know which given individuals or agencies may be allowed such **access** to patient information. Workers' compensation statutes usually allow for access to medical records once a claim has been filed. If such a statute does not exist, the courts may rule that the filing of such a claim is a waiver under common law of the right of confidentiality in such health-related information.

Access laws seldom involve staff and mid-management nurses. Usually, the medical records department and/or the administrative staff of the institution are apprised by the hospital attorney when charts may be accessed by law. Mid-management nurses might become involved if access is sought to ongoing or current medical charts. This type of review of current records may be done in conjunction with the institution's Medicare and Medicaid reimbursement program. Before allowing access to medical records, nurses should take some precautions. First, they should receive written confirmation of such reviews from the hospital administration or the nursing service administration prior to the review. Then they should ascertain that the persons asking for access to the charts are the persons listed in the written confirmation, and ask for proof of identification as necessary. If any doubt persists concerning such a chart review, the nurses should contact their supervisors before allowing the charts to be seen. Finally, they should remain accessible to answer questions as needed. The reviewers may not clearly understand the nurse's system of charting, and nurses could be invaluable in interpreting the system to them.

Qualified Privilege

The defense of **qualified privilege** prevails when the person making the allegedly defamatory statements has a legal duty to do so, such as when a nurse manager reports, in good faith, on the professional performance of a staff nurse. Qualified privilege legally negates any inference of malice because of the overriding public policy interest. When the quality of medical care is at issue, the reputation rights of health care professionals must concede to the greater social need.

Liability will not be imposed, even if the communications are false, as long as there is no malice and the communications are made in good faith to those persons who need to know such facts. The court, in the precedent-setting case of *Wynn v. Cole* (1979), found no liability on the part of a director of a health department who provided a prospective employer with information concerning a specific nurse's abilities. Such privileged communications exist for assessments provided by former employers to prospective employers. The caveat to be watchful is threefold:

1. The communications must be made through appropriate channels to persons needing the information.
2. Liability may be granted for untruthful communications released with malice.
3. The communications should be worded in objective and observable behavioral terms rather than judgmental descriptions.

In *Haynes-Wilkinson v. Barnes-Jewish Hospital* (2001), the court extended this concept, noting that statements to boards of nursing are also protected by law. In *Kevorkian v. Glass* (2007), the court noted that a privileged communication cannot be grounds for a civil defamation lawsuit, even if the employee's personal reputation or job prospective is hurt.

Defamation may be mitigated (lessened or reduced) by such factors as retraction (one did all he or she could to rectify the previous statement) or by whether it was provoked or not. For example, the nurse may be provoked into a given statement by the anger and hostility aimed at the staff member by the patient or family. Although not an excuse for the defamation, such mitigating factors may serve to lessen the damages awarded the plaintiff.

EXERCISE 7.2

Interview nurse managers in hospital and community settings about privileges and qualified privileges. How do the nurse managers use these doctrines in their respective clinical settings? Discuss the issue that the doctrine of privilege creates from an ethical perspective. Does the doctrine of privilege either enhance or compromise an individual nurse's ethical rights?

DEFENSES AGAINST NONINTENTIONAL TORTS

Defenses against negligent actions include (1) release, (2) contributory or comparative negligence, (3) assumption of the risk, (4) unavoidable accident, (5) defense of the fact, and (6) immunity statutes.

Release

A **release** may be signed during the process of settling a claim to prevent any and all future claims arising from the same incident. Once signed, the release bars (prohibits or prevents) future suits. In medical malpractice claims, a release is frequently a part of the out-of-court settlement. In effect, the plaintiff states that the settlement is the only compensation that will be sought for the negligent action.

Releases are distinguished from exculpatory clauses or exculpatory contracts, which are signed before care is given and seldom serve as a successful defense. Usually, **exculpatory contracts** are signed to limit the amount of damages one receives in a suit or to prevent a future lawsuit based on the individual health care giver's actions. Such contracts usually fail on the grounds that they violate public policy. The court in *Cudnick v. William Beaumont Hospital* (1994) held that **exculpatory agreements,** which completely release a hospital from liability for an employee's negligence and which are signed by patients prior to receiving therapy, are against public policy and thus are invalid and unenforceable. The court further identified two exceptions to the rule invalidating exculpatory agreements for medical malpractice: (1) experimental procedures are exempted because "they inherently require a deviation from generally accepted medical practices" (at 897), and (2) agreements releasing medical care providers from liability after treatment, pursuant to a lawsuit settlement agreement, are valid and enforceable.

Contributory and Comparative Negligence

Contributory and comparative negligence both serve as defenses and in essence hold injured parties accountable for their fault in the injury. Such fault by the plaintiff may occur for failure to follow prescribed treatments, if incorrect treatment is given based on the patient's false information to the physician/primary health care provider, or for extended delays in seeking appropriate medical care.

Many states once used an all-or-nothing **contributory negligence rule:** Patients who had any part in the adverse consequences were barred from any compensation, even if their contribution was as small as 1%. Only five states or territories still recognize strict contributory negligence: Alabama, District of Columbia, Maryland, North Carolina, and Virginia. Today, most jurisdictions use comparative negligence, and recovery by the injured party is reduced based on the percentage of fault attributed to the plaintiff. For example, in a $500,000 reward, if the plaintiff is found to be 30% responsible for the negligence, then the plaintiff will be allowed a $350,000 award for damages.

Legislatures and courts have adopted varying types of comparative negligence. Some jurisdictions apply **pure comparative negligence,** wherein the plaintiff is allowed to recover the portion of the injury attributable to the defendant's negligence, even if the plaintiff was 99% at fault. Thirteen states recognize pure comparative fault: Alaska, Arizona, California, Florida, Kentucky, Louisiana, Mississippi, Missouri, New Mexico, New York, Rhode Island, South Dakota, and Washington State. The majority of jurisdictions recognize **modified comparative negligence,** wherein the plaintiff whose negligence is found to exceed that of the defendant is barred from recovery. Twelve states allow for recovery under this latter rule using a 50% bar, meaning that an injured party cannot recover if he or she is 50% or more at fault. These states include: Arkansas, Colorado, Georgia, Idaho, Kansas, Maine, Nebraska, North Dakota, Oklahoma, Tennessee, Utah, and West Virginia. The remainder of the states follow a 51% bar, meaning that an injured party cannot recover if he is 51% or more at fault.

Recent cases involving comparative negligence include *Caraballo v. Lehigh Valley Hospital* (2007), *Dubreuil v. Foucauld* (2007), and *Feher v. Genesee Medical Group* (2007). In *Caraballo,* a lawsuit filed in Pennsylvania, the patient was pregnant and diagnosed with gestational diabetes. Three months into her prenatal care, she weighed 305 pounds and her blood glucose was 218. She was referred to a diabetes clinic for care, and a medical plan to lower her blood glucose level with glyburide was initiated. The medication was to be taken twice daily. Counseling was done about the risks of gestational diabetes, particularly the fact that she could have an abnormally large infant.

Three weeks after the institution of the glyburide therapy, an ultrasound indicated that the fetus was in the 95th weight percentile, and the patient was again counseled about the risks she was facing, including the fact that the baby could be stillborn. Two weeks later, she was counseled at the diabetes clinic about the need for compliance with the medication. Her blood glucose level a week later was 231, and the electronic memory in her glucose meter revealed that she was sporadically testing her blood glucose level. Eating habits were reviewed and the patient admitted that she frequently skipped meals during the days, eating the majority of her calories late in the evening.

A stillborn infant was delivered by cesarean section and she filed a lawsuit against the health care providers and the hospital. The court determined that there was no liability on the part of the health care providers or the hospital, as the patient was greater than 51% responsible for the outcome in this case.

In *Dubreuil,* a Florida case, a 51-year-old male patient was admitted on a Sunday for possible cardiac symptoms. He was scheduled to have a stress test on Monday, but the patient declined to remain in the hospital overnight as he did not have health insurance. He was discharged with instructions to return the next day for the stress test, to fill some prescriptions, including one for nitroglycerine, and to begin taking the medications as prescribed. These instructions were repeated by the discharge nurse. The patient did not fill the prescriptions nor return for the scheduled stress test and died 6 months later. The subsequent lawsuit was returned with a directed verdict for the defendants. *Feher* reached a similar conclusion when the patient and wife failed to comply with direct medical instructions.

Harvey v. Mid-Coast Hospital (1999) remains an exception to the preceding cases. In that case, a 19-year-old was treated for bipolar disease with Tegretol. He was found unconscious in his dorm room and was admitted through the emergency center to the intensive care unit. During the initial blood analysis at the time of admission, it was found that he had a toxic level of Tegretol in his blood.

While in the intensive care unit, he began having seizures and developed status epilepticus. The intensive care unit nurses did not notice the status epilepticus in time to intervene and avert neurological damage. The hospital's defense to a subsequently filed malpractice action was to assert a comparative negligence defense, alleging that the patient's self-inflicted overdose was the primary cause of the permanent neurological damage. In rejecting this defense, the court noted that in a professional malpractice suit the patient's own negligence could fall into one of four hypothetical categories:

1. A patient could refuse to follow advice or instructions.
2. A patient could delay seeking treatment or returning for follow-up.
3. A patient could furnish false, misleading, or incomplete information to a health care provider.
4. A patient's own self-injurious behavior could have caused the need for the medical treatment.

According to the court, the first three are situations in which the patient's own negligence can diminish or bar outright the patient's chances of success with a malpractice suit, because of comparative negligence. However, "when a patient's own negligent or intentional self-harm occurred before care was sought and only provided the occasion for needing care, the legal system does not apply the concept of contributory or comparative negligence" (*Harvey v. Mid-Coast Hospital,* 1999, at 37).

Assumption of the Risk

A defense similar to contributory and comparative negligence, **assumption of the risk** states that plaintiffs are partially responsible for consequences if they understood the risks involved when they proceeded with the action. A case example of this concept is *Lopez v. State of Louisiana Health Care Authority/University Medical Center* (1998). The patient was in his 4th day in the alcohol detoxification center of a state hospital. After breakfast, he and others lined up to be escorted outside for a smoke break. It was the 18th time since his admission that the patient had waited to be escorted for a smoke break.

The patient was leaning against a wall that had a door but no door handle. He stood right in front of the doorstop. All the other persons waiting for the smoke break were standing by the wall on the opposite side. A nurse opened the door from the other side and the patient was struck. He was immediately examined by the facility's physician and found to be unhurt, but sued the nurse and the facility for negligence.

The court ruled that the nurse, and thus the facility, was not negligent. If anything, the court said, it was the patient who was negligent. He knew that the door could and would open directly toward him. The patient was ambulatory, and he elected to walk outside for a smoke break, demonstrating that he was not physically or mentally handicapped. There was an indication in his chart 2 hours before the incident that noted that the patient was "calm, steady, and aloof." The court concluded with the statement: "Healthcare facilities do not have to protect patients from risks which patients who are aware of their surroundings and mentally capable should realistically anticipate and avoid on their own" (at 522).

Note that an opposite conclusion will be reached when the person is not able to appreciate the danger or severity of a situation. In *Kremerov v. Forest View Nursing Home, Inc.* (2005), the recreational coordinator set up a makeshift bowling alley in the adult daycare center, using plastic bowling pins and a five-pound rubber ball. An 85-year-old Russian immigrant, who had never bowled before, fell and twisted her ankle. Though there was a safety warning about "wearing comfortable shoes," the court determined that the plaintiff, who had never bowled before, would not have known that it is customary to wear bowling shoes when bowling. She wore her 1¼-inch heels.

Sometimes both assumption of the risk and contributory/comparative negligence can be raised in a single case. An example of such a case is *Lyons v. Walker Regional Medical Center, Inc.* (2003). In this case, the patient left the hospital against medical advice, after signing the blanket release form the hospital provided. The question raised at court was the issue of competency of advice and whether the patient fully comprehended the severity of his condition when he signed the forms and left the emergency center. The court noted that the reason the case centered on the competency of the advice was because critical laboratory values were not charted correctly and thus the patient was not appropriately informed of the severity of his condition prior to leaving the institution. Though the "panic levels exceeded" notation was on the laboratory forms themselves, the hospital's policy of placing a "panic level exceeded" label on the front of the chart was not followed. The physician was not verbally apprised of these results and did not discover the laboratory values until after the patient left the hospital. The court noted in its deliberations that both assumption of the risk and contributory negligence are predicated on truthfulness, and in order to use these common law defenses, the patient must fully appreciate his or her true medical condition.

Unavoidable Accident

This defense comes into play when nothing other than an accident could have caused the person's injury. For example, a staff member slips and falls in a patient's room. There is nothing on the floor that could have caused the accident, and no one is at fault.

Defense of the Fact

This defense is used when there is no indication, direct or otherwise, that the health care provider's actions were the cause of the patient's injury or untoward outcome (e.g., the patient who receives an injection in the left arm and then begins to experience numbness and tingling in the right leg). When there is no connection in the two events, the defense to be pled is defense of the fact.

Immunity

Some states have enacted **immunity** statutes that serve to dismiss certain causes of action. The best example of a state immunity statute is the Good Samaritan statute. Because of Good Samaritan laws, discussed next, negligent actions against health care providers at scenes of accidents are rare.

Good Samaritan Laws

Legislation was at one time needed to encourage medical personnel to stop at the scene of an accident and render appropriate medical care. In response to this need, all states have enacted **Good Samaritan laws,** which abrogate common law rescue doctrines in an effort to encourage health care providers to risk helping strangers in need of assistance, even when the health care providers have no duty to render such aid (*Jackson v. Mercy Health Center, Inc.*, 1993). While individual provisions of Good Samaritan laws vary greatly from state to state, the laws have been instrumental in procuring necessary health care in emergency situations.

A Good Samaritan is one who compassionately renders personal assistance to others in need. Good Samaritan laws are enacted to allow health care personnel and citizens trained in first aid to deliver needed medical care without unnecessary fear of incurring criminal and civil liability. The uniqueness of Good Samaritan laws is that they insulate a health care practitioner from his or her liability for rendering care at the scene of an accident. Three elements necessary for a Good Samaritan defense are:

1. the care rendered was performed as the result of an emergency,
2. the initial emergency or injury was not caused by the person invoking the defense, and
3. the emergency care was not administered in a grossly negligent or reckless manner.

Dispute exists over which persons should be protected, the extent to which the protection extends, and the type of emergency that qualifies for Good Samaritan protection. Some states extend protection merely to licensed health care providers. Other states allow ordinary citizens to be covered under the legislation along with licensed health care providers.

Court cases that have extended protection to individuals who volunteer to assist in emergencies include *Boccasile v. Cajun Music Limited* (1997) and *McDaniel v. Keck* (2008). In *McDaniel*, a school nurse accompanied her students to a farm that was located in another school district. While there, the farm owner's 7-year-old son was poked in the eye. The school nurse volunteered to look at the injured eye and told the parents to put some ice on the eye until the swelling subsided. Two days later, the parents took the child to a pediatrician, who found a piece of wire in the eye and sent the child to an ophthalmologist. After several surgeries, the eye was removed. The court, in dismissing the school nurse from the subsequent lawsuit, noted that unless there is gross negligence, the person rendering first aid or emergency treatment at the scene of an accident or emergency, if done voluntarily and without expectation of compensation, and not done in a doctor's office, hospital, or clinical location that has proper medical equipment and/or supplies, is not liable under Good Samaritan laws. Note, though, that this is a New York case and that many states still hold that the emergency forming the basis of a Good Samaritan defense must be a roadside occurrence.

Vermont remains the one state requiring individuals to assist others exposed to grave physical harm as long as the assistance can be given without endangering themselves. Reasonable assistance should be given, and violation of the statute is punishable by fines (*Vermont Statutes Annotated*, 1968).

The need for Good Samaritan laws becomes apparent because there is no legal duty to render assistance to a stranger in times of distress, unless so mandated by statute or unless the individual caused the stranger's distress. While one could argue that a moral or ethical duty should exist, no legal duty arises until the individual first initiates the giving of emergency care. Then the legal duty becomes one of reasonable or emergency care. Only when a person renders grossly negligent or willful and wanton negligent care is the health care provider not protected by the Good Samaritan immunity. As a practical matter, malpractice suits against Good Samaritans are relatively rare.

Before proceeding under a Good Samaritan law, nurses must recognize that the acts vary greatly among states. Consequently, they must be aware of exactly what is covered by an individual state act. Nurses should look for the following information when reviewing an individual state act:

1. Who is covered as part of the protected class? Some states cover all persons who give emergency care, some cover only physicians and nurses, and a few state acts cover only in-state physicians and nurses.

2. Where does the coverage extend? All state acts allow for aid at the scene of an accident, emergency, or disaster, with some states mandating that such accidents, emergencies, or disasters be roadside occurrences. Other states allow for emergency care wherever the need is, be it in a hospital, doctor's office, or outside of a medically equipped place. Still other states specifically limit coverage under Good Samaritan laws to areas outside the workplace. The nurse must know what qualifies as the scene of an emergency before rendering aid under the Good Samaritan laws.

3. What is covered? Some states protect the individual during transportation to a medical facility. Another group of states protects against failure to provide for further assistance.

Most states require that the care be given in good faith and that it be gratuitous. Unfortunately, the acts may not define criteria to determine whether an emergency actually exists and what constitutes the scene of an emergency. Because of this, protection is uncertain in some states.

GUIDELINES

Good Samaritan Laws

1. Make your decision quickly as to whether you will stay and help. Remember, there is no common law duty to stop and render aid. Once you begin to provide care, you incur the legal duty to maintain a standard of reasonable emergency care.

2. Ask the injured person or family members for permission to help. Do not force your services once refused.

3. Care for the injured party where you can do so safely. This includes in the vehicle or at the exact site where the victim is found. Move the injured party only if you must do so without causing further harm and as needed to prevent further harm (e.g., off a major highway).

4. Apply the rules of first aid: Assess for and prevent bleeding, assess for the need to initiate cardiopulmonary resuscitation, cover the injured party with a blanket or coat, and so forth.

5. Continuously assess and reassess the person for additional injuries, and communicate findings of your assessment to the person or family members.

6. Have someone call or go for additional help while you stay with the injured party.

7. Stay with the person until equally or more qualified help arrives. Prevent unskilled persons from treating or moving the injured party.

8. Give as complete a description as possible of the care that you have rendered to the police and emergency medical personnel so that continuity of care exists. Give family members or police any personal items such as dentures, eyeglasses, and the like.

9. Do not accept any compensation (e.g., money or gifts) offered by the injured party or family members. Acceptance of compensation may change your care into a fee-for-service situation and cause you to lose your Good Samaritan protection.

10. Should you choose not to stop and render aid, stop at the nearest phone and report the accident to proper authorities so that the injured party may be aided.

EXERCISE 7.3

Explore your own state laws regarding Good Samaritan statutes. Are all health care providers included in the statutes? Are other qualified persons covered? How do the statutes ensure that persons needing assistance will receive the needed help?

Recognizing that there may be no legal duty to stop and aid accident victims, is there an ethical duty to stop and render aid? Which ethical principles guide your answer to the question? Is there ever a time when you would be ethically bound *not* to stop and render care?

STATUTE OF LIMITATIONS

Statutes of limitations specify time limits for initiating claims. Unless specific exceptions apply, a suit must be filed within the time limit or the cause of action is barred (prohibited by law). Typically, individual states allow 1 to 2 years as the time frame for the filing of a malpractice suit. Therefore, injured parties must bring the suit within 1 to 2 years after they knew of the injury or had reason to believe that an injury was sustained. In the case of a minor, the statute of limitations may not begin being calculated until the child reaches the age of majority, though a few states restrict this approach. For those states, the statute of limitation is calculated the same for all individuals within the state. Review Chapter 3 for case examples of statutes of limitations.

PRODUCTS LIABILITY

Products liability refers to the liability of a manufacturer, processor, or nonmanufacturing seller for injury to a person or person's property by a given product. This includes the manufacturer of component parts, the assembling manufacturer, the wholesaler, and the retail store owner (here the health care institution). Under this type of action, the injured party may sue the maker of the product, or the seller of the product, or the intermediary distributors of the product, or all three entities. The landmark and leading case for imposing liability in this area of the law, irrespective of fault, is *Caprara v. Chrysler Corporation* (1981). In that case, the court declared that "the one in the best position to know of potential dangers and to have eliminated the same should respond to the injured party in damages" (at 124).

Theories of recovery for such products liability suits can be based on negligence, breach-of-warranty of fitness, or strict liability, depending upon the jurisdiction in which the claim is made. Under breach-of-warranty liability, the patient contends that the manufacturer or others in the chain of distribution breached either an expressed or implied warranty of fitness of the product. In a strict liability action, the plaintiff contends that the product is unreasonably dangerous due to a defect in the manufacturing process, a mistake or oversight in the design of the product that renders the product dangerous when used as intended or when used for another reasonably foreseeable purpose, or inadequate warning labels or instructions.

This area of law is really a mixture of tort and contract law. The expressed and implied warranties of fitness for a particular purpose and of merchantability are based in contract law. Tort law concerns the liability of a person in a civil action against the person or property of another and the violation of a duty owed to the injured party. The warranties (from contract law) form the basis for finding liability without fault (from tort law) for injuries caused by the use of products.

The first hurdle for the plaintiff in products liability cases is to prove that there has been a sale of a product rather than the mere delivery of a service. The distinction is crucial because a products liability action does not exist if there is no sale of a product. Some courts have held there was no responsibility because there was service, not the sale of a product (*North Miami General Hospital v. Goldberg*, 1993), whereas other courts have suggested that the hospital owes a higher duty of care to the patient because the patient has no voice in the equipment or products used.

A second issue for products liability cases concerns defining products as opposed to services. A product has been defined as a "thing produced by labor" or "something produced by nature or the natural process" (Boyer, Ellis, Harris, & Soukhanov, 1991, p. 492). For years, debate has centered around blood transfusions and whether they are products or services of a hospital. While some initial cases determined that blood transfusions were products for purposes of products liability cases, all jurisdictions, either by decisional law or by legislative statutes, have determined that blood transfusions by a hospital are a service incident to treatment and not a product sold by the hospital. More recent developments in this area concern whether a blood bank is a health care provider for purposes of statutes of limitations. In *Smith v. Paslode Corporation* (1993), the eighth circuit held that a blood bank was a health care provider in that the blood bank "provides health care services under the authority of a license or certification" (at 3). This minority opinion illustrates the difficulty courts have with determining the status of blood banks and blood products.

A third issue concerns unavoidably unsafe products. To be considered unavoidably unsafe, a product must contain the following three criteria:

1. Its benefits must greatly outweigh its risks.
2. Its risks cannot be eliminated.
3. No safer product exists as an alternative.

If these three elements are proven, the manufacturer will be held liable for injuries only if there was failure to adequately warn of the risks. Prescription drugs usually are considered unavoidably unsafe, and case law concerns negligence for failure of adequate warning rather than for product liability. One of the more interesting cases to date, *Detwiler v. Bristol-Meyers Squibb Company* (1995), found liability against a physician who implanted a silicone breast implant. While the majority of the decision concerned statutes of limitations, the court held that silicone implants failed to meet the standard of unavoidably unsafe.

As a general rule, proper warning to the physician will satisfy the manufacturer's duty to warn, since patients can obtain the device or medication only upon the orders of the prescribing health care provider. For example, in *Ellis v. C. R. Bard, Inc.* (2002), a patient's estate sued the manufacturer of a patient-controlled analgesia pump (PCA). The court ruled there was no liability on the part of the manufacturer and held that the "learned intermediary" rule applies. That rule states that a manufacturer of a prescription drug or prescription medical device does not have the responsibility for warning the patient of potential dangers. Instead, the manufacturer must warn the health care provider who prescribes the drug or device and the nurses who will provide the drug or the device to the patient. Doctors and nurses are responsible for knowing the potential dangers and for including warnings in their instructions to the patients.

Exceptions to this requirement, when the patient must be directly warned (as through mass media newspaper communications), include situations in which (1) the drug may be given without an individual prescription (e.g., with mass inoculation for polio), and (2) federal Food and Drug Administration regulations require package inserts (*Lukaszewicz v. Ortho Pharmaceutical Corporation*, 1981). The majority of state laws now require that pharmacists have this same duty to warn when a prescription is filled for an individual patient.

COLLECTIVE AND ALTERNATIVE LIABILITY

Currently, two theories are emerging to aid plaintiffs who previously could not prove which manufacturer was at fault. **Collective liability** stems from cooperation by several manufacturers in a wrongful activity that by its nature requires the participation of more than one wrongdoer (concert of action). All the wrongdoers' actions result in an inadequate industry-wide standard of safety as to the manufacture of a product (enterprise liability). **Alternative liability** applies when two or more manufacturers commit separate wrongful or unreasonable acts, only one of which injures the plaintiff, but the plaintiff cannot identify the actual cause-in-fact defendant.

These theories rapidly emerged in light of the diethylstilbestrol (DES) lawsuits. Women injured by the drug directly and through their offspring attempted to sue manufacturers for failing to adequately test and label the drug and thus to warn of its risks. But it was virtually impossible to identify the manufacturer of the particular DES they took. This occurred because of (1) inadequate long-term record keeping by pharmacies, (2) the widespread practice of prescribing generic drugs, and (3) failure of the DES tablets to identify the manufacturer. Under these newer liability theories, injured women and their daughters gained compensation for the industry's failure to adequately test the drug on fetuses and to warn of its risks.

CAVEATS IN PRODUCTS LIABILITY LAWSUITS

Several issues influence whether a products liability action will be brought and whether it will succeed.

1. States often follow strict liability in medical or health-related causes of actions. Not to allow a strict liability cause of action would place an unfair burden on the plaintiff. Indeed, even with such a cause of action, compensation has been denied persons injured in health care settings.
2. The defendant must be a commercial supplier or be determined to be a commercial supplier for a products liability cause of action to exist in most jurisdictions.
3. The cause of action must be based on a sold product and not a service, or no action will exist under products liability.
4. There may also be a negligence cause of action. If the defendant passes all the hurdles and successfully defends against a products liability cause of action, the plaintiff may still be able to prove negligence.

EXERCISE 7.4

Think of all the equipment and products you use daily in the care of patients and the pharmaceutical agents you give to patients during the course of an average day or shift. What precautions or teachings do you take to further ensure safe, competent patient care?

SUMMARY

- Defenses are "arguments in support of or used for justification" and may be based on statutory law, common law, or the doctrine of precedent.
- Defenses to intentional torts include consent, self-defense, defense of others, necessity, access laws, duty to disclose laws, and qualified privilege.
- Defenses to quasi-intentional torts include consent, truth, privilege, disclosure statutes, and immunity statutes.

- Defenses to nonintentional torts include release, contributory negligence, comparative negligence, assumption of the risk, and statute of limitations.
- Additional types of defenses include products liability, collective liability, and alternative liability defenses.

APPLY YOUR LEGAL KNOWLEDGE

1. Which of the available defenses are more commonly used by professional nurses? Why?
2. How do statutes of limitations protect professional nurse-defendants? Do they also protect the injured parties?

3. Can products liability defenses prevent injured parties from showing negligence and liability against professional nurse practitioners?

YOU BE THE JUDGE

The 85-year-old resident in a long-term care facility repeatedly told the certified nurse's aide (CNA) that she wanted to leave some of her nicer possessions, primarily several pieces of furniture, to the CNA in appreciation of the excellent care she had been given over the past few years. Following her death, the CNA took possession of several pieces of furniture that had belonged to the resident and the CNA was subsequently dismissed from the long-term care facility for theft.

The CNA filed a lawsuit against the long-term care facility for defamation of character, noting that she has not stolen the furniture and that labeling her as a thief was totally untruthful on the part of the facility. The long-term care facility countered that acceptance of such a gift from a resident was totally in violation of company policy and was a valid reason to terminate the CNA.

QUESTIONS

1. Was termination of the employee for violating the policy against accepting such a gift from a deceased patient reasonable given the circumstances?
2. Was the long-term care facility correct in stating that the employee had stolen the furniture in question and was therefore a thief?
3. Did the fact that the family allowed the employee to take the furniture support the employee's contention that she was entitled to possession of the deceased resident's furniture?
4. How should the court decide the defamation of character cause of action?

REFERENCES

Board of Trustees v. Martin, 2003 WL 40790 (Wyoming, January 6, 2003).

Boccasile v. Cajun Music Limited, 694 A.2d 686 (Rhode Island, 1997).

Boyer, M., Ellis, K., Harris, D. R., & Soukhanov, A. H. (Eds.). (1991). *The American heritage dictionary* (2nd ed.). Boston: Houghton Mifflin.

Caprara v. Chrysler Corporation, 52 N.Y.2d 114 (New York, 1981).

Caraballo v. Lehigh Valley Hospital, 2007 WL 4863898 (Ct. Com. Pl. Lehigh Co., Pennsylvania, December 19, 2007). `

Cudnick v. William Beaumont Hospital, 525 N.W.2d 891 (Mich. Ct. App., 1994).

Detwiler v. Bristol-Meyers Squibb Company, 884 F. Supp. 117 (DSNY, 1995).

Dubreuil v. Foucauld, 2007 WL 684317 (Cir. Ct., Palm Beach Co., Florida, January 23, 2007).

Ellis v. C. R. Bard, Inc., 2002 WL 31501163 (11th Cir., November 12, 2002).

Estate of Klein v. North Shore University Hospital, 2007 WL 1247192 (Sip. Ct. New York Co., New York, March 29, 2007).

Feher v. Genesee Medical Group, 2007 WL 4208505 (Sup. Ct. San Diego Co., California, September 25, 2007).

Gunnells v. Marshburn, 578 S.E.2d 273 (Ga. App., 2003).

Harvey v. Mid-Coast Hospital, 36 F. Supp.2d 32 (D. Maine, 1999).

Haynes-Wilkinson v. Barnes-Jewish Hospital, 131 F. Supp.2d 1140 (E.D. Mo., 2001).

Heinrich v. Conemaugh Valley Memorial Hospital, 648 A.2d 53 (Pennsylvania, 1994).

Jackson v. Mercy Health Center, Inc., 884 P.2d 839 (Oklahoma, 1993).

Kempster v. Child Protection Services of the Department of Social Services, 515 N.Y.S.2d 807 (New York, 1987).

Kevorkian v. Glass, 913 A. 2d 1043 (Rhode Island, January 22, 2007).

Kremerov v. Forest View Nursing Home, Inc., 2005 WL 3485838 (N.Y. App., December 19, 2005).

Landeros v. Flood, 551 P.2d 389, 17 Cal.3d 399 (California, 1976).

Lopez v. State of Louisiana Health Care Authority/ University Medical Center, 721 So.2d 518 (La. App. 1998).

Lukaszewicz v. Ortho Pharmaceutical Corporation, 510 F. Supp. 961 (E.D. Wisc., 1981).

Lyons v. Walker Regional Medical Center, Inc., 2003 WL 1861023 (Alabama, April 11, 2003).

Mattocks v. Bell, 194 P.2d 307 (D.C. App., 1963).

McDaniel v. Keck, 2008 WL 2756498 (N.Y. App., July 17, 2008).

Merriam-Webster online dictionary. (2008). Available online at http://www.merriam-webster.com/dictionary/defenses

National Childhood Vaccine Injury Act of 1986, 42 U.S.C., Section 300aa-25.

North Miami General Hospital v. Goldberg, No. 87-337 (Fla. App. Ct., February 23, 1993).

Perez v. Bay Area Hospital, 829 P.2d 700 (Or. App., 1992).

Sager v. Rochester General Hospital, 647 N.Y.S.2d 408 (N.Y. Sup., 1996).

Smith v. Paslode Corporation, WL 392245 (8th Cir., July 13, 1993).

State v. Cummings, 2008 WL 2940817 (Ohio App., August 1, 2008).

State v. Welch, 140 P. 3d 1061 (Kan App., 2006).

United States v. Clay, 2006 WL 2385353 (E. D. Ky., August 17, 2006).

Vermont Statutes Annotated, Title 12, Chapter 23, Sec. 519 (1968).

Wyatt v. Department of Human Services, 2008 WL 162243 (Iowa, January 18, 2008).

Wynn v. Cole, 284 N. W. 2d 144 (Mich. App., 1979).

CHAPTER 8

Informed Consent and Patient Self-Determination

PREVIEW

In the past, informed consent was a matter concerning the patient and the physician, a concept capable of being delegated to the nurse as the physician thought best. Too often, the consent was automatic and uninformed, with patients and their loved ones asking far too few questions. Fortunately, this trend has changed, and nurses must understand the concept of informed consent to ensure that patient consent is truly valid and informed. Extensions of the concept of informed consent are patients' rights in research, genetic testing, and patient self-determination. This chapter explores the essential characteristics of consent, the power to consent, and the multiple documents that assist individuals with decision-making at the end of life.

LEARNING OUTCOMES
After completing this chapter, you should be able to

8.1 Define *informed consent,* comparing and contrasting it with consent.

8.2 Describe means of obtaining informed consent, including expressed, implied, oral, written, complete, and partial.

8.3 Compare and contrast standards of informed consent.

8.4 Describe four exceptions to informed consent.

8.5 Describe who has responsibility for obtaining informed consent.

8.6 Describe types of consent forms in use in health care settings.

8.7 Analyze whose signature must be obtained to ensure informed consent.

8.8 Describe one's right to refuse consent for medical care.

8.9 Describe the patient's right to either consent to or deny consent for research.

8.10 Discuss the issue of health care literacy as it pertains to informed consent.

8.11 Discuss the various issues that arise with informed consent and genetic testing.

8.12 Describe advance directives, including living wills, natural death acts, and durable power of attorney for health care and do-not-resuscitate directives.

8.13 Discuss the purpose of the Physician Order for Life-Sustaining Treatment and its implementation.

8.14 Discuss legal issues surrounding assisted suicide.

KEY TERMS

best interest standard
consent
court order
de-identified information
do-not-resuscitate directives
durable power of attorney for health care (DPAHC)
emergency consent
expressed consent
Genetic Information Nondiscrimination Act of 2008
genetic testing
health literacy
hospice center
implied consent

in loco parentis
informed consent
informed refusal
legal guardian or representative
living wills
medical durable power of attorney (MDPA)
medical illiteracy
medical or physician directive
minor
natural death act
patient self-determination
patient-based standard of informed consent

physician-assisted suicide
Physician Orders for Life-Sustaining Treatment (POLST)
physician-based standard of informed consent
prior patient knowledge
protected health information (PHI)
right of refusal
shared medical decision making
standards of disclosure
substituted judgment
therapeutic privilege
waiver

ROLE OF CONSENT

Generally, the health care provider's right to treat a patient, barring true emergency conditions or unanticipated happenings, is based on a contractual relationship that arises through the mutual consent of parties to the relationship. Informed consent is the voluntary authorization by a patient or the patient's legal representative to do something to the patient. Informed consent is based on the mutual consent of all parties involved, and the key to true and valid consent is patient comprehension.

Consent becomes an important issue from a legal perspective in that patients may sue for battery (unconsented touching) if they did not consent to the procedure or treatment and the health care provider proceeded with the procedure or treatment. Thus, patients may bring a lawsuit and be awarded damages even if they were helped by the procedure or treatment. The therapy was performed correctly and the patient's health actually improved because of the therapy. The more current trend, however, is to argue consent under a negligence or malpractice cause of action.

Consent is an issue in its own realm. Consent does not always become a factor in a malpractice suit, although it may be a concurrent issue. Consent concerns the health care provider's right to treat a given individual, not the manner in which the treatment was delivered. Thus, one can deliver safe, competent care and still be sued for lack of consent.

The right to consent and the right to refuse consent are based on a long-recognized, common law right of persons to be free from harmful or offensive touching of their bodies. In a landmark case during the early part of the last century, the court declared the reason for consent, and that case is still quoted today when referring to the consent doctrine. "Every human being of adult years has a right to determine what shall be done with his own body, and a surgeon who performs an operation without his patient's consent commits an assault for which he is liable in damages" (*Schloendorff v. Society of New York Hospitals*, 1914, at 93).

Thus, two concepts are involved: (1) the prevention of a battery and (2) the person's right to control what is done to his or her body. Because of these rights, the health care provider has an affirmative duty to obtain consent prior to treating a patient. Consent, therefore, is not contingent on a request for information or clarification by the patient, but must be actively sought by the health care practitioner.

CONSENT VERSUS INFORMED CONSENT

Consent, technically, is an easy yes or no: "Yes, I will allow the surgery" or "No, I want to try medications first, then maybe I will allow the surgery." Patients may not understand or may understand only vaguely what they are allowing, yet valid consent has been given.

The law concerning consent in health care situations is based on informed consent, which mandates to the physician or independent health care practitioner the separate legal duty to disclose needed material facts in terms that patients can reasonably understand so that they can make an informed choice. There should also be a description of the available alternatives to the proposed treatment and the risks and dangers involved in each alternative. Failure to disclose the needed facts in understandable terms does not negate the consent, but it does place potential liability on the practitioner for negligence. In other words, without any consent given, practitioners may be sued for battery, an intentional tort. Without informed consent, practitioners open themselves to potential lawsuits for negligence.

Wells v. Storey (1999) reiterated this concept. In that case, the court noted that before a patient undergoes a surgical procedure, the patient must give **informed consent.** There are two components: the patient must be fully informed and there must be voluntary consent. "Lack of informed consent is a separate and distinct basis for a lawsuit. Theoretically, a patient can sue for lack of informed consent even when there has been no malpractice" (*Wells v. Storey*, 1999, at 1037).

The doctrine of informed consent has developed from negligence law as the courts began to realize that, although consent may have been given, not enough information was imparted to form the foundation of an informed decision. The right to informed consent did not become a judicial issue until 1957. In a landmark decision, the California courts found a doctor negligent for failing to explain the potential risks of a vascular procedure to a patient subsequently paralyzed by the procedure (*Salgo v. Leland Stanford, Jr. University Board of Trustees*, 1957).

Some courts have extended the right to informed consent to what might be called **informed refusal.** The practitioner may be liable for failure to inform the patient of the risks of not consenting to a therapy or diagnostic screening test. *Truman v. Thomas* (1980) was one of the first cases to recognize this important corollary to informed consent. In that case, the court awarded damages against a physician for failure to inform the patient of the potential risks of not consenting to a recommended Papanicolaou (Pap) smear.

INCLUSIONS IN INFORMED CONSENT

To be informed, patients must receive, in terms they can understand and comprehend, the following information:

1. A brief but complete explanation of the treatment or procedure to be performed (*Anderson v. Louisiana State University*, 2006).

2. The name and qualifications of the person to perform the procedure and, if others will assist, the names and qualifications of those assistants (*Grabowski v. Quigley*, 1996; *Luettke v. St. Vincent Mercy Medical Center*, 2006; *Lugenbuhl v. Dowling*, 1996).

3. An explanation of any serious harm that may occur during the procedure, including death if that is a realistic outcome. Pain and discomforting side effects both during and following the procedure should also be discussed (*Caldwell v. Anekwe*, 2008).

4. An explanation of alternative therapies to the procedure of treatment, including the risk of doing nothing at all (*Hinman v. Russo*, 2006; *Wecker v. Amend*, 1996).

5. An explanation that the patient can refuse the therapy or procedure without having alternative care or support discontinued (*Matter of Anna M. Gordy*, 1994).

6. The fact that patients can still refuse, even after the procedure or therapy has begun. For example, all radiation treatments need not be completed.

FORMS OF INFORMED CONSENT

Consent may be obtained in a variety of ways. Consent may be expressed or implied, written or oral, complete or partial.

Perhaps the easiest means of obtaining informed consent is when the consent is expressed. **Expressed consent** is consent given by direct words, written or oral. For example, after the nurse informs the patient that he or she is going to start an intravenous infusion, the patient states, "Okay, but could you put the needle in my left hand, since I am right handed?" As a rule, expressed consent is the type most often sought and received by health care providers.

Implied consent is consent that may be inferred by the patient's conduct or that which may legally be presumed in emergency situations. Implied consent has its foundation in the classic case of *O'Brien v. Cunard Steamship Company* (1899). In that case, a ship's female passenger joined a line of people receiving vaccinations. She neither questioned nor refused the injection. In fact, she willingly held out her arm for the vaccination. Later, she unsuccessfully sued for battery.

In the preceding example, rather than saying that he or she would allow an intravenous infusion to be started, suppose the patient merely extended the left arm and said nothing. The reasonable practitioner would infer from the conduct that the patient both understood the therapy and consented by action. Implied consent is frequently obtained by health care practitioners for minor procedures and routine care. Implied consent may be presumed to exist in true emergency situations. For **emergency consent,** patients must not be able to make their wishes known, and a delay in providing care would result in the loss of life or limb. An important element in allowing emergency consent is that the health care provider has no reason to know or believe that consent would not be given were the patient able to deny consent. For example, the health care provider may not wait until the patient loses consciousness to order treatment that the patient had previously refused, such as a blood transfusion for a known Jehovah's Witness patient.

Allen v. Rockford Health Systems (2006) clarified the need to proceed using implied consent in a medical emergency. The police had stopped an individual driving 5 miles per hour on the wrong side of the road at 2:45 A.M. A breathalyzer test was negative, and the individual was taken to the local emergency center. At the emergency center, the patient was hostile, verbally abusive to staff members, could not walk a straight line, was drowsy, and had slurred speech. She had a prescription bottle, labeled for another person, for 20 Soma tablets. The prescription had been filled the previous day and there were seven tablets in the bottle.

Suspecting a drug overdose, the physician ordered blood work, a straight catheterization for a urine sample, Narcan, and activated charcoal. The patient vehemently fought against these treatments, stating she wanted none of them. After her release from the institution, she sued the staff and institution for assault and battery as there was no consent.

The court, in discounting any liability on the part of the health care providers and institution, noted that it is not possible to obtain consent from a patient when the patient is mentally incompetent to make medical decisions. The caregiver is not required to obtain consent to treatment if the treatment is necessary to protect the patient's health and it is impossible or impractical to obtain consent from the patient or from a family member of another individual authorized by law to consent on the patient's behalf.

Consent may be implied by law, as in the instance in which the patient is a minor and the parent, or state standing in the place of a parent, consents to treatment. The law implies the minor's consent for the treatment.

Consent may be given orally or may be reduced to writing. Unless state law mandates written consent, the law views oral and written consent as equally valid. As a precaution, health care providers should recognize that oral consent is much more difficult to prove should consent or lack of consent become a legal issue. To prevent such court issues, most health care institutions require written consent.

Health care providers should also recognize that the signed consent form takes precedent over any oral statements that an individual may have made (*Tobin v. Providence Hospital*, 2001). In *Tobin*, a patient had three units of his own blood drawn and stored before he had hip replacement surgery. Complications following the surgery caused him to require a fourth unit of blood; an hour after the fourth unit of blood was started, the patient experienced complications. His blood pressure dropped, and he became hemodynamically unstable and began bleeding. He died the following morning. The autopsy revealed that he had disseminated intravascular coagulation (DIC), a rare complication caused by the blood transfusion.

The family sued and prevailed at the lower-court level. The appellate court rejected the verdict. The patient in this case had signed a surgical consent form allowing other donors' blood to be used if additional blood was required. Even though the patient had indicated to family members that he did not want a stranger's blood, the court ruled that his earlier signed consent form was valid and superceded any oral statements.

Consent may be partial or complete. The patient may authorize the entire treatment or procedure or only part of the proposed therapy. For instance, if the patient authorizes a breast biopsy, but refuses to sign the consent form for a mastectomy based on the biopsy results, only a biopsy may be performed. The health care practitioner would then need to have a separate consent form signed before performing the mastectomy, should such surgery prove necessary.

STANDARDS OF INFORMED CONSENT

The various jurisdictions apply **standards of disclosure** for informed consent in one of two ways. These tests or standards of disclosure have evolved to ensure that patients are informed in their decisions and to allow a means of determining the adequacy of the disclosure.

Currently, the states are almost evenly divided between two types of standards for informed consent. Twenty-five states follow the **physician-based standard** and 23 states plus the District of Columbia follow a **patient-based standard.** The remaining three states either have no stated standard for informed consent (West Virginia) or use a hybrid of the physician-based and patient-based standards as determined by case law (Minnesota in *Kinikin v. Heupel*, 1981, and New Mexico in *Gerety v. Demers*, 1978). Physician-based standards generally require the physician to disclose the risks, benefits, and alternatives to a treatment in the same manner that other "reasonable prudent practitioners" would employ. Patient-based standards hold the practitioner responsible for disclosing information on the risks, benefits, and alternatives to a treatment that other "reasonable patients" would need in order to make an informed decision.

A new standard for informed consent that has been emerging over the past few years is termed shared medical decision making. **Shared medical decision making** is a process in which the primary health care provider gives a patient the relevant risks and benefits for all treatment alternatives pertinent to the patient's disease or condition and the patient shares with the primary health care provider all relevant personal information that might make one treatment or therapy more appropriate for the specific patient. Both parties then use this information to come to a mutual decision regarding the appropriate course of therapy or treatment plan. Advocates of shared medical decision making see this type of standard as preferred because of improvements in patient autonomy and comprehension, the ability to reduce unwanted medical procedures and services, and its potential for increased communication and trust between primary health care providers and patients. Given the current movement in U.S. health policy toward increased consumer responsibility in funding medical treatments, considering whether patients receive sufficient information and decision support to enable them to meaningfully participate in their health care has taken on new importance.

To bring a successful malpractice suit based on informed consent, the plaintiff must be able to show, by a preponderance of the evidence, all of the following:

1. There was a duty on the part of the health care provider to know of a risk or alternative treatment.
2. There was a duty on the part of the health care provider to disclose the risk or alternative treatment.
3. There was a breach of the duty to disclose.
4. If the health care occurs in a state where the reasonable patient standard is used, a reasonable person in the plaintiff's position would not have consented to the treatment if he or she had known of the outstanding risk.
5. The undisclosed risk caused the harm, or the harm would not have occurred if an alternative treatment plan was selected.
6. The plaintiff suffered injuries for which damages can be assessed.

EXERCISE 8.1

Explore your own state requirements for standards of informed consent. How did you go about discovering these standards? Do elective procedures and emergency situations use the same standard of informed consent? Are ethical principles evident in these standards for informed consent? Which of the standards gives the most ethical rights to patients?

EXCEPTIONS TO INFORMED CONSENT

The courts recognize the following four exceptions to the need for informed consent in circumstances in which consent is still required:

1. Emergency situations
2. Therapeutic privilege

3. Patient waiver
4. Prior patient knowledge

From a practitioner standpoint, consent is still needed to prevent charges of a battery, but the informed consent requirements are eased.

Emergencies give rise to implied consent. Some courts have recognized that if there is time to give information, a limited disclosure may be valid. If no time exists or the patient is incapable of understanding by virtue of the physical disability, then no information need be given.

Therapeutic privilege, sometimes referred to as therapeutic exception, which has its origins in the common law defense of necessity, allows primary health care providers to withhold information that a patient is not mentally or emotionally stable to handle. The detrimental nature of the information must be more than fear that the information would lead to the patient's refusal. "The disclosure of the information should pose serious and immediate harm to the patient, such as prompting suicidal behavior" (van den Heever, 2005, p. 420). In using this defense, the primary health care provider justifies its use as based on danger or patient incompetence, not merely on the principle of beneficence.

Therapeutic privilege is not favored by the courts, and some courts have held that a relative must concur with the patient decision to consent and that the relative must be given full disclosure, whereas other courts have held that no relative need give concurrent consent. If the risk to the patient abates, the primary health care provider should fully disclose the previously withheld information to the patient.

The patient may also agree to a **waiver** of the right to full disclosure and still consent to the procedure. The caveat to be avoided in this instance is that the health care provider cannot suggest such waiver. The waiver, to be valid, must be initiated by the patient.

Prior patient knowledge involves the patient to whom the risks and benefits were fully explained the first time the patient consented to the procedure. Liability does not exist for nondisclosure of risks that are public or common knowledge or that the patient had previously experienced.

Obtaining informed consent is a two-step process: communicating information to patients so that they can make informed decisions and documenting that decision. Communicating the plan of care is typically the role of the primary health care provider who performs the procedure or treatment. However, most nurses participate in the documentation phase.

ACCOUNTABILITY FOR OBTAINING INFORMED CONSENT

The physician or independent practitioner has the responsibility for obtaining informed consent (*Anderson v. Louisiana State University*, 2006). Individual hospitals have no responsibility for obtaining informed consent unless (1) the primary health care provider is an employee or agent of the hospital, or (2) the hospital knew or should have known of the lack of informed consent and took no action. Court cases and individual state statutes have upheld this second principle.

The institution becomes responsible for informed consent only if those primarily responsible for ensuring that informed consent is obtained are employed by the hospital or institution or only if the hospital fails to take appropriate actions when informed consent is not obtained and the hospital is aware of that omission (*Anderson v. Louisiana State University*, 2006). In *Anderson*, the court restated the position that it was not relevant that the nurse was the individual who asked a patient to sign the informed consent form. "The physician has the legal responsibility to communicate with the patient about the benefits, risks and alternatives of the proposed procedure and to obtain the patient's consent. The physician may delegate to a nurse the task of properly completing the consent form and obtaining the patient's signature" (*Anderson v. Louisiana State*

University, 2006, at paragraph 6). Courts and health care providers feel that to allow liability and thus to allow the hospital to monitor consent procedures and the actual disclosure of material facts upon which to base informed consent would destroy the health care provider's professional relationship with the patient.

Nurses can, though, create accountability for informed consent through their actions. In *Rogers v. T. J. Samson Community Hospital* (2002), a nurse took upon herself the task of explaining a surgical procedure, the possible complications of the procedure, and available alternatives. This, said the court, opened the hospital and the nurse to liability. By taking on this task, which is the physician's responsibility, nurses expose the hospital as well as themselves to potential liability. The court also noted that the information that was given to the patient did not need to be incorrect; the giving of information exposed the potential liability of the nurses and hospital.

Contrast the *Rogers* case with *Hinman v. Russo* (2006). In *Hinman,* the nurse explained Lasik eye surgery to a patient, ensuring that the patient read, initialed each page, and signed the final page of the standard patient consent form, which fully advised the patient of the side effects that could occur. She did not discuss with the patient alternative therapies to Lasik vision-correction surgery, as the physician had previously determined that this patient was not a viable candidate for either radial keratotomy or clear lensectomy. When the patient sued for poor vision following the procedure, the court of appeals found no liability on the part of the nurse or her employer. It was irrelevant, stated the court, that alternative procedures unsuited to the patient were not discussed with her.

Nurses' Role in Obtaining Consent

Nurses who are not independent practitioners may become involved in the process of obtaining informed consent in one of several ways. Given that consent must be obtained for all procedures and treatments, not just medical procedures, one realizes the vast impact of this doctrine. This does not mean that nurses obtain written consent each time they give an injection or turn a patient. Most nursing interventions rely on oral expressed consent or implied consent that may be readily inferred through the patient's actions.

What the doctrine of informed consent means is that nurses must continually communicate with a patient, explaining procedures and obtaining the patient's permission. It also means that the patient's refusal to allow a certain procedure must be respected. Know the state laws on allowing the patient to refuse life-sustaining treatment. Even if the patient validly refuses life-sustaining treatment, the nurse could face charges for honoring or failing to honor this request. Each state has its own laws and applications of the laws. If the patient is unable to communicate, permission may be derived from the patient's admission to the hospital or obtained from the patient's legal representative.

A very real concern for nurses is in obtaining consent for the nursing aspects of medical procedures in which the primary procedure is performed by another practitioner. An example of such a concern is with post-operative care. Should the patient be taught about post-operative care before surgery, or should the nurse wait until after the surgery has been performed? Who is responsible for teaching post-operative care—the primary practitioner or the nursing staff? The answers from a legal perspective are far from clear. Possibly the best way to handle this dilemma is for the nurse to wait until after the patient has consented to the surgical procedure to give post-operative care information. This approach prevents interference with the physician–patient relationship and avoids potential conflicting explanations.

Another approach is to have post-operative teaching materials and films developed to orient the patient to the entire procedure. This approach may be augmented by having a nurse available for questions or clarifications as needed. Many hospitals have implemented this approach with major procedures and operations such as heart catheterizations, vascular arteriography, and open-heart surgery.

A third area of concern for the nurse is in obtaining informed consent for medical procedures provided completely by another practitioner. This obvious area of concern was perhaps the first one identified by most nurses. Nurses traditionally have been the health care providers obtaining the patient's signature on consent forms for surgical or medical therapies performed by physicians. Some hospitals continue to permit nurses to obtain the patient's signature on the consent form. Other hospitals, to avoid this potential liability, prohibit nurses from obtaining signatures on consent forms.

It is important that nurses understand that the primary health care providers may legally delegate the responsibility of obtaining the patient's informed consent to nurses. As the *Anderson* case illustrates, physicians retain their accountability for informed consent even if they delegate responsibility for having the patient sign the consent form. Most hospitals have begun to prohibit primary care practitioners from delegating the accountability for obtaining informed consent to nurses. Once nurses become an integral part of the informed consent process, then the hospital may also assume liability under the doctrine of respondent superior. The doctrine of respondeat superior is described in depth in Chapter 13.

Nurses also have an important role if patients subsequently wish to revoke their prior consent or if it becomes obvious that a patient's already-signed informed consent form does not meet the standards of informed consent. Most nurses have been faced with the problem of what to do when it becomes all too clear that the patient does not understand the procedure to be performed or believes that there are no major risks or adverse consequences inherent in the procedure. Nurses then have an obligation to inform the primary health care provider that informed consent is lacking. This may be done by contacting both the immediate supervisor and the primary health care provider.

The court in *Muskopk v. Maron* (2003) outlines what can happen when the nurse fails to bring such information to the physician's attention. In that case, the patient had been diagnosed with carpal tunnel syndrome in both hands. She was at that time asymptomatic on the left hand, and the surgery was scheduled for a right-hand correction of the carpal tunnel syndrome. The paperwork and the surgical preparations were for surgery on the patient's left hand. The patient told the nurse in the preoperative area that she was having surgery on her right hand, as that was the side where the patient was experiencing the most pain and limitations. The nurse informed no one of this conversation, and the surgery was done on the patient's left hand. The court ruled that the patient could proceed with her lawsuit against both the surgeon and the nurse for malpractice.

In its holding, the court noted that a nurse has a legal duty to investigate in this type of situation. The nurse must first review the paperwork with an open mind to the possibility that the paperwork could be wrong and the oral comments of the patient correct. If the paperwork does not match what the patient is saying, the nurse has the duty to contact the physician and explain the issue. Second, all efforts to correct the situation should be noted in the patient record.

CONSENT FORMS

Essentially two types of consent forms are presently in use. The blanket consent form that is required prior to admission is sufficient for routine and customary care. Routine and customary care may also be implied from the patient's voluntary admission into the hospital; therefore, this initial blanket consent form is needed only for insurance coverage and assignment of benefits.

EXERCISE 8.2

A patient is admitted to your surgical center for a breast biopsy under local anesthesia. The surgeon has previously informed the patient of the procedure, risks, alternatives, desired outcomes, and possible complications. You give the surgery permit form to the patient for her signature. She readily states that she knows about the procedure and has no additional questions; she signs the form with no hesitation. Her husband, who is visiting with her, says he is worried that something may be said during the procedure to alarm his wife. What do you do at this point? Do you alert the surgeon that informed consent has not been obtained? Do you request that the surgeon revisit the patient and reinstruct her about the surgery? Since the patient has already signed the form, is there anything more you should do?

Specific consent forms provide information, such as the name and description of the procedure to be performed. Usually, the form also includes a section stating that (1) the person who signed the form was told about the medical condition, risks, alternatives, and benefits of the proposed procedure, and (2) any and all questions have been answered. With this type of form, the physician and hospital could show that no battery occurred because consent was given. However, the plaintiff may still be able to convince a court that informed consent was not given.

A second type of specific consent form attempts to prevent this latter possibility. This second specific type of form is a detailed consent form that lists the procedure, consequences, risks, and alternatives. Many states are now mandating this type of form through statutory medical disclosure panels.

Most of the latter forms have the following elements:

1. Signature of the competent patient or a legal representative
2. Name and full description of the proposed procedure
3. Name of the person or persons to perform the procedure
4. Description of risks and alternatives of the proposed procedure, including no treatment
5. Description of probable consequences of the proposed procedure
6. Signatures of one or two witnesses according to state law

With such detailed forms, nurses should remember the following. First, witnesses are not required to make the consent valid. Witnesses merely attest to the competency of the patient signing the form and to the genuineness of the signature, not that the patient had all the information needed to make an informed choice. Although nurses need not be witnesses for the consent form to make it valid, if they observe the signature and chart that such information was given at the time of the signing of the consent form, they would make excellent witnesses in an ensuing medical malpractice case (*Anderson v. Louisiana State University*, 2006).

A case that illustrates the fact that nurses signing the informed consent form as witnesses do not make the hospital more liable in resulting malpractice lawsuits is *Auler v. Van Natta* (1997). The patient had signed a consent form for a modified radical mastectomy and immediate reconstruction with a latissimus dorsi flap. When the patient later learned that a saline implant had been used, she sued the physician and the hospital. Before going to trial, the hospital asked to be nonsuited in the case, and the court agreed. The hospital, the court held, did not gratuitously take upon itself the duty to inform the patient and get her consent merely because a registered nurse signed her name on the informed consent form as a witness to the patient's signature.

Second, consent may be withdrawn at any time. Nothing in the written form precludes the patient's right to withdraw his or her consent at will. Third, consent forms, although strong evidence of informed consent, are not conclusive in and of themselves. Several challenges have surfaced, including:

1. Technical language precluded reasonable patients from understanding what they actually signed.
2. The signature was not voluntary, but was coerced or forced.
3. The signer was incompetent due to impairment by medications previously received.

Note, though, that state legislatures lean toward decreasing the person's traditional common law right to sue for lack of informed consent in cases where there is no medical negligence. In cases tried in court, the patient has the burden of proof to show that he or she did not understand and thus did not give valid consent. The significance is that burden of proof is shifted from the defendants, thus removing the difficult burden of proof as to the patient's state of mind on the issue of whether the patient gave informed consent (*Anderson v. Louisiana State University*, 2006).

Fourth, consent forms may be absent or the form may not address the performed procedure, and the nurse then has a duty to ensure that the physician and hospital administrative staff are knowledgeable of the deficiency. In a case from the Court of Appeals of Wisconsin, the physician performed an intraoperative tubal ligation during a cesarean section (*Mathias v. St. Catherine's Hospital, Inc.*, 1997). When the surgeon asked for the instrument to do the tubal ligation, two nurses circulating in the delivery room looked for a signed consent form in the patient's chart and told the surgeon there was no consent form for a tubal ligation. The surgeon performed the tubal ligation despite the lack of a signed consent form. Three days later, one of the nurses who had been in the delivery room brought the patient a standard consent form for tubal ligation and asked her to sign it "just to close up our records."

The patient filed suit on the grounds of lack of informed consent. Nevertheless, the court held that the hospital and nurses faced no legal liability for the patient's civil lawsuit. To be able to rule in favor of the hospital, the court needed only to judge the nurses' actions at the time of the tubal ligation. The nurses in the delivery room checked the patient's chart to ascertain whether the appropriate signature was present on the informed consent form. One of the nurses informed the physician that there was no consent form for the procedure and observed the physician acknowledging hearing that fact.

At this point, the court said, the nurses had no legal duty to take further action. The court noted it may have been a clerical mistake that the form was absent or there may have been some other valid reason the surgeon continued with the operation. It is not necessarily true that the surgeon was performing an unauthorized procedure merely because there was no consent form on the chart. In any event, the nurses were not at fault. What happened was beyond the scope of their legal liability. The hospital also was not to blame, either as the nurses' employer or for having provided the operating room to this surgeon, who practiced independently.

A recent case, *Beeman v. Covenant Health Care* (2006), illustrates that hand-written notations may also be binding on consent forms. In this case, the patient was scheduled for a diagnostic arteriogram. During the procedure, the surgeons opted to perform an interventional angioplasty and stent placement because of the degree of arterial occlusion. The interventional procedures resulted in an arterial tear and the patient sued for lack of informed consent.

The presurgical consent form that the patient had signed included a handwritten notation that angioplasty and stent placement would also be possible during the procedure. The patient testified that the nurse explained the forms to him and asked if there were questions. The physician testified that the patient had spoken to the physician about the procedure and that the patient then signed the consent form. The Court of Appeals upheld the lower-court verdict finding no liability on the part of the defendants.

Consent forms are considered to be valid until withdrawn by the patient or until the patient's condition or authorized treatments change significantly. Some hospitals use a 30-day guideline, but most hospitals prefer to have no set guidelines. Such guidelines could become cumbersome for the patient with a chronic, disabling diagnosis or for a patient who gave valid consent and then became incompetent to renew or sign new consent forms.

WHO MUST CONSENT

Equally important to giving patients all material facts needed on which to base an informed choice is that the correct person(s) consent to the procedure or therapy. Informed consent becomes a moot point if the wrong signature is obtained.

Competent Adult

The basic rule is that if the patient is an adult according to state law, only that adult can give or refuse consent. Most states recognize 18 as the age at which one becomes an adult, although some actions, such as marriage, might serve to classify the person as an adult prior to the legal age. The adult giving or refusing consent must be competent to either sign or refuse to sign the necessary consent forms. Competency at law means that (1) the court has not declared the person to be incompetent, and (2) the person is generally able to understand the consequences of his or her actions. There is a strong legal presumption of continuing competency.

The actual determination of legal competency is not necessarily the function of the psychiatric medical staff. It is usually made based on the assessment of the person by a physician or other member of the health care profession. This assessment is often performed at the time informed consent is requested. Consultation with other health professionals is always a possibility and should be performed if there is (1) underlying mental retardation, (2) an obvious mental disorder, or (3) a disease that affects the patient's mental functioning.

Courts generally have held that there is a strong presumption of continued competency. Such cases involved persons whose minds sometimes wandered or who were disoriented at times; in one case, an individual was confined to a mental institution. In each case, the court sought evidence to show that the person was capable of understanding the alternatives to the procedure as proposed and could fully appreciate the consequences of refusing consent to the procedure (*Matter of Roche*, 1996).

There are two exceptions to the legal adult's right to give or to refuse informed consent. The hospital must seek and abide by the decision of (1) a court-appointed guardian and (2) a person with a valid, written power of attorney. Such persons will present themselves to the hospital administration if they have previously been appointed and if the adult patient is incapable of giving or refusing consent.

In a lengthy and interesting decision, the Supreme Court in California also ruled that family members cannot make decisions for patients who are conscious:

> If the patient is conscious, not terminally ill, not comatose, not in a persistent vegetative
> state and the patient has not previously signed a medical directive or durable power
> of attorney for health care decisions expressing the patient's will in this situation,
> there must be clear and convincing evidence that the patient wants to die or that

allowing the patient to die is in the patient's best interests. (*Conservatorship of Wendland*, 2001, at 158)

The case was unique in that the patient's wife, acting as his legal guardian, had requested the court to order the hospital not to replace the patient's nasogastric tube, but instead allow the patient to die. The patient had been severely injured in a single-vehicle rollover accident. He was initially in a coma for several months, but had regained consciousness by the time this court action was heard. Though the patient was unable to orally communicate, he was able to follow simple commands and appeared to be able to answer questions appropriately. The physician caring for the patient testified that the patient did not respond one way or the other when asked if he wanted to die. The court concluded, since there was no evidence that the patient had expressed a will to die if he were in such a physical and mental state, that it would follow the precedent that this patient was mentally competent and able to accept or decline for himself life-sustaining treatment.

Incompetent Adult

The **legal guardian or representative** is the person who is legally responsible for giving or refusing consent for the incompetent adult. Because the law is allowing someone other than the adult to make decisions for the adult, guardians and representatives have a narrower range of permissible choices than they would if deciding for themselves. Some states insist that the known choices of the patient be considered first. Any expressed wishes concerning therapy or refusal of therapy made while the patient was still fully competent should be evaluated and followed if at all possible.

In re Easly (2001) made it clear, though, that the court-appointed guardian does have an important role in determining the care the patient will receive. In that case, to conform with the Americans with Disabilities Act (ADA), a 71-year-old mentally retarded individual was being considered for placement in a community group home. Her nephew, who was her legal guardian, vigorously objected to any plan that would remove his aunt from the institution in which she had lived for the past 56 years. The court concluded that placement of persons who themselves lack the capacity to consent or refuse consent to changes in their placements are not governed solely by the judgment of their treatment professionals. Their legal guardians' preferences must be considered as the patients' own preference.

To be appointed as a legal representative or guardian, the court must first declare the adult incompetent. The court will then appoint a guardian, either temporarily or permanently. If the court has reason to believe the adult is only temporarily incapacitated, then it will appoint a guardian until the adult is able to once again manage his or her affairs.

Guardians are usually selected from family members because the law holds that such persons will have the patient's best interests at heart and are in a position to best know the patient's desires. If the spouse of the incompetent adult is also elderly and ill, an adult child may be the appointed guardian.

Some persons are never adjudicated as incompetent by a court of law, and in selected states the family is asked to make decisions for the incompetent patient. For example, an automobile accident may render the patient incapable of making decisions and giving consent, and the physician will frequently ask the family about medical matters for the unconscious patient. The order of selection is generally (1) the spouse, (2) adult children or grandchildren, (3) parents, (4) grandparents or adult brothers and sisters, and (5) adult nieces and nephews.

The practitioner is cautioned to validate state laws and judicial decisions because family consent may not be valid consent in a handful of states. Lack of valid consent may lead to a court battle, especially if the practitioner acts on family consent and there was disagreement among family members as to the course of action to take.

Minors

Most states recognize a child under 18 as a **minor.** Parental or guardian consent is necessary for medical therapies unless:

1. The emergency doctrine applies.
2. The child is an emancipated or mature minor.
3. There is a court order to proceed with the therapy.
4. The law recognizes the minor as having the ability to consent to the therapy.

The court in *HCA, Inc. v. Miller* (2000) acknowledged that parents not only have the right to control their children's health care, they also have an obligation to see that it is provided. Unless the need for treatment is too urgent for a parent or family member to be contacted and asked to give consent, parental consent must be obtained before treatment can be given.

Some states also allow **in loco parentis,** or the ability of a person or the state to stand in the place of the parents. Look to statutory law to see who may consent in the absence of a parent. If there is a family consent doctrine, it will be a grandparent, adult brother or sister, or adult aunt or uncle. A newer trend is allowing minor parents to consent for their children's medical and dental treatments.

As with adults, the law applies the doctrine of implied consent for minors with medical emergencies, unless there is reason to believe that the parents would refuse such therapy. For example, if the patient were the child of Jehovah's Witness parents, medical personnel would have reason to believe that the parents might not consent to the giving of blood. The best course for the medical staff to follow if there is doubt about whether consent would be forthcoming is to seek a **court order** for the therapy unless there is a true emergency or life-threatening condition.

If the child's parents are married to each other or have joint custody, most states allow either parent to sign the consent form or make treatment decisions. Unless the divorce results in a sole custody arrangement or in total abrogation of parental rights, the parent with custody is generally considered the party to give or deny consent. Such issues are state specific, and health care providers are cautioned to know their individual state law.

Emancipated minors are persons under the legal age who are no longer under their parents' control and regulation and who are managing their own financial affairs. Some states continue to require parents to completely surrender the right of care and custody of the child to prevent "runaway" children from coming under this classification. Such emancipated minors may validly consent to their own medical therapies. Examples of emancipated minors are married persons, underage parents, or those in the armed service of their country. Some states allow college students, living away from their parents, to fall in this category.

Mature minors may also consent to some medical care. This is a newer concept that is gaining legal recognition. Its origin is in family law and involves the right of the child to make a choice as to which parent will have custody of the child following a divorce. The concept of a mature minor was recognized as early as 1957 (*Madison v. Harrison*). States that recognize the mature minor generally define the mature minor as a teenager between the ages of 14 and 17 who is able to understand the nature and consequences of the proposed therapy and who independently makes his or her own decisions on a daily basis.

Obtaining valid informed consent when minors declare themselves to be emancipated or sufficiently mature to consent in their own stead can be problematic. The best course of action when there is a question of valid consent is to temporarily postpone any elective procedure or treatment until it is determined if the minor can consent within state law. If a true emergency presents, then the practitioner may proceed under an emergency consent doctrine. The practitioner should carefully document in the medical record existence of valid informed consent or the need for emergency care. The best course of action may be to seek parental consent as well as the consent of the mature minor.

The law also recognizes the right of minors to consent for some selected therapies without informing parents of the treatment. The reason for these exceptions is to encourage minors to seek needed treatment. Informing parents of the treatment might prevent minors from receiving the necessary therapy. Instances for which minors may give valid consent include:

1. The diagnosis and treatment of infectious, contagious, or communicable diseases (all states and the District of Columbia)
2. The diagnosis and treatment of drug dependency, drug addiction, or any condition directly related to drug usage
3. Obtaining birth control devices (25 states and the District of Columbia allow minors 12 and older to consent to contraceptive services; 21 states limit which minors may consent to contraceptive services; 4 states have no relevant policy or case law)
4. Treatment during a pregnancy as long as the care concerns the pregnancy (32 states and the District of Columbia allow all minors to consent to prenatal care; 3 states allow a minor to be considered "mature" to consent; 15 states have no relevant policy or case law)
5. Medical care for a child (30 states and the District of Columbia allow all minor parents to consent to medical care for their child; 20 states have no relevant policy or case law)

Court orders may be obtained for the care of minors if the parents refuse to consent to needed procedures or treatment, although there is a trend toward nonintervention unless treatment is needed to save a life. For example, hospitals have obtained court orders for blood transfusions when the parents have refused consent for the transfusion. In *In re Hamilton* (1983), the court ordered chemotherapy for a 12-year-old girl when the parents refused consent based on religious grounds. That court overruled the parents to improve the quality of the child's life during her final days.

EXERCISE 8.3

Jimmy Chang, a 20-year-old college student, is admitted to your institution for additional chemotherapy. Jimmy was diagnosed with leukemia 5 years earlier and has had several courses of chemotherapy. He is currently in an acute active phase of the disease, though he had enjoyed a 14-month remission phase prior to this admission. His parents, who accompany him to the hospital, are divided as to the benefits of additional chemotherapy. His mother is adamant that she will sign the informed consent form for this course of therapy, and his father is equally adamant that he will refuse to sign the informed consent form because "Jimmy has suffered enough." You are his primary nurse and must assist in somehow resolving this impasse. What do you do about the informed consent form? Who signs and why?

Using the MORAL model, decide the best course of action for Jimmy from an ethical perspective rather than a legal perspective. Did you come to the same conclusion using both an ethical and a legal approach?

RIGHT TO REFUSE CONSENT

The right of consent involves the **right of refusal.** If persons have the right to consent, they also have the right to refuse to give consent. The right to refuse continues even after primary consent is given. Patients or their guardians need only to notify the health care giver that they no longer wish to continue with the therapy. In some limited circumstances, the danger of stopping therapy poses too great a harm for the patient, and the law allows its continuance. For example, in the immediate post-operative period, the patient cannot refuse procedures that assure a safe transition from anesthesia. Likewise, the patient may not refuse immediate care for life-threatening arrhythmias following a myocardial infarction if that refusal would worsen the patient's condition. After the arrhythmias have abated, the patient may refuse further therapy.

The right for such refusal may be based on the common law right of freedom from bodily invasion or the constitutional rights of privacy and religious freedom. This right extends to the refusal to consent for lifesaving treatment in most states. In *Shine v. Vega* (1999), a young adult patient came into the emergency center for treatment for an acute asthmatic attack. She had a history of asthma dating back to her early childhood. The nurse began to monitor her, drawing and sending blood to the laboratory for blood gas analysis. When the results of the blood gas analysis came back, the nurse decided that the oxygen mask was not sufficient and the nurse convinced the physician to intubate the patient. The patient and her older sister both voiced adamant disapproval of the plan to intubate her, and they ran from the emergency center. They were chased through the hospital's corridors by security guards. The patient was caught, returned to the emergency center, strapped down in four-point restraints, and forcibly intubated. She recovered and was later discharged from the hospital.

Two years later, the patient died after refusing to go to the hospital for an asthma attack. The family filed a lawsuit, alleging that her death was attributable to fear of hospitals, doctors, and nurses stemming from the forced intubation incident. The court agreed and upheld their right to sue for wrongful death.

The court, in its decision, noted that a medical emergency justifies nonconsensual treatment only when it is not possible or feasible to obtain informed consent from a person legally entitled to provide or withhold consent. Even in a life-threatening situation, care providers cannot substitute their own judgment for that of a mentally competent adult patient or family member. An earlier case had similarly held that the patient's right to refuse treatment outweighed the physician's duty to treat (*Daniel Thor v. Superior Court of Solano County,* 1993).

The right of refusal is not without some potential consequences. The patient or guardian must be informed that the right of refusal may mean, and most often does mean, that the patient's physical condition continues to deteriorate and may actually hasten death. The right of refusal may also mean that third-party reimbursement may be denied, because most insurance policies have a clause that denies or limits reimbursement for refusing procedures that would aid in the diagnosis or reduction of the injury or illness.

Limitations on Refusal of Therapy

In some limited instances the state may deny a patient's right of refusal. These state rights exist to prevent committing crimes and to protect the welfare of society as a whole. Limitations on refusal center on three points:

1. Preservation of life if the patient does not have an incurable or terminal disease
2. Protection of minor dependents
3. Protection of the public's health

In cases filed to enforce the right to refuse care, the courts balance individual rights against societal rights (*Daniel Thor v. Superior Court of Solano County,* 1993; *Jefferson v. Griffin Spalding County Hospital Authority,* 1981; *Leach v. Akron General Medical Center,* 1984). In *Leach,* the court found that a patient has the right to refuse therapy based on a privacy right. In this case, the patient was incompetent, and the issue was allowing the patient to forgo life-sustaining treatment.

A more recent case that specifically addressed the right of parents to refuse life-sustaining procedures is *HCA, Inc. v. Miller* (2000). The case involved the care of a neonate who was born weighing less than 500 grams. On the advice of their obstetrician, the mother and father did not desire a neonatologist to attend at the time of the birth, as the parents were of the opinion that the child, if he or she survived, would be severely impaired. At the time of the delivery, a neonatologist was summoned as the child was born alive. This neonatologist believed that there was a legal and moral duty to take measures to ensure this neonate's survival. The child did survive, but was severely disabled. The parents sued the hospital for treating the child without their consent.

In a lengthy decision, the court determined that the basic premise is that parents have the right of consent for their children. For a parent to allow a child to expire, this court held that there must be a medical certification as to the child's terminal state. Such a certification was not available in this case; in fact, the neonatologist at the time of the birth believed the child was viable. That meant the parents had no legal right to refuse treatment as a means of allowing the child to die and the hospital was not wrong in providing treatment against the parents' wishes.

The government, said the court, "has a compelling interest in seeing that children are cared for properly, notwithstanding the wishes of the parents. When a parent neglects to provide for a child's needs, child protection authorities can intervene" (*HCA, Inc. v. Miller,* 2000, at 193). Note that not all jurisdictions may follow this particular ruling; readers are urged to seek legal advice in their specific jurisdiction.

LAW ENFORCEMENT

Medical personnel are often requested by the police and other law enforcement personnel to draw blood, remove stomach contents, remove bullets, and the like for the purpose of gathering evidence to be used against a suspect. The suspect will often refuse to give consent to the proposed treatments and procedures. As a health care provider, can you legally do as requested? Or will you open yourself to a potential lawsuit for battery?

The Supreme Court of the United States attempted for several years to answer these questions for the health care provider. In *Rochin v. California* (1950), the court ruled that the "removal of stomach contents shocks the conscience" and refused to permit the test results on the stomach contents from being introduced into evidence (at 757). Seven years later, the court ruled that blood drawn from an unconscious person could be introduced into evidence, showing that the driver was legally intoxicated (*Breithaupt v. Adams,* 1957).

Finally, with the landmark *Schmerber v. California* decision in 1966, the court gave the health care provider some criteria for cooperating with law enforcement officials while staying relatively liability free. Five conditions must be present and documented:

1. The suspect must be under formal arrest.
2. There must be a likelihood that the blood drawn will produce evidence for criminal prosecution.
3. A delay in drawing the blood would lead to destruction of the evidence.
4. The test is reasonable and not medically contraindicated.
5. The test is performed in a reasonable manner. (*Schmerber v. California,* 1966, at 763)

Remember, though, that state law may supersede the law enforcer's request; that is, in most states, the hospital or health care provider has no legal duty to perform the test as requested by the law enforcement official. State law may dictate who and under what circumstances blood may be involuntarily drawn.

Ruppel v. Ramsever (1999) illustrates these points. In that case, the patient agreed to be brought in by paramedics to the hospital's emergency center after she hit a parked car. Once at the hospital, she refused care and demanded to leave. She was detained for 10 minutes by the hospital security guard while the police were called. They arrived, placed her under arrest for driving under the influence (DUI), and requested the physician and nurse to draw a blood sample for an alcohol level. The patient adamantly refused her consent to the drawing of blood.

The patient later filed a civil rights lawsuit against the hospital, which was dismissed by the court. Health care professionals, wrote the court, who are directed by law enforcement officers to collect samples of blood or urine for evidence, and who do so in good faith and with due care, cannot be sued for their actions. There is no requirement for health care professionals to second-guess whether the officer has probable cause.

These same principles were reinforced by the court in *Hannoy v. State* (2003). That court concluded that so long as the nurse is ordered by law enforcement to draw a blood sample or has consent from the patient, he or she has committed no wrong.

INFORMED CONSENT IN HUMAN EXPERIMENTATION

Using vulnerable groups of people for research poses many potential problems because of the ease with which the subjects can be coerced. This is especially true of the mentally disabled, children, and prisoners. The major issue, other than coercion, seems to be that of informed consent.

Whenever research is involved, be it a drug study or a new procedure, the investigator(s) must disclose the research to the subject or the subject's representative and obtain informed consent. Federal guidelines have been developed that specify the procedures used to review research and the disclosures that must be made to ensure that valid, informed consent is obtained.

Since 1974, the Department of Health and Human Services (HHS) has required that an institutional review board (IRB) examine and approve the research study prior to any funding from HHS. Specific requirements the IRB must ensure before approving the research study are:

1. Risks to the subjects are minimized.
2. Risks to subjects are reasonable in relation to anticipated benefits, if any, to the subjects and to the importance of the knowledge that may reasonably be expected to result.
3. Selection of subjects is equitable.
4. Informed consent will be sought from each prospective subject or the subject's legally authorized representative.
5. Informed consent will be appropriately documented.
6. Where appropriate, the research plan makes adequate provision for monitoring the data collected to ensure the safety of the subjects.
7. Where appropriate, there are adequate provisions to protect the privacy of subjects and to maintain the confidentiality of data.

Where some or all of the subjects are likely to be vulnerable to coercion or undue influence, such as children, prisoners, pregnant women, mentally disabled persons, or economically or educationally disadvantaged persons, additional safeguards have been included in the study to protect the rights and welfare of these subjects (56 *Federal Register* 28012-22, Section 46.111).

The federal government has also mandated the basic elements of information that must be included to meet the standards of informed consent. These basic elements include the following:

1. A statement that the study involves research, an explanation of the purposes of the research and the expected duration of the subject's participation, a description of the procedures to be followed, and identification of any procedures that are experimental.
2. A description of any reasonably foreseeable risks or discomforts to the subject.
3. A description of any benefits to the subjects or others that may reasonably be expected from the research.
4. A disclosure of appropriate alternative procedures or courses of treatment, if any, that may be advantageous to the subject.
5. A statement describing the extent, if any, to which confidentiality of records identifying the subject will be maintained.
6. For more than minimal research, an explanation as to any compensation and an explanation as to whether any medical treatments are available if injury occurs, and, if so, what they consist of or where further information may be obtained.
7. An explanation of whom to contact for answers to pertinent questions about the research and research subjects' rights and whom to contact in the event of a research-related injury to the subject.
8. A statement that participation is voluntary, refusal to participate will involve no penalty or loss of benefits to which the subject is otherwise entitled, and the subject may discontinue participation at any time without penalty or loss of benefits to which the subject is otherwise entitled (56 *Federal Register* 28012-22, Section 46.116).

The information given must be in language that is understandable by the subject or the subject's legal representative. No exculpatory wording may be included, such as a statement that the researcher incurs no liability for the outcome to the subject. When appropriate, one or more of the following elements of information should be provided to subjects:

1. A statement that the particular treatment or procedure may involve risks to the subject that are currently unforeseeable
2. Anticipated circumstances under which the subject's participation may be terminated by the investigator without regard to the subject's consent
3. Any additional costs to the subject that may result from participation in the research
4. The consequences of a subject's decision to withdraw from the research and procedures for orderly termination of participation by the subject
5. A statement that any significant new findings developed during the course of the research that may relate to the subject's willingness to continue participation will be provided to the subject
6. The approximate number of subjects involved in the study (56 *Federal Register* 28012-22, section 46.116)

The advent of the Health Insurance Portability and Accountability Act of 1996 (HIPAA) has affected how medical record information can now be used in research studies. The Privacy Rule, which became effective April 14, 2003, addresses specific safeguards for research. No separate patient permission to use medical record information is required if de-identified information is used. **De-identified information** is health information that cannot be linked to an individual; most of the 18 demographic items constituting the **protected health information (PHI)** must be removed before researchers are permitted to use patient records without obtaining individual patient permission to use/disclose their PHI. The de-identified data set that is permissible for usage may contain the following demographic factors: gender and age of individuals and a three-digit ZIP code. Note that if individuals are 90 years of age or older, they are all listed as 90 years of age.

To prevent the onerous task of requiring patients who have been discharged from health care settings to sign such permission forms, researchers are allowed to submit a request for a waiver. The waiver is a request to forgo the authorization requirements based on two conditions: (1) the use and/or disclosure of PHI involves minimal risk to the subject's privacy, and (2) the research cannot be practically done without this waiver. Additional information about HIPAA and confidentiality is covered in Chapter 9.

Concerns over past abuses in the area of research with children have led to the adoption of federal guidelines specifically designed to protect children when they are enrolled as research subjects. Before proceeding under these specific guidelines, state and local laws must be reviewed for laws regulating research on human subjects. Proposals involving new investigational drugs or devices must meet Food and Drug Administration regulations (21 *Code of Federal Regulations*, Parts 50, 56, 312, 314, and 812).

In 1998, Subpart D: Additional Protections for Children Involved as Subjects in Research was added to the code (45 *Code of Federal Regulations* 46.401 *et seq.*). These sections were added to give further protection to children when they are subjects of research studies and to encourage researchers to involve children, where appropriate, in research. The sections present guidelines for involving children in research that:

1. does not involve greater than minimal risk
2. involves greater than minimal risk, but presents the prospect of direct benefit to the individual subjects
3. involves greater than minimum risk and no prospect of direct benefit to the individual subject, but is likely to yield generalizable knowledge about the subject's disorder or condition
4. is not otherwise approvable, which presents an opportunity to understand, prevent, or alleviate a serious problem affecting the health or welfare of children.

Since adopting these new guidelines, two federal agencies proposed further broadening the use of children as a research subjects. The National Institutes of Health (NIH) and the Federal Drug Administration (FDA) have taken action that was designed to increase the role of the child as a research subject (45 *Code of Federal Regulations*, Section 46.101[a][2]; National Institutes of Health, 1998). The goal of both these actions was to ensure that drugs that are being used and those proposed to be used in a pediatric population be properly labeled for pediatric indications and dosages. The NIH policy is that "children . . . must be included in all human subjects' research . . . unless there are scientific and ethical reasons not to include them" (National Institutes of Health, 1998, p. 1).

GUIDELINES

Informed Consent

Two criteria must be satisfied:

1. The consent is given by one who has the legal capacity for giving such consent:
   a. Competent adult
   b. Legal guardian or representative for the incompetent adult

    c. Emancipated, married minor

    d. Mature minor

    e. Parent, state, or legal guardian of a child

    f. Minor for the diagnosis and treatment of specific disease states or conditions

    g. Court order

2. The person(s) giving consent must fully comprehend:

    a. The procedure to be performed and by whom the procedure will be performed

    b. The risks involved

    c. Expected or desired outcomes

    d. Any complications or untoward side effects

    e. Alternative therapies, including no therapy at all

GUIDELINES

Rights of Patients in Research

1. Informed consent is the first hurdle to valid human experimentation. The nurse must ascertain that the patient or legal representative understands that a research study will be involved and that the patient or legal representative has a basic understanding of the research to be performed (nature of the study, expected results of the study, and the like).

2. The patient or legal representative must be given the choice to participate or not. This entails giving information in understandable terms and in sufficient quantity so that the patient or legal representative can make an informed choice of participation.

3. The patient or legal representative must know that he or she can choose to terminate participation at any point in the research study. This may be done without penalty, forfeiture of quality care and treatment, or loss of dignity.

4. The patient or legal representative should be aware of who is conducting the research study and how to contact this person(s) at any given time. All questions should be answered for the patient or legal representative as needed by the principal investigator.

5. The patient should be free from any arbitrary hurt or intrinsic risk of injury. Any physical or mental risks to which the patient may be exposing himself or herself should be explained as fully as possible when the initial informed consent is obtained. Likewise, medical care or treatment for such incurred risks should be made available to the patient by the researcher, and the patient or legal representative should be aware of these considerations at the time of the initial informed consent.

6. The patient always retains his or her right to privacy and confidentiality. If at all possible, the patient should never be capable of being identified through the research study. A coding system should be devised and followed. If not possible, the patient should be known to as few persons as can be allowed by the research design.

7. The quality of research in which human subjects are involved is important. Institutional review boards exist for all institutions in which human subjects are used for ongoing research studies. Institutional review boards should look first to the expected outcomes of the study and to that which is being studied in deciding if human persons may be used as subjects.

8. While the rights of the minor and of the mentally or developmentally disabled person are no greater than those of the competent adult subject in a research study, the need to protect

these rights is greater. These persons are more likely not to understand the nature of the research or the fact that they can terminate their participation at will; they are also more easily coerced into becoming subjects for the proposed research study. The nurse must guard against such happenings and ascertain that valid legal representation exists for such underage or disadvantaged persons.

HEALTH LITERACY

A major issue with informed consent today concerns health literacy, also referred to as **medical illiteracy,** information literacy as it pertains to health issues, and functional health literacy. **Health literacy** concerns the degree to which individuals have the capacity to obtain, process, and understand basic health information and the services needed to make appropriate health decisions (Department of Health and Human Services, 2000), while functional health literacy is "the ability to read, understand and act on health information" (Andrus & Roth, 2002, p. 282). Included in this ability to understand and act on health information is the ability to comprehend prescription bottles, printed health care instructions, and the other essential health-related materials.

Whatever the term used, the issue concerns the inability of a growing number of individuals to understand medical terms and instructions. Comprehending medical jargon is difficult for well-educated Americans; it is virtually impossible for approximately 90 million Americans who have "limited health literacy" (Maniaci, Heckman, & Dawson, 2008). Comprehending medical instructions and terms is almost impossible for individuals whose first language is not English, who are unable to read at greater than a second-grade level, or who have vision or cognitive problems caused by aging. These individuals have difficulty following instructions printed on medication labels (both prescription and over-the-counter), interpreting hospital consent forms, and even understanding diagnoses, treatment options, and discharge instructions. Studies show that poor health literacy may be a stronger predictor of one's health than income, level of education, employment status, race, culture, and age (Lauder & Gabel-Jorgensen, 2008; Maniaci et. al, 2008; Roberts, 2008). Not surprisingly, the main focus of the studies concerned health literacy and correct medication comprehension compliance.

Nurses play a significant role in addressing this growing problem. The first issue to address is awareness of the problem, as many patients and their family members hide the fact that they cannot read or do not understand what health care providers are attempting to convey. Professional schools are beginning to address this concern in the classroom, and health care institutions address this issue through multiple types of educational programs. A second issue involves ensuring that the information and words nurses use to communicate with patients are at a level they can comprehend. One means of assuring that patients and family members understand what was addressed might be to hand a bottle of medication to the patient and ask him or her to show the nurse how he or she would take the medication and when the medication should be taken. Remember that merely handing a person printed information may not be appropriate for comprehension. Institutions are beginning to use a variety of means to ensure comprehension of health information, including audio/visual presentations, use of short instructional periods followed by additional instruction immediately prior to discharge, follow-up phone calls within a day or two of discharge, ensuring that patients know how to contact institution personnel and whom to contact if problems arise, and development of standards for communication within the institution. A final issue concerns the area of research on how to most effectively convey health information and patient instructions.

GENETIC TESTING

Rapid scientific advances in the area of genetics, including scientists' ability to clone sheep and to create artificial human chromosomes, have created challenges for health care providers. Among these challenges are the questions of informed consent for **genetic testing,** discrimination against persons with less than perfect genes, and the confidentiality of genetic testing. The first issue is addressed here, and the confidentiality issue is addressed in Chapter 9.

Genetic testing is beginning to reveal whether symptomatic patients have a suspected genetic disorder and whether asymptomatic patients are predisposed to developing a genetic disease later in life or will pass the genetic disposition to their offspring. To prevent some children from developing later illnesses, several states mandate that all newborns be screened for certain genetic disorders. The screening of newborns varies greatly by state. For example, states may mandate screening for cystic fibrosis or may allow parents the right to refuse the test for cause, such as religious grounds. The majority of states ensure that parents are informed about the testing prior to taking a blood sample.

The issue of informed consent remains the same, whether the informed consent concerns a surgical procedure, an invasive piece of monitoring, or evaluation of a genetic trait. Though a simple blood test, with minimal risks to the patient, is needed for the testing, the implications of this test are immense. All future life events may be affected by this simple test, including family planning, career choices, health insurance coverage, and the psychological well-being of the person and family.

The Institute of Medicine and the American Nurses Association continue to recommend that the following elements be included when informed consent is sought for genetic testing from either patients or parents. These elements include:

1. Nature of the disorder. How the condition may affect the individual, whether it is treatable, and what the treatment entails should be addressed. Patients and parents may choose not to have the test performed if no treatment is available.
2. Efficacy of the test. Patients and parents should be informed of the rate of false negatives and false positives with the test and whether further testing will be done based on a positive result. They should also be informed about the difference between the probability of developing the condition or a certainty of developing the disease. Included in the discussion should be the ratio percentage of the probability of developing the condition, if such figures are known.
3. Decisions that will follow if the test is positive. For example, the pregnant patient who is positive for a genetic abnormality may be asked to decide whether to carry the fetus to term. Those attempting to conceive may be asked to decide about permanent sterility.
4. Support services. Several agencies offer support to patients and parents, and they should be informed of these potential services as part of the informed consent process.
5. Disclosure and confidentiality issues. The question of whether the patient wants to reveal positive test results to other family members who may have inherited or may be at risk for the same genetic marker should be discussed. The patient or parent should also know that the insurance carriers and other health care providers may have access to the test result (Andrews et al., 1994; Scanlon & Fibison, 1995).

The Health Insurance Portability and Accountability Act of 1996 (HIPAA) provides some protection on a national perspective to prevent the possibility of discrimination in insurance coverage. Portions of the act prevent using genetic information to determine insurance eligibility as well as preventing the limitation or denial of benefits using a preexisting exclusion clause. There are, though, no provisions to prevent plans from requiring genetic testing of those enrolled, excluding coverage for a particular condition, or charging higher premiums to those with genetic mutations.

The **Genetic Information Nondiscrimination Act of 2008,** better known as GINA, is a new federal law that begins to address these shortcomings (GINA, 2008). Signed into law on May 21, 2008, GINA protects Americans from being treated unfairly because of differences in their DNA that may ultimately affect their health status. This law prevents discrimination from health insurers and employers. Parts of the law that relate to health insurers will take effect in May 2009 and those relating to employers in November 2009. Individuals not covered by the law are those in the military. The law also does not cover life insurance, disability insurance, and long-term care insurance policies.

The law was proposed to ease concerns about discrimination that might have kept some individuals from obtaining genetic tests. The law also enables individuals to take part in research studies without fear that their DNA information might be used adversely for insurance purposes or in the workplace.

Prior to GINA, a minority of states had passed legislation to prevent against genetic discrimination. The federal law sets a minimum standard of protection that must be afforded in all states. Should individual states set a higher minimum standard, the state standard is to be upheld for citizens within the state.

Patient Education in Genetic Testing

The implications for patient education in this area of the law are immense. The nurse's knowledge of such issues may be limited because information in this area is literally exploding every day. Nurses will undoubtedly be asked many questions from frightened and concerned parents and patients, and they must first understand genetic testing, its limitations, and its potential for enhanced health care. Nurses must also understand and apply mental health interventions, since patients and parents are most vulnerable to self-doubt, guilt, hopelessness, and powerlessness at this time. Nurses can best meet the patients' and parents' needs by incorporating all members of the interdisciplinary health care team—specialists in genetics, social workers, mental health practitioners, religious counselors, and staff nurses.

The advocacy role of the nurse is extremely important during genetic testing and following positive test results. Nurses may need to assist the patients or parents in asserting their rights to all knowledge currently known about the condition/trait, in voicing their fears, and in facing some of the hard decisions that result from positive test results.

PATIENT SELF-DETERMINATION

Patient self-determination involves the right of individuals to decide what will or will not happen to their bodies. Usually, the right of self-determination is addressed in issues surrounding death and dying, but self-determination concerns all aspects of consent and its refusal.

THE ISSUE OF CONSENT

Before one can discuss the patient's right to die or to forgo life-sustaining procedures, one must consider the issue of informed consent. Competent adults have long been recognized as having the right to refuse medical treatment, unless the state can show that its interests outweigh that right. Examples of such overriding state interests include:

1. Protecting third parties, especially minor children
2. Preserving life, especially that of minors and incompetents
3. Protecting society from the spread of disease

Competent adults may decide which treatments they will receive and which medical procedures they will refuse. Often the decision to forgo medical treatment must survive a period in which the health care receiver is incompetent. Many states have attempted to assist individuals in attaining their wishes through statutory enactments.

Patients generally express their desires in oral form. In some states, these oral wishes have been upheld by the judiciary. The courts examine documentation of these wishes and determine if the person knew of the terminal condition when expressing his or her wishes or whether the person was talking, in general terms, about future care when he or she became terminally ill. The courts have been reluctant to enforce generalities, and vague talk about potential happenings in the future have been held to have little weight by the court.

For years, legal experts have concluded that competent adults have the right to refuse medical treatment, even if the refusal is certain to cause death, a view that is consistent with the majority of states to decriminalize suicide. But it was not until 1984 that an appellate court directly confronted an issue in which a clearly competent patient refused necessary life-sustaining treatment. In *Bartling v. Superior Court* (1984), the decision of the California Court of Appeals was eased because the patient died before the case was resolved. That tentativeness of the court was overcome by the next case to present itself, *Bouvia v. Superior Court* (1986).

The issue addressed in *Bartling* concerned the right of a competent adult patient, with a serious illness that was probably incurable but not necessarily terminal, over the objections of his physicians and the hospital, to have life-support equipment disconnected despite the fact that the withdrawal of such devices would hasten his death. Mr. Bartling, a severe emphysemic patient, entered the hospital for depression. While hospitalized, a tumor was noted on x-ray, and during the subsequent biopsy, his lung collapsed. Despite aggressive therapy, Mr. Bartling was trached and ventilator-dependent at the time this cause of action was heard. Though Mr. Bartling died during the course of the appeal, the appellate court did hold that the "right of a competent adult to refuse medical treatment is a constitutionally guaranteed right which must not be abridged" (at 192).

In *Bouvia v. Superior Court* (1986), the court addressed many of the same issues. Ms. Bouvia, a 28-year-old patient with severe cerebral palsy, sought removal of a nasogastric tube, inserted and maintained against her will for the purpose of involuntary feedings. Here, the court wrestled not only with the right of a competent adult to refuse medical therapy, but also with the facility's obligation to serve the autonomous interests of patients, as defined by those patients. In *Bouvia,* the autonomous decisions included medical support to prevent further pain and suffering during the dying process. The legal history of the right of competent patients to forgo life-sustaining treatment is provided in a clear and accurate way through these two California opinions. The very strong unanimous court in *Bouvia* also demonstrates the consensus absent in 1984 that was beginning to solidify by 1986.

Incompetent patients present a totally different picture. The first court case to challenge the judiciary in this respect was *In re Quinlan* (1976). In a lengthy decision, the New Jersey Supreme Court held that although patients generally have the right to refuse therapy, guardians for the incompetent do not. "The only practical way to prevent destruction of the (privacy) right is to permit the guardian and family of Karen to render their very best judgment . . . as to whether she would exercise it in these circumstances" (at 664).

That court allowed the father of Karen Quinlan to authorize the withdrawal of life-support systems for Karen. The decision was a difficult one to reach because Karen did not meet the Harvard criteria for brain death. While she was ventilator-dependent at the time of the court case, she did have some brain activity on the electroencephalogram and some reflex movements. The decision was also difficult because it conflicted significantly with a precedent-setting

New Jersey case that held that one should always save a life, even if the patient's objection to lifesaving procedures was based on religious beliefs (*John F. Kennedy Memorial Hospital v. Heston*, 1971).

The decision reached by the court in *Quinlan* was based on the **best interest standard.** Essentially, this objective standard examines the personal preferences made while the now-incompetent patient was capable of stating what he or she would want in the event of a catastrophic happening. Evidence was presented by friends of Karen Quinlan, noting that she had frequently stated that she did not want to be kept alive in a comatose state. The court determined that to allow Karen's father the right to remove Karen from life-support systems was in her best interest. It should be clear, however, that the father made the final decision. The court system gave him the right to make the ultimate decision, but did not influence that decision.

The next significant decision in this area of the law was *Superintendent of Belchertown State School v. Saikewicz* (1977). Here, the Massachusetts Supreme Court deviated from the *Quinlan* case in two significant ways:

1. This court used the doctrine of **substituted judgment** (subjective determination of how persons, were they capable of making their opinions and wishes known, would have chosen to exercise their right to refuse therapy) to decide what Joseph Saikewicz would have wanted to be done with his right to refuse therapy.
2. No ethics committee was suggested by the court. Unlike *Quinlan*, the *Saikewicz* opinion met with general disfavor because the court totally rejected the notion that these types of decisions should be made by families and physicians with the aid of ethics committees. Indeed, the *Saikewicz* court held that the decision to discontinue therapy "must reside with the judicial process and the judicial process alone" (at 475).

Eichner v. Dillon (1980), the third case to further define allowing patients the right to forgo life-sustaining procedures, restricted the termination of extraordinary life-support treatments to the patient who was terminally ill or in a "vegetative coma characterized as permanent or irreversible with an extremely remote possibility of recovery" (at 468). *Eichner* also combined the substituted judgment doctrine as followed in *Saikewicz* with the best interest (personal preferences made while the now-incompetent patient was rational and capable of stating what he or she would want in the event of a catastrophic happening) test as derived from *Quinlan*. Although not a perfect solution, the decision did seem to soften the negative impact of *Saikewicz*.

The final decision concerning the incompetent patient's right to die seemed to be settled in 1990. In *Cruzan v. Director, Missouri Department of Health* (1990), the court made explicit that right-to-die issues will be decided on a state-to-state basis and that there will be little, if any, U.S. constitutional limits on what states may do. Following the *Cruzan* decision, cases have allowed more latitude to family members, and courts have struggled to find instances in which patients had made some expression, however fleeting, about their desires for sustaining life with artificial or life-support measures.

Two more recent cases exemplify those points. In *In re Fiori* (1995), a Pennsylvania court held that a hospital may terminate life-support treatment for a patient in a persistent vegetative state without a court order if the hospital obtained the consent of close family members and the consent of two physicians. The court limited this holding to patients in a persistent vegetative state with no cognitive powers and no chance of recovery and who never clearly expressed a preference for termination. In a previous case, *Grace Plaza of Great Neck, Inc. v. Elbaum* (1993), the court had held that where doubt exists as to an incompetent's desired course of treatment, a judicial determination is necessary before life support can be terminated. The court further stated that proof of a patient's desires, such as through a living will or prior statement, will serve to limit a provider's autonomy in denying termination of treatment.

LIVING WILLS

Living wills, initiated in the 1960s, about the same time that hospitals approved policies stating that all patients would be afforded cardiopulmonary resuscitation measures, gained popularity following these court cases. **Living wills,** created in attempt to dictate future actions, are directives from competent individuals to medical personnel and family members regarding the treatment they wish to receive when they can no longer make the decision for themselves. The living will is not necessary if the patient is competent and capable of making his or her wishes known. It becomes important when the previously competent person becomes seriously ill and unable to give or deny informed consent.

Usually, the language of a living will is broad and vague. It gives little direction to the health care provider concerning the circumstances and actual time the declarant wishes the living will to be honored. There is typically no legal enforcement of the living will, and medical practitioners may choose to abide by the patient's wishes or to ignore them as they see fit. There is also no protection for the practitioner against criminal or civil liability, and many primary health care providers have been afraid to proceed under a living will's direction for fear that family members or the state will file charges for wrongful death.

A case example outlining the various problems surrounding living wills is *Haymes v. Brookdale Hospital Medical Center* (2001). The patient's sister called 911 after the patient self-inflicted a cerebral gunshot wound. The emergency medical technicians transported the patient to the hospital. The sister provided the hospital with a document that she claimed was the patient's living will, and the sister demanded that all treatment be ceased. The hospital refused to follow the document and continued treatment. The patient was intubated, successfully weaned from the respirator, and now has permanent brain injuries that require continuous medical care.

The sister sued the hospital. The court, in dismissing the case, noted that in the absence of a valid advance directive, a direct physician's order not to resuscitate, or a court order, health care providers cannot be sued for treating an unconscious patient. In denying acceptance of the living will document, the court noted that there was only one signature on the document and state law mandated that two signatures were required. Additionally, the document did not clearly indicate the expressed wishes of the patient for this particular situation.

NATURAL DEATH ACTS

To protect practitioners from potential civil and criminal lawsuits and to ensure that patients' wishes are followed when they are no longer able to make their wishes known, a special type of living will, known as the **natural death act,** was enacted into law. These natural death acts are legally recognized living wills in that they serve the same function as living wills but with statutory enforcement. Recognizing that the physician may be unwilling to follow the directive, several of these laws require a reasonable effort on the part of the physician to transfer the patient to a physician who will abide by the patient's expressed wishes.

Statutory provisions for natural death acts vary from state to state. Generally, persons over 18 years of age may sign a natural death act. Such persons must be of sound mind and capable of understanding the purpose of the document they sign. The natural death act document is usually a declaration that withholds or withdraws life-sustaining treatment from the patient should he or she ever be in a terminal state. The natural death act ideally is in written form, signed by the patient, and witnessed by two persons, each of whom is 18 years or older. Recognizing that patients may not be physically capable of written enactments, a newer trend is to allow oral enactment of natural death acts.

Some states also specify that the witnesses to the natural death act not be:

1. Related to the patient by blood or marriage
2. Entitled to any portion of the estate of the patient by will or intestacy
3. Directly financially responsible for the patient's medical care
4. The attending physician, his or her employee, or employee of the facility in which the declarant is a patient
5. The person who, at the request of the patient, signed the declaration because the patient was unable to sign

Other states incorporate some of these restrictions.

The form of the natural death act also varies from state to state. Some states provide no suggestion as to the contents of the document, whereas other states have a mandatory form that must be filled in by the declarant. Still other states suggest a form but provide that additional directions may be added if they are not inconsistent with the statutory requirements. For states that have no set form, private organizations have suggested formats for these special living wills. Some states also have a clause stating that the declarant must have discussed these issues with the designated surrogate.

Once signed and witnessed, most natural death acts are effective until revoked, although some states require that they must be reexecuted every 5 or 10 years. In some states, the patient who is pregnant may not benefit from the provisions of the natural death act during the course of the pregnancy. It may be advisable for the declarant to review, redate, and re-sign the natural death act every year or so. This assures family members and health care providers that the directions contained in the natural death act reflect the current wishes of the patient.

The natural death act may be revoked by physical destruction or defacement, by a written revocation, or by an oral statement indicating that it is the person's wish to revoke the previously executed natural death act. Some states have less restrictions on revocation; for example, the revocation may take place without regard to the mental condition of the patient or the revocation is ineffective until the attending physician is notified of the revocation.

Once a valid natural death act exists, it is effective only when the person becomes qualified; that is, the person is diagnosed to have a terminal condition and the removal or withholding of life-support systems would merely prolong the patient's process of dying. Most states require that two physicians certify in writing that any procedures and treatments will not prevent the ultimate death of the patient but will serve only to postpone death in a patient with no chance of recovery. Medications and procedures used merely to prevent the patient's suffering and to provide comfort are excluded from this definition.

Today, many states also allow an oral invocation of a natural death act and/or another person to invoke a natural death act for the patient. States were exploring a variety of options to ensure that natural death acts met the needs of patients when the durable power of attorney for health care became more prominent.

Enforcement of these natural death acts is illustrated by *Estate of Neumann v. Morse Geriatric Center* (2007) and *Scheible v. Morse Geriatric Center* (2007). In the first case, a 92-year-old patient with advanced Alzheimer's disease had a living will that prohibited the use of any artificial life-saving devices. When she became seriously ill, she was intubated by paramedics called to the nursing home; the endotracheal tube was continued for an additional six days. It was finally removed at her family's insistence and she died shortly after its removal.

The family first brought suit for nonconsensual medical treatment, which was upheld by the trial court. In a separate finding a week after the first verdict, the court additionally found for the family for the pain and suffering that the patient had endured while the endotracheal tube was in place, noting that the current trend is to allow recovery for pain and suffering when living wills are not honored.

The facts in the *Scheible* case are similar. A 92-year-old resident's granddaughter had provided the facility with an advance directive that she had signed as the resident's surrogate decision maker. When the patient suffered a seizure, paramedics were summoned, the patient was entubated, and she was transported to an acute care facility where she remained ventilator dependent for six days. She expired four days after the endotracheal tube was discontinued. The family was awarded $150,000 for the resident's pain and suffering after her life was prolonged contrary to the living will and advance directive.

DURABLE POWER OF ATTORNEY FOR HEALTH CARE

The **durable power of attorney for health care (DPAHC)** or the **medical durable power of attorney (MDPA)** allows competent patients to appoint a surrogate or proxy to make health care decisions for them in the event that they are incompetent to do so. These legislative enactments were the next logical step following limitations with living wills and natural death acts. No longer does the family or health care provider need to guess if this is the time the patient would want the living will to be followed, as a person has been given the authority of the patient to either accept or refuse care and to speak for the patient.

Power of attorney is a common law concept that allows one person (an agent) to speak for another (the principal), a concept of the agency relationship. At common law, the power of attorney terminates upon the death or incapacity of the principal. To prevent this occurrence when the patient most wants the power of attorney to be effective, legislatures adopted the Uniform Durable Power of Attorney Act. This act sanctions the right of an individual to grant a durable power of attorney, which would be valid even if the principal was incapacitated and legally incompetent. Referred to as a "springing" right, the DPAHC assures that the individual retains his or her right of informed consent while competent while allowing this right of informed consent to "spring" to another when the individual becomes incompetent.

Under most of the DPAHC statutes, individuals may designate an agent to make medical decisions for them when they are unable to make such decisions. The power includes the right to ask questions, select and remove physicians from the patient's care, assess risks and complications, and select treatments and procedures from a variety of therapeutic options. The power also includes the right to refuse care and/or life-sustaining procedures. Health care providers are protected from liability if they abide, in good faith, by the agent's decisions.

Agents further have the authority to enforce the patient's treatment plans by filing lawsuits or legal actions against health care providers or family members. Agents have the right to forgo treatment, change treatment plans, or consent to additional treatment. In short, they have the full authority to act as the principal would have acted. Thus, the DPAHC is the best form of substituted judgment currently available for an otherwise incompetent patient.

Patients are cautioned to appoint persons as agents who understand what the patient would want and are capable of making those hard decisions. Friends, relatives, or spouses may be appointed as agents. As with natural death acts, some states mandate that the principal and the surrogate have discussed potential health care needs and options, at least superficially. Most states allow the patient or potential patient to appoint subsequent agents. In the event the first named person cannot serve or is unwilling to serve in this capacity, then a second or third person has the principal's authority. Without this latter provision, patients' wishes might still not be honored.

Once appointed by the principal, surrogate decision makers have the ability to act as the now-incompetent person would have acted if he or she were able to communicate with health care providers. Though there is no absolute right to this status, courts now seem to favor noninterference with an appointed surrogate. In *In re Nellie G.* (2007), an elderly patient had signed a power of attorney giving her daughter authority to manage her affairs should she become incapacitated. The patient subsequently suffered a stroke, was admitted to a rehabilitation center, and was later transferred to a nursing home. Given the fact that the patient was completely incompetent to handle her affairs, the facility petitioned the court for the appointment of an independent guardian.

The court ruled that the facility had acted improperly. The court held that as long as the family member designated by the patient in her health care directive was managing the patient's affairs competently and was not using his or her position to profit at the patient's expense, intervention into her actions was not appropriate.

Note, also, that most courts debate at some length to ensure that the best interests of incapacitated patients are upheld. In *In re Susan Jane G.* (2006) the court invalidated an advance directive when the patient's daughters were able to show that the document had been signed, naming the patient's husband as the surrogate decision maker, after their mother had already become incompetent. The issues arose in this case when the daughters wanted to move their mother to a nursing home where she would receive better care and the patient's husband refused the move.

In *Guardianship of Baker* (2006), the patient's wife wanted to remove the patient from a nursing home because the physician prescribed antipsychotic medication. She had already had him moved 14 times for the same reason. The nursing home contacted the state long-term care ombudsman's office and also filed an application for guardianship with the court. The court appointed a second attorney to represent the patient and secured a second medical opinion, which supported the need for antipsychotics for this patient's care. The court appointed a guardian for the patient when it was determined that without his medications he was combative and that it was very difficult for caregivers to meet his basic care needs. With the medications his quality of life was significantly better.

MEDICAL OR PHYSICIAN DIRECTIVES

Some states allow for a directive that lists a variety of treatments and lets patients decide what they would want, depending on the patient's condition at the time. For example, the patient can select to allow life-sustaining therapy if the condition is not terminal or to disallow life-sustaining therapy if the condition is terminal and irreversible. Generally known as a **medical or physician directive,** this document has legal worth comparable to the living will.

UNIFORM RIGHTS OF THE TERMINALLY ILL ACT

The act, first adopted in 1985 and amended in 1989, is narrow in scope and limited to treatment that is merely life prolonging and to patients whose terminal condition is incurable and irreversible, whose death will occur soon, and who are unable to participate in treatment decisions. The act's sole purpose is to provide alternative ways in which a terminally ill patient's desires regarding the use of life-sustaining procedures can be legally implemented. The majority of states have not yet signed this act.

This act was passed because no two states have living will or natural death act provisions that are identical. Perhaps the act was passed because the political nature of the right to die had driven the legislature to enact virtually meaningless statutes to avoid political fallout.

Many of the provisions of the act look identical to some state natural death act provisions. For example, the qualified patient must be diagnosed as terminal and life-sustaining procedures would only prolong the dying of the patient. Physicians who are unwilling to comply with patients' requests not to begin or continue life-support procedures should take all necessary steps to transfer the patient to a physician who will comply with the provisions of the declaration. Patients diagnosed as being in a persistent vegetative state are not qualified patients.

SUMMARY OF ADVANCE DIRECTIVE DOCUMENTS

All states and the District of Columbia have enacted some form of advance directive. Three states recognize solely the natural death act or statutory living will documents, though all three allow for appointment of a health care agent for limited end-of-life decisions. An additional three states solely recognize durable power of attorney for health care documents, 32 states allow both statutory living wills and durable power of attorney for health care documents, and 13 states have passed legislation that combines these two documents into a sole document.

All states and the District of Columbia allow the naming of a proxy in at least one of the state documents, though in three states (Louisiana, Montana, and Pennsylvania) the proxy is limited to circumstances of terminal illness and/or persistent vegetative states. Approximate 37 state statutes include forms for appointing proxies or for creating comprehensive advance directives. In 18 states, the forms must be "substantially followed" or certain information disclosure must be included in the form. Generally, changes or additions to the standard language are allowable. At least 90% of the legislative acts address personal instructions for care, general life-sustaining procedures, and terminal illness. Given the mobility of Americans today, an issue that remains to be addressed concerns the need for national conversation regarding standardization of these documents.

PHYSICIAN ORDERS FOR LIFE-SUSTAINING TREATMENT

A unique application similar to advance directives is the **Physician Orders for Life-Sustaining Treatment (POLST)** form, previously known as an Emergency Medical Service No Cardiopulmonary Resuscitation (EMS-No CPR) form. The POLST form is intended for use by any person 18 years of age or older who has a serious health condition. The form contains information about the person's end-of-life directives, including cardiopulmonary resuscitation, medical interventions, antibiotics, and artificially administered nutrition. The POLST is not technically an advance directive, but a physician's or other primary health care provider's orders regarding treatment that the person will accept or refuse to accept.

The program began in Oregon in 1991. Initially developed for use by emergency medical service (EMS) personnel, the main purpose of the POLST was to provide these initial responders with written physician orders that gave specific instructions concerning medical interventions that the EMS personnel were to implement. These mandatory orders allowed the EMS personnel to honor the person's end-of-life treatment preferences either to have or to limit treatment, even when the person was transferred from one care setting to another. This latter provision accomplishes a secondary purpose of the form in that it is portable and may be used from one setting to another.

The need for such a readily accessible form arose because advance health care directives do not give guidance to EMS personnel because they are not physician's orders and because no state forces a physician or other primary health care provider to comply with an advance directive. The POLST form is easy to complete, requiring only that the physician or other primary health care provider sign the form, and there is no witness to the signature or notarization of the form required. The POLST form is generally brightly colored so that it is easily recognizable by both the patient and the health care provider.

Persons who complete the POLST are advised to also complete an advance directive. The POLST merely outlines the person's preferences for end-of-life care and does not give guidance regarding who the person would select to have as his or her surrogate decision maker or guidance about issues outside the four categories on the form itself. A POLST may be the initial orders that accompany the patient who is newly admitted to a health care facility, and the advance directive form gives more detailed information about the patient's long-term care.

Currently, the POLST is an endorsed program in a few states, including Oregon, Washington State, Pennsylvania, West Virginia, and New York and in some communities in Wisconsin. Another 20 states are developing programs, either for the entire state or for communities within the state (POLST State Programs, 2008).

Advance directives and the POLST have some similarities. They are designed to assist persons with making their final wishes known so that these wishes and desires can be followed even if the person cannot speak for himself or herself. They encourage open and frank conversations with health care providers and among family and close friends. They also encourage this communication to take place at a time when the patient is competent to understand the ramifications of alternative options and can execute advance directives and POLSTs.

PATIENT SELF-DETERMINATION ACT OF 1990

In November 1991, the Patient Self-Determination Act of 1990 was enacted into law as part of the Omnibus Budget Reconciliation Act of 1990. This act was in direct response to the Nancy Cruzan case in Missouri, and it mandates that patients must be queried about the existence of advance directives and that such advance directives be made available to them, if they so wish.

In 1983, Nancy Cruzan was involved in a one-car automobile accident. She was discovered lying face down in a ditch without cardiac or respiratory functioning, and life support was started. She eventually was diagnosed as being in a persistent vegetative coma, and her parents requested the removal of artificial hydration and nutritional support. The trial court allowed such removal because Cruzan "expressed thoughts at age 25 in a somewhat serious conversation with a friend that if sick or injured she would not wish to continue her life unless she could live at least halfway normal" (*Cruzan v. Director, Missouri Department of Health,* 1990, at 2843). The Supreme Court of Missouri reversed that decision, stating that such statements were unreliable for the purpose of determining her intent, and further held that the family was not entitled to direct the termination of her treatment in the absence of a living will or "clear and convincing, inherently reliable evidence absent here" (at 2844).

The U.S. Supreme Court held that states had the authority to impose legal requirements on decisions to discontinue therapy for incompetent patients. The case was then remanded back to the trial level in Missouri and, on retrial, the court concluded that the friend's statement of Nancy Cruzan's desires was sufficient to allow the removal of the feeding tube. Ms. Cruzan died on December 16, 1990.

Justice Scalia, in his separate concurrence, praised states for beginning to grapple with the issue of terminating medical treatment through legislation. Almost every state recognizes some form of advance directive, from living wills to durable powers of attorney for health care. The problem, though, is that few people prepare advance directives. Thus, the Patient Self-Determination Act was passed to ensure that persons did know about such advance directives and that they would be assisted in making such directives, if they so desired.

The Patient Self-Determination Act is based on three basic premises:

1. Patients who are informed of their rights are more likely to take advantage of them.
2. If patients are more actively involved in decisions about their medical care, then that care will be more responsive to their needs.
3. Patients may choose care that is less costly. (Rouse, 1991, p. 21)

The act merely lets people know about existing rights and does not create any new rights for patients, nor does it change state law. Perhaps the act has served as incentive for more states to pass durable powers of attorney for health care statutes, but it does not mandate such passage. The act does not require that patients execute advance directives. It merely provides for patient education about such directives and provides assistance for those patients wishing to execute such directives. The legislation specifically states that providers may not discriminate against a patient in any way based on the absence or presence of an advance directive. Nor does the act legislate communication or conversation. Yet one of the purposes of the act is to encourage communication and conversation about existing directives, at a time when the patient is competent to understand and to execute advance directives.

To make the Patient Self-Determination Act a reality, health care providers must themselves understand the act and its purposes, and they should know how to answer patients' and families' questions. Quality care could be enhanced with this act, as health care providers often struggle to determine appropriate courses of care complicated by lack of knowledge about patients' preferences for treatment. Patient education about advance directives should ideally take place outside the acute care setting, and nurses may become involved in consumer education programs. Nurses can also become involved in assessing patients' readiness to prepare an advance directive in the acute care setting.

The most challenging aspect of the process of preparing an advance directive is assisting patients to identify their preferences for treatment. Some individuals have clear opinions, while other patients are more comfortable trusting future choices to family members without articulating specific wishes. It is also important for health care providers and patients to remember that preferences change over time and that the willingness to undergo aggressive treatment is in large part dependent on perception of the likely outcome of that treatment.

An expression of patient wishes for or against treatment choices is important. If these preferences are known, then the standard one applies in life-threatening situations is that of substituted judgment, which holds that the decision is the one the patient would have made if competent to make such a decision. If the preferences are not known, then the standard becomes one of best interests in light of everything that is known about the patient. Often, it is helpful to the patient's family and friends to articulate this latter standard, because they may be experiencing denial, guilt, or attachment.

Early in this inception, Lynn (1991) listed three types of patients for which advance directives are the most important. These individuals include:

1. Patients for whom a legally designated surrogate does not exist or could be controversial, such as an acquired immune deficiency syndrome (AIDS) patient who chooses to designate a long-term mate rather than a parent or sibling

2. Patients with unusual or highly specific preferences
3. Patients and families for whom the existence of a document will reduce anxiety

The Patient Self-Determination Act offers nurses an opportunity for greater participation in decision making. Nurses may enter discussions with patients about their hopes and fears that can be the basis for planning future care. Although one may not always understand the treatment preferences expressed by patients and family members, one can respect the courage required to confront the issues.

GUIDELINES

Advance Directives

1. Nurses should review the state statutes and provisions for durable powers of attorney for health care, natural death acts, and living wills. Realize that the requirements may vary greatly state to state, and have the in-hospital attorney hold classes for nurses so that the nursing staff is fully aware of any statutory requirements and the means by which these advance directives are enforced.
2. Review the hospital policy and procedure manual for any hospital guidelines in this area. If no policies exist, suggest to the committee or persons responsible for such policies the need for guidance in this area.
3. Should the patient or family tell you that a signed advance directive exists, you should make that known to the physician and hospital administration immediately. Document the existence of the declaration in the patient's medical record, and ask for a copy of the declaration for the medical record.
4. Should the patient revoke the declaration or tell the nurse that he or she desires to revoke the declaration, the nurse is obligated to document such in the record and to immediately notify the attending physician and hospital administration. This is true even if the competency of the patient is questionable because some statutes allow for revocation even if the declarant is not of sound mind.
5. It is advisable that the nurse not be a witness to the living will or natural death act because many natural death acts forbid a witness from being employed by the attending physician or facility in which the patient is hospitalized. Usually, a friend or someone unrelated to the patient serves as the witness for this declaration.
6. Should the patient have a copy of the living will or natural death act in his or her medical record, read it carefully to ascertain the scope of its provisions. It is much easier to clarify the declaration while the patient is still competent than to try to clarify directives in the document. Document in the medical record any clarification that the patient gives to you, and ensure that the attending physician also understands the scope of the patient's declaration.
7. In most states, the nurse or another person may write and sign advance directives as proxy of the competent patient. Here, the nurse must be sure that the patient is of sound mind, because competency is an important issue in the execution of such a directive. Document in the record what occurred and the circumstances that made it necessary for a second person to sign for the patient (partial paralysis or whatever the medical reason for the competent patient to be unable to sign).
8. Assist the family members in this time of crisis by being available and by answering as many of their questions as possible. Tell the family members of any existing ethics committee or

other persons available to talk with them. Remember that they need time to internalize what is happening, especially if they are called on to concur with the patient's directive or to insist on the implementation of the patient's directive.

DO-NOT-RESUSCITATE DIRECTIVES

Health care organizations across the nation have initiated **do-not-resuscitate directives** that patients may execute upon admission to health care institutions. Per the patient's request, the physician will then follow hospital policy in attaching such orders to the patient record. Most institutions require documentation that the patient's decision was made after consultation with the physician regarding the patient's diagnoses and prognosis. The order should then be reevaluated according to institution policy.

Selected states are also enacting legislation addressing do-not-resuscitate orders in acute care and long-term care facilities. New York, one of the first states to enact such a law, recognized the need to allow patients and surrogate decision makers the ability to state their preferences for or against resuscitative measures. Other states have followed this lead, with some states enacting laws under the title of "comfort measures only" rather than the harsher do-not-resuscitate verbiage. *Payne v. Marion General Hospital* (1990) represents the first case in this area of the law.

Some states, including New York, in an attempt to balance the competing needs between primary health care providers and surrogate decision makers, require that physicians who disagree with a surrogate decision maker's request for a full code must petition the court to overturn the resuscitation request. Other states, including Texas, handle such disagreements by immunizing the physicians from litigation if the physician enacts a do-not-resuscitate order for patients for whom cardiopulmonary resuscitation would be futile.

Recent cases give some guidance regarding resuscitation issues. *Terry v. Red River Center Corporation* (2006) involved a lawsuit that was filed by the family of a patient who was resuscitated in a nursing home despite three advance directives in her chart, admitted to an acute care facility, and allowed to die based on the hospital's interpretation of the advance directives. The court ruled that the hospital was not at fault for resuscitating the patient. One of the three directives, dated six years earlier, noted that two physicians needed to sign in order for the document to be valid. The directive was only signed by one physician. A second directive allowed the patient to be admitted to an intensive care unit, but disallowed cardiopulmonary resuscitation, which the court noted was an absurd contradiction. The third directive was signed by a family member rather than the patient, thus invalidating the directive. The final holding of the court was that patients should be resuscitated whenever there is doubt as to the patient's true wishes.

Blanchard v. Regency Nursing Home (2007) concerned a 63-year-old patient who sustained a cardiopulmonary arrest; the staff, believing that he was a no-code patient, did not begin cardiopulmonary resuscitation for 15 minutes. Subsequently, it was noted that the patient's directive required a full code. The court upheld the family's award for wrongful death.

King v. Crowell Memorial Home (2001) involved the death of an 84-year-old resident of a nursing home. The son filed this lawsuit, alleging that the patient was improperly classified as a no-code patient by the physician at the nursing home. The son alleged that his father would still be alive if cardiopulmonary resuscitation had been attempted by members of the staff who were present at the time his father coded. The son had previously been named his father's durable power of attorney for health care, and the son claimed that he had instructed the nursing home about his father's desire to be coded in the event such action was necessary. As there was no evidence the son had taken any action toward this end, the court determined that no such request had been made. Additionally, the son offered no proof that his father would not have died, but would have survived if cardiopulmonary resuscitation had occurred.

MATURE MINORS AND THE RIGHT TO DIE

In 1989, the Illinois Supreme Court became the first court in the United States to rule that a minor patient should be permitted to refuse medical treatment necessary to save her life. *In re E. G.* (1989) involved a 17-year-old leukemia patient whose doctors recommended a course of treatment that included a series of blood transfusions. She objected to these blood transfusions based on her religious convictions, and the court upheld this right of refusal. The court stated:

> Although the age of majority in Illinois is 18, that age is not an impenetrable barrier that magically precludes a minor from possessing and exercising certain rights normally associated with adulthood. . . . If the evidence is clear and convincing that the minor is mature enough to appreciate the consequences of her actions . . . then the mature minor doctrine affords her the common law right to consent to or refuse medical treatment. (*In re E. G.*, 1989, at 327–328)

To a great extent, the court in reaching that momentous decision carefully weighed the fact that E. G. was a very mature teenager, and that her religious convictions were based on deeply held, family-shared values. The psychologist testified at court that she had the maturity of a 22-year-old.

The stakes are extraordinarily high in these cases, and legal authorities continue to contend that these issues must be addressed. This is especially true in light of the various standards adopted by states concerning mature minors and their right in deciding issues that concern their welfare. Much of the argument has centered on an agreed definition of maturity, especially in the medical realm. Many courts still rely on the parents and their decision-making capacity. Thus, the question remains whose voice would have the most weight with the courts, those of the mature minors or the parents.

There are two possible answers to this dilemma. One would be to lower the age of medical competency, identifying an age at which minors could either give consent or refuse to give consent. Research indicates that between the ages of 12 and 14, adolescents undergo a major shift in cognitive functioning that enables them to reason abstractly, as well as to consider cause-and-effect relationships (Millstein & Halpern-Felsher, 2002). Thus, there is reason to advocate a standard treating 14-year-olds as competent in health care decision making.

Unfortunately, such an age-based standard creates several problems. It is no less arbitrary than the current standard of 18 as the age of majority. The same research that establishes the adolescent onset of cognitive functioning also recognizes that these abilities are acquired gradually and that they reflect both a biological and an environmental component. Moreover, it is likely that some minors younger than the age of competency will seek to consent to their own health care treatment, reinforcing the same process now in place through the courts.

A second alternative is to adopt a uniform best interest approach, denying all adolescents autonomy until they reach the age of maturity. This standard has the advantage of not having to discern the adolescent's competency or maturity, but also has the disadvantage of taking decision making away from competent minors. Neither of these two approaches is likely to prevail, and the courts will continue to debate such issues.

EXERCISE 8.4

Find out what your hospital does about advance directives. How is the patient apprised of these options, and who assists the patient desiring to complete such a directive? If patients come to your institution with advance directives, how are staff members alerted to their existence? Are any provisions taken to ensure the validity of advance directives prior to a patient's death? Give suggestions you might have for a more effective usage of such documents.

HOSPICE CARE

Some terminally ill patients prevent the need for natural death acts and living wills by entering hospice centers. A **hospice center** allows patients to receive the nursing and medical care that is required and to be kept comfortable, without the fear that they will be resuscitated or placed on life-support systems when death occurs. Most hospice centers and health care facilities have home hospice care that allows patients to receive the benefits of hospice centers in their own homes.

Congress recognized the need for such terminal care apart from the hospital setting and authorized Medicare reimbursement for hospice care (Tax Equity and Fiscal Responsibility Act, 1982). Medicare reimbursement is limited to a 6-month time interval, and this does not indicate that Congress meant that patients with a longer life expectancy should seek or accept more aggressive care.

The problem encountered with hospice centers is that the usual patients seeking such care are competent—the very same patients who could refuse heroic care if they were in a formal hospital setting. Problems encountered with allowing a patient to die are usually confined to incompetent, hospitalized patients.

ASSISTED SUICIDE

Although suicide as a crime has been abolished in all states, most states still prohibit assisted suicide. Some states treat assisted suicide harshly, whereas other states prohibit only causing suicide, not assisting it. Though selected states have tried unsuccessfully through legislation to pass physician assisted suicide (PAS) statutes, Oregon was the first to pass such a statute. A second state has now also voted to adopt such a statute. In November 2008, the citizens of Washington State passed Initiative 1000, which permits **physician-assisted suicide** in the state, effective March 2009. Proposals to consider assisted suicide were considered in California, Vermont, and Hawaii during the 2007 calendar year, though none of these proposals were formally on the 2008 November ballot. Opponents to this type of legislation include the Roman Catholic Church and the American Medical Association as well as the American Nurses Association. The debate against assisted suicide is likely to be rekindled following the report of a 79-year-old German woman who took her life recently not because she was terminally ill, in pain, or suffering, but because she did not wish to be moved to a nursing home ("German Woman's Assisted Suicide," 2008).

The Oregon Death with Dignity Act (DWDA) was first narrowly passed by voters in November 1994, with a 51.3% majority. A ballot measure to seek its repeal, Measure 51, was defeated by a 60% vote on November 4, 1997. The first patients to request life-ending medications did so in 1998. In 2002, United States Attorney General John Ashcroft attempted to suspend the drug-prescribing licenses of physicians who prescribed life-ending medications under the DWDA. In October 2005, the United States Supreme Court heard arguments in the case of *Gonzales v. Oregon*, and on January 17, 2006, that court ruled in favor of Oregon, again upholding the law. There have been no more legal challenges to the law since the *Gonzales* case.

Since its enactment, 341 patients have died under the terms of the law (Summary of Oregon's Death with Dignity Act, 2005). The most frequently cited reasons for obtaining physician-assisted-suicide means were loss of autonomy, decreasing ability to participate in activities that made life enjoyable, and loss of dignity. Additionally, there was a significant increase in the numbers of patients indicating that fear of inadequate pain control prompted their desire for medications to terminate their lives (White, 2007). Table 8.1 recounts case law and major legislative decisions that have led to assisted-suicide standards that currently exist in the United States.

The act allows physicians who choose to participate to write lethal drug prescriptions for competent, terminally ill adults who are residents of the state. Other provisions that must be met before the prescription is written include:

1. Both the attending physician and a consulting physician must certify that the patient is in a terminal state, understands his or her prognosis, and understands feasible alternatives, including, but not limited to, comfort care, hospice care, and pain control.
2. The patient must make an oral and written request for the prescription, signed and dated by the patient and witnessed by at least two individuals who, in the presence of the patient, attest that to the best of their knowledge and belief the patient is capable, acting voluntarily, and is not being coerced to sign the request. Note that the witnesses may not be related in any manner to the patient nor may they be recipients under the patient's will. This must be followed by a second oral request 15 days or more after the first request.
3. The attending physician must determine that the patient is making an informed and voluntary request, verify that the patient has documentation evidencing Oregon residency, can

TABLE 8.1 Rights of the Terminally Ill: Case Law and Major Legislative Decisions

Year	Case/Legislation	Description
1976	*In re Quinlan`*	Right to remove person in prolonged vegetative state from ventilator
1990	*Cruzan v. Director, Missouri Department of Health*	Right given to states to decide whether families can remove artificial feeding tubes from persons in prolonged vegetative states
1991	Patient Self-Determination Act	Requires health care facilities receiving Medicare funds to provide information to patients at the time of admission about advance directives
1994	Oregon Death with Dignity Act	Allows competent terminally ill adult patients to obtain prescriptions for lethal drugs
1995	*Compassion in Dying v. Washington*	Court decision stating that the Washington State ban on the right of terminally ill adult patients to request assistance in committing suicide from a qualified professional was unconstitutional
1997	*Vacco v. Quill* and *Compassion in Dying v. Glucksberg*	Supreme Court rulings that states can ban physician-assisted suicide; states may also legalize and regulate physician-assisted suicide

rescind the request at any time and in any manner, and must offer the patient an opportunity to rescind the request at the end of the 15-day waiting period.

4. If in the opinion of either the attending or consulting physician a patient may be suffering from a psychiatric or psychological disorder or depression causing impaired judgment, either physician shall refer the patient for counseling and no medication to end the patient's life shall be prescribed until the counseling determines that the patient is not suffering from a psychiatric or psychological disorder or depression causing impaired judgment (Oregon Death with Dignity Act, section 127.800 et seq, 2005).

The question of whether mentally competent, terminally ill patients have a constitutional right to seek a physician's aid in ending their lives was answered by the U.S. Supreme Court in 1997. Both Washington and New York state courts had held that their states' attempt to ban physician-assisted suicide violated the constitutional due process rights of terminally ill patients who seek to hasten their deaths by using physician-prescribed medications. At the core of the matter is whether states may distinguish between patients who choose to refuse or withdraw medical treatment (allowing to die) and those who choose to extend this right to include medication-assisted suicide (assisting to die).

The U.S. Supreme Court, in one of the most important decisions of the 1990s, rejected the challenge to the constitutional right of the person to die, and, in essence, said that courts could ban physician-assisted suicides (*Compassion in Dying v. Glucksberg,* 1997; *Vacco v. Quill,* 1997). Although finding no constitutional right to die, the court explicitly left open the door for states to legalize and regulate physician-assisted suicide, if they choose to do so. This decision by the Supreme Court came just months before the Oregon voters passed the Death with Dignity Act for the second time. A Model State Act to Authorize and Regulate Physician-Assisted Suicide was developed to prevent potential managed-care abuses with physician-assisted suicide. The model act requires that four conditions be met before one can receive assistance. These requirements, all having the effect of limiting managed-care abuses, include:

1. The patient must be competent, defined as "based on the patient's ability to understand his or her condition and prognosis, the benefits and burdens of alternative therapy, and the consequences of suicide."
2. The patient must be fully informed.
3. The choice must be voluntary, one that is made independently, free from coercion or undue influences.
4. The choice must be enduring, in that the request must be stated to the responsible physician on at least two occasions that are at least 2 weeks apart, without self-contradiction during that interval (Baron et al., 1996, p. 20).

To date, no states have enacted the model act.

Despite the controversy surrounding this legislation, Oregon's experience with assisted suicide has raised awareness of end-of-life care. Oregon has the largest percentage of in-home hospice deaths, and the majority of individuals who die in Oregon have a written directive or other end-of-life planning in place (Skidmore, 2007).

The nurse's role in this area is still developing. The American Nurses Association (ANA) opposes the movement and opposes nurses' participation either in assisted suicide or active euthanasia because they violate the ethical traditions embodied in the *Code of Ethics for Nurses* (ANA, 1994, 2001). If nurses are asked directly by patients to assist with their suicide, they must refuse. But, before closing the door to open communications, look beyond the request to what the patients may be saying. They may be expressing a need for greater pain control or for someone to talk to about the fears of a terrible death. At this time, nurses must be clear that they cannot assist patients in this aspect, but may be able to assist with procuring medications for more effective pain control or by supplying needed forms to assist patients with advance directives. Another avenue may be to ensure that patients speak with a chaplain or representative of their faith or with a social worker. Ensure that the patients know that someone cares and will assist them in ways that nursing can intervene.

In recognition of the universal need for humane end-of-life care, the American Association of Colleges of Nursing (AACN), supported by a Robert Wood Johnson Foundation grant, convened a roundtable of nurse experts and other health care providers to begin communications surrounding this area. This roundtable was in accord with the 1997 International Council of Nurses mandate that nurses have a unique and primary responsibility for ensuring that individuals at the end of life experience a peaceful death. This group of experts in health care ethics and palliative care developed the End-of-Life Competency Statements (AACN, 1999). While developed as terminal objectives for undergraduate nursing students, they apply to all nursing professionals.

ETHICAL ISSUES

A variety of ethical issues underlie content in the area of informed consent and patient self-determination. Informed consent involving adolescents is but one issue that has legal and ethical components for health care providers who treat adolescents as well as for legislators who formulate and implement consent policies for adolescents. The American Medical Association (AMA) has long advocated the need for health care providers to involve adolescents in the decision-making process, especially when the decisions concern care for the adolescent (AMA, 2003). Though the parents generally have the legal right to either consent or not to consent for their child, there is a "need to respect the rights and autonomy of every individual, regardless of age" (Kunin, 1997, p. 44). Implications for expanding the consent rights of minors are immense, especially as states consider expanding the right of mature minors to consent for needed medical therapies and those states that have already expanded the mature minors' right of consent have done so with adequate research regarding how adolescents reach health care treatment decisions in real-life situations.

A second issue with informed consent relates to the concept that merely because an individual has reached the age of maturity within a given state, that individual is able to either consent to or refuse consent for medical care and treatments. One of the hallmarks of informed consent is comprehension by the individual from whom consent is requested. Over the years, it has been suggested that for elective procedures one should give the person all the information needed for informed consent and then wait at least 24 hours before securing the consent. The premise is that a 24-hour delay in signing informed consent forms allows the person sufficient time to better understand what is being requested and sufficient time to have his or her questions answered. How do health care providers begin to determine the level of comprehension needed to assure that informed consent is truly informed? Does the fact that one is 18 years of age enhance his or her comprehension of needed medical facts?

Ethical issues also surface in the use of the best interest test for persons who are incompetent to either consent to or refuse medical interventions. Health care providers and the courts view the substituted judgment test for determining how an incompetent person would have consented or not consented as more tolerable because it is predicated on what a person actually said and/or did while he or she was still in a competent state. The whole issue of advance directives is predicated on this type of substituted judgment. The best interest test, an objective means of viewing what another thinks is the best choice for an incapacitated person, has no such guidance, as the person for whom the decision is made often never reached the age of competency. Scholars continue to debate the issue of best interest and how one begins to address what is truly better for an incompetent person who was never competent (Baumrucker, Sheldon, Stolick, & vandeKieft, 2008).

A final ethical question that is paramount today involves the entire question of physician-assisted death. As additional states attempt to expand the Oregon experience, ethical questions have surfaced regarding the need for such legal measures given the advances made during the past 5 to 10 years. Quill (2008) notes that there are four other last-resort options available to persons in the final stages of their lives:

- Right to intensive pain and symptom management
- Right to forgo life-sustaining therapy
- Voluntary stopping eating and drinking
- Sedation to unconsciousness (pp. 18–19)

Additionally, the prospect that palliative care and hospice care will further expand to more completely assist patients and families during the final stages of life is quite possible. Hospice, the gold standard for care at the end of life, has as its challenge the design of programs "that would allow patients to simultaneously continue some disease-directed therapies in order to serve a wider range of dying patients" (Quill, 2008, p. 19).

EXERCISE 8.5

Select one of the four ethical issues discussed in the previous section and describe how therapeutic jurisprudence could begin to resolve this issue. Review Chapter 2 for a discussion on therapeutic jurisprudence.

SUMMARY

- Informed consent involves two separate components: the person must be fully informed so that he or she can make an informed choice and the consent must be voluntary.
- Informed refusal mandates that the patient be fully informed of the risks of not complying with recommended interventions.
- Elements of informed consent include:
  - Brief explanation of the intervention
  - Name and qualifications of the persons performing the procedure
  - An explanation of any serious harm that might occur
  - An explanation of alternative therapies to the intervention
  - Right to refuse the proposed intervention

- Right to refuse further treatment even after the intervention is started
- Forms for informed consent are expresses, implied, written or oral, complete, and partial.
- Standards of informed consent are the physician-based and patient-based standards, though a newer shared medical decision-making model is emerging.
- There are four exceptions to informed consent: emergency situations, therapeutic privilege, patient waiver, and prior patient knowledge.
- The primary health care provider has the responsibility for obtaining informed consent, though others can create accountability through their actions.

- Specific and blanket consent forms describe the two types of forms that exist in health care institutions today.
- Competent adults are generally the individuals from whom consent is requested.
- Legal guardians or representatives have the ability to consent for incompetent adults.
- Parents have the right of consent for their children except in the few instances where laws give the minor the right to consent for himself or herself.
- There are three limitations on the right of the person to refuse consent:
  - Preservation of life
  - Protection of minor dependents
  - Protection of the public's health
- Informed consent is required for research studies and is governed by federal statutes.
- Health literacy concerns the degree to which individuals have the capacity to obtain, process, and understand basic health information.
- The Patient Self-Determination Act involves the right of individuals to decide what will or will not happen to their bodies.
- The best interest test is an objective test that allows a person to determine what one thinks would be in the best interest of another person and then pursue a plan of care.
- Substituted judgment, a subjective test, attempts to determine how persons, were they capable of making their opinions and wishes known, would have chosen to exercise their right to refuse therapy.
- Types of advance directives include living wills, natural death acts, durable powers of attorney for health care, medical or physician directives, and do-not-resuscitate directives.
- The Physician Orders for Life-Sustaining Treatment was developed to assure that patients' wishes concerning resuscitation, life-sustaining treatments, and hydration and nutrition would be honored by responding emergency medical personnel and acute care facilities.
- Oregon and Washington State are the only states that allow physician-assisted suicide.
- Some of the ethical issues concern informed consent for adolescents, how to ensure that the patient fully comprehends proposed therapies, and use of the best interest test for incompetent adults.

APPLY YOUR LEGAL KNOWLEDGE

1. Does the distinction between consent and informed consent have implications for professional health care providers?
2. What should the nurse do when told by a patient that he or she has an advance directive?
3. How does the nurse decide if a patient's consent is truly voluntary and informed?
4. What type of role should nurses have in securing informed consent? In assisting with research studies? In assisting with genetic testing?
5. How do you incorporate end-of-life competencies in your daily nursing practice?

YOU BE THE JUDGE

The patient was to undergo a fundoplication surgery to repair an esophageal hernia. This procedure involves the insertion of an esophageal dilator, which at this institution is performed by the anesthesia team. In this particular instance, the dilator was to be inserted by a nursing anesthesia student. The student introduced herself to the patient immediately before the procedure. She used her first name only and stated that she was a registered nurse who would be working with the nurse anesthetist and the anesthesiologist. The student referred to the nurse anesthetist by first and last names and to the anesthesiologist using the term *doctor* and his last name.

During the insertion of the dilator, the student tore the lining of the esophagus. This required an open procedure to be performed, which resulted in complications for the patient. The patient sued for lack of informed consent, inadequate supervision, and negligence. Specifically, the patient argued that he had the right to know if a student was to perform any part of the procedure and that he had the right to refuse such participation.

The court returned a verdict in favor of the patient on the part of inadequate supervision. As stated in the institution's written policies, the student was to be supervised by an anesthesiologist, not merely a nurse anesthetist.

QUESTIONS

1. Is the patient correct in asserting that he has a right to know the names and status of individuals who will be performing this procedure?
2. Does the manner in which the student introduced herself and the two other team members have relevance in this case?
3. Was the informed consent deficient to the degree that there was a lack of informed consent by the patient?
4. How would you decide this case?

REFERENCES

Allen v. Rockford Health Systems, Inc., 2006 WL 1195525 (Ill. App., May 2, 2006).

American Association of Colleges of Nursing. (1999). *Peaceful death: Recommended competencies and curricular guidelines for end-of-life nursing care.* Washington, DC: Author.

American Medical Association. (2003). *Confidential care for minors.* Chicago, IL: Author.

American Nurses Association. (1994). *Position statement on active euthanasia.* Washington, DC: Author.

American Nurses Association. (2001). *Code of ethics with interpretive statements.* Washington, DC: Author.

Anderson v. Louisiana State University, 2006 WL 2956492 (La. App., October 17, 2006).

Andrews, L. B., Fullarton, J. E., et al. (Eds.). (1994). *Assessing genetic risks: Implications for health and social policy.* Washington, DC: National Academy Press.

Andrus, M. R., & Roth, M. T. (2002). Health literacy: A review. *Pharmacotherapy, 22*(3), 282–302.

Auler v. Van Natta, 686 N.E.2d 172 (Ind. App., 1997).

Baron, C. H., et al. (1996). A model state act to authorize and regulate physician-assisted suicide. *Harvard Journal on Legislation, 33*, 1–34.

Bartling v. Superior Court, 163 Cal. App.3d 186, 209 Cal. Rptr. 220 (Cal. App. Ct. 2d Dis., 1984).

Baumrucker, S. J., Sheldon, J. E., Stolick, M., & vandeKieft, G. (2008). The ethical concept of "best interest." *American Journal of Hospice and Palliative Medicine, 25*(1), 56–62.

Beeman v. Covenant Health Care, 2006 WL 3733259 (Mich. App., December 19, 2006).

Blanchard v. Regency Nursing Home, 2007 WL 4616732 (Sip. Ct, Pierce Co., Washington, June 14, 2007).

Bouvia v. Superior Court, 179 Cal. App.3d 1127, 225 Cal. Rptr. 297 (Cal. App. Ct. 2d. Dis., 1986).

Breithaupt v. Adams, 352 U.S. 432 (1957).

Caldwell v. Anekwe, 2008 WL 3497829 (Ind. App., August 14, 2008).

Compassion in Dying v. Glucksberg, 117 S. Ct. 2258 (1997).

Compassion in Dying v. Washington, 49 F. 3d. 586 (1995).

Conservatorship of Wendland, 28 P.3d 151 (California, 2001).

Cruzan v. Director, Missouri Department of Health, 497 U.S. 261, 110 S. Ct. 2841, 111 L.E.D. 2d 224 (1990).

Daniel Thor v. Superior Court of Solano County, 855 P.2d 375, 21 Cal. Rptr. 2d 357 (Cal., 1993).

Department of Health and Human Services. (2000). *Healthy people 2010.* Washington, DC: Government Printing Office Publishers.

Eichner v. Dillon, 73 App. Div.2d 431, 426 N.Y.S.2d 517 (2d. Dept., 1980).

Estate of Neumann v. Morse Geriatric Center, 2007 WL 1828700 (Cir. Cy. Palm Beach Co., Florida, March 7, 2007); second hearing WL 1159236 (March 16, 2007).

56 *Federal Register*, 28012-22, June 18, 1991, as amended at 70 *Federal Register* 36328, June 23, 2005.

45 *Code of Federal Regulations* 46.401 et seq. (1998).

Genetic Information Nondiscrimination Act of 2008, Public Law 110-233, 122 *Statutes* 881, May 21, 2008.

Gerety v. Demers, 589 P. 2d 180 (New Mexico, 1978).

German woman's assisted suicide fuels debate. (2008). Reuters Communications. Available online at http://www.msnbc.msn.com/id/25482205/print/1/displaymode/1098/

Gonzales v. Oregon, 546 U. S. 243 (2006).

Grabowski v. Quigley, 684 A.2d 610 (Pa. Super., 1996).

Grace Plaza of Great Neck, Inc. v. Elbaum, 82 N.Y.2d 10 (New York, 1993).

Guardianship of Baker, 2006 WL 2875822 (Ohio App., October 5, 2006).

Hannoy v. State, 2003 WL 21321386 (Ind. App., June 10, 2003).

Haymes v. Brookdale Hospital Medical Center, 731 N.Y.S.2d 215 (N.Y. App., 2001).

HCA, Inc. v. Miller, 36 S.W.3d 187 (Tex. App., 2000).

Health Insurance Portability and Accountability Act of 1996, Public Law 104-191 (1996).

Hinman v. Russo, 2006 WL 2226333 (D. N. J., August 2, 2006).

In re E. G., 4549 N.E.2d 322 (Illinois, 1989).

In re Easly, 721 A.2d 844 (Pa. Cmwlth., 2001).

In re Fiori, 652 A.2d 1350 (Pennsylvania, 1995).

In re Hamilton, 657 S.W.2d 425 (Tenn. App., 1983).

In re Nellie G., 2007 WL 678256 (N.Y. App., March 6, 2007).

In re Quinlan, 70 N.J. 10, 335 A.2d 647 (1976).

In re Susan Jane G., 2006 WL 2925210 (N.Y. App., October 10, 2006)

Jefferson v. Griffin Spalding County Hospital Authority, 247 Ga. 86, 274 S.E.2d 457 (1981).

John F. Kennedy Memorial Hospital v. Heston, 58 N.J. 576 (1971).

King v. Crowell Memorial Home, 622 N.W.2d 588 (Nebraska, 2001).

Kinikin v. Heupel, 305 N. W. 2d 589 (Minnesota, 1981).

Kunin, H. (1997). Ethical issues in pediatric life-threatening illnesses: Dilemmas of consent, assent, and communication. *Ethics and Behavior, 7,* 43–57.

Lauder, B., & Gabel-Jorgensen, N. (2008). Recent research on health literacy, medication adherence, and patient outcomes. *Home Healthcare Nurse, 26*(4), 253–257.

Leach v. Akron General Medical Center, 13 Ohio App.3d 393, 469 N.E.2d 1047 (Ohio, 1984).

Luettke v. St. Vincent Mercy Medical Center, 2006 WL 2105049 (Ohio App., July 28, 2006).

Lugenbuhl v. Dowling, 676 So.2d 602 (La. App., 1996).

Lynn, J. (1991). Why I don't have a living will. *Law Medicine and Healthcare, 19,* 101–104.

Madison v. Harrison, #68651 (Massachusetts, 1957).

Maniaci, M. J., Heckman, M. G., & Dawson, N. L. (2008). Functional health literacy and understanding of medications at discharge. *Mayo Clinical Proceedings, 83*(5), 554–558.

Mathias v. St. Catherine's Hospital, Inc., 569 N.W.2d 330 (Wis. App., 1997).

Matter of Anna M. Gordy, 658 A.2d 613 (Delaware, 1994).

Matter of Roche, 687 A.2d 349 (N.J. Super. Ch., 1996).

Millstein, S. G., & Halpern-Felsher, B. L. (2002). Judgments about risk and perceived invulnerability in adolescents and young adults. *Journal of Research on Adolescence, 12*(4), 399–422.

Muskopk v. Maron, 2003 WL 22257518 (N.Y. App., October 2, 2003).

National Institutes of Health. (1998). *NIH policy and guidelines on the inclusion of children as participants in research involving human subjects.* Rockville, MD: Author.

O'Brien v. Cunard Steamship Company, 154 Mass. 272, 28 N.E. 226 (1899).

Oregon Death with Dignity Act. (2005). *Oregon Revised Statutes.* Sections 127.800–127.995.

Patient Self-Determination Act, Sections 4206 and 4751 of the Omnibus Reconciliation Act of 1990, Public Law 101-508, November 1990.

Payne v. Marion General Hospital, 549 N.E.2d 1043 (Ind. App. 2d Dis., 1990).

Physician orders for life-sustaining treatment state programs. (2008). Available online at http://www.ohsu.edu/ethics/polst/programs/state+programs.htm.

Protection of Human Subjects, 45 *Code of Federal Regulations,* Sec. 46.111, 46.101(b), 46.110, 46.116 (1991).

Protection of Human Subjects, 45 *Code of Federal Regulations,* Sec. 46.101(a)(2) (1997).

Protection of Human Subjects, 45 *Code of Federal Regulations,* Sec. 46.401 *et seq.* (1998).

Quill, T. (2008). Physician-assisted death in the United States: Are the existing "last resorts" enough? *Hastings Center Report, 38*(5), 17–22.

Roberts, D. (2008). Nursing antidotes for poor health literacy. *MedSurg Nursing, 17*(2), 75.

Rochin v. California, 342 U.S. 165 (1950).

Rogers v. T. J. Samson Community Hospital, 276 F.3d 228 (6th Cir., 2002).

Rouse, F. (1991). Patients, providers, and the Patient Self-Determination Act. *Hastings Center Report, 21*(1), S2–S3.

Ruppel v. Ramsever, 33 F. Supp.2d 720 (C.D. Ill., 1999).

Salgo v. Leland Stanford, Jr. University Board of Trustees, 317 P.2d 170 (Cal. Dis. Ct. App., 1957).

Scanlon, C., & Fibison, W. (1995). *Managing genetic information: Implications for nursing practice.* Washington, DC: American Nurses Association.

Scheible v. Morse Geriatric Center, 2007 WL 4523047 (Cir. Ct. Palm Beach Co., Florida, March 16, 2007).

Schloendorff v. Society of New York Hospitals, 211 N.Y. 125, 105 N.E. 92 (1914).

Schmerber v. California, 384 U.S. 757 (1966).

Shine v. Vega, 709 N.E.2d 58 (Massachusetts, 1999).

Skidmore, S. (2007, October 27). A decade later, Oregon still only assisted suicide state. *The Columbian.* 116 (179), A3.

Summary of Oregon's Death with Dignity Act. (2007). Available online at http://www.oregon.gov/DHS/ph/pas/docs/year10.pdf

Superintendent of Belchertown State School v. Saikewicz, 373 Mass. 728, 370 N.E.2d 417 (1977).

Tax Equity and Fiscal Responsibility Act of 1982, Public Law 97-248 (September 3, 1982).

Terry v. Red River Center Corporation, 2006 WL 3307399 (La. App., November 15, 2006).

Tobin v. Providence Hospital, 624 N.W.2d 548 (Mich. App., 2001).

Truman v. Thomas, 27 Cal.3d 285, 611 P.2d 902 (1980).

21 Code of Federal Reglations, Parts 50, 56, 312, 314, and 812 (2001).

Vacco v. Quill, 117 S. Ct. 2293 (1997).

van den Heever, P. (2005). Pleading the defense of therapeutic privilege. *South African Medical Journal, 95*(6), 420–421.

Wecker v. Amend, 918 P.2d 658 (Kan. App., 1996).

Wells v. Storey, 792 So.2d 1034 (Alabama, 1999).

White, H. (2007). Eighth annual Oregon assisted suicide report shorter with more ambiguous language. Available online at http://www.lifesite.net/ldn/printerfriendly.html

CHAPTER 9

Documentation and Confidentiality

PREVIEW

A major responsibility of all health care providers is that they keep accurate and complete patient medical records. Much of what is collected and recorded remains sensitive information. Understanding the need for clear and concise records and knowing which portions of the record may be discovered and introduced during trials enables nurses to be proficient recorders of patient care in all health care settings. The newer areas of confidentiality concern computer documents, electronic resources, and the multiple applications of the Health Insurance Portability and Accountability Act of 1996. This chapter presents guidelines for documentation in patient records and incident reports, and presents pointers for assuring patient confidentiality.

LEARNING OUTCOMES
After completing this chapter, you should be able to:

9.1 Discuss purposes of the medical record.

9.2 Define and describe basic information to be included in the medical record.

9.3 List and give examples of guidelines for accurate documentation.

9.4 Analyze the concepts of:
   a. Alteration of records
   b. Retention of records
   c. Ownership of the medical record
   d. Access to medical records
   e. Computerized charting

9.5 Describe important aspects of incident reports.

9.6 Compare and contrast charting by exception to traditional charting.

9.7 Define *confidentiality* and relate that concept to:
   a. Substance abuse conferences
   b. AIDS/HIV conferences
   c. Access laws
   d. Child/elder abuse conferences
   e. Electronic mail and Internet service

9.8 Define and analyze applications of the Health Insurance Portability and Accountability Act of 1996 (HIPAA).

9.9 Describe reporting and access laws, including the common law duty to disclose and limitations to disclosure.

9.10 Analyze some of the ethical issues involved in documentation and patient confidentiality.

KEY TERMS

alteration of records

charting by exception

common law duty to disclose

computerized charting

confidentiality of medical
    records

covered entities

effective documentation

electronic health record

electronic medical record

Health Insurance Portability
    and Accountability Act
    (HIPAA)

incident, variance,
    situational, or unusual
    occurrence report forms

medical records

omnia praesumuntur contra
    spoliatorem

patient access to medical
    records

patient's right to privacy

protected health information
    (PHI)

retention of records

MEDICAL RECORDS

Medical records and a medical records library are mandated by federal governmental and non-governmental agencies. Additionally, agencies such as the Joint Commission (JC) and state and local rules and regulations further define this complex area.

From a nursing perspective, the most important purpose of documentation is communication. Among the purposes for the medical record are to:

1. Assist in planning and evaluating patient care and recommending a patient's continuing treatment.
2. Document the course of the patient's care, including responses to treatment, and communications among health care providers responsible for the patient's care.
3. Protect legal interests of the patient, health care facility, and health care providers.
4. Provide data for use in continuing education and in research.

Thus, these records not only record what has transpired, but also serve as a vital communication link among members of the health care team and a resource for further educational and research programs.

Contents of the Record

Basic information that should be recorded for any patient includes:

1. Personal data such as name, date of birth, gender, marital status, occupation, and person(s) to be contacted for emergencies
2. Financial data such as health insurance carrier with assignment of rights, patient employer, and person responsible for payment of the final bill
3. Medical data

These final data entries form the bulk of the record and include, but are not limited to, a history of signs and symptoms, diagnoses, treatments, medical tests, laboratory results, consultation reports, anesthesia and operating room records, signed informed consent forms, progress notes, nurses' notes, and records of a variety of departments such as respiratory therapy, dietary consultations, occupational therapy, and physical therapy.

Documentation of nursing care should be reflective of the individual patient status. Thus, nurses' notes should address patient needs, problems, limitations, and patient responses to nursing interventions. Individualized, goal-directed nursing care is provided to patients. Each patient's nursing needs are assessed by a registered nurse at the time of admission or within the period established by the nursing department/service policy. Patient education and patient/family knowledge of self-care are given specific consideration in the nursing plan. Pertinent patient quotes about symptoms and feelings should be included in the medical record. It is advisable to use some form of nursing process in charting so that no pertinent information is overlooked or forgotten.

Documentation must show continuity of care, interventions that were implemented, and patient responses to the therapies implemented. Nurses' notes are to be concise, clear, timely, and complete. Even if the patient condition does not change, that absence of change should be recorded at least once per shift. The complete patient assessment performed by the nurse caring for a selected patient should be reflected, in its entirety, in the patient's medical record.

EFFECTIVE DOCUMENTATION

The American legal system has helped nurses recognize what must be included in charting and, through case law, has given tips on how to chart entries correctly. These tips for **effective documentation** are enumerated in the following paragraphs.

Make an Entry for Every Observation

If no mention has been made of a change in a patient's condition, the jury can infer that no observation of the patient was conducted. In *Columbia Medical Center v. Meier* (2006), an elderly patient was admitted to the hospital's intensive care unit for adult respiratory distress syndrome (ARDS) and septic shock. He was sedated, given paralytics, intubated, and placed on a ventilator. During this admission, he developed a serious decubitus ulcer on his coccyx. Four weeks after his admission, he was transferred to a rehabilitation facility. While in the rehabilitation center, he developed decubitus ulcers on both of his heels. Two months later, he was again transferred, this time to a Veterans Administration facility, specifically for treatment of the decubitus ulcer on his coccyx. After several months, the ulcer was fully healed.

The patient sued the first hospital for failure to prevent and/or adequately treat his developing decubitus ulcer. The legal focus was whether the development or progression of a skin lesion was avoidable or was unavoidable because of the patient's medical condition despite the health care providers being able to show that all necessary care and treatment for skin integrity was given to the patient. The court first examined the various means by which an ulcer could have been avoided or treated, including skin assessment, frequent repositioning of the patient and use of foam pads to provide pressure relief. If the patient cannot tolerate turning due to adverse changes in his medical condition, then that fact must be carefully documented.

In this case, there was no documentation that the nurses implemented any of the interventions that would have prevented the pressure ulcer from becoming more severe once it was discovered. The physician was informed of the developing pressure sore the next day rather than when first discovered. A wound-care nurse consultation was ordered as well as a special bed. The only follow-up to these orders were that the nurse consultant saw the patient three days later and there was no notation that orders she gave were ever incorporated into the care plan or were being implemented. Absence of documentation, said the court, leads to only one conclusion, and that is that the care was not performed, and failure to provide care is negligence. The patient was awarded a jury verdict of $240,000.

In *Sam v. State of New York* (2007), a 1-month-old premature infant in the hospital's neonatal intensive care unit had IV fluid infusing through an IV site on her right calf. The night nurse noted at midnight that the IV was infusing well and a nursing note written at 1:00 A.M. did not mention the IV or the site of the IV. At 2:30 A.M., the nurse found the IV site swollen and discolored from the infiltration of fluid in the surrounding tissue. The IV was discontinued and the child now has a permanent residual cosmetic deformity on her right lower leg.

Hospital policy stated that the IV site for these patients was to be checked every 30 minutes. An expert was to testify that the site should be checked at least every 60 minutes, which is the national standard of care for such patients. There was evidence that the nurse had initialed the IV flow sheet every 30 minutes, though it was inconclusive if the initials indicated the amount of fluid received or that the IV site was checked. The hospital settled the case for $650,000.

The lesson from this case is that even routine checks of patients must be recorded, because failure to record such data leads to the inference that the patient had not been checked. The nurse attempted to show that there had been some patient assessment, but it was clear from the nursing notes that this patient was not adequately assessed.

A similar finding occurred in *Webb v. Tulane Medical Center Hospital* (1997). In this case, a 23-year-old man had been diagnosed with sickle cell anemia when he was less than a year old. He had suffered poor health throughout his short life, with continued bouts of pneumonia and repeated sickle cell crises. He was admitted to the acute care setting for intravenous antibiotics and pain medications and discharged on oral antibiotics after 7 days. He was told to report for a follow-up visit in the hospital's sickle cell clinic 6 days after discharge.

On the morning of his clinic visit, he came in, stating that he had chest and abdominal pain. He was not immediately seen by the physician, but was admitted to the acute care setting through the emergency center with a diagnosis of multiple pulmonary infarcts. The patient continued to deteriorate. His chest pain continued, he developed a low-grade fever, and antibiotics had little effect on his overall condition.

At midnight, the physician ordered and the nurses started two units of packed cells to transfuse over a total of approximately 8 hours, and they were completed about 8:00 A.M. By noon, the patient's temperature was 103.8°F, and he was having more severe chest and abdominal pain. The physician was notified, blood gases were drawn, and the patient was coded about 10 minutes later.

A visiting friend had called for help. The patient was revived after a lengthy code but remained comatose in the intensive care unit until his death 7 days later.

At trial, the patient's mother prevailed against the hospital. The Court of Appeals agreed with the trial judge's belief that there was evidence of nursing negligence. The court agreed that, once the blood transfusion was begun, the patient should have been observed frequently and carefully monitored for potential complications. Failure to do so, said the court, is a breach of the legal standard of care for nursing practice.

The court also believed that, although the blood transfusion had been completed for more than 4 hours, his continued high fever, chest pains, labored breathing, and abdominal pain warranted close monitoring by the nurses. Failure of nursing staff to provide such close monitoring was also a breach of the nursing standard of care. The courts found a serious problem with the fact that there were no nursing notes charted after 10:00 A.M. that any nurse had checked on the patient. Thus, the court concluded that no care had been given for the 2 to 3 hours just prior to this patient's arrest.

Ultimately, the nurses were found not to be liable for the patient's death because an autopsy revealed that the cause of death had been a cardiopulmonary infarct acutely precipitated by aspiration of vomitus, a sudden event that could have happened even with the closest of monitoring and the best nursing care possible. The court believed that this was the end stage of a tragic progression of the sickle cell disease.

Conversely, the court also accepts charted notes as true indications of interventions and the patients' reactions to these interventions. *Pludra v. Life Care Center of America, Inc.* (2004) illustrates this concept. An 83-year-old man was admitted to the nursing home with a diagnosis of terminal cancer. In the nursing home, nursing assistants three times found him on the floor in his room. The third time he broke his left femur and was readmitted to the hospital. He coded three days later and died.

The family sued the nursing home, alleging negligence in that the patient's bed rails were not raised as per policy, nor was a bed alarm used for this patient. This allegation was discounted in favor of the nursing flow charting and progress notes. In those documents, the flow charting clearly showed that the bed rails were up consistently and the nursing progress notes indicated that the patient himself had continuously disconnected the bed alarm. The court believed what was charted, and the case was dismissed.

Bogner v. Rahway Hospital (2008) and *Persing v. Unnamed Hospital* (2007) both illustrate that nursing documentation can accurately dispute a patient's testimony. In the first case, the patient testified that she rang her call buzzer for 30 to 45 minutes for assistance to help her to the bathroom, then arose on her own and leaned on her bed-side table, which rolled and caused her to fall. She sustained a hip fracture.

The nurse had spoken to the patient soon after the fall and documented the fall and what the patient had said at the time of the fall. The patient said she wanted to get up and see what was happening on the other side of the room and tripped on the leg of the tray table. She never mentioned that the call bell was not working or had not been answered. Though the patient had been a high-risk fall precaution, the physician had ordered that she could be up ad lib for bathroom privileges and the high-risk fall precautions had been discontinued.

In *Persing*, a 60-year-old patient was in a transitional care unit for rehabilitation following a pelvic fracture at home. He fell while in the hospital and suffered a new right hip and right femur fracture. The patient claimed his medications made him disoriented and that his nurses knew he had been trying to get out of bed by himself. He claimed he used his call light to call for help getting to the bathroom and, when no one responded, he got up on his own and fell. Additionally, he testified that he was supposed to have nonslip hospital slippers, but instead was wearing ordinary socks at the time he fell.

The nurses caring for him had documented their assessment of his mental status relative to fall risk. He had sufficient safety awareness to know he needed to call and wait for assistance before trying to get out of bed. Restraints were not used, as they were not appropriate for a patient with his level of adequate safety awareness. Further, the nursing notes documented that the patient did not call for assistance before his fall. The courts in both of these cases found no liability on the part of the nursing staff.

Follow-Up as Needed

Merely charting changes in patient status may not be adequate. The landmark decision of *Darling v. Charleston Community Memorial Hospital* (1965) showed that follow-up measures must be taken. James Darling, an 18-year-old high school football player, had broken his leg during a Saturday afternoon game and had the leg casted at the local hospital. Following the casting, he was admitted for observation. The nursing staff continued to assess Darling's casted leg, noting repeatedly in the patient record his deteriorating condition, the foul odor being emitted from the casted extremity, and the patient's ever-increasing pain. The nurses did share their observations with the primary physician, but took no further action when the primary physician failed to take corrective action.

EXERCISE 9.1

The patient died at age 83 due to complications associated with her diagnosis of Huntington's Chorea. The court noted that this particular disease is a progressive genetic disorder for which there is no cure and the patient is at risk for skin breakdown. When she entered the rehabilitation center, her skin was essentially intact. Her care plan included frequent repositioning, daily monitoring of skin integrity, and for her physician and family to be notified of redness or any skin breakdown.

She was subsequently transferred to an acute care facility. On admission, the nursing assessment noted that the patient had lacerations on her toes and feet with poor skin condition on both buttocks. Her right heel was bruised and there were areas of redness on both heels. The family brought a lawsuit against the rehabilitation facility for negligence.

How should the court rule in this case? What evidence would be most relevant for the court to examine in determining its findings?

The court concluded that the follow-up and evaluation of the patient's responses were equally important to the initial assessment. The nurses had a further duty to the patient, the court said, and merely assessing and charting Darling's condition were insufficient. The court also inferred that proper documentation, no matter how accurate and timely it is, can never be a substitute for quality nursing care. Rather, the nursing staff should have reported their observations and lack of subsequent medical interventions to the nursing supervisor. The supervisor should have consulted the medical chief for the service.

Complete records, though, may help to protect the staff from legal liability. In *Anderson v. United States* (2006), an elderly gentleman fell at home, breaking his hip. He was initially treated at a Veterans Administration (VA) hospital and then a nursing home. At some point in his care, he also sustained a wrist fracture. He filed lawsuits against both the VA facility and the nursing home. The nursing home settled out of court.

The court found that there was no negligence on the part of the VA facility based on the completeness of the nursing documentation. The patient's thorough initial assessment on arrival included complaints of hip pain but no left-sided wrist symptoms. The nurse made specific note of his age, fall history, mobility problems, generalized weakness, medications, and substance abuse, all of which indicated that he was a high risk for falls. The 24-hour nursing flow sheet was carefully and completely documented each day he was in the facility. Early flow sheets documented reports of pain and signs of edema in his left wrist, for which he was treated, and nursing progress notes for the same time interval noted that the edema had abated within a 2-day period.

A few days after admission, he developed dementia and required restraints. While in restraints, he was checked frequently by the staff and the flow sheets include having a nurse check the tightness of the restraints at least every hour to ensure proper positioning, circulation, and skin integrity. The daily flow sheets during this time made no mention of any pain, swelling, deformity, or instability of either wrist.

In contrast, the court noted, there was an 11-day period after his initial admission to the nursing home for which the nursing notes and order sheets were totally blank. On the 12th day, there was a nursing note stating that the patient was complaining of left-wrist pain, his left forearm was swollen, and there was a definite deformity of the wrist. The note also indicated that the patient was a poor historian and the nurse was not able to determine when or how this wrist injury had occurred.

Read Nurses' Notes Before Giving Care

Few nurses have been encouraged to read the nurses' notes prior to caring and/or charting for a patient. By taking the time to read the entry prior to the current one, it is possible to determine whether there has been a change in the patient's condition. Even physicians have a duty to read nurses' notes, the court concluded in *Garcia v. San Antonio Community Hospital* (2002). There, a newborn and his mother were dismissed from the hospital 23 hours after his birth. The infant had not passed a stool during the time he was hospitalized and the nurse instructed the mother to contact the physician if the infant did not pass stool within a day. The mother called the physician several times over the next 5 days. She told the physician that the infant had not passed a stool, was irritable, and had a decreased appetite. The physician, rather than having the infant brought to the office for a physical examination, told the mother to give him laxatives and over-the-counter medications for flatus.

At 6 days of age, the infant was diagnosed with an obstructed and perforated bowel. The court ruled that the nurses had not deviated from the standards of care, but had followed hospital protocol. They had charted that the infant had no stool. The infant was not in the hospital for 24 hours, and all of the information was in the record if the physician had read it.

Two additional court cases also concluded that physicians have a duty to read nursing notes (*Estate of Mahunik v. Hebron*, 2007; *Ploch v. Hamia*, 2006). In this latter case, the court concluded that it was below the legal standard of care for a physician not to read the nursing notes before discharging a patient.

A case that specifically mandates that the chart be reviewed by the nurse prior to beginning a surgical case is *Fox v. Department of Health* (2008). In *Fox*, the surgeon began a hysterectomy on a patient, unaware that the patient was pregnant. He was subsequently censured by the state medical board. In his defense, the circulating nurse testified at court that it is routine for the nurse to review the patient's record before the case is started. Any information that needs to be brought to the surgeon's attention should be done prior to beginning the case, including critical tests that may be missing from the record.

In this case, the court held that it was not below a physician's standard of care to rely on the preoperative nurse for results of preoperative tests. In this case, there was no printout of the pregnancy test in the patient's record and the circulating nurse reportedly told the surgeon that the patient's pregnancy test was negative.

Always Make an Entry, Even If It Is Late

Record entries must be timely, charted as close to the happening as possible. Time dulls even the best memories, and a nurse may have to strain to recall what actually transpired. Too often, valuable information is then omitted for lack of recall. If one must chart after the fact, it is more important that all pertinent data are included rather than preserving the chronological order of the chart. To show timeliness, remember to include the complete date and time of charting in the entry. The use of military or 24-hour time has aided in accuracy of timed entries.

Davis v. Montgomery County Memorial Hospital (2006) illustrates the difficulty with late entries. In this case, a patient had been transferred for skilled rehabilitation following hip replacement surgery. During her stay at the skilled facility as she was being assisted to the bathroom, she fell and was injured. The certified nursing aide (CNA) testified that he had placed a gait belt around the patient's waist before he helped her to stand and then assessed the patient for dizziness. The patient stated that she was not dizzy, but on her way to the bathroom she lost her balance and fell. The patient testified that the CNA had come to assist her and placed his arm around her waist and then helped her walk toward the bathroom. When he reached his arm out to move the privacy curtain, she lost her balance and fell.

A nurse had actually documented the incident with a late entry into the patient's record. The late entry did not mention a gait belt and the nurse could not remember later in court if a gait belt was used. The court ultimately ruled in favor of the patient and against the facility.

There is no rule against charting out of time sequence, and a late entry is far superior to no entry at all. However, the longer the time interval between the actual patient care and the charting of that care, the more likely it is that the court may become suspicious that the additional entry was done merely to prevent liability.

If a late entry is made, never try to squeeze the information into a small space or along the margins of the chart. Such crowding in data often is perceived in a courtroom as an attempt to cover up information. The nurse may want to add a note stating why the entry was late or somehow to explain why the charting had not been done earlier. Such a note could be as simple as "first day back from three scheduled days off" or "patient chart unavailable at 03:00 P.M." Likewise, never leave several blank lines for a colleague to enter notes. The colleague should make his or her entry as a late entry.

In *Gorcey v. Jersey Shore Medical Center* (2006), a patient was admitted to the emergency department with severe injuries that he had sustained in an automobile accident. The paramedics were initially unable to obtain a blood pressure, but then recorded a pressure of 146/50 once they had initiated infusion therapy. The patient was treated at the hospital for 2 hours before he died. In the lawsuit that was filed, the family asserted that the patient had died of internal bleeding and that the lack of blood pressure recordings during the 2 hours he was treated at the hospital contributed to the physician's failure to appreciate the true nature of the patient's condition.

In court, the nurse was allowed to testify that she had taken vital signs, including blood pressures, every 15 minutes and scribbled them on pieces of paper that she put in her pocket and was not able later to record in the chart. The appellate court mandated the case back to the trial court for a rehearing, but the lesson to be learned is that one should always record such vital information in the chart, whether at the time of the occurrence, which is the preferred time to chart, or as a late entry with an explanation of why the entry was made after the fact.

An interesting case that concerned late entries is *Ross v. Redding Medical Center* (2003). In that case, the physician dictated and dated a patient's admitting history and physical and the operative report more than 3 weeks after the surgical procedure and 3 days after the patient died. The court found no liability on the part of the defendants, but did note that such late charting can raise serious suspicions when the charting is done so far after the fact.

Remember, too, that after a certain time period, most states hold that the chart must be "complete." This usually occurs 30 to 60 days after the patient's discharge from an acute care setting or an ambulatory surgical setting. After that time period, no further changes may be made.

Make the Chart Entry after the Event

Never chart in advance of a happening, treatment, or medication. The patient may not tolerate the procedure as had been intended or take the medication, or the nurse may have been unable to complete what he or she had intended to do. For example, another patient on the unit may have arrested or needed assistance immediately and the already-charted procedure was never completed, or the patient may be in a full code and the vital signs as recorded show an acceptable heart rate, respiratory rate, and blood pressure. Although it seems a small issue, if it can be shown that the nurse charted in advance, an attorney may be able to lessen the nurse's credibility in the eyes of a jury.

A case that validates why one should never chart in advance is *Kivalu v. Life Care Centers of America* (2005). At the beginning of his 10-hour shift, the licensed practical nurse (LPN) pre-completed a patient's chart, showing that he had given the patient morphine at 4:00 A.M. and 6:00 A.M. However, the patient expired at 3:15 A.M., before either dose of morphine could be given. The LPN was fired for violation of the facility's policies and procedures and applicable state statutes. There is no room for deviation from the policy manual, the court ruled, based on a nurse's own judgment of how to save time on a busy work shift.

Accurate nurses' notes form the basis of the patient medical record. Too often, this charting reflects the expected as opposed to the actual. In *Genao v. State* (1998), a nurse documented a sedated psychiatric patient's condition three times without ever seeing the patient. When the patient was finally "seen," she was found after being raped by another patient.

Use Clear and Objective Language

For years, nurses have been taught to use somewhat vague terminology in charting rather than drawing conclusions. Entries might have noted "appears to be asleep" or "seems to be resting comfortably" or, even more vaguely, "had a good night." These types of entries were thought to protect the nurse against drawing conclusions or being accused of making medical diagnoses. Today's attorney looks at such vague verbiage and is inclined to ask questions that cast doubt on the nurse's observational powers or that serve to imply that what the nurse actually saw was quite different from what was charted. Thus, the nurse should chart using objective, definite terms so that there is no doubt about the certainty of the entry.

A case that speaks directly to the clarity of the entry is *Shahine v. Louisiana State University Medical Center* (1996). The patient sued the surgeon and the hospital over persistent numbness in her right hand, which she first noticed after her total right hip replacement. Her suit alleged that the numbness was an ulnar nerve injury from improper positioning or from the surgeon's pressing against her arm or hand during the surgery.

The Court of Appeals exonerated all defendants from liability. The reason for this favorable result was the effort the circulating nurse made to document in precise detail how the patient had been positioned, stabilized, and padded before surgery, and specifically her documentation of the steps taken to extend the patient's arms out of harm's way and to pad her arms and hands to avoid pressure- or positioning-related injuries.

The court found it was critical that the nurse wrote a detailed factual statement describing to the smallest detail how the patient had been positioned and that she refrained from unsubstantiated judgmental assertions such as stating that the patient was positioned properly or in a manner designed to avoid injury.

A similar conclusion was drawn in *Anderson v. Beth Israel Medical Center* (2006). The patient developed blood clots in his left arm and shoulder following sinus surgery. He contended that the blood pressure cuff was erroneously placed on his left arm where he had a peripherally inserted central catheter. The court concluded that the blood pressure cuff was on the right arm, based on the circulating nurse's notes. She, said the court, was apparently the only one in the room who had noted which arm was used for taking the patient's blood pressure.

Estate of Maxey v. Darden (2008) illustrates how important it is to know what must be accurately documented and then document accordingly. This case concerned the withdrawal of life support by a patient's surrogate decision maker. Consent, in this particular state, requires the signature of two witnesses to attest to the signature of the patient's surrogate in such circumstances. It also requires that any witness to such a surrogate's signature must indicate that he or she actually witnessed the signature; that is, that he or she was in the presence of the signatory when he or she signed the form and actually saw the person sign the form. In this case, the chart merely noted that the person had signed the form, not that she witnessed the signature nor that she was actually in the room when the form was signed.

Mental capacity can also be established by the factual charting of nurses. In *Mitsinicos v. New Rochelle Nursing Home, Inc.* (1999), a nursing home resident had filed a lawsuit against the nursing home. The court had to decide if the resident had sufficient mental capacity to file a lawsuit or whether a guardian was necessary. To resolve the issue, the court read nursing documentation to conclude that the resident's intermittent confusion did not render him legally incompetent.

When charting is not specific, the court may find against the hospital and staff. In *Griffin v. Methodist Hospital* (1997), the court stated that to defend against malpractice, it is not good enough to generalize about whether the standard of care has been met. An expert witness must be able to find in the chart what specific examinations and treatments were performed. Saying after the fact that a patient was monitored appropriately is useless without nursing notes of the specific actions that constituted monitoring of the patient's condition.

Time of occurrences has always caused some confusion, especially when trying to discover if a code has been called in a timely manner or if the appropriate treatment has been initiated in a timely way. Two court cases have addressed time confusion as being detrimental to the defense of a filed lawsuit.

In *Landry v. Clement* (1998), the issue concerned the time a physician was notified of late decelerations on a fetal heart monitor strip. The nurses' notes said that the physician phoned at 4:30 P.M. and was notified of the late decelerations. But the fetal heart monitor strip clock noted that the deceleration occurred at 5:30 P.M. At trial, a nurse testified that the fetal heart monitor clock was fast by one full hour and that the actual time of the deceleration was 4:30 P.M. Although the court did not say that the time discrepancies directly affected the quality of the patient's care, the legal record was seriously compromised by the fact that the fetal heart monitor clock was set an hour ahead of the real-time clock.

In *Hutchins v. DCH Regional Medical Center* (2000), the patient developed an infection a few days following surgery for hemorrhoids. The patient then developed respiratory complications traced to beta hemolytic strep. He expired from respiratory complications 34 days after the surgical procedure. In the subsequent lawsuit, the preparation of the patient's skin prior to the hemorrhoid surgery was questioned. The nurse's notes indicated that the surgical preparation took exactly 8 minutes, which would not have allowed sufficient time for the required 5-minute Betadine scrub to be completed. At trial, the nurse testified that her note meant that she had spent 8 minutes alone on the Betadine scrub, not on the whole procedure.

The court ruled in favor of the hospital, noting that the nurse's documentation was ambiguous on a critical point. The recommendation was that the hospital and nurse reexamine the way documentation was completed in the future.

Be Realistic and Factual

Nurses are cautioned to chart exactly what happened to the patient to prevent a lawsuit for attempted concealment or minimization of an injury. In *Kodadek v. Lieberman* (2001), the surgeon broke the tip of the needle that he was using to suture a bleeding vessel during a young child's tonsillectomy. The bleeding worsened as the surgeon probed for the needle tip, and a decision was made not to retrieve the needle tip. An x-ray was done to determine that the needle tip was not a threat to the patient, and the surgery was concluded.

Following the procedure, the surgeon and the hospital's director of perioperative services informed the parents what had occurred during the surgery. They admitted that a small portion of the needle was still in the patient's tonsil fossa, that this was a common occurrence, and that the needle tip would not cause the patient any problems. When the patient experienced problems, the needle tip was removed by a second surgeon and the parents sued the hospital, original surgeon, and nurses involved in the surgical procedure.

The court noted that there was no mention made in the nurses' records that a needle had broken during the tonsillectomy, that an x-ray had been taken, that the surgeon decided to leave the needle tip in the tonsil fossa, or that the nurse had given the surgeon other than the requested size needle for suturing. The court stated that patients can sue a nurse or physician who fraudulently misinforms the patient or tries to conceal the fact that a mistake has been made. The special relationship that patients have with their health care providers makes such conduct wholly inappropriate and actionable.

Nurses should also chart a realistic picture of the patient, particularly patients who refuse to comply with therapeutic regimes or are difficult to care for because of abusive and threatening language. These patients may well have a less-than-satisfactory outcome, especially if they are noncompliant. Charting what the patient said, instances of noncompliance, and threats against nursing personnel helps to prevent such a case from coming to court. Prospective attorneys will be hesitant to represent clients who caused or contributed to their unsatisfactory outcome.

A case that illustrates how documenting a patient's anger, acting out, and continuous verbalizations of threats assists in preventing liability is *Greywolf v. Carroll* (2007). The patient, who had a longstanding history of voluntary and involuntary psychiatric admissions for repeated self-harm behaviors, filed a lawsuit against her psychiatrist for malicious prosecution, abuse of legal process, invasion of privacy, and medical malpractice. The case was dismissed based on the nurses' progress notes that documented the patient's behaviors during the time that the patient was in the inpatient psychiatric unit.

Noted observations should be factual and should describe objectively the patient's symptoms, appearance, and behaviors. Avoid any language of blame or negligence in charting. If needed, use quotation marks to include actual patient statements. Never use statements that draw conclusions without giving supportive objective data, such as "patient states he was trying to climb over the bedrail and that is why he fell."

EXERCISE 9.2

The patient was admitted involuntarily to a psychiatric facility based on her behavior, mental status, and questionable indications that she might be suicidal. On admission, the nurse noted that the patient was confused, disoriented, and unable to remember her own address. Her memory was assessed as fair to poor, she was argumentative, and she displayed paranoid behaviors. This behavior and mental status was judged to be a sharp deterioration of her mental status post-operatively and, in the opinion of her physicians, required her to be held and treated as a psychiatric patient even though she denied consent for this therapy and confinement.

Following her eventual dismissal from the facility, she filed a lawsuit against the physicians, nurses, and hospital alleging that the pain medications she received post-operatively caused her mental condition. How should the court rule and why?

Chart Only Your Own Observations

It is advisable that nurses refrain from charting for other nurses, unless absolutely necessary. For example, the physician insists on giving a particular injection, and the nurse notes the medication received by the patient and the person who administered the medication. Because patient records may be used in a variety of courts, the nurse doing the charting will be unable to remember particulars about the patient, diagnoses, and nursing care. Yet the nurse will be called to testify because his or her name appeared on the chart. For the same reason, chart only what is observed or assessed.

Lemoine v. Arkansas Department of Workforce Services (2008) portrays what can happen when a nurse charts other than her own observations. The nurse in this case worked as a home health hospice nurse. She visited terminally ill patients in their homes, monitoring their conditions, recording vital signs, providing palliative care measures, and obtaining needed medications. She would report her findings to a central office and had been assigned a laptop computer for documentation of her assessments, interventions, and findings.

For one client, she filed a report several hours before actually visiting the patient. The report included chronic findings that had been previously reported and most certainly would still apply for this individual patient. The nurse claimed that she had assessed the data via a telephone call she made to the patient. The nurse was subsequently dismissed from her position.

The issue for the court was not the accuracy of the information or whether she actually received the data via a telephone call to the patient. Deliberate, intentional falsification of a patient assessment is grounds for dismissal, said the court. Even if the data were accurate, she still was falsifying a report of a home visit to a patient.

Some institutions still require that professional nurses chart for nonlicensed personnel or "co-sign" charts for these personnel, though this practice is abating. Charting for others or co-signing notes makes the charting nurse potentially liable for care, observations, or omissions as charted. Always read and investigate what has been charted before co-signing. Nurses should further investigate ways of changing such policies.

Chart Patient's Refusal for Care

If the patient refuses care or ordered treatment, ensure that the refusal is documented timely. Remember, too, that patient education about the consequences of that refusal must be included in the medical record. In a case that illustrates this principle, the patient refused a mammogram after a lump had been discovered in her breast. The court noted that the standard of care requires that a physician recommend a mammogram, and if the patient refuses, the physician should explicitly chart that refusal. The physician should also insist that the patient return for a follow-up examination no later than 1 month and that refusal should also be charted, if the patient indicates that she needs no further care (*May v. Jones,* 1996).

Clearly Chart All Patient Education

Nurses inevitably combine patient education with a variety of other physical tasks, such as teaching the patient proper foot care while bathing the diabetic patient, instructing about meal plans while assisting with the feeding of a newly diagnosed congestive heart failure patient, or demonstrating how to correctly change a toddler's dressing while showing the parents how to observe for signs of wound infection. Some of this patient education is carefully documented, especially if the patient is to be discharged later that day or early the next morning. All patient education must be documented in the patient record, with an evaluation of the teaching also documented.

To document patient comprehension, ask pertinent questions about material that was just taught. Another strategy is to have the patient perform a demonstration of the task or select appropriate foods from the daily menu selection to verify that learning has occurred. Finally, listen carefully to the patient's questions for appropriateness and content mastery. When documenting, reference that teaching has been done, rather than "discussed with the client how he would select low-sodium foods." Include all teaching that is done for reinforcement of needed knowledge and revalidation that the patient is retaining the information. If printed materials are sent home with the patient, retain a copy of the information sheet for the medical record.

Correct Charting Errors

The legal system has also given guidance in the area of how to rectify charting errors. There is adequate case law to support the contention that if there are errors in part of the record, the jury could find that errors might just as easily exist elsewhere as well, and thus the entire record could be found to be erroneous. Recognizing that anyone could make an error or misspell a word, the error in question should have a single line drawn through it with the correct entry placed above the error or next to the erroneous entry. Also include the time and date of the correction, and initial or sign the correction to show by whom, when, and why a new notation was made. The nurse may explain the correction with an entry such as "Entry made on wrong chart" or "Spelling error." To avoid charting on another patient's chart, each page of the patient's medical record should be imprinted with the patient's name, medical record number, and other institution identifiers.

If the reason for striking a portion of charting is self-evident, no additional note need be made and the nurse should just initial the cross-out. For example, if a misspelled word is crossed out and the correctly spelled word is the next entry, it is obvious why the correction was made. Frequently, this is seen when "right" is crossed out and "left" inserted or vice versa. It is obvious that the wrong extremity was first charted and then the correct extremity was identified.

In *Terajima v. Torrance Memorial Medical Center* (2008), the patient sued the hospital claiming failure of the post-operative nursing staff to obtain and record vital signs in a timely manner, leading to post-operative complications. The court found no liability against the institution or its staff despite the fact that a nurse's aide had made mistakes in her charting. Specifically, the nurse's aide overwrote some of the blood pressure readings instead of crossing them out, initialing them, and then writing the correct blood pressure readings next to the crossed-out blood pressure entries or writing them in a separate portion of the flow sheet. The hospital's own nursing expert witness admitted that overwriting any chart entry is never correct procedure. The court examined the entire record for the time interval in question and concluded that the nurse and the nurse's aide were, in fact, monitoring the patient very closely and appropriately conveyed essential information to other members of the health care team. There was no basis, concluded the court, to equate mistakes in charting to negligent care.

Many institutions discourage the use of the word *error* (such as "spelling error" or "error in charting") when correcting a chart entry. There is some concern that using the word *error* may be interpreted as though the entire entry is in error.

Nurses should never, under any circumstance, totally obliterate the entry, tape a new entry over the erroneous entry, or use a more imaginative way to prevent the reading of the error in their charting. Correction fluid was not invented to obliterate a medical record entry and should not be used for this purpose. Such obliterations or erasures serve only to raise suspicion in the minds of others, and questions of what was hidden arise. Innocent though the entry may have been, it is hard to defend a lawsuit with altered records. In *Ahrens v. Katz* (1984), white-outs of part of the nursing notes in the original chart were discovered and the records x-rayed so that the injured party's counsel could determine what the nurse had originally written. In *Phillips v. Covenant Clinic* (2001), the court specifically noted that "common sense says that someone who destroys or loses a document relevant to litigation must have felt threatened by the contents of the record" (at 719). In that case, the clinic records were unavailable and there was no means to locate the original chart.

For the same reason, charts should never be destroyed or recopied, for the question is always asked about what it was that the nurse or other health care provider was trying to hide. Additionally, records should not be altered if the nurse knows that a lawsuit is pending. The attorney for the patient already has a copy of the record, and additions or changes will not be on his or her copy. Thus, the attorney for the patient will introduce that a new version of the chart has been made.

Physicians do not have the right to demand that nurses alter records, nor may physicians alter nurses' notes. In *Henry v. St. John's Hospital* (1987), a patient in active labor was administered 6 cc of Marcaine intramuscularly in each hip by the resident, and the nurse recorded the drug, dosage, and person administering the medication in the nursing notes. After the neonate was born with fetal distress, the resident went back and amended the dosage to a lesser amount. The court found against the resident and defendant hospital.

Attorneys for injured patients examine charts for evidence that later materials have been included or that there has been a total substitution of a part of the record. Examples of such alterations include:

1. Writing crowded around existing entries
2. Changes in slant, pressure, uniformity, or other differences in handwriting
3. Use of different pens to write a single entry
4. Additions of different dates written in the same ink, while original entries were written in a separate but consistent ink
5. Differences between pages as to folds, stains, offsets, holes, tears, and type of paper used
6. Use of forms not in use at the purported time of entry
7. Use of later years (2004 for 2003), especially if corrected

A different color of ink was the clue that the record had been altered in *Rotan v. Greenbaum* (1959). In *Rothstein v. Orange Grove Center. Inc.* (2001), a handwriting expert was employed by the plaintiff to show that portions of the medical record were created after the original entries. The handwriting expert noted that some entries on the same page actually made different impressions due to different materials being used when they were written, showing that the entries were not made on the same dates as indicated.

Above all, the record must be readable and charted in ink. One of the primary purposes of charting is to communicate with other health care workers about the patient's condition, response to therapies, and progress. If nurses cannot write clearly and their writing cannot be read, then they should print the entry. There is no communication if the primary entry maker is unable to read the entry.

Writing should be legible and only standard, institution-approved abbreviations used. If nurses have difficulty remembering an abbreviation or frequently confuse the abbreviation among several meanings, they should not use it. It is far better to spell out an entry than to be unable to explain the abbreviation to the jury. Counsel for the injured party frequently review the records with the author during deposition, insisting that each illegible word and comment be explained.

Nurses' notes should be organized and written as neatly as possible. Although writing sloppy notes has no bearing on the quality of care delivered, opposing attorneys will make the observation if the nurse is disorganized and sloppy in charting, then he or she is most likely disorganized and sloppy in the delivery of nursing care. Many jurors will accept these statements as true and find against the health care provider and for the injured patient.

Since documentation is done to communicate to other health care deliverers the status of the patient, never invent new abbreviations that have meaning to only one or two persons or to one nursing unit in the hospital. Such self-coined abbreviations hinder rather than assist the communication process. A second and equally valid reason not to coin new abbreviations is that the nurse is likely not to remember what the abbreviation meant when asked by opposing counsel. It is difficult to show quality, competent care when the primary nurse is unable to ascertain what happened to the patient.

Perhaps the best reason not to use self-coined abbreviations is how they appear to the patient or what they signify. In a 1990 case, the family had been concerned about the quality of health care delivery during the elderly patient's hospital stay. The family brought suit, especially after they discovered the "PBBB" notation in the physician's progress note stood for "pine box by bedside." The case settled before going to court (Mangels, 1990).

Never Alter a Record at Someone Else's Request

Never alter a record at someone else's request, even if the request seems harmless. Seasoned malpractice or personal injury attorneys will be able to see that the record has been altered, alerting them that something irregular has happened. At trial, the attorney may well use this irregularity to bolster the case. This brings into question both your credibility and behavior for the judge and jury. Deliberately altering a medical record could also be grounds for disciplinary action by the state board of nursing and termination of employment by the facility.

Identify Yourself after Every Entry

At the conclusion of all entries, nurses identify themselves by full name and title. This is true whether or not the nurse has been previously identified. Some institutions allow the nurse to use initials at the conclusion of a page entry if the nurse has signed the bottom portion of the page where all personnel charting are identified by name and status.

Use Standardized Checklists or Flow Sheets

To prevent routine care from being omitted from the chart and to ensure that frequent observations are both performed and charted, many hospitals have adopted graphic sheets or flow sheets. Even checking that patients have received take-home instruction sheets is significant in preventing subsequent liability (*Roberts v. Sisters of St. Francis*, 1990). These simple checklist approaches to charting are legally valid and prevent the need for long chart entries. This method also seems to prevent some of the shorthand charting that leaves large gaps in the chart.

Leave No Room for Liability

One last point to remember is that the nurse should chart on all lines in sequence and should ensure that additional entries cannot be squeezed in later. Blank spaces allow others to enter information over the previous nurse's signature, in which case the previous nurse may then be legally liable for the entry.

Likewise, the patient record is no place to record employee complaints. In *Claim of Rice* (2001), a social worker noted in a medical record that the patient was not having his therapy sessions because the social worker was too overworked to see the patient. The court noted three issues with such charting:

1. The entry was false, as there were other social workers who could have seen the patient.
2. The statement was potentially detrimental to the hospital, as it exposed the organization to liability.

3. Patient records are not the place for caregivers to express complaints against their supervisors about staffing or other employment issues, even if their complaints are legitimate.

GUIDELINES

Charting—What the Record Should Contain

1. All the information that is necessary to communicate the patient's progress:
   a. Initial assessment data
   b. Description of actual and/or potential problems
   c. Record of all procedures, treatments, medications, and care
   d. Record of health teaching
   e. Description of patient reactions to treatments, procedures, medications, and teaching
   f. Record of actions taken and persons contacted
2. Information presented in a form that communicates the patient's progress:
   a. Notes made at the time of or immediately following the event recorded, with correct time and date
   b. Notes written and properly signed by the person doing or observing the event being recorded
   c. Notes made in chronological order
   d. Notes free of omissions, personal opinions, generalizations, and ambiguous abbreviations
   e. Notes that are concise, precise, spelled correctly, accurate, and unambiguous
   f. Notes that are legible and neat
   g. Notes that have no unused spaces or blank lines
3. Information that is recorded from a legal perspective:
   a. Record the obvious: Record what you actually saw, did, or communicated to another.
   b. Do not allow inaccuracies to be charted: Record what actually happened, even if you wish you had done something differently.
   c. Do not obliterate an entry: Draw a single line through an error, mark it "mistaken entry," and sign it using your first initial, last name, and correct title.
   d. Do not destroy parts of the record: Follow the same advice as for obliteration of an entry.
   e. Describe events and behaviors: Do not use labels or medical terms you are unsure of in charting.
   f. Document all communications to others and any intermediary steps taken; if you question an order, document that you recontacted the physician and clarified the order.
   g. Record all routine assessments and nursing care; help develop a flow sheet for more accurate records if needed.

EXERCISE 9.3

For your last two patients (or any two patients), compare the nursing notes against the guidelines presented in this chapter. Can they be written more completely to adhere to the guidelines? If the answer is yes, do so. Has this exercise changed your opinion of the importance of nursing documentation? Explain your answer.

ELECTRONIC MEDICAL RECORDS (COMPUTERIZED CHARTING)

Many institutions have now adopted, either in part or in whole, **electronic medical records,** sometimes referred to as **electronic health records** or **computerized charting.** The use of computers in compiling the patient's medical record increases accurate recording of facts and allows for prompt charting, particularly when bedside and/or laptop computers are used. Nursing information systems (NISs) allow for accuracy at all stages of the nursing process, from assessment to evaluation. Most systems prompt the nurse if a portion of the nursing process is omitted, and many will not allow you to continue until the omitted data are added. Perhaps one of the more important reasons for computers in hospitals is the improved patient care that results with computers. Necessary test and laboratory results can be instantly available, medication errors are reduced, and problems with charting, such as illegible writing, misspellings, unapproved abbreviations, and time needed for writing entries, are eliminated by computers.

With electronic records, documentation is readily available and easy to retrieve, review, and amend as needed, especially for patients readmitted to the same institution. Data can be viewed and edited by all members of the health care team, including those on site and, in many institutions, those at remote locations. Additionally, better quality control occurs with computerized charting as Joint Commission (JC) and state requirements are individualized into facility systems. Security is tightened because whenever a patient's record is accessed, the name of the person accessing the record is automatically inserted, as is the time and date of the access. Most programs are also interactive, posing questions and suggestions to keep errors at a minimum, eliminating redundancies, and enhancing the quality of the recording. The final "selling-point" for computerized charting is that it should allow health care providers to decrease charting time, thus allowing for greater time with patients.

Issues of concern with using computers for hospital records usually focus on privacy and confidentiality rights of the patient. With a properly designed and implemented computer program, there can be more security than in current, more traditional charting procedures. Security is enhanced because:

1. There are fewer points of access into the system.
2. Each person's access can be restricted to a limited scope of information, with only those portions of the records that are relevant for one's functioning being accessible. The person can be "locked out" if violations occur.
3. The information sought through individual access codes can be monitored, making misuse easier to detect.
4. Passwords are changed on a regular basis.
5. Access to the system is terminated when the employee resigns his or her employment status.
6. Confidentiality statements are signed by users to acknowledge their awareness of legal and institution requirements for usage.

The desire for privacy and confidentiality is well founded. An early Supreme Court case addressed medical information privacy. *Whalen v. Roe* (1977) determined that a New York State database of lawful users of abusable medications was allowable, because the prohibitions on public disclosure of the information in the database were adequate to prevent any constitutional harms to the persons listed in the database. The court considered all provisions that were in place to protect the database. The stringent physician and administrative procedures protecting the patient's interest in privacy also played a part in the court's ultimate ruling. Interestingly, the court did not address whether compilation of the information was itself a violation of privacy, nor did it question whether adequate security measures were present.

There are some privacy measures in effect, primarily because the U.S. Constitution contains certain privacy rights. The Privacy Act of 1974 prevents the federal government from collecting private information for one purpose and then using it for another purpose (5 U.S.C., Section 552a, 1974). The Computer Fraud and Abuse Act of 1986, amended as part of the Patriot Act of 2001 (section 1030, 2001), defines a federal fraud offense as an offense for the alteration, damage, or destruction of information contained in a computer used by or for the government of the United States. The act made it a crime to traffic in computer passwords and declared that tampering with computerized medical records warrants punishment without a showing of monetary loss or any showing of incorrect or harmful treatment (42 U.S.C., Section 290dd-3, 1988). Security measures regarding patient data and privacy are covered under the Health Insurance Portability and Accountability Act of 1996 (HIPAA), discussed later in this chapter.

An issue that still remains concerns the machines themselves. Computer-based records can be altered, destroyed, or rendered inaccessible by computer viruses or other acts of sabotage. Technology changes can render a record storage system obsolete long before the need for the records stored in them has ended. Thus, hospitals continue to strive for alternate means of storing records so that they remain retrievable.

CHARTING BY EXCEPTION

This abbreviated system of charting, initiated in the 1980s, differs from the more traditional methods of charting. **Charting by exception** requires documentation of only significant or abnormal findings, and previously entered standardized or expected results are not reentered into the chart. Heralded as a means of reducing charting time and making abnormal data more obvious, the charting by exception format relies upon the use of preprinted guidelines, such as nursing-diagnosis-based standardized care plans and protocols, flow sheets, critical pathways, and graphic records to show the patient's progress or lack of progress. Bedside charting is increased, so that there is immediate access to patient data by health care workers. Charting by exception streamlines documentation by combining three essential elements:

1. Standards of nursing care
2. Flow sheets
3. Bedside access to chart forms

Institutions can personalize charting by exception to fit their own needs. For example, they can use only the preprinted guidelines, or allow for individualization of patient care within the preprinted guidelines. To be successfully used, though, the institution must establish standards that are uniformly used by all health care personnel and establish normal findings and expected outcomes so that all significant data are considered when assessing patient outcomes. With the advent of the total electronic record, there is some support for institutions to move to a charting by exception format.

Charting by exception is not without some legal perils. Charting by exception may fail to provide enough information to alert practitioners to potential problems. *Lama v. Borras* (1994) remains the leading and only available appellate-level case regarding charting by exception. In *Lama,* the patient underwent surgery for a herniated disk. Two days later, there was an entry noting that the surgical dressing was "very bloody," and pain at the site of the incision was noted on the following day. By the fourth day post-operatively, the surgical dressing was again "soiled," and severe incisional pain was noted on the fifth day post-operatively. On the sixth day after surgery, the physician diagnosed diskitis and began antibiotic therapy.

Review of the patient's chart failed to show what happened during the time that the patient's dressing became bloody and he experienced increasing pain. Vital signs and medications were charted, but important details such as the status of the incision and duration and intensity of pain were not charted. Lacking, too, were possible nursing and medical interventions that accompanied the changing surgical drainage and pain or any communications that occurred between the nursing and medical staffs.

The jury in this case concluded that more complete charting could have answered questions that charting by exception failed to answer. The jury also concluded that the infection might have been diagnosed sooner if more traditional charting methods had been followed. "Intermittent charting failed to provide the sort of continuous danger signals that would be the most likely to spur early intervention by a physician" was the final holding of this court (at 477). The court further found that this type of charting failed to meet the regulations of the Puerto Rico Department of Health, which requires that qualitative nurses' notes be recorded for each patient by each nursing shift.

Charting by exception may make it impossible to show the attentiveness of the nursing staff to patients, particularly patients in whom complications develop. Charting by exception may not assist nurses in being able to defend themselves, because even they cannot re-create what was done and not done for an individual patient. Remember that it may be 2 years before the nurse knows that a lawsuit is filed. Though charting by exception remains a viable option, institutions are cautioned to ensure that this system of charting is well developed before its implementation and that quality controls are added to ensure its success.

ALTERATION OF RECORDS

Essentially two types of **alterations of records** may be necessary to ensure a truthful, accurate record. The first concerns minor errors, such as those that occur in spelling, notations of laboratory data, incorrect phraseology, and the like. These types of errors are usually corrected by the person making the entry at the time of the entry or shortly after the entry was made. The error should be marked through with a single line and the correct information entered, timed, dated, and signed. Incorrect entries should never be erased or obliterated, because such actions raise suspicion in the jurors' minds.

The second type of alteration concerns substantive errors, such as incorrect test data, omitted progress notes, incorrect orders, and the like. Only administrative staff or the primary health care provider should correct such substantive errors, and all persons misled by the error should be contacted and advised of the correct information. Correction for these types of errors includes the addition of new materials with the explanation of why they were necessitated, who made the addition, the date, and the time.

An addendum to the record by a physician or other health care provider should not be seen as proof of an error. Occasionally, an addendum may be written based on new information that was just received. However, because a patient's record should reflect as closely as possible concurrent treatment and observation, adding information at a later date is unusual. The further away in time the charting occurs, the more suspicious a reviewer can be about the provider's purpose.

Patients may wish to correct or modify an entry in the medical record. Usually, the patient is permitted to add to the original chart a letter of explanation regarding the modification or addition. Staff agreeing with the letter of modification or addition may also add their own letters of support. This approach preserves the original document while clarifying the source and nature of the change.

Alteration of medical records without justification places the credibility of the entire record in question. Additionally, deliberately altering a medical record or writing an incorrect record may subject the health care provider to statutory sanctions, such as licensure revocation for unprofessional behavior.

RETENTION OF RECORDS

Health care facilities have a responsibility to maintain and protect patient records (*Fox v. Cohen,* 1980). This obligation, **retention of records,** is codified in state statutes that impose a clear duty on facilities not to lose or destroy records within certain time frames. The time frame usually co-incides with state statutes of limitations for medical negligent causes of action. There are also some retention recommendations published by the federal government as part of Medicare guidelines.

Record retention varies according to state law, with the majority of states preserving the record for the period of time in which suits may be filed (state statutes of limitations) or for between 5 and 10 years. For example, Colorado has adopted the federal statute for retention of medical records in long-term care facilities, which is 5 years (Standards for Hospitals and Health Care Facilities, 2008). Approximately half the states have legal requirements regarding the length of time to retain records when the patient is a minor. For states that do not have this legal require-ment, the recommended time interval is until the minor reaches majority plus the statute of lim-itations. As a practical matter, most institutions save records for longer periods of time.

The impact of lost medical records can be devastating to meeting the burden of proof. If records are lost, are incomplete, or have disappeared, a tendency by the court is to presume negligence, and juries have no difficulty finding for the injured party. Known as **omnia praesumuntur contra spoliatorem** (all things are presumed against a despoiler), courts have al-lowed such disappearances and lack of records to suggest a presumption of guilt. In *May v. Moore* (1982), the Alabama Supreme Court held that even testimony about a physician's lost records (and this physician had a record of losing charts when there was a bad outcome) was admissible and was sufficient to create an inference of negligent treatment.

The court in *Stokes v. Spartanburg Regional Medical Center* (2006) held that the plaintiff's lawyer has the right to request that the judge instruct the jury that the health care facility must present a plausible reason why critical information from a patient's medical record is not avail-able. If the reason is not satisfactory, the jury is allowed to conclude that the evidence would have been damaging to the health care provider's case and that is the reason for its destruction or unavailability. In this case, an adult post-operative patient was admitted to a pediatric unit because the adult unit had no available space. He had undergone surgery for removal of a cancerous thyroid and selected lymph nodes from his neck. In the post-operative care unit, he had received oxygen per mask and a pulse oximeter was used. When transferred, he had no supplemental oxy-gen and a pulse oximeter was not used. He died from respiratory failure due to post-operative neck-swelling less than 3 hours after he was transferred to the pediatric unit.

The family asserted that the patient died because the pediatric nursing staff were unfamil-iar with the care of an adult post-thyroidectomy patient, failed to appreciate the possibility that a hematoma at the surgical site could obstruct his breathing, failed to closely monitor him, and failed to have an adult tracheostomy tray available for such an emergency. At trial, the facility was unable to produce the laboratory results from the blood gases that were done during the code and the vital signs nursing flow sheet from the less than 3 hours he was in the pediatric unit. This Court of Appeals of South Carolina remanded the case back to the trial court, with the stipula-tion that the jury be instructed that the missing data could be viewed detrimentally against the facility and the health care providers named in this lawsuit.

Conversely, the court may rule that there was no legal duty to preserve the record. This was the finding in *Thornton v. Shah* (2002) when the court concluded that a health maintenance organization had no legal duty to preserve nurses' triage records for a 5-year period. The court in *Phillips v. Covenant Clinic* (2001) held that though spoilage of evidence is a valid legal concept, there is also the possibility that medical records from a clinic could be inadvertently lost, with no intent to destroy records so as to prevent liability. This is especially true when the facts support an emergency admission of a critically ill individual.

A newer interpretation of acceptable loss of original medical record data may be seen as a direct result of the advent of electronic medical records. The court in *Chobanian v. Meriter Hospital, Inc.* (2008), reviewing the impact of spoilage of the evidence, ruled that it had not occurred in this particular case. "Spoilage does not occur, however, and no particular inferences can be drawn one way or another when original chart notes, monitor strips, films, etc., are copied on microfilm or stored in an electronic digital format and the originals are destroyed. Originals may be copied and disposed of in the institution's usual and customary method in the ordinary course of business without legal prejudice" (*Chobanian v. Meriter Hospital, Inc,* 2008, at 4426747). In this particular case, the original data that were destroyed included fetal monitoring strips, as they were electronically stored within the computer's memory from which full sets of duplicated monitor tracings could be generated.

A case that defines the four elements that are required before the plaintiff can prevail in a lawsuit when spoilage is a factor is *Proske v. St. Barnabas Medical Center* (1998). Here the patient sued her physician for failure to diagnose her breast cancer more quickly. The patient's hospital records contained all her mammography reports, and the earlier reports contained indeterminable findings or concluded there were calcifications present that appeared benign. The court was unable to decide either for or against the plaintiff because all of her mammography films had disappeared. The plaintiff then added allegations against the hospital where the films had been taken. These additional allegations were for spoilage of the evidence.

The Superior Court of New Jersey ruled in favor of the hospital on the patient's allegations of spoilage. The films, they said, were innocently misplaced while being removed for storage at a remote location by an outside medical records services vendor. There was no proof of actual intent to tamper with or to destroy the evidence. The court would have ruled for the plaintiff if there had been evidence of deliberate tampering with the evidence.

The court ruled that a patient can sue a health care provider for spoilage of the evidence when:

1. The provider, who may or may not be a defendant or potential defendant, knows malpractice litigation is pending or probable.
2. The provider intentionally tampers with or destroys evidence to try to disrupt the patient's legal case.
3. The patient's malpractice case is compromised.
4. The patient suffers a monetary loss. (*Proske v. St. Barnabas Medical Center,* 1998, at 1210)

Because the patient could not prove these four elements, the court ruled for the defendant.

Destruction of medical records may be performed to protect confidentiality, and destruction should be complete. Should a patient request the destruction of his or her medical record prior to the retention interval lapsing, many courts favor sealing the record over total destruction. Sealing preserves the record while preventing its discovery.

OWNERSHIP OF THE RECORD

Because the chart is the business record of the institution, the health care facility is the rightful owner of the entire record. Correspondingly, the individual physician owns the chart records of patients seen in the physician's office. Courts have recognized this right of hospital ownership by declaring that since hospital records are essential to proper administration, hospital records become the property of the hospital. *Beason v. State* (2008) reinforces this right of ownership.

In that case, a patient had an emergency cardiac catheterization after an apparent heart attack. He was informed that he needed open-heart surgery immediately and he was scheduled for surgery the following morning. He requested a copy of his chart so that he could obtain a second opinion.

Because it was late in the day, the medical records department was not open and would not be open the next day until after his scheduled surgery would already be started. The medical records department was the only authorized department to assist him in obtaining the chart copy and no one else was willing to copy his medical record for him. The patient grabbed the chart and left the facility. On his way off the facility's property, he struck a security guard during a scuffle in the parking lot.

The Court of Appeals of Texas ruled that the patient was guilty of stealing hospital property. His use of force, as demonstrated by hitting the security guard, elevated the seriousness of the offense from simple theft to robbery. He was sentenced to 2 years of supervised probation.

This ownership right of health care providers to their business records does not preclude the patient's property rights in the same records. The patient generally has the right to all the information contained within the record and to a copy of the original record. The facility may charge the patient a reasonable fee for the copy of the record. Some exceptions are made for certain psychiatric records, and state law may forbid the patient access to some psychiatric records.

A recent case defined patients' and providers' rights and responsibilities as they pertain to the medical record (*Cornelio v. Stamford Hospital,* 1998). According to the court, the law allows a patient, a patient's physician, or a patient's legal representative to examine any and all materials contained in the patient's medical record. This includes original pathology specimens, pathology slides, x-ray films, lab specimens, physicians' notes, reports, correspondence, bills, insurance forms, and the like. The patient does not have to first file a lawsuit against the health care provider to be entitled to access the materials contained in the patient's medical record. A patient or patient's representative seeking access to a patient's health care record does not need to have a subpoena or even a reason for desiring access to the chart. However, the individual requesting access to another's medical record must have proper authorization (*In re Gould,* 2003).

Copy expenses for materials that can be copied are the patient's or patient's representative's responsibility. Patients may have the right to copies of the medical records they need in order to pursue disability or industrial insurance claims at a reduced cost or at no cost. Providers must consult their own attorneys to make themselves aware of how their state laws cover this special circumstance. Using an outside photocopy vendor, rather than making copies of the patient's chart in-house, is not a violation of a patient's right to medical confidentiality.

Certain materials cannot be copied, but the patient still has rights of access to examine them, as in the case of pathology slides. The originals stay in the custody of the health care provider. Once pathology specimens or smear slides are obtained by the health care provider, they are no longer part of the patient's personal property, but remain with the health care provider. Even though the patient may have a copy of medical records, health care providers are still required by law to keep the original records and pathology materials.

The court noted that the right to access and the right to copy materials that can be copied are two separate or independent rights. The patient has the right to come to the health care facility and view the original, not be placated with copies. When the patient or representative comes to view the chart, the person can be seated in a designated area and closely supervised while in possession of the chart. The hospital should make available x-ray viewers and microscopes for examination of the originals.

ACCESS TO MEDICAL RECORDS

In addition to a legal right to the health care record, there are some practical reasons for allowing **patient access to medical records.** Allowing patients access to their medical records helps to dispel feelings that the physician was lying about the severity of the illnesses or that the physician was unsympathetic to their illnesses. Allowing access helps reassure patients that their care was based on actual medical findings.

Most states require that the record be completed prior to the patient's right of access, and statutes have been enacted to establish procedures for such patient access. For example, the policy may provide that access be between the hours of 9 A.M. and 5 P.M. Monday through Friday and only when a hospital representative is present to answer questions. It is also generally recognized that the competent patient can authorize this right of access to others. These others include insurance carriers, legal representation, and outside professionals acting on behalf of the patient. Generally, this facility must allow the person access to the medical record within 30 days of the request for access, and this request for access must be in writing.

One of the problems concerning access of patients to their medical records arises when patients are incompetent or minors or when they die prior to exercising their right. In such instances, others may be able to authorize access to a patient record. As a general rule, a guardian of an incompetent patient stands in the place of the patient and can authorize access. If there is no court-appointed guardian, hospitals may rely on the authorization of the next of kin or the person responsible for authorization and payment of the medical treatment. Access may be refused if family confidences or information about other than the patient would be needlessly disclosed through access to a mentally incompetent patient's medical record. *McDonald v. Clinger* (1982) denied access of a patient record to a spouse with a showing that such disclosure would cause a danger to the patient, spouse, or other person.

Access to charts of minors also presents a recurring problem, especially in the event of treatment for sexually transmitted diseases, pregnancy, or substance abuse. Generally, if minors are authorized under state law to consent to their own care, then parents will not have a right to access the record. Additionally, payment of care may help to decide access questions. If minors, even mature minors, rely on their parents for payment of care, then the parents may have right to access the record or of disclosure from the primary health care provider.

In the event of a patient's death, the next of kin or the executor of the estate may authorize access to the record. If the spouse has predeceased the patient, it would be advisable to obtain the authorization of all adult children rather than rely on the authorization of only one of the adult children, though this may not be required by individual state laws.

Access may be gained to a patient record by law. Examples of access by law include subpoenas of records of a party if the party's mental or physical condition is relevant to the lawsuit, subpoenas of records for suspected billing fraud by the health care provider, and when there is a statutory duty of disclosure.

In *Florida Department of Health and Rehabilitative Services v. V. M. R., Inc.* (1991), a warrant was issued allowing the Florida Department of Health and Rehabilitative Services to enter a women's medical center and inspect the clinic's premises and records. The clinic and two patients moved to quash the warrant, claiming that the medical records could not be released without written authorization from patients. The court agreed and noted that, although there may be an exception to the privacy provisions in limited circumstances, no such exception had been accorded this agency. Additionally, the court found that the agency's right to examine records did not extend to such personal information as a patient's name, address, and medical history. The impact of such decisions respects the state's authority to regulate, but the power does not allow a governmental agency to make public private medical records.

A second major area of concern with access problems is the **patient's right to privacy** and confidentiality. Such privacy rights encourage candor by the patient and optimize proper medical treatment and diagnosis. Privacy rights also allow nurses to be truthful and open in their assessments and recording of patient care. For example, in *Head v. Colloton* (1983), the Iowa Supreme Court held that the records of a potential donor for a bone marrow transplant were hospital records and, as such, were exempt from release as public records under the state's freedom of information law.

In general, health care providers involved in the direct care of the patient have access to the record, and records should be housed where they will be the most accessible for patient care providers. This encourages prompt recording as well as quality patient care. Administrators and hospital staff members have access for auditing, billing, quality assurance purposes, and defending potential claims.

Exceptions to the preceding statement include substance abuse treatment or substance abuse treatment records. In *Lugar v. Baton Rouge General Medical Center* (1997), a man who had previously been treated for alcohol abuse applied for life insurance from the same company with whom he was working as an insurance agent. He indicated that he had never received alcohol treatment or been arrested for alcohol abuse.

In doing the background check, the company knew the man had been treated at a certain hospital, but did not know for what he had been treated. The insurance company asked the man to sign a release for medical records. The hospital released his confidential medical records to the insurance company. The records showed that he had sought treatment and had been admitted for a long history of alcohol abuse. He lost his job with the insurance company and brought suit against the hospital for breach of medical confidentiality.

Under state and federal law, a general release for medical records does not authorize the provider to divulge the fact of substance abuse treatment or substance abuse treatment records. That requires a written release, signed by the patient, which specifically applies to such information and records. Unfortunately, the man had signed such a release when he signed the insurance company's legal release form.

Researchers may also have access to medical records. Staff members and qualified students generally may review charts for research purposes without prior patient consent. An internal or external review panel to protect the rights of human subjects is required prior to allowing researchers access to medical records if the institution receives federal funding. As noted in Chapter 8, the Health Insurance Portability and Accountability Act of 1996 (HIPAA) has greatly limited this right of access for research.

INCIDENT REPORTS

Incident, variance, situational, or **unusual occurrence report forms** were originally designed to be part of the overall risk management or quality assurance effort of any health-oriented institution. Federal and state standards dictate the establishment of an incident reporting system, with the main functions of incident reports being the review and evaluation of patient care. If one uses the definition of an incident to be an unfavorable deviation of expectations involving patient care that may be the result of medical management, it is easy to see that incident reports were devised to augment and improve the quality of patient care. Other obvious uses of such forms are to enhance the hospital's in-service educational offerings, to alert hospital administrative staff to potential problem areas, to minimize injuries from the incident, and to decrease the likelihood of similar incidents in the future.

Incident reports may serve to aid the hospital attorney in planning defense strategy and in deciding whether a case should be litigated or settled out of court. The hospital's liability carrier frequently asks for such reports when investigating claims. Because of their confidential status in most states, nurses traditionally have been instructed to be candid in their remarks on incident reports so that the quality of care can be upgraded.

The root of the confidential nature of incident reports lies in a hospital or business record privileged communication doctrine. Although not a common law right, hospitals have long declined to divulge such reports, arguing that disclosure would make the incident report virtually useless.

Today, the right to discover incident reports is dependent upon individual courts. Declaring that plaintiffs still must show the need for their right to incident reports, some courts have allowed such discovery (*Johnson v. University Hospitals of Cleveland*, 2002) while others have denied the access of these reports (*Lindsey v. St. John Health System*, 2007; *Quinton v. Medcentral Health System*, 2006; *1620 Health Partners, L. C. v. Fluitt*, 2002; *Smith v. Manor Care of Canton, Inc.*, 2006; *Tenet Health System v. Taitel*, 2003).

In re Intracare Hospital (2007) outlines the steps that a health care facility should take to ensure the confidentiality of an incident report. Incident or occurrence reports must be labeled as such and must be noted as confidential. Merely labeling a document as confidential, though, is not sufficient. A privilege log should be maintained by the risk management or legal department, listing and identifying in general terms all incident or occurrence reports as they are received for which the privilege of confidentiality might later be asserted. To be confidential, the report must be transmitted to an appropriate committee, considered by the committee, and acted on by the committee in the regular course of its operations. Bylaws or other pronouncements by the facility establishing committees must define the scope of responsibility and specify that the committee's deliberations and conclusions will be confidential. Finally, the committee must be mandated to meet and actually meet on a regularly defined basis and must consider and make recommendations to hospital management within the scope of its responsibility.

Nurses must exercise caution in completing such reports and should always fill out the forms as though they are discoverable. No language that admits liability should be included, and there should be no mention of the incident report form having been completed in the patient's chart. Indicating that there is an incident report incorporates by reference the incident report into the chart and makes it as discoverable as the original patient chart. The ideal incident report is a check-off list, with a limited area for a brief, written description of the occurrence.

Nurses must include in the chart relevant documentation concerning the underlying event that mandated completion of an incident report. For example, if the patient is found on the floor, the medical record should note that fact as well as all measures that were performed to ensure appropriate treatment was initiated.

It is also advisable to abandon multiple copies of the form because such copies tend to deny a privileged communication. For an incident report to be considered privileged under the attorney–client privilege, it ideally will be completed and forwarded directly to the hospital attorney or the in-house representative.

GUIDELINES

Incident Reports

1. The incident report should be initiated by the one who directly observes the incident or by the first person to arrive at the site of the incident.
2. Incorporate the patient's account of the happening into the incident report and state these comments as direct quotes. If the patient is unable to give an account, describe exactly what

you witnessed or discovered. For example, "the patient fell out of bed" is appropriate if you actually saw the fall. Statements such as "Patient found on floor at foot of bed" or "Patient states, 'I was trying to get up and lost my balance'" are more appropriate if you were the first person to discover the patient on the floor.

3. Write only the facts. Do not infer assumptions or draw conclusions. Do not add what you would like to have done after the fact. Above all, never imply liability. A question such as, "How could this incident have been prevented?" should be left unanswered or answered in the negative.

4. Have other witnesses assist you in preparing the report and have them co-sign the final report.

5. If appropriate, have the patient or injured party seen by a physician and document any actions taken and treatment given.

6. Avoid writing in the medical record that an incident report was completed, or else it will become incorporated by reference into the total patient chart. Document what happened and the actions taken if the incident report involved a hospitalized patient.

7. Forward the report to the nursing service, the hospital attorney, the quality assurance committee, and anyone else so designated by hospital policy.

8. Ensure that only one copy of the report exists. If other departments or committees would like to see the report, the original may be forwarded to them in succession.

9. Should your hospital require multiple copies of incident reports, initiate action to reduce the number of copies to one, as it is difficult to show how multiple copies maintain confidentiality.

EXERCISE 9.4

Mrs. Johnson, 76 years old, was admitted to the acute care facility for hip replacement surgery. She became extremely short of breath and a pulse oximeter reading of 76% on room air was obtained. She was scheduled for an emergency scan to rule out a pulmonary embolus. While in the radiology department, she fell from the stretcher and struck her head on the floor. Documentation in her patient record revealed that Mrs. Johnson had a head laceration and was vomiting during the procedure. This documentation was noted in the records of the attending physician, nurse, and the imaging technician.

Following her successful recovery from the pulmonary embolism, Mrs. Johnson remarked to her daughter that she still had a large lump on her head from the fall in radiology. The daughter, acting as her mother's representative, filed a lawsuit for negligence. In the precourt review of the case, the attorney for Mrs. Johnson requested a copy of the institution's incident report for this event, claiming that he could not adequately represent Mrs. Johnson without full details of the fall.

How would you advise the judge to rule in this instance?

FAXING OF MEDICAL RECORDS

Using fax machines to send health information is another way to ensure that material is received promptly and accurately. Difficulty arises in assuring the patient's right to privacy. Multiple regulations, including HIPAA standards, affect the faxing of medical records and mandate safeguards that protect the security and confidentiality of computerized and paper-based records.

Medical information should be faxed only if urgently needed and must be accompanied by a signed release form. Prior to faxing the material, it is advisable that a verification of fax numbers is performed and recorded; some institutions send a blank record if this is the first time they have faxed to a given number/institution. A cover sheet indicating the confidentiality of the material and to whom it is to be given must accompany all medical faxes. The cover sheet should also note what an unintended receiver should do with the faxed information, if it is inadvertently received. Faxed materials should only be handled by authorized individuals and the originals should be immediately returned to the patient record. Additionally, fax machines must be located in an area with restricted access.

CONFIDENTIALITY OF MEDICAL RECORDS

The primary reason for **confidentiality of medical records** is to promote candor by patients and health care providers to optimize medical and nursing treatment. Violation of a patient's right of confidentiality opens the health care provider to a potential lawsuit. Several lawsuits support this statement. In *Claim of Gilbert* (1998), the court upheld the firing of an AIDS program coordinator at a community health center for violating her employer's confidentiality policy. The program coordinator had divulged information about a prospective client to a colleague who was not a co-worker.

Howard v. Milwaukie Convalescent Home (2008) concerned a charge nurse who copied pages from charts for more than a year and forwarded them to the director of nursing and an administrator to support concerns that she had about the performance of a staff licensed practical nurse that she supervised. Performance review is a legitimate concern and does not violate medical confidentiality, ruled the court, as quality review and performance assessments are necessary and legitimate functions for the facility. When she began copying material from patient records to protect herself in the event that she was reported to the board of nursing, she did violate the patients' right of confidentiality. These latter records were not given to her superiors, no effort was made to conceal the identities of the patients, and the records were taken out of the facility by the nurse in question. The nurse kept these records at her home, a gross breach of the patient's confidentiality. The court supported the dismissal of this nurse from the facility.

Similarly, in *Vaughn v. Epworth Villa* (2008), a nurse's aide photocopied and sent the local office of the United States Equal Employment Opportunity Commission (EEOC) pages from patient medical records in an attempt to show that she was disciplined for charting errors when other employees in the same institution, younger and nonminorities, made similar errors and were not disciplined. When the facility where she worked became aware of what the nurse's aide had done, she was terminated for violation of medical confidentiality. The court upheld this termination, whether or not there was a valid discrimination cause of action.

In *United States v. Occident* (2007), a nurse's aide used her employment position to obtain confidential information from patient hospital records and co-worker pay-stubs. She sold this information to an accomplice who fraudulently applied for credit cards and used the credit cards to purchase approximately $250,000 in merchandise. The United States Court of Appeals for the Fourth Circuit upheld the aide's conviction and 2-year prison sentence for violation of the United States identity-theft statute.

In *Hurchanik v. Swayze* (2007), a patient's personal information was stolen from her physician's office by an unnamed person. The patient learned that an imposter had used her name and employment information to open a residential service account with the phone company. When the impersonator was identified, the patient testified that she had seen the person in the doctor's office during a patient visit. Though the patient could not prove how the impersonator had acquired her personal information, the court was satisfied that there had to have been a breach of her confidential information, as the phone number that the impersonator used was the identical incorrect phone number that was recorded in the patient's medical record. That, said the court, could only have happened if the impersonator had viewed the patient's record.

EXERCISE 9.5

The parents of a premature neonate admitted to the neonatal intensive care unit brought suit against the facility for medical and nursing negligence that resulted in repeated episodes of hypoxia and ischemia resulting in permanent brain injuries to their child. The preliminary issue for the court was whether the attorneys for the parents could acquire data from other patient charts to establish that this was a continuing rather than isolated event. Specifically, they requested data showing the numbers of neonates weighing less than 1,000 grams that were admitted, the number of such infants transferred to other facilities, and the number of such infants who were not transferred and died in the hospital. The admission logs for the facility were kept at this institution for internal quality review.

How should the court act on this request? Explain why the attorneys should be able to have such information or why they should be denied access to these records.

Disclosure of a roommate's name is not protected, but the roommate's confidential medical information is protected. In *Foley v. Samaritan Hospital* (2006), the family of a deceased patient filed a lawsuit for negligence against the hospital in which she had received care. She was treated at the facility's emergency center for severe abdominal pain. The lawsuit alleged that the nurse obtained vital signs but did not timely report significant drops in the patient's blood pressure and that the radiologist obtained the CT scan, but likewise did not report significant findings to the attending physician.

Lawyers for the family requested the names of two patients who were also being treated in the emergency center during the same time interval. The court ruled that HIPPA does not protect their names, but does protect their medical information, and thus their names could be revealed to the family's legal counsel.

Similarly, in *Docherty v. Unemployment Board* (2006), the court found that there was limited expectation to confidentiality in semi-private patient rooms. In that case, a phlebotomist was to draw blood from one of two pediatric patients who shared a semi-private room. At the time of the incident, both patients had parents visiting with them. The mother of the patient whose blood was being drawn asked the purpose of the blood test. The other patient's mother overheard the response, which indicated that the blood was being drawn to test for HIV and hepatitis. The phlebotomist was fired after the patient's mother complained to hospital administration about the lack of confidentiality.

The court concluded that there was no expectation of privacy in this instance, given the hospital's practice of placing patients in shared rooms, requiring hospital personnel to perform medical treatments in these shared rooms, allowing visitors during treatment periods, and failing to provide alternative locations for hospital employees to discuss sensitive patient information. Thus, there was no reasonable expectation that all of the patient's information would remain totally confidential. A family member made a legitimate request for information and the employee had to respond. He had no control over the fact that the patients' beds were only 8 feet apart in a small room or that others were present in the room.

HEALTH INSURANCE PORTABILITY AND ACCOUNTABILITY ACT OF 1996

In August 1996, President Clinton signed the **Health Insurance Portability and Accountability Act (HIPAA)** into law (Public Law 104-191). This act mandates the development of a centralized electronic database containing all health records for every patient in the United States as a means of administrative simplification. The act is sweeping legislation that provides for:

1. The portability of health care coverage
2. An antifraud and abuse program
3. The streamlining of the transfer of patient information between insurers and providers
4. Tax incentives toward the acquisition of health insurance and accelerated benefits
5. The establishment of the federal government as a national health care regulator

Prior to the enforcement date of this act, federal law did not protect patient confidentiality in medical records. Protection was given through limited federal law and a patchwork of state laws, varying in degrees of protection. Under this act, the Secretary of the Department of Health and Human Services has promulgated comprehensive standards facilitating the transmission of medical data, administrative records, and financial records. Significant fines and penalties are included in the act to enable the Secretary to enforce the act against those who violate its provisions.

The first issue to understand is that the HIPAA rule applies to "covered entities." **Covered entities** include health plans such as Medicare and Medicaid, and commercial health plans such as Blue Cross and Blue Shield, Aetna, SIGNA, Indian Health Service, and the Veterans Administration health program (Standards for Privacy of Identifiable Health Information, sections 160.102 and 103). By definition, providers are covered only if they transmit protected health information in an electronic form. Not covered are health plans that have less than 50 participants, self-administered plans, law enforcement officials, schools, and employers, although an employer's health plan is a covered entity.

The second issue to understand concerns **protected health information (PHI).** These are individually identifiable health information indicators, and the list includes 18 such indicators. PHI is collected from the individual by the covered entity and relates to past, present, or future physical or mental health or condition of the individual, or the past, present, or future payment for the provision of health care to an individual. PHI identifies the individual, or there is a reasonable expectation to believe that the information can be used to identify the individual (Standards for Privacy of Identifiable Health Information, section 160.103).

PHI includes the following: name of the individual or initials; addresses (street address, e-mail, or Internet addresses); dates (including birth date and dates of services received); telephone and fax numbers; Social Security or other personal identification numbers; medical record numbers; health plan account numbers; license or certificate numbers; medical device identifiers; biometric identifiers such as fingerprints or photographic images; or any other unique identifying characteristic or code.

For example, the disclosure that Mr. John Jones is covered under a CIGNA policy is protected health information because it contains both demographic information (his name) and information about present or future payment for health care services (insurance company name). To be PHI, the information does not need to concern a particular diagnosis or treatment received for a medical condition.

Information may be disclosed to assist in health care (Standards for Privacy of Identifiable Health Information, section 164.510). A covered entity may disclose to a family member, other relative, or close personal friend of the patient, or any other person identified by the individual, the PHI directly relevant to the person's involvement with the individual's care or payment related to the individual's health care. This allows family members or friends to obtain needed prescriptions or medical supplies for an individual.

This disclosure of information to assist in health care extends to directory information, including the individual's name, location in the facility, condition described in general terms, and religious affiliation. A covered entity may also disclose or use PHI to notify or assist in the notification of a family member, personal representative of the individual, or another person responsible for the care of the individual in the case of serious injury or death. For example, a covered entity may disclose to law enforcement officers the address of a patient who died in the facility as a result of a car accident or serious accident (Standards for Privacy of Identifiable Health Information, section 164.510 [b]).

Similarly, a covered entity may disclose PHI in response to law enforcement requests for the purpose of locating a suspect, fugitive, material witness, or missing person. Descriptive characteristics may be disclosed in this instance, such as height, weight, scars, tattoos, and presence or absence of facial hair. Disclosure as required by law, such as reporting contagious diseases, certain chronic illnesses, and gunshot or knife wounds, are also permitted under the HIPAA standards.

The privacy standard limits how this information may be used or shared, mandates safeguards for protecting the health information, and shifts the control of health information from providers to the patient by giving patients significant rights. Health care facilities must provide patients with a document entitled Notice of Privacy Practices, which explains how their PHI will be used or shared with other entities. This document also alerts patients to the process for complaints if they determine that their information rights have been violated.

HIPAA standards allow information to be shared or used for treatment, payment, and limited operations (TPO) purposes. Communications may occur between providers without having to obtain a number of signed forms from the patient or their authorized representatives. The caveat is that those providers sharing information have a relationship with the patient. Under this part of the act, information may be shared with both covered and noncovered entities. Much of the information that nurses require or share with other providers comes under the treatment purposes, including providing or coordinating the provision of services.

Patient rights included under the privacy rule allow the right to request restrictions on the use and sharing of PHI, the right to request alternate communications, such as asking to be contacted only at home rather than at work, and the right to obtain a list of disclosures for purposes other than PTO or for which special authorization has been obtained. Alternate communication requests, if reasonable, must be respected.

If a disclosure of PHI is not for PTO and/or is not required by law, a valid authorization must be obtained. Such an authorization must contain the following:

1. A description of the information to be used or disclosed
2. Identification of the person(s), or class of persons, authorized to make the requested disclosure
3. The name or other specific identification of the person(s) to whom the covered entity makes the requested disclosure
4. A description of each purpose of the requested use or disclosure (noting that the statement "At the request of the individual" is sufficient)
5. An expiration date or an expiration event that related to the individual or the purpose of the use or disclosure (such as "end of research study" or "none")
6. Signature of the individual or personal representative and date (Standards for Privacy of Identifiable Health Information, section 164.508 [c][1])

Note that the authorization must have three required statements: the individual's right to revoke the authorization in writing; the ability or inability to condition treatment, payment, enrollment, or eligibility for benefits on the authorization; and the potential for disclosure pursuant to the authorization to be subject to redisclosure by the recipient and no longer be protected by this rule (Standards for Privacy of Identifiable Health Information, section 164.508[c][2]).

If the authorization is a valid authorization, it should be accepted by the covered authority. There is no requirement that the authorization must only be on an individual covered entity's form. HIPAA specifically notes that the demand that each authorization be only on a specific form is a game that hinders the lawful disclosure of PHI.

Violators of the act may incur either fines or penalties. There are some provisions for the individual who discloses PHI in violation of the act, but did not know and would not have known by exercise of reasonable diligence that he or she had violated the act. Also, penalties may be excused if the failure to comply was due to reasonable cause, not willful neglect, and the failure to comply is corrected within 30 days (HIPAA: Administrative Simplification, section 1320d). In an unpublished case, an employee of a Wisconsin health care facility was terminated from employment because she had accessed the medical records of her significant other's former wife. When the former wife's records were introduced into evidence, the former wife asked the hospital to investigate. Computer records clearly showed the employee who was dismissed had obtained the records and given them to the attorney (personal communication, M. J. Mullen, North Dakota Asst. Attorney General, March 24, 2004).

A Minnesota case extended the right to terminate an employee for misuse of medical records to denial of the ability to collect unemployment benefits following the termination (*Pribble v. Edina Care Center*, 2003). In this case, the nurse, to show that she was being unfairly treated by her employer, began photocopying patient records so that she could show her charting was not "substandard." She faxed these photocopied records to her attorney. The court affirmed that such photocopying was a violation of patient records confidentiality and that she had been terminated for cause; thus she was ineligible to collect unemployment compensation.

GUIDELINES

HIPAA Compliance

1. Restrict the posting of patient information, such as on white boards or other signage where it can be viewed by other patients and visitors to an institution. Ideally, such patient information should be placed in areas accessible only to health care providers who have a need to know such information.
2. Restrict overhead paging, particularly if the paging announces information about specific patients. Instead of a page that states "Code Blue, Room 304," consider changing the paging system so that only internal systems are used. Conversely, announce "Code Blue, 3 Southwest."
3. Leave no message for patients on answering machines or with family members. Ask for a return call only. Additionally, do not initiate phone calls to patients' employment sites, unless specifically requested by the patient.
4. Shred all papers that have PHI or ensure that such papers are locked in files/offices where others cannot see the information. For example, merely tossing such papers in open trash containers, even if the trash container is in a locked office, may allow the janitorial staff access to PHI.
5. Use cover sheets when faxing information, ensure that the fax numbers are correct before faxing the PHI, and list how the recipient is to handle the faxed information should it be received by other than the intended recipient.

6. Ensure that fax machines and computers are located in areas where other parties may not view the PHI.
7. Secure computer identifications and establish policies for automatic or required periodic changing of passwords.
8. Develop a secure method of transporting PHI. This entails identifying who can transport PHI and how the information will be protected during transport. If envelopes are used to transport PHI, ensure that they are sealed and that no tampering of the seal occurs during transport.
9. Know the institution's policies and procedures for protection of PHI. Report any violations of the privacy rules to supervisory personnel immediately.

Electronic Mail and the Internet

The age of information presents some unique challenges. The increasing use of electronic mail (e-mail) via the Internet is an area of potential liability for health care providers. Communicating patient care in a paper world is fraught with potential for wrongful disclosures. Although safety measures can be used with e-mail, such as encryption or an electronic "lock and key" system, security is not perfect. Messages are "locked" by the sender, making the message unreadable except by the intended recipient, who has a "key" or electronic password to decrypt the message. Thus, there is some measure of privacy. The danger lies in the possibility of an unauthorized decryption of the message by hackers or others intending to commit identify theft or another form of fraud.

Similar issues arise with Internet messages, because there is no greater security when Internet communication is in transit over phone lines than there is with an ordinary phone call. Messages can be intercepted and read as they pass through routers. Although federal laws give some protection in this area, privacy issues for messages sent via the Internet remain a hotly debated topic.

A case that illustrates the extent to which courts hold e-mails confidential is *Woodson v. Scott and White Memorial Hospital* (2007). A hospital nurse was instructed to cease from continuing with some unacceptable conduct. Hospital policy dictated that employee e-mails and e-mail accounts are confidential and not to be accessed by co-workers without permission from the author and recipient. The nurse in question was warned to stop using her co-workers computers without their consent, stop accessing their e-mail accounts, stop printing out their e-mails, and stop gossiping about what she found in their e-mails. Additionally, the nurse was informed that she was not to access the medical records of her co-workers. When she continued to access her co-workers e-mails, spread gossip about these same co-workers, and access their personal medical records, she was terminated with cause.

REPORTING AND ACCESS LAWS

The law compels disclosure of medical information in contexts other than discovery or testimony. Reporting laws require that information be given to governmental agencies, both federal and state. Examples include vital statistics, child abuse, elder abuse, public health, and wounds.

Some statutes do not mandate reporting but allow access to medical records without the patient's permission. Examples of such access laws include workers' compensation, state public records laws, and the federal Freedom of Information Act.

COMMON LAW DUTY TO DISCLOSE

The **common law duty to disclose** recognizes a duty to disclose medical information in limited circumstances. Generally, public safety concerns underlie these disclosure rights.

Contagious Diseases

With contagious diseases, there is a duty to warn others at risk of exposure unless forbidden by statute. This includes family members and health care providers, as well as others at risk. In most states, there is no duty to warn all members of the public individually, but states vary on this requirement.

Threats to an Identified Person

Some courts have ruled that there is a duty to warn identified persons when a patient has made a credible threat against them. The first decision to affect this duty was *Tarasoff v. Board of Regents of the University of California* (1976). In that case, a nonhospitalized psychiatric patient told his psychiatrist that he would kill his former girlfriend. The threat to kill was made more than once, and there was no doubt in the psychiatrist's mind that the patient could make good on his threat. After Miss Tarasoff was killed, her parents brought this lawsuit for wrongful death, and the court concluded that the psychiatrist or his employer did have a duty to either warn the potential victim or to warn others who could have advised the victim of her potential danger. In a later decision, *Thompson v. County of Alameda* (1980), the same court clarified the scope of this duty to warn by ruling that only threats to readily identifiable persons created a duty to warn, and there is no corresponding duty to the public at large.

A more recent case, *Godinez v. Siena College* (2001), reinforced the ability to warn against possible threats to a specific group of individuals. In *Godinez*, a college student who was receiving mental health treatment told his parents that he was planning to "act out violently" at the college graduation ceremonies. His parents called the nurse where their son was receiving therapy, who in turn notified mental health authorities and they called the local police. The son was questioned by college officials, who let him participate in the ceremonies.

The son filed suit, claiming that the mental health nurse released confidential mental health information, but the court noted that his parents, not the professional staff, had released confidential information. Thus, the issue of medical confidentiality was a moot issue. The court praised the staff for their quick response to what could have been a dangerous situation.

Courts have slowly applied the duty to warn principle, and most courts are now holding that there is a duty to warn identifiable individuals. For example, in *State v. Bright* (1996), the court ruled that it is not a breach of medical confidentiality for a health care professional to warn a potential victim of a patient's dangerous propensities. "Courts around the United States are not just overlooking the traditional definition of medical confidentiality to protect potential victims, but are imposing an affirmative duty on psychiatrists, psychologists, therapists, and other mental health workers, in inpatient and outpatient settings, to warn identifiable victims when patients make threats toward them" (at 1057).

In *Bright,* an armed forces veteran was receiving outpatient therapy for chronic alcohol abuse. Over the past 20 years, he had been considered bipolar. His therapist knew the patient had killed his brother some years before but was found not guilty by reason of insanity. During the course of the therapy, the patient repeatedly voiced an intention to kill his ex-wife. The ex-wife had left the state and was living in hiding because of the patient's harassment, intimidation, and threatening conduct.

Finally, the patient stated that he was leaving town that evening to find his ex-wife and kill her. The therapist called the local police and the police in the county where the ex-wife lived. Working together, the two police agencies apprehended the man 1 1/2 miles from the intended victim's residence. The patient had with him a newly purchased hunting knife and a roll of duct tape in his trunk. He was charged with making terrorist threats and attempted murder. The court had nothing but praise for the therapist's actions.

A trend seems to be emerging to extend this duty to warn to the general public. For example, in *Kathleen K. v. Robert B.* (1984), the court allowed a woman to sue her sexual partner for deliberate and/or negligent failure to warn her that he had genital herpes. A later case, *Reisner v. Regents of the University of California* (1995), held that a man who discovered in 1990 that he had contracted the acquired immune deficiency syndrome (AIDS) virus from his girlfriend may sue a physician for failing to inform the girlfriend that she had received contaminated blood in 1985.

A further trend in the duty to warn concerns genetic diseases. The court in *Safer v. Pack* (1996) held that the physician has a duty to warn individuals, including the patient's immediate family members, who are at risk of avoidable harm from a genetically transmitted condition. This holding was based on the premise that a genetically transmissible condition is sufficiently similar to a contagious disease.

Robert Batkin, the father of plaintiff Donna Safer, was diagnosed in 1956 with multiple polyposis and colorectal cancer. Despite Dr. Pack's efforts to excise the cancer, Mr. Batkin died of metastatic disease in 1964. In 1990, Safer, then 36 years old, was diagnosed with a cancerous blockage of the colon and multiple polyposis. After undergoing a colectomy with ileorectal anastomosis, it was discovered that the cancer extended beyond her bowel. The finding of the additional metastases led to removal of her left ovary and a regimen of chemotherapy.

In 1991, Ms. Safer obtained her father's medical records. They revealed that he had suffered from multiple polyposis, which she claimed is a hereditary disease leading to colorectal cancer. She filed a complaint alleging that Dr. Pack had been professionally negligent by failing to warn her of the risk posed to her health. Safer further contended that the medical standards prevailing at the time required Dr. Pack to inform her of the risk so that she could benefit from early diagnosis and treatment.

The lower court found for Dr. Pack, and Safer appealed. The superior court said:

> We see no impediment, legal or otherwise, to recognizing a physician's duty to warn those known to be at risk of avoidable harm from a genetically transmissible condition. In terms of foreseeability especially, there is no essential difference between the type of genetic threat at issue here and the menace of infection, contagion, or a threat of physical harm. . . . The individual or group at risk is easily identified, and substantial future harm may be averted or minimized by a timely and effective warning. (*Safer v. Pack*, 1996, at 1192)

The superior court then decided that a physician must reasonably attempt to inform those likely to be affected or to make the information available. This duty, the court held, extends beyond the patient to members of the immediate family, who may be adversely affected by the failure to warn. The court did note in its discussion that there may be some confidentiality issues if the father in this case had specifically asked that his family not be informed of his genetically transmissible disease.

Since the incidents of 2001, terrorist threats may also affect this area of the law. In *Davis v. Allen Parish Service District* (2006), the nurse at the change of shift informed the oncoming nurse to watch carefully a certain psychiatric patient of Middle Eastern descent who had been verbalizing threats about the U.S. president and government facilities and property. The patient was being held involuntarily in a locked psychiatric unit, but he had phone privileges. That evening the patient

used the phone and began speaking in an agitated tone in English and in Arabic a
his friends killing the president and blowing up petroleum facilities on the Texas G

The nurse phoned a nursing supervisor and the assistant administrator a
then phoned the U.S. Secret Service. She informed the agent of what the patient w
then elaborated on the patient's psychiatric condition and the fact that he was i
admitted to the psychiatric service. The next day the hospital administrator found ou
phone call to the Secret Service. After conferring with the hospital legal staff, he tern
nurse for violation of patient confidentiality, and the nurse sued for wrongful discharg

The nurse was found to have violated hospital policy by disclosing the patient's confidential
medical information without his express consent. Only the hospital administrator could authorize
release of confidential information without the patient's express consent. Though the court did not
discount the right to alert the Secret Service, it was up to the hospital administrator to make that call.

LIMITATIONS TO DISCLOSURE

Several statutory and common law limitations on disclosure have evolved that assist in preserving
confidentiality and impose sanctions for some violations of confidentiality.

Substance and Alcohol Abuse Confidentiality

The Department of Health and Human Services (HHS) first issued the Standards for Privacy of
Individually Identifiable Health Information pursuant to provisions of HIPAA (45 *Code of Federal
Regulations* Parts 160 and 164) in 2000, amending these standards in 2002 and 2003. Substance
abuse treatment programs that are subject to HIPAA must comply with these standards.

Information may be released with the patient's consent, if the consent is written and contains all of the following elements:

1. Name or general designation of the program or person permitted to make the disclosure
2. Name or title of the individual or name of the organization to which disclosure is to be made
3. Name of the patient
4. Purpose of the disclosure
5. How much and what kind of information to be disclosed
6. Signature of the patient and, in some states, a parent or guardian
7. Date on which consent is signed
8. Statement that the consent is subject to revocation at any time except to the extent that the
   program has already acted on it
9. Date, event, or condition upon which the consent will expire if not previously revoked.
   (45 *Code of Federal Regulations*, 2000, amended 2002 and 2003)

The Privacy Rule defers to requirements in other applicable laws regarding the disclosure of
health information relating to minors. A minor must always sign the consent form for a program
to release information even to his or her parent or guardian, and some states require programs to
obtain parental permission before providing treatment to a minor.

HIV/AIDS Confidentiality

Special characteristics of HIV and AIDS and of the AIDS epidemic present new and unique challenges
to health care providers trying to maintain patient confidentiality while meeting their obligations to
disclose medical information. First, widespread fear of AIDS and ignorance about its transmission

have made concerns of privacy and confidentiality even more important and urgent. If information about a person's AIDS infection or HIV positivity reaches employers, insurers, schools, or friends, it may have disastrous effects. Confidentiality is at the heart of HIV and AIDS testing, for most individuals will not submit to HIV testing and counseling unless they are assured of confidentiality.

Second, the fact that the transmission of AIDS and HIV is not through close proximity or casual contact limits the need for disclosure of information about infection. Third, with the increased life expectancy for patients with AIDS/HIV, post-positive blood screens have strengthened the case for confidentiality.

States have adopted a variety of legislative and administrative approaches to confidentiality and disclosure of information regarding AIDS and HIV. All 50 states require reporting of AIDS cases, without the patients' consent, to the Centers for Disease Control and Prevention or to the state health department for epidemiological purposes. The states are divided, though, on whether the reporting is anonymous or entails more descriptive demographics. The majority of states have adopted statutes maintaining the strict confidentiality of AIDS-related information, while some states have passed statutes permitting disclosure of AIDS testing to certain persons or under certain circumstances.

There is also some limited movement toward mandatory testing for HIV/AIDS. In July 1996, the American Medical Association endorsed the mandatory testing of all pregnant women and newborns. In February 1997, New York became the first state to mandate the screening of all newborns for HIV and the disclosure of the test results to the newborns' mothers. Connecticut has followed this lead and now requires that all newborns are tested for AIDS unless the mother had an AIDS test during the pregnancy. Supporters of the bill argued that early identification and treatment of HIV are saving lives. As newer research studies are now supporting that infants need not be born with HIV with proper prenatal care, there is a renewed effort to test all pregnant women for HIV/AIDS (National Institute of Allergy and Infectious Diseases, 2004).

A number of states permit the state health department to engage in contact tracing or partner notification. Some states notify all sexual and needle-sharing contacts, while others have chosen a more limited means of notifying contacts, such as the contact of all individuals who have received infected blood products. Health care providers are urged to investigate their state statutes in this regard.

Because standards of care are constantly evolving in patients with AIDS, issues of liability often depend on when the care of the patient actually occurred. For example, in *Doe v. Johnson* (1991), the issue centered on a blood transfusion the patient received in 1985 and whether there was a duty to inform patients about the possibility of contracting AIDS from the blood supply. Since this was not a standard of care at the time of the blood transfusion, the court said the jury should decide if the blood transfusion was a reasonable treatment alternative at the time the patient underwent surgery.

Almost uniformly, courts have upheld privacy rights when disclosure of test results have been made without the patient's consent (*Biddle v. Warren General Hospital,* 1998; *Doe v. High-Tech Institute, Inc.,* 1998; *In re Sealed Case,* 1995; *Jane Doe v. Marselle,* 1996).

SELECTED ETHICAL CONCERNS

To assess the ethical advisability of mandatory HIV testing, one must first examine some general ethical principles regarding public health screening. Traditionally, screening may be ethically justified when:

1. An important health issue is at stake,
2. Acceptable treatment modalities exist and are accessible to the general public,

3. Accurate diagnostic procedures are available,
4. Tests are cost effective in terms of containing or preventing the spread of disease,
5. Fundamental ethical rights are not transgressed by screening, and
6. The overall benefits of screening outweigh the harms.

The argument concerns whether the fundamental ethical rights of confidentiality, autonomy, and informed consent are transgressed through mandatory HIV testing. With mandatory screening during pregnancy, the argument that a second human being could be infected through no fault of his or her own adds appeal for the need for such testing.

The ethical arguments supporting mandatory testing of the newborn are the Harm Principle and the principle of beneficence. The Harm Principle is defined as a liberty-limiting principle where "a person's liberty is justifiably restricted to prevent harm to others caused by that person" (Beauchamp & Walters, 2003, p. 31). The ethical principle of beneficence "requires us to abstain from injuring others and to help others further their important and legitimate interests, largely by preventing or removing possible harms" (Beauchamp & Walters, 2003, p. 23). An ethical issue yet to be address concerns mandatory testing of other than newborns. Can one also use these ethical arguments, now that we have better genetic markers, to argue that individuals have an obligation to undergo genetic testing for the sake of their offspring or others that may be harmed in the future?

A second ethical issue that pervades this area of the law concerns the duty to warn, whether it is to a known person or the public at large. This duty directly confronts an individual's right to know with the ethical obligation that primary health care providers have to hold patient information confidential. Additionally, it directly asks the question of whose rights take precedent, those of the individual or the health care provider. Codes of ethics for nurses, physicians, and other members of the interdisciplinary team have provisions regarding the confidentiality of patient information and the importance of honoring this confidence. Each individual health care practitioner thus has the ethical responsibility of questioning whether to hold information confidential or allow the information to be discussed with others.

EXERCISE 9.6

You have been appointed to a panel to establish a national standard for nursing documentation. It is hoped that this will assist in preventing future litigation that involves documentation. What types of uniform charting forms should be developed and why? Can one form or one set of forms be developed for national use? List the pros and cons of a national standard for documentation.

Are there ethical principles involved in documentation, especially confidentiality and truthfulness in documentation? From an ethical perspective, would a national standard for documentation more completely protect the ethical principles involved in documentation? Why or why not?

SUMMARY

- From a nursing perspective, the most important purpose of documentation is communication.

- Basic information contained in the patient's medical record includes personal data, financial data, and medical data.

- Effective documentation includes:
  Making an entry for every observation
  Following up as needed
  Reading nurses' notes before giving care to patients
  Making an entry into the chart, even if the entry is late
  Charting the entry after the event
  Using clear and objective language
  Being realistic and factual
  Charting only your own observations; never alter a record at another's request
  Charting patient's refusal of care
  Charting all patient education
  Correcting chart errors correctly
  Identifying yourself after every entry
  Using standardized checklists or flow sheets
  Leaving no room for liability
- Charting by exception requires documentation of only significant or abnormal findings, and previously entered standardized or expected results are not reentered in the chart.
- Alteration of records may be performed by the primary writer for minor mistakes; substantive errors are corrected by administrative personnel or the primary health care provider.
- The time frame for retention of records is codified in state statutes, imposing a clear duty on facilities not to lose or destroy records within certain time frames.

- The record is owned by the institution as a business document, though patients have a right of access to the record.
- Incident reports may be discoverable in some states, though the purpose of such reports is for the overall risk management or quality assurance efforts of the organization.
- Confidentiality of medical records primarily exists to promote candor by patients and health care providers so that medical and nursing interventions may be maximized.
- The Health Insurance Portability and Accountability Act of 1996 (HIPAA) was enacted to begin to address the issue of portability of health care coverage, streamline the transfer of patient information, and assure additional confidentiality of patient data.
- Protected health information (PHI) describes 18 individually identifiable health information indicators that are protected under the HIPAA law.
- There are some exceptions to reporting laws, including a common law duty to disclose medical information in limited circumstances, such as for contagious diseases, threats to identifiable persons, and abuse cases.
- Ethical concerns in this area of the law are numerous and varied.

APPLY YOUR LEGAL KNOWLEDGE

1. How can a staff member ensure confidentiality in clinical settings?
2. What makes charting effective, and how can professional nurses ensure that their charting is effective?
3. After learning the purposes and guidelines for documentation, how might one design a better chart?
4. What safeguards can be used to ensure confidentiality when sending medical information by fax or by e-mail?

YOU BE THE JUDGE

The patient, on the first day post-operative for a transurethral prostate resection, received a unit of whole blood early in the morning on the supposition that he was bleeding internally. That afternoon at 3:22 P.M., the

patient's wife informed the nurse that her husband was breathing "heavily" and requested that the nurse assess him. The nurse, according to the testimony of the wife, informed her that the doctor was aware of the patient's breathing pattern and that there was nothing about which she should worry. The nurse did not leave the nursing station. The patient subsequently died related to shock from the internal bleeding complicated by a reaction to the whole blood.

In court some years later, this same nurse testified that she had called the surgeon immediately to report that the patient's respirations were 50, that she had taken vital signs that were within the normal limits for this patient, and that she had obtained a pulse oximeter reading that was acceptable. She also testified that she kept calling the physician's office to report these findings.

None of this nursing care was documented in the progress notes that the patient's nurse placed in the patient's chart the next day. She testified that she had compiled the progress notes from scratch notes she had written during the previous afternoon. The nurse further testified that it was her practice to make handwritten notes during the time that she worked and then to type her progress notes on the hospital system the next day. Additionally, this nurse never documented taking vital signs during the critical 2 hours between the spike in the patient's respirations and the time he was pronounced dead.

The surgeon's office nurse testified that a call was received from the hospital at 4:00 P.M. and that the surgeon immediately left the office for the hospital. The surgeon testified that he called the hospital from his car phone and that he immediately called a code as soon as he reached the patient's room.

QUESTIONS

1. Did the lack of documentation affect the ultimate outcome of this case?
2. Was there negligence on the part of the nursing staff in the care of this patient?
3. How does the obvious contradiction in the testimony between the patient's hospital nurse and the office nurse and physician's account of what happened affect your decision in this case?
4. What standards for documentation did the patient's nurse breach?
5. How would you decide this case?

REFERENCES

Ahrens v. Katz, 595 F. Supp. 1108 (N. D. Ga., 1984).

Anderson v. Beth Israel Medical Center, 2006 WL 1913413 (N.Y. App., July 13, 2006).

Anderson v. United States, 2006 WL 862860 (N. D. Ill., March 30, 2006).

Beason v. State, 2008 WL 82225 (Tex. App., January 9, 2008).

Beauchamp, T. L., & Walters, L. (2003). *Contemporary issues in bioethics* (6th ed.). Belmont, CA: Thompson Wadsworth Publishers.

Biddle v. Warren General Hospital, No. 96-T-5582 (Ohio App., 1998).

Bogner v. Rahway Hospital, 2008 WL 89944 (N. J. App., January 10, 2008).

Chobanian v. Meriter Hospital, Inc., 2008 WL 4426747 (Wisc. App., October 2, 2008).

Claim of Gilbert, 679 N.Y.S.2d 452 (N.Y. App., 1998).

Claim of Rice, 735 N.Y.S.2d 637 (N.Y. App., 2001).

Columbia Medical Center v. Meier, 2006 WL 2036574 (Tex. App., July 21, 2006).

Computer Fraud and Abuse Act of 1986, 42 U.S.C. Section 290dd-3 (1988); amended as part of the U.S.A. Patriot Act of 2001, 18 U.S.C., section 1030 (2001).

Cornelio v. Stamford Hospital, 717 A.2d 140 (Connecticut, 1998).

Darling v. Charleston Community Memorial Hospital, 33 Ill.2d 326, 211 N.E.2d 253 (1965), cert. den'd. 383 U.S. 946 (1965).

Davis v. Allen Parish Service District, 2006 WL 3780540 (5th Cir., December 18, 2006).

Davis v. Montgomery County Memorial Hospital, 2006 WL 1896217 (Iowa App., July 12, 2006).

Docherty v. Unemployment Board, 2006 WL 1226578 (Pennsylvania Commonwealth, May 9, 2006).

Doe v. High-Tech Institute, Inc., No. 97CA0385, 1998 WL 379926 (Colo. Ct. App., 1998).

Doe v. Johnson, 476 N.W.2d 28 (Iowa, 1991).

Estate of Mahunik v. Hebron, 2007 WL 1296848 (Com. Pl., Allegheny Co., Pennsylvania, March 30, 2007).

Estate of Maxey v. Darden, 187 P. 3rd 144 (Nevada, July 3, 2008).

Florida Department of Health and Rehabilitative Services v. V. M. R., Inc., No. 90-2779, 1991 Fla. App. LEXIS 6122 (July 2, 1991).

Foley v .Samaritan Hospital, 2006 WL 4313368 (N.Y. Supp., February 3, 2006).

Fox v. Cohen, 406 N.E.2d 178 (Ill. App. Ct., 1980).

Fox v. Department of Health, 2008 WL 4643822 (Fla. App., October 22, 2008).

Garcia v. San Antonio Community Hospital, 2002 WL 31478236 (Cal. App., November 6, 2002).

Genao v. State, 679 N.Y.S.2d 539 (New York, 1998).

Godinez v. Siena College, 733 N.Y.S.2d 262 (N.Y. App., 2001).

Gorcey v. Jersey Shore Medical Center, 2006 WL 533379 (N.J. Super., March 6, 2006).

Greywolf v. Carroll, 2007 WL 30097 (Alaska, 2007).

Griffin v. Methodist Hospital, 948 S.W.2d 72 (Tex. App., 1997).

Head v. Colloton, 331 N.W.2d 870 (Iowa, 1983).

Health Insurance Portability and Accountability Act of 1996, Public Law 104-191 (1996).

Health Insurance Portability and Accountability Act: Administrative Simplification, 42 U.S.C. Sections 1320d-5(b)(2), 1320d-5(b)(3), 1998.

Henry v. St. John's Hospital, 512 N.E.2d 1044 (Illinois, 1987).

Howard v. Milwaukie Convalescent Hospital, 2008 WL 4117167 (D. Oregon, August 25, 2008).

Hurchanik v. Swayze, 2007 WL 4099511 (Ohio App., November 19, 2007).

Hutchins v. DCH Regional Medical Center, 770 So.2d 49 (Alabama, 2000).

In re Gould, 2003 WL 21976113 (La. App. August 20, 2003).

In re Intracare Hospital, 2007 WL 2682268 (Tex. App., September 13, 2007).

In re Sealed Case, 67 F.3d 965 (D.C. Cir., 1995).

Jane Doe v. Marselle, 675 A.2d 835 (Connecticut, 1996).

Johnson v. University Hospitals of Cleveland, 2002 WL 31619030 (Ohio App., November 21, 2002).

Kathleen K. v. Robert B., 198 Cal. Rptr. 273 (Cal. App., 1984).

Kivalu v. Life Care Centers of America, 2005 WL 3535063 (Idaho, December 28, 2005).

Kodadek v. Lieberman, 545 S.E.2d 25 (Ga. App., 2001).

Lama v. Borras, 16 F.3d 473 (1st Cir. [PR], 1994).

Landry v. Clement, 711 So.2d 829 (La. App., 1998).

Lemoine v. Arkansas Department of Workforce Services, 2008 WL 4425580 (Ark. App., October 1, 2008).

Lindsey v. St. John Health System, 2007 WL 397075 (Mich. App., February 6, 2007).

Lugar v. Baton Rouge General Medical Center, 696 So.2d 652 (La. App., 1997).

Mangels, L. (1990). Chart notes from a malpractice insurer's hell. *Medical Economics, 67*(22), 120–121.

May v. Jones, 675 So.2d 276 (La. App., 1996).

May v. Moore, 424 So.2d 596 (Alabama, 1982).

McDonald v. Clinger, 84 A.D.2d 482, 446 N.Y.S.2d 801 (4th Dept., 1982).

Mitsinicos v. New Rochelle Nursing Home, Inc., 685 N.Y.S.2d 758 (N.Y. App., 1999).

National Institute of Allergy and Infectious Diseases. (2004). *HIV infection in infants and children.* [Fact Sheet]. Washington, DC: National Institutes of Health.

Persing v. Unnamed Hospital, 2007 WL 4590654 (Sup. Ct. Los Angeles Co., California, December 12, 2007).

Phillips v. Covenant Clinic, 625 N.E.2d 714 (Iowa, 2001).

Pludra v. Life Care Center of America, Inc., 2004 WL 42247 (Mass. App., January 8, 2004).

Ploch v. Hamai, 2006 WL 16634 (Mo. App., December 19, 2006).

Pribble v. Edina Care Center, 2003 WL 945792 (Minn. App., March 11, 2003).

Privacy Act of 1974, 5 U.S.C. Section 552a (1974).

Proske v. St. Barnabas Medical Center, 712 A.2d 1207 (N.J. Super., 1998).

Quinton v. Medcentral Health System, 2006 WL 2349548 (Ohio App., August 11, 2006).

Reisner v. Regents of the University of California, 37 Cal. Rptr. 518 (California, 1995).

Roberts v. Sisters of St. Francis, 566 N.E.2d 662 (Illinois, 1990).

Ross v. Redding Medical Center, 2003 WL 21246105 (Cal. App., May 29, 2003).

Rotan v. Greenbaum, 273 F.2d 830 (D.C. Cir., 1959).

Rothstein v. Orange Grove Center, Inc., 60 S.W.3d 807 (Tennessee, 2001).

Safer v. Pack, 677 A.2d 1188 (N.J. Super. Ct App. Div., 1996).

Sam v. State of New York, 2007 WL 2175371 (N.Y. Ct. of Claims, May 9, 2007).

Shahine v. Louisiana State University Medical Center, 680 So.2d 1352 (La. App., 1996).

1620 Health Partners, L. C. v. Fluitt, 2002 WL 31557951 (Fla. App., November 20, 2002).

Smith v. Manor Care of Canton, Inc., 2006 WL 636975 (Ohio App., March 13, 2006).

Standards for Hospitals and Health Care Facilities, 6 CCR 1011-1 Chapter V, Part 14, Long Term Care Facilities (amended June 18, 2008; effective July 30, 2008).

Standards for Privacy of Identifiable Health Information, 45 CFR Sections 160.102, 160.103, 164.510, 164.508(a)(1), 164.508 (c)(1), 164.508(c)(2), (2000, amended 2002, 2003).

State v. Bright, 683 A.2d 1055 (Del. Super., 1996).

Stokes v. Spartanburg Regional Medical Center, 2006 WL 3692613 (South Carolina App., January 23, 2006).

Tarasoff v. Board of Regents of the University of California, 17 Cal.3d 425, 551 P.2d 334 (1976).

Tenet Health System v. Taitel, 2003 WL 22336129 (Fla App., October 15, 2003).

Terajima v. Torrance Memorial Medical Center, 2008 WL 192650 (Cal. App., January 24, 2008).

Thompson v. County of Alameda, 27 Cal. 3d 741, 614 P 2d. 728 (1980).

Thornton v. Shah, 2002 WL 1822126 (Ill. App., August 8, 2002).

United States v. Occident, 2007 WL 1988454 (4th Cir., July 6, 2007).

Vaughn v. Epworth Villa, 2008 WL 3843340 (10th Cir., August 19, 2008).

Webb v. Tulane Medical Center Hospital, 700 So.2d 1141 (La. App., 1997).

Whalen v. Roe, 429 U.S. 589 (1977).

Woodson v. Scott and White Memorial Hospital, 2007 WL 3076937 (5th Cir., October 22, 2007).

CHAPTER 10

Professional Liability Insurance

PREVIEW

With the advent of the malpractice crisis of the 1970s, health care providers rapidly became acutely aware of the vast scope of potential lawsuits that could be filed against them, either individually or collectively. This malpractice scare served to alert health care providers of their unique vulnerability. Lawsuits could be filed by any health care consumer or employer at almost any time. The majority of physicians quickly acquired and increased their liability coverage. For multiple reasons, nurses, like their physician counterparts, should not be without professional liability insurance. This chapter explores issues nurses should consider and investigate when choosing a policy that will give them the best protection should a subsequent lawsuit be filed against them.

LEARNING OUTCOMES
After completing this chapter, you should be able to:

10.1 List elements common to all professional liability insurance policies.

10.2 Differentiate types of professional liability insurance policies available commercially to professional nurses.

10.3 Identify issues to be considered when deciding between individual coverage, group coverage, and employer-sponsored coverage.

10.4 Compare and contrast the various arguments that arise when deciding about having individual coverage.

KEY TERMS
certificate of insurance
claims-made policies
coverage agreements
coverage conditions
coverage extensions
covered injuries
declarations
deductibles
defense costs

employer-sponsored coverage
exclusions
indemnity
insurance policy (insuring
    agreement)

limits of liability
occurrence-based policies
policy period
policyholder

professional liability
    insurance
reservation of rights
supplementary payments

PROFESSIONAL LIABILITY INSURANCE

Professional liability insurance protects nurses against lawsuits that arise from real or alleged errors or omissions, including negligence, in the course of delivering nursing care in clinical settings. Professional liability insurance benefits include payment for the cost of expert legal advice and representation, including representation in trial courts and before nursing licensing boards; payment for court costs and settlements, including appeals; and reimbursement for the nurse, to a limited extent, for lost wages incurred in defending the lawsuit. Additionally, some professional liability insurance covers volunteer work and Good Samaritan activities. If these latter activities are covered in the policy, there will be a separate section specifying the limits for such covered activities and any restrictions that may pertain.

INSURANCE POLICIES

An **insurance policy,** sometimes called an **insuring agreement,** is a formal contract between the insurance carrier and an individual or corporation. For a stated premium (fee per year), the insurance policy will provide the insured party, or **policyholder,** with a specific dollar amount of protection when certain injuries are caused by the person(s) insured by the policy. The conditions of the coverage and the extent of coverage are detailed in the policy itself.

Regardless of the policy chosen, there are some common elements of all professional liability policies. The policies provide payment for a lawyer to represent the insured nurse in the event of a claim or lawsuit. Most insurance carriers insist that the nurse use a lawyer the insurance company has on retainer, because this assures both the nurse and the insurance carrier that the selected lawyer will be well versed in medical malpractice issues. All policies specify the limits of legal liability. Insurance carriers will pay settlements or jury awards but will not cover the cost of any moral obligations that nurses might feel they owe the injured party.

TYPES OF POLICIES

There are essentially two ways of classifying types of insurance policies. The first way is as either occurrence-based or claims-made insurance coverage. **Occurrence-based policies** cover the nurse for any injuries arising out of incidents that occurred during the time the policy was in effect, known as the **policy period**. This holds true even if the subsequent lawsuit is filed after the policy has expired and the policy was not renewed by the policyholder. Language that indicates that a policy is an occurrence-based policy includes such statements as "This policy applies only to those claims which are the result of medical incidents that occurred on or after the effective date of coverage, and before the expiration date stated on the certificate of insurance."

Claims-made policies provide coverage only if the claim for an injury that has occurred is filed with the courts and is reported to the insurance company during the active policy period or during an uninterrupted extension of that policy period. The uninterrupted extension allows the claims-made policy to be enforced for a specific period of time following the policy period. One way to ensure this uninterrupted extension is to purchase a policy tail. A policy tail converts the original policy so that the policy includes a clause or clauses that the policyholder wishes to add to the current language of the policy. Language that indicates that a policy is a claims-made policy includes "This policy applies only to those claims which are the result of medical incidents happening on or subsequent to the prior acts dates stated on the certificate of insurance and which are first made against you while the insurance is in force."

The occurrence-based policy is preferable for most nurses because lawsuits may not be filed immediately, particularly in cases involving children, neonates, and conditions that arise months to years after the triggering event. Claims-made coverage is adequate if the policy is continuously renewed and kept active or if a policy tail is purchased for extended coverage. If there is doubt regarding coverage needed, consult the insurance agent or an attorney.

A second way of classifying types of insurance policies is individual, group, or employer-sponsored coverage. Individual coverage is the broadest type of coverage and is specific to the individual policyholder. This type of policy covers the named policyholder (professional nurse) on a 24-hour basis, as long as actions fall within the scope of professional nursing practice, including both paid services and voluntary services. This type of policy is tailored to meet the needs of the individual nurse. Group coverage involves insuring a group of similarly licensed professionals and may be advantageous in some private clinics or businesses. Group coverage is frequently obtained by professional practitioners where all of the insured individuals practice during office hours and have essentially the same job descriptions.

Employer-sponsored coverage, which is obtained by institutions, is perhaps the narrowest of coverage for individual nurses since they must first show that they are practicing within the scope of their employment as well as within the scope of professional nursing practice. Those covered are called the *insureds,* or they may be legally referred to as "former insureds for acts committed while insured." Employer-sponsored coverage is favored by the institution because the coverage is written specifically for the business and its major concerns.

Institutions that have coverage for their nurses should supply the individual nurse with written verification that the institution does have an active policy and that individual nurses are covered under the policy. Called a **certificate of insurance,** such a document alerts the nurse to specifics about the institution's policy and assists the nurse in knowing what type of coverage he or she needs to secure in an individual policy.

EXERCISE 10.1

Using your own professional clinical area, list arguments for purchasing either occurrence-based or claims-made insurance policies. Determine which coverage would be best for you as an individual policyholder. What type of coverage is most often written within your state? Is this type of coverage adequate for your potential needs? If not, are there additions to the policies that could add needed coverage for nurses in your geographical area?

DECLARATIONS

The first part of the policy is known as the **declarations.** Included under this section are the policyholder's name, address, covered professional occupation (such as general staff nurse, advanced family nurse practitioner, or emergency center staff nurse), and the covered time period. Most insurance policies cover a calendar year, and the exact dates of coverage will be listed in the declarations section. For example, the policy period may be from April 1, 2009, through March 31, 2010. This section also lists the company's limits of liability coverage and state requirements for information that may modify the policy. If Good Samaritan activities are covered by the policy, the limits of liability coverage will be included in this section.

COVERAGE AGREEMENTS

Coverage agreements outline the types of claims that will be covered by a given policy. Generally, there is language that speaks to medical injury, either through errors or omissions, arising during the policy period, by the individual insured, or by any person for whose acts or omissions such insured is legally responsible. This section will also include injury arising out of Good Samartian or volunteer activites. In some policies, there may also be coverage for personal injuries, though this type of policy coverage is not often seen.

There may also be **coverage extensions** in some policies. Coverage extensions outline additional protections that a policy affords the policyholder, such as license protection, including representation before a board of nursing during a disciplinary hearing or proceeding or legal representation at a deposition hearing. If there is a coverge extension clause, the limits of liability for each of these additional coverages will be included.

LIMITS AND DEDUCTIBLES

The insurance policy should have a section marked **limits of liability.** This section usually has language about two separate dollar figures. For example, it could read $500,000 each claim, $1,000,000 aggregate, or $1,000,000 each claim, $3,000,000 aggregate. These dollar figures indicate what the insurance company will pay during a given policy period. The insurance company will pay up to the lower limits for any one claim or lawsuit and up to the upper limits during the entire policy period.

All claims arising from the same incident or occurrence are considered a single claim for purposes of the insurance coverage. For example, if a professional nurse inadvertently gave patient A the medications that were ordered for patient B, both patients could file suit for injuries caused by this single medication error. Most insurance companies would consider these two separate lawsuits as a single claim arising from the same incident and would pay up to the lower limits of the policy. The upper-limit figure or aggregate figure is the total amount that the insurance carrier will pay for all claims made in a calendar year or policy period.

Deductibles include any amounts that the insurance carrier deducts from the total amount available to pay for plaintiff damages. Some policies deduct the amount paid for the nurse's legal defense from the total limits of liability.

ADDITIONAL CLAUSES IN INSURANCE POLICIES

Exclusions are items not covered in the insurance policy. In professional liability policies, such exclusions frequently describe circumstances or activities that will prevent coverage of the insured party. Exclusions also include the absence of appropriate licensure or certification. These exclusions may be covered in the policy under the general title **reservation of rights,** so entitled because the company reserves the right to deny coverage once the facts are known. When and if it is determined that a restricted activity has been involved, the insured nurse must reimburse the insurance company for incurred expenses for any legal defense that addressed these specific exclusions. Other insurance companies insist that the insured nurse pay all expenses out of pocket until it is shown that an excluded activity has not been involved.

Some of the more common examples of excluded activities involving inappropriate behavior include:

1. Criminal actions
2. Incidents occurring while the insured was under the influence of either drugs or alcohol
3. Physical assault, sexual abuse, molestation, habitual neglect, or licentious and immoral behavior toward patients whether intentional, negligent, inadvertent, or committed with the belief that the other party was consenting
4. Actions that violate state nursing practice acts

In recent years, more insurance policies are covering, up to the limits of the policy, damages that are awarded as punitive damages. The rationale for this inclusion is that the policyholder purchased the policy to cover damages in the event that an event occurred and damages were awarded by a jury/judge. Not to cover punitive damages when all other types of damages were allowable seemed to negate the purposes for which one purchased such a policy.

More recent additions to the preceding list include exclusion for the transmission of AIDS/HIV from the health care provider to a patient and exclusions for expanded roles in nursing. Sometimes, this last exclusion is worded as "exclusions for liability incurred in the position of proprietor, superintendent, or executive officer of a clinic, laboratory, or business enterprise."

Exclusions also include any claims or suits resulting from the practice of a profession that does not appear on the certificate's declarations. Nurses should alert their insurance company when there is a change in professional status to ensure that the nurse is fully covered during the policy period.

Terms in the coverage section indicate when the insured is actually covered and for what activities. Policies that have fairly broad coverage will include language similar to the following: ". . . professional services by the individual insured, or by any persons for whose acts or omissions such insured is legally responsible." Such verbiage indicates that insureds are covered both for their own actions and for actions performed by nurses under their direct and indirect supervision. This coverage is vital for nurses who hold supervisory positions, such as nursing supervisors, charge nurses, and nursing faculty. This clause is also necessary given the issues surrounding delegation.

Defense costs are included in most policies. These include all reasonable and necessary costs incurred in the investigation, defense, and negotiation of any covered claim or suit. Most companies pay these in addition to the limits of liability. Additionally, if the nurse is required to appear before the state board of nursing or a governmental regulatory agency, the company will pay attorney fees and other costs resulting from investigation or defense of the proceeding, up to $1,000 per policy period. This latter amount is in addition to the coverage limits.

The section on **covered injuries** outlines the types of injuries and provisions that the insurance company will honor. Usually, insurance companies include personal (bodily) injury; mental anguish; property damage; personal injury to a patient such as invasion of privacy, libel, and slander; and economic damages as covered injuries. The lawsuit must specifically note that the suit is for monetary damages. In other words, the insurance company will cover the cost of litigation and awards if money damages are involved. The insurance company will not cover the cost of litigation if the action sought is a specific performance, as in the instance of a lawsuit brought to prevent a nurse practitioner from performing medical acts. *Sermchief v. Gonzales* (1983) is an example of such a specific performance lawsuit.

Supplementary payments include provisions for additional payments to the insured party. Most policies supplement lost earnings or reasonable expenses incurred by the insured as well as the cost of appeal bonds and costs of litigation charged against the insured. These latter provisions may also be classified as defense costs.

Conditions or **coverage conditions** outline the insured nurse's duties to the insurance carrier in the event a claim or lawsuit is filed, provisions for cancellation of the policy, prohibition of assignment of the policy, and subrogation of rights. Many insurance policies will cover policyholders only if they give written notice to the insurance carrier immediately upon the filing of a claim or lawsuit and forward to the insurance carrier every demand, notice, summons, or other process received.

A case that illustrates this point is *Beverly Enterprises v. Jarrett* (2007). In that case, a deceased resident's probate administrator filed suit on behalf of the family against a nursing home for negligence and violations of the nursing-home residents' rights law. The court papers for the lawsuit were either misplaced or misdirected at the nursing home, and the legal counsel for the nursing home was not able to file a formal response within the state-mandated time frame for answering a complaint. Without the needed response, the court decided the case in favor of the patient's family by default. The court of appeals reviewed the case and upheld the default judgment of the lower trial level.

The case illustrates the fact that prompt notification of an impending lawsuit to one's insurance carrier is critical. Without such notification, the insurance carrier cannot adequately defend the lawsuit, and coverage under the policy can be voided under the insured's obligation to promptly notify the insurance carrier of any and all impending lawsuits.

Also in this section are the nurse's right to select counsel and the right to request a settlement. Generally, the insurance company will pay up to the single claims amount if the case is settled out of court. In *General Hospital of Passaic v. American Casualty Company* (2007), the parents brought suit against a physician and two nurses for injuries caused their newborn infant. The case was settled out of court, and the insurance company was ordered to pay $100,000 for one of the nurse's errors that ensued during the delivery of the infant. That amount of damage was the maximum that her policy would pay for injuries arising out of a single claim.

Most policies allow the insurance carrier to settle without the policyholder's consent and deny the policyholder the right to retain counsel apart from the insurance company. As explained in the general provisions section, most insurance companies prefer to retain attorneys known to have expertise in medical matters, rather than allow the insured the right to obtain attorneys unknown to them.

Included in the policy is a clause that the insurance company will proceed in good faith in reaching a fair decision in lawsuits that are filed against an insured. A case that illustrates this point is *New England Insurance Company v. Healthcare Underwriters Mutual Insurance Company* (2002). In that case, a lawsuit was allowed to proceed against an obstetrician and the hospital's labor and delivery nurses for negligence in delaying securing a pediatric specialist to attend a neonate following an emergency cesarean section. The hospital's primary malpractice insurance had a limit of $1 million, and the hospital's excess carrier insurance company paid the additional $1.5 million awarded the claimants. The excess carrier then sued the primary insurance company for bad faith—that is, for breach of the legal duty to make a reasonable attempt to settle the case for $1 million or less. The family's attorney indicated that he would have recommended to his clients that they accept the $1 million in damages had that amount been offered during the trial.

The court reiterated that the insured is entitled to a good-faith effort to settle a liability claim. The insured can write to the insurance company and insist on a good-faith settlement offer to pay within the policy limits, as needed.

GUIDELINES

Professional Liability Insurance Policies

1. Read the policy carefully before purchasing it and ask for explanations as needed. Make sure that the policy will augment an employer-sponsored policy or will adequately protect your interests if you are independently employed. Ensure that you are purchasing a policy from a reputable company.

2. Make sure that the per-claim and aggregate coverage limits are adequate for your specific nursing needs. As a double check, scan your geographic area for the tendency of nurses to be named in lawsuits and the average dollar damages being awarded plaintiffs in lawsuits that name nurses as defendants.

3. Check on any information that relates to malpractice claims in your area. Resources to be explored include the local law library, insurance carriers, health claims arbitration boards, and hospital attorneys.

4. Assess whether the policy gives you optimal coverage. Ideally, it should be occurrence-based coverage and include protection for both your direct professional actions as well as the professional actions of those you supervise. If your geographical area allows only the purchase of claims-made coverage, investigate the availability and cost of a policy tail. Investigate other options that are covered by the policy. Does this policy cover appeal bonds or supplementary benefits? Can you select your own counsel or request a settlement out of court?

5. Understand the exclusions of the policy. Will you still be covered if you accept a job as an independent practitioner? If the exclusions also exclude your job description, as in the instance of advanced practice nurses, investigate additional insurance policies.

6. Be aware that there are areas of nursing practice in which the risk of lawsuits is higher. These areas include, but are not restricted to, critical care areas, home health care, emergency centers, the operating room, and maternal and child health areas. Thus, the need for individual coverage is most acute.

7. Above all, remember that you are a member of a profession with the potential to have lawsuits constantly filed against its members. Do not consider practicing professional nursing without the valuable protection provided by liability insurance.

 EXERCISE 10.2

Using the sample policy found in Figure 10.1, find the various provisions that were just discussed, including:

1. Limits of liability
2. Declarations
3. Deductibles
4. Exclusions
5. Reservation of rights
6. Covered injuries
7. Defense costs
8. Coverage conditions and supplementary payments

Did you have difficulty finding some sections? Would this be a policy that you would consider purchasing for your own liability coverage? Why or why not?

DECLARATIONS

Policyholder's Name: ___Judy Doe _____

Covered Professional Occupation: Registered Nurse; Staff position
Acute care institution or community health/home health

Coverage Period: May 1, 2008 through April 30, 2009

Duties in Event of a Claim: If there is a claim, you must do the following:

1. notify us and our program administrator, in writing, as soon as possible;
2. specify the names and addresses of the injured party(s) and any witnesses, information on the time and place of the event;
3. verbally discuss the nature of the event with our claims representative;
4. immediately forward all documents that you receive in connection with the claim to us:
5. fully cooperate with us, or our designee, in the consummation of settlements, the defense of suits or other proceedings, enforcing any right of contribution or indemnity against another who may be liable to you because of injury or damage. You shall attend hearings and trials, assist in securing and giving evidence, and obtaining the attendance of witnesses;
6. refuse, except at your own cost, to voluntarily make any payment, assume any obligation, or incur any expense.

Limits of the policy: $1,000.000 per claim/$3,000,000 aggregate

In consideration of payment of the premium, in reliance upon the statements in the declarations and subject to all of the terms of this policy, agrees with the named insured as follows:

COVERAGE AGREEMENTS

The company will pay on behalf of the insured all sums that the insured shall become legally obligated to pay as damages because of:

COVERAGE—INDIVIDUAL PROFESSIONAL LIABILITY

Injury arising out of the rendering of or failure to render, during the policy period, professional services by the individual insured, or by any person for whose acts or omissions such insured is legally responsible, except as a member of a partnership, performed in the practice of the individual insured's profession described in the declarations including service by the individual insured as a member of a formal accreditation or similar professional board or committee of a hospital or professional society.

EXCLUSION

This insurance does not apply to:

1. Liability of the insured as a proprietor, superintendent, or executive officer of any hospital, sanitarium, clinic with bed and board facilities, laboratory or business enterprise other than as stated in the above declarations;
2. Liability of the insured as a nurse-anesthetist or as a nurse midwife.

LIMITS OF LIABILITY

Individual Professional Liability

The limit of liability stated in the declarations as applicable to each claim is the limit of the company's liability for all damages because of each claim or suit covered hereby. All claims arising from the same rendering of or failure to render the same professional services shall be considered a single claim for the purposes of this insurance. The limit of liability stated in the declarations as aggregate is, subject to the above provision respecting each claim, the total limit of the company's liability under this coverage for all damages. Such limits of liability shall apply separately to each insured.

SUPPLEMENTARY PAYMENTS

The company will pay, in addition to the applicable limit of liability:

FIGURE 10.1 Sample professional liability insurance policy. (continued)

1. All expenses incurred by the company, all costs taxed against the insured in any suit defended by the company, and all interest on the entire amount of the judgment therein that accrues after entry of the judgment and before the company has paid or tendered or deposited in court that part of the judgment that does not exceed the limit of the company's liability thereon.

2. Such premiums on appeal bonds required in any such suit, premiums on bonds to release attachments in any such suit for an amount not in excess of the applicable limit of liability of this policy, and the cost of bail bonds required of the insured because of accident or traffic law violations arising out of the use of any vehicle to which this policy applies, not to exceed $250 per bail bond, but the company shall have no obligation to apply for or furnish such bonds.

3. Reasonable expenses incurred by the insured at the company's request in assisting the company in the investigation or defense of any claim or suit, including actual loss of earnings not to exceed $25 per day.

DEFINITIONS

"Insured" means any person or organization qualifying as the policy holder in the person's insured provision of this policy. The insurance afforded applies separately to each insured against whom claim is made or suit is brought, except with respect to the limits of the company's liability.

"Damages" means all damages, including damages for death, that are payable because of injury to which the insurance applies. "Named insured" means the person or organization named in the declarations of this policy.

CONDITIONS

Insured's duties in the event of occurrence, claim, or suit:

1. Upon the insured's becoming aware of any alleged injury to which this insurance applies, written notice containing particulars sufficient to identify the insured and also reasonably obtainable information with respect to the time, place, and circumstances thereof, and the names and addresses of the injured and of available witnesses, shall be given by or for the insured to the company or any of its authorized agents as soon as practicable.

2. If claim is made or suit is brought against the insured, the insured shall immediately forward to the company every demand, notice, summons, or other process received by him or his representative.

3. The insured shall cooperate with the company and, upon the company's request, assist in making settlements, in the conduct of suits and in enforcing any right of contribution or indemnity against any person or organization who may be liable to the insured because of injury or damage with respect to which insurance is afforded under this policy; and the insured shall attend hearings and trials and assist in securing and giving evidence and obtaining the attendance of witnesses. The insured shall not, except at his own cost, voluntarily make any payment, assume any obligation, or incur any expense.

SUBROGATION

In the event of any payment under this policy, the company shall be subrogated to all of the insured's rights of recovery therefore against any person or organization, and the insured shall execute and deliver instruments and papers and do whatever else is necessary to secure such rights. The insured shall do nothing after loss to prejudice such rights.

ASSIGNMENT

The interest hereunder of any insured is not assignable.

CHANGES

Notice to any agent or knowledge possessed by any agent or by any other person shall not effect a waiver or change in any part of this policy or stop the company from asserting any right under the terms of this policy; nor shall the terms of this policy be waived or changed, except by endorsement issued to form a part of this policy, signed by a duly authorized representative of this company.

FIGURE 10.1 Sample professional liability insurance policy. (continued)

INDIVIDUAL VERSUS EMPLOYER LIABILITY COVERAGE

Should a nurse have individual professional liability coverage, or should the nurse rely on the employer's insurance policy in the event of a malpractice action? Many nurses have been assured by hospital administrative staff and by competent lawyers that they can depend on the hospital's insurance policy to cover them in the event of a subsequent legal action. However, the actual truth is that nurses who relied on hospital policies most often were not adequately protected monetarily, nor were they adequately represented by legal counsel in the lawsuit.

There are several reasons for this situation. First, many institutional liability insurance policies have limited coverage and cover employees only while they are performing work as hospital employees. Thus, private-duty nurses and off-duty employees are automatically excluded from coverage. Nurses who volunteer their professional services likewise are frequently not covered under standard policies. School nurses and community or home health care nurses may not be covered at all in most medical insurance policies, though the newer trend is to protect these nurses in the performance of their employment.

Second, the hospital's policy is designed to meet the needs of the large institution, and hospital attorneys may not be able to protect the individual nurse's best interests. For example, the hospital may elect to settle out of court rather than pursue a particular case, even though the nurse's best interests can be served only through a court hearing. Also, should the hospital wish to bring an indemnity claim against the nurse for the incident that triggered the lawsuit, the hospital policy will not cover the nurse nor will it pay for his or her legal representation. **Indemnity** claims are those brought by the employer for monetary contributions from the nurse or nurses whose actions or failure to act caused the original patient injury.

A case illustration of this concept of indemnification is *Patient's Compensation Fund v. Lutheran Hospital* (1999). In that case, the fund paid a $10 million settlement to a patient and then attempted to recover this amount from the nurse and her individual policy. The patient was admitted to the facility for treatment of ureteral stenosis, for which morphine sulfate and belladonna suppositories were prescribed post-operatively. The morning following the surgery, the patient sustained a cardiac arrest and was resuscitated, though he sustained permanent brain injury due to hypoxia.

Only one of the nurses named in the suit had professional liability insurance, though all the nurses who cared for the patient in the early post-operative period were named in the lawsuit. The nurses prevailed on a technicality in that they were not valid "health care providers" as defined in the Patient Compensation Fund. However, this case serves to illustrate that insurance companies and other health care agencies can and do file lawsuits for expenses incurred on behalf of nurses and other health care providers.

Finally, most hospital insurance policies do not have supplementary payments for the nurse-defendant. This means that if nurses incur additional expenses in investigating the claim or lose days of work defending the claim, then they must cover the expenses out of pocket.

Employer-based coverage, though, is a good starting point for prudent nurses. They should ask to either see or read the hospital policy or ask about specific provisions in the employer-sponsored coverage and then acquire their own individual coverage to augment the employer's policy. Nurses should also take into consideration the following factors:

1. The type of nursing that they normally perform (staff versus charge versus supervision)
2. The dollar amount of the average awards in their particular geographic area
3. The unit or type of nursing care they normally provide (critical care versus general medical-surgical nursing)
4. The propensity for lawsuits against nurses in that geographic area

The hospital attorney can provide nurses with information regarding trends in malpractice in their locality. Then nurses should find a policy that provides the necessary coverage. They can extend coverage as their job status changes or as they expand practice roles.

EXERCISE 10.3

Consult with your risk manager or institution's legal counsel. What types of provisions are made in the institution policy for individual nurses? What type of coverage would be advisable for nurses working in the institution to purchase?

REASONS TO PURCHASE INDIVIDUAL LIABILITY INSURANCE

Nurses should procure professional liability insurance for several reasons:

1. Perhaps the most convincing reason is that defending against a lawsuit, no matter what the merit of the case, is costly. There are attorney fees, court costs, and costs of discovery, not to mention the actual award (or settlement) if the nurse is found negligent. Few nurses can sustain such financial strain without insurance coverage. Judgments that are not paid by insurance coverage can lead to garnishment of wages, the inability to obtain loans and/or mortgages, and bad credit ratings. Also, the nurses' personal assets, including bank accounts, individual property, as well as one's home, can be used to satisfy the court-ordered judgment.

2. Nurses who have professional liability insurance are not "targets" and are not sued more frequently than nurses who choose not to have individual professional liability insurance coverage. Plaintiffs do not know if the individual has professional liability insurance until after the lawsuit is filed. The reason that plaintiffs sue is because of negligence and personal injury.

3. Professional liability insurance is relatively inexpensive for individuals who are employed in acute care settings. Costs vary according to the type of nursing one performs, such as working on a general medical-surgical unit as opposed to in an emergency center or working in an advanced practice role as opposed to a staff nurse position. Costs also vary by geographic region.

4. A popular reason for insurance coverage is the assurance of adequate protection should a lawsuit be filed. Malpractice is not synonymous with incompetence or guilt; even the most conscientious nurses could be sued for performing their actions below the acceptable standard of care if an untoward happening occurs and they are in the direct line of causation. For example, even though nurses are covered during patient transfers from one facility to a second facility, events happen that place nurses at risk. What if, during the transfer, the nurse temporarily leaves the side of the patient to speak with the pilot or driver? Is this abandonment of the patient, and thus not within the scope of the nurse's authority? One's mental health is well worth the cost of the insurance policy.

5. Having one's own professional liability insurance does not automatically trigger an employee indemnity lawsuit. But should the institution choose to sue the nurse for reimbursement, he or she is protected.

6. The fact that professionals assume accountability for their own actions or omissions is an additional reason for acquiring such liability coverage. Inherent in accountability is responsibility (and ability to pay) should the plaintiff be negligently injured by the professional's actions or omissions.

7. Malpractice insurance premiums are currently a tax-deductible business expense.

ARGUMENTS FOR HAVING PROFESSIONAL LIABILITY INSURANCE

There are no valid reasons for nurses to be without professional liability insurance. A favorite argument of many in-hospital attorneys is to remind nurses that they are more lawsuit prone if they have an individual insurance policy. However, in today's society the nurse is, in essence, the conduit either to the hospital's potential liability or to the physician's potential liability through the doctrine of respondeat superior or through a dual servant role. The nurse's expanding role, with its autonomy and advocacy components, has led to heightened legal accountability and increased potential for being named in lawsuits.

A second favorite argument is that the monetary award, if one is found to have liability, will be greater because of the fact that the nurse is insured. In reality, the judge and jury conclude their deliberations based on the facts of the case. Juries, because of possible prejudice, cannot be informed about insurance coverage in deciding the case.

In selected states, tort reform acts have limited the amount of economic liability against individual defendants, particularly physicians and health care corporations. Thus, nurses may find themselves named in more, not fewer, lawsuits as attorneys seek means to find additional sources of revenue for injured clients.

It is immaterial to the patient bringing the lawsuit whether or not the nurse has insurance. But it should matter greatly to nurses, since the cost of defense could destroy them financially. In most states, the judgment remains open until satisfied or dropped. That means that a nurse may be paying on a prior judgment for several years after the judgment; in states that allow garnishment of wages for adjudicated debts, one's wages may be garnished for several years after the initial judgment.

Finally, no specialty in nursing is immune to lawsuits. Though there are some specialties where more lawsuits are filed, such as obstetrics, critical care, and emergency nursing, all nurses are at risk for being named in a malpractice lawsuit. Having professional liability insurance will not prevent the lawsuits, but it will greatly assist the nurse in his or her defense of the lawsuit.

EXERCISE 10.4

Poll nurses with whom you work about the advantages of professional liability insurance. Do those you interviewed have individual policies? List the reasons they gave for having or not having individual policies. Which reasons are listed most frequently? Were the reasons valid as opposed to mere guesses by the nurses you interviewed? List arguments you could use to educate these nurses about the value and necessity of having individual professional liability insurance coverage.

Using ethical principles, list reasons why nurses should have professional liability insurance. Does having such coverage make nurses more autonomous in their practice? Are the ethical rights of patients better met if nurses have professional liability coverage? Do any of the ethical principles negate having such coverage?

SUMMARY

- Professional liability insurance protects nurses against lawsuits that arise from real or alleged errors or omissions, including negligence, in the course of delivering nursing care in clinical settings.
- The two primary ways of classifying professional liability insurance are as occurrence-based or claims-made policies.
- Occurrence-based policies cover the insured for injuries arising out of incidents that occurred during the time the policy was in effect.
- Claims-made policies provide coverage only if the claim for an injury that has occurred is filed with the courts and is reported to the insurance company during the active policy period or an uninterrupted extension of the policy period.
- A second way of classifying insurance policies is as individual, group, or employer-sponsored policies.
- Clauses in an insurance policy include limits of liability, declarations, deductibles, exclusions, reservation of rights, covered injuries, defense costs, and coverage conditions and supplemental payments.
- Though health care institutions give multiple reasons for not having an individual professional liability policy, there are no good reasons for a nurse not to have an individual policy.

APPLY YOUR LEGAL KNOWLEDGE

1. What do the terms and language in insurance policies mean to the policyholder?
2. Are certain insurance policies more desirable for nurses who work in different clinical areas in acute care settings? Do these policies differ for nurses working in home care settings or in ambulatory settings?
3. Are there times when it would be advisable to have no individual professional liability coverage?

YOU BE THE JUDGE

During an unexpected heat wave, the administrator of a nursing home decided against turning on the air conditioner, which resulted in the death of four of the residents of the home. One of the deceased resident's daughters brought a lawsuit against the home for a wrongful death suit. She was awarded a judgment of $275,000. She then filed a second lawsuit against the nursing home's insurance company to collect payment on the judgment.

The insurance company refused to pay, stating that the judgment underlying the lawsuit was professional liability and the insurance company did not cover the nursing home for professional judgment. The nursing home then filed a lawsuit against the insurance company for payment of this judgment.

QUESTIONS

1. What provisions of an insurance policy would you consult to determine if an insurance company should pay such a claim, and what would the limits of the liability be?
2. Is the nursing home insurance company correct in saying that this is a professional judgment issue?
3. Which insurance company (the nursing home's or that of the administrator of the nursing home, assuming she has coverage) should pay the court-ordered judgment?
4. How would you decide the case?

REFERENCES

Beverly Enterprises v. Jarrett, 2007 WL 466810 (Ark. App., February 14, 2007).

General Hospital of Passaic v. American Casualty Company, 2007 WL 2814655 (D. N. J., September 24, 2007).

New England Insurance Company v. Healthcare Underwriters Mutual Insurance Company, 2002 WL 1467282 (2nd Cir., July 9, 2002).

Patient's Compensation Fund v. Lutheran Hospital, 588 N.W.2d 8880 (Wisconsin, 1999).

Sermchief v. Gonzales, 600 S.W.2d 683 (Mo. en banc, 1983).

PART FOUR

IMPACT OF THE LAW ON THE PROFESSIONAL PRACTICE OF NURSING

CHAPTER 11

Nurse Practice Acts, Licensure, and the Scope of Practice

PREVIEW

Throughout the years, an elaborate system of licensure and credentials for health care providers has evolved to ensure that only qualified individuals deliver health care. Both licenses and credentials have as their primary purpose the protection of the public at large. Through proper issuance of licenses and credentials, qualified health care providers are distinguished from unqualified persons. The first group is given a license to practice, whereas the latter group is prohibited from harming society in a health care role. This chapter outlines the relationship between state nurse practice acts, entry into professional practice, educational issues, and the scope of practice issues. The chapter also discusses complementary and alternative medicine (CAM), medical cannabis, and multistate licensure.

LEARNING OUTCOMES

After completing this chapter, you should be able to:

11.1 Define *licensure*, including mandatory, permissive, and institutional licensure.

11.2 Describe the process for creating state boards of nursing and their authority, including limitations on their authority.

11.3 Describe the process of how state nursing acts define the professional scope of practice.

11.4 Describe entry into practice in relationship to state nurse practice acts.

11.5 Analyze the impact of education on nursing practice issues.

11.6 Describe the legal ramifications of complementary and alternative medicine, including the medical use of cannabis (marijuana).

11.7 Discuss the status of multistate licensure and mutual recognition compacts today.

11.8 Analyze some of the ethical issues surrounding licensure, certification, and scope of practice.

KEY TERMS

articulation with medical
    practice acts
certification
complementary and alternative
    medicine (CAM)
continuing education
credentials
disciplinary actions
diversion programs
endorsement

grandfather clause
institutional licensure
joint statements
licensure by examination
licensure by waiver
mandatory licensure
medical cannabis
mutual recognition
National Practitioner Data
    Bank (NPDB)

nurse licensure compact
nurse practice acts
permissive licensure
professional licensure
reciprocity
scope of practice
standing orders
temporary licenses

CREDENTIALS

Credentials are proof of qualifications, usually in written form, stating that an individual or an organization has met specific standards. Two types of credentials are used in health care that affect nursing: licensure and certification.

PROFESSIONAL LICENSURE

Professional licensure is the legal process by which an authorized authority grants permission to a qualified individual or entity to perform designated skills and services in a jurisdiction in which such practice would be illegal without a license. Licenses are issued by governmental agencies and are enforced by the police power of the state. For nurses, the authorized authority is the state board of nursing or the state board of nursing examiners. The qualified individual is the candidate for licensure, and this candidate is a graduate nurse who has successfully completed all requirements for licensure or a nurse with licensure in another state. The designated skills and services are professional nursing actions.

Licensure is enacted through state legislative action. Licensure statutes measure minimum competency of the person licensed and are primarily intended to protect health care consumers. Licensure laws, an example of a state's exercise of its police power, exist to protect the public against unqualified practitioners.

Individual state legislative bodies enact into law their specific licensing procedures, stating which professions must be licensed to practice within the state. In most states, physicians and dentists were the first professionals to be licensed, with nurses generally the next licensed professional. Part of the statutory law in all jurisdictions of the United States is the state nurse practice act. Each state, the District of Columbia, and territories of the United States have individual nurse practice acts. Additionally, some states have separate acts for registered nurses and licensed practical nurses; thus the total number of individual nurse practice acts is 60.

State Boards of Nursing

Individual legislators do not directly enforce statutory law. The means of ensuring enforcement of nurse practice acts is through the state board of nursing or the state board of nurse examiners. This board is created by language in the selected nurse practice act, and is ultimately accountable to the legislators for professional nursing within a given jurisdiction. A board of nursing has no greater authority than that which the statute, enacted by the legislature, grants to it. Therefore, the board of nursing is limited by the language of the given nurse practice act.

State boards of nursing are mandated in the state nurse practice acts. The specific act sets the number of members of the board, qualifications for membership, and the term of appointment. States vary in the numbers of persons on the board, and currently there are 7 to 17 members on state boards of nursing. The individual nurse practice act may allow for legal or expert members, or for election (for example, North Carolina) rather than appointment of the members.

Boards of nursing have an executive director who is responsible for administering the work of the board and seeing that the nurse practice act provisions as well as rules and regulations of the board are followed. Generally, boards of nursing:

1. govern their individual operation and administration.
2. approve or deny approvals to schools of nursing.
3. examine and license applicants.
4. review licenses, grant temporary licenses, and provide for inactive status for those already licensed.
5. regulate specialty practice.
6. discipline those who violate provisions of the licensure law.

The board is given the authority to set standards by promulgating rules and regulations and has as a charge the enforcement of such rules and regulations. Most state boards of nursing have published standards of professional conduct and guidelines for unprofessional conduct, with enforcement assured by the board's ability to revoke, stipulate, or suspend a previously granted license or to deny licensure.

The board's authority arises from various sources of law. Its authority may be: legislative, through the promulgation of rules and regulations; quasi-judicial, through hearings; or administrative, through licensure control. State legislatures may also require that licensure be either mandatory or permissive.

The state board of nursing may have as its concern only the professional practice of nursing or may incorporate both professional and practical licensed nurses, and 46 states now have joint boards. If the charge of the state board of nursing is merely professional licensure, then a separate board of nursing for the practical nurse will also exist within the same jurisdiction. States that currently have separate boards of nursing for registered nurses (RN) and practical licensed or vocational nurses (LPN or LVN) are California, Georgia, Louisiana, and West Virginia. Texas had separate boards of nursing until 2007, when new rules were adopted incorporating the two previous nurse practice acts into one act and renaming the Texas Board of Nurse Examiners the Texas Board of Nursing.

Mandatory Licensure

Mandatory licensure requires that all persons who are compensated as a member of a licensed profession obtain licensure prior to practicing actions of the profession. Mandatory licensure regulates the practice of the profession and requires compliance with the statute if an individual engages in activities defined within the scope of that profession. Thus, both the title of registered nurse and the professional actions are protected. All states have mandatory licensure for RNs.

A case that illustrates the power of the board of nursing to regulate nursing practice is *People v. Stults* (1997). In that case, a nonlicensed medical assistant obtained a position in a medical clinic that had previously been held by a registered nurse with a pediatric specialty. The medical assistant had worked in pediatric clinics for nearly two decades after completing a college-level medical assistant program with an emphasis in pediatric care. She knew the pediatric nurse who had the position and was contacted by the physician and asked to take the position when the pediatric nurse resigned.

The physician assumed that the medical assistant was a registered nurse. Three years later, a new office manager asked for the medical assistant's license, which was conspicuously absent from the clinic's files. The medical assistant had no license and was reported to the state board of nursing.

It could not be proven in court beyond a reasonable doubt that the medical assistant had ever claimed or pretended to be a registered nurse. To uphold her conviction for unlicensed nursing practice, however, the court did not need proof that she had misrepresented her licensure status. In the clinic, the medical assistant had performed tasks that required a nursing license within the state of Illinois. Falsely claiming or leading others to believe one is a licensed nurse is illegal, but is not the only way to violate the nursing practice act and the law. The medical assistant was performing nursing functions illegally without a registered nurse or practical nurse license, said the court. Giving injections and immunizations to pediatric clients and performing physical assessments cannot be done by a nonlicensed person. She had also been doing phone triage of patients, giving specific medical advice to mothers about their sick children, and offering general advice to patients, such as how to manage feeding problems and when to switch babies from formula to solid foods. The ultimate holding of the court was that a nonlicensed person cannot counsel patients about their health care concerns. Direct physician supervision of a nursing function being carried out by a nonlicensed person does not take nonlicensed nursing practice out of the scope of the nursing practice act or make it legal, the court ruled. Thus, the appellate court upheld her conviction.

Generally, there are several exceptions to mandatory licensure within a jurisdiction that requires it. These exceptions may include all or most of the following:

1. Performance of nursing actions by unlicensed practitioners in emergency conditions
2. Practice by nursing students incidental to their current course of study, including students who are licensed and those who are not licensed
3. Nursing actions by employees of the federal government, provided the nurse holds a valid and current license in a U.S. state or territory
4. Practice by graduate nurses for a specific length of time during which licensure is being processed, provided the nurse has been issued a temporary permit to practice nursing within the state
5. Nursing care given to patients by qualified nurses during transportation of the patient through a given state
6. Unpaid persons caring for family members or friends
7. Nurses working for the Red Cross during a disaster
8. Caregivers who conduct religious services and rites and who do not purport to be registered nurses

As noted in the third exception, nurses in the armed services or nurses employed by federal agencies must hold a current state license, but not necessarily from the state in which they are currently employed or assigned.

Permissive Licensure

Permissive licensure regulates only the use of the title and does not protect nursing actions. With permissive licensure, nurses cannot use the title "RN" unless duly licensed, but they can perform many or all of the same nursing actions as long as they do not call themselves an RN. For example, if a state had permissive licensure, LPNs or LVNs, working under the supervision or through direct orders of a physician, could perform most of the same actions that an RN performs, as only the title is protected, not the nursing actions.

Permissive licensure correlates best with the initial registration acts of the early 1900s. The term *registered nurse* was defined as a person who had graduated from an acceptable school of nursing and had passed an examination, rather than a person engaged in a specific type of practice. These first registration acts provided for permissive licensure. Beginning in 1938, all states have moved from permissive to mandatory licensure for RNs.

Institutional Licensure

Institutional licensure is the process by which a state government regulates health institutions. Institutional licensure is the alternative to individual licensure. Most government agencies issue licenses to health care facilities, granting permission for the facility to operate, and the issuing body holds the facility responsible for maintaining sanitation, fire safety, staffing, and equipment. Institutional licensure of individuals gives these facilities the added right to decide who is qualified to perform what tasks and duties, and awards licenses as the facility deems appropriate.

Institutional licensure grants the institution authority to directly regulate staff members' practice as well as requirements for administration, equipment specifications, fire safety, footage regulations, and minimal nursing staff requirements. Usually, the process is implemented, not controlled, by individual state monitoring agencies or national organizations, such as the Joint Commission (JC). Theoretically, institutional licensure gives nonprofessionals the regulation of a given profession without standard criteria for such regulation.

Advocates of institutional licensure note that allowing nurses more flexibility in their practice and the opportunity to more effectively expand the practice of nursing are valid reasons to allow institutions the right to license individuals. Proponents also claim that institutional licensure will allow professionals to be more responsive to changing needs, that such licensure will allow providers to take on and relinquish activities as the situation and their abilities demand, and that it will be more cost-effective, thus saving consumers money.

Perhaps the crucial differences between institutional and individual licensure are more philosophical than practical. Individual licenses reinforce the responsibility of the professional to the individual patient rather than to the employer. In an environment that often sacrifices quality in an attempt to lower costs, this would seem a most fundamental argument against institutional licensure. Would nurses feel they could speak against an employer who is also a regulator?

EXERCISE 11.1

Make a list of the pros and cons of institutional versus state licensure for nursing. Now repeat that list from the perspective of a consumer rather than that of a professional. How does institutional licensure undermine professional nursing? How do ethical principles and the American Nurses Association *Code of Ethics for Nurses* (2001) impact the issue of institutional licensure? Can one truly be a patient advocate under institutional licensure?

NURSE PRACTICE ACTS

Nurse practice acts, which originated to protect the public at large, define the practice of nursing, give guidance within the scope of practice issues, and set standards for the nursing profession. The state nurse practice act is the single most important piece of legislation for the nurse because the practice act affects all facets of nursing practice. The nurse practice act is the law, and state boards of nursing cannot grant exceptions or waive its provisions. For example, if licensure can be granted only to individuals who graduate from an approved school of nursing, then the board must refuse licensure to a candidate who did not graduate from an approved school of nursing even if the candidate can show evidence of competency and equivalency.

By the early 20th century, the minimum requirements for nursing practice were beginning to take shape. Nurse registration acts, permissive precursors to nurse practice acts, were emerging, and in 1901 the state nurses associations adopted proposals supporting commitment to passage of state laws to control the practice of nursing. North Carolina was the first state to pass a permissive nurse practice act in 1903. By 1923, every state had passed some type of nurse registration act, and New York in 1938 was the first state to enact a mandatory nurse practice act, establishing two levels of nursing practice: licensed RNs and LPNs/LVNs. Other states followed suit, and by 1952 all states, the District of Columbia, and the U.S. territories had enacted nurse practice acts.

The early acts mainly regulated registration and fee structures. With the advent of mandatory acts, only licensed professionals could practice nursing. Some states enacted definitions of professional nursing, whereas other states had no formal definition. In 1955, the American Nurses Association (ANA) approved a model definition for nursing practice and continued through the years to broaden the definition, amending it in 1970 to incorporate nursing diagnosis and further allowing for an expanded scope in 1979. To provide for some consistency in individual state nurse practice acts, the ANA published a model act for state legislators in 1980 and again in 1990. This latest model nurse practice act incorporates the advanced nurse practitioner as well as the registered nurse (ANA, 1990). The National Council of State Boards of Nursing (NCSBN) also has introduced model nurse practice acts. The Model Nursing Practice Act and Model Nursing Administrative Rules were revised by the 2004 Delegate Assembly and further revised in 2006. The latest revison addressed delegation and assistive personnel issues.

All nurse practice acts are worded in fairly general terms defining professional nursing, and there is no laundry list of specific actions to ensure that the nurse stays within the given act. Rather, the acts' general provisions should give guidance as to acceptable actions. For example, one reason that specific actions are not listed is that, as statutory law, the nurse practice acts are slow in changing to conform to modern practice and technological advances. If actions were specifically enumerated, one would be required to follow the nurse practice act exactly, even though current practices might have changed.

An example may assist with understanding this last statement. Imagine that the state nurse practice act has no provision for nursing diagnosis, yet the JC standards require that nursing diagnoses be written for each patient within hospitals that have JC accreditation. If enumerated actions in the nurse practice act specifically omitted nursing diagnoses as part of the professional practice of nursing within the state, the professional nurse would run the risk daily of violating the act or of working in a nonaccredited institution.

Further, suppose that the institution's policies and procedures mandate that nursing diagnoses are part of the assessment due each patient, just as the patient's progress, response to nursing interventions, and nursing care needs are part of the nursing protocol. Now the dilemma would concern the nurse practice act and one's livelihood. Does the individual nurse violate the nurse practice act or ignore the hospital's policy and procedure manual and refrain from making a nursing diagnosis? Such a scenario could happen if nurse practice acts were checklists for approved nursing actions.

Thus, nurse practice acts are not checklists. The practice acts contain general statements of appropriate professional nursing actions. Nurses must incorporate the nurse practice act with their educational background, previous work experience, institutional policies, and technological advancements. If the main purpose of nurse practice acts is to protect the public from unsafe practitioners, then the ultimate goal of nurse practice acts must be to provide competent, quality nursing care by currently qualified practitioners.

EXERCISE 11.2

Read your state's nurse practice act, emphasizing the general provisions defining nursing actions. Does the act give sufficient guidance for nurses to know if an action is either within the act or outside its scope? Where would you seek guidance if you were unsure that a specific action was either within or outside the state nurse practice act? How would you proceed if you determined that an action was outside the act?

ELEMENTS OF NURSE PRACTICE ACTS

Definition of Professional Nursing

All state nurse practice acts define nursing. As previously stated, some state definitions include nursing diagnoses and speak of collaboration with other professionals. Some nurse practice acts allow for individual treatment, while others specify nursing interventions and therapies. Basically, there are three approaches to statutory definitions of professional nursing:

1. The traditional approach is based on the ANA's original model definition. This approach does not include diagnosis, treatment, or prescription.
2. The transitional approach allows some expanded roles beyond those described in the nurse practice act through the use of standing orders and through supervision by a responsible physician. Some states with transitional approaches add an additional action for nurses, such as the legal permission to diagnose and evaluate patients, but not to treat them.
3. The administrative approach is seen in the majority of states. This approach uses a broader definition of nursing and allows additional acts as may be authorized by appropriate state agencies.

Advanced nurse practitioners and expanded nursing roles are incorporated, relying on the authority granted to the state board of nursing to promulgate rules for such advanced roles. These rules and regulations are then administered and enforced through the state board of nursing. This approach may also allow for overlap between physician and professional nursing roles and functions. For example, this approach allows both physicians and nurses to diagnose and treat patients, within the respective realms of their disciplines.

Requirements for Licensure

Requirements usually center on personal characteristics and educational requirements to ensure that the candidate is at least minimally competent to practice professional nursing. These criteria include academic and clinical performance, a passing score on the licensing examination, and personal qualities.

Academic and clinical performance are validated by transcripts from approved schools of nursing. The state board may use its own criteria for approval or may rely on national accreditation agencies such as the National League for Nursing Accreditation Commission (NLNAC) and the Commission on Collegiate Nursing Education (CCNE).

All states administer licensing examinations and use a standardized, nationally normed test. With the advent of computers and the availability of computer-generated examinations, states have exclusively moved to this venue for completion of the national examination. Provisions are made for handicapped candidates in accordance with the Americans with Disabilities Act (ADA). With the increasing numbers of nurses seeking reciprocity or endorsement (recognition of licensure from one state to another state) from other state boards, states have elected to continue the practice of national norms for successful passage of the examinations.

Personal qualifications and attributes screened generally include citizenship or visa permits, physical and mental health fitness, minimal age requirements, fluency in English requirements, and moral character references.

Payment of fees is another area to meet licensure requirements. These fees include processing and administration fees for the licensure examination, interim work permit fees, and temporary licensure fees.

Exemptions

Most states allow exemptions from state licensure in very few circumstances. Some of the valid exemptions have previously been enumerated, such as exemptions for professional students in current coursework and for graduate nurses during the application process.

Another form of exemption is the **grandfather clause,** sometimes called a grandmother clause. The term describes an exemption for persons who were working within the profession prior to a deadline date. These individuals may be granted the privilege of applying for a license without having to meet all the requirements for licensure or without having to take the licensing examination. Such a grandfather clause was used to allow World War II nurses, those with on-the-job training and expertise, licensure even though they had not graduated from an approved school of nursing or passed the licensure examination.

The grandfather clause was projected to be used if the ANA proposal for professional entry into practice for baccalaureate nurses was ever fully implemented. In 1964, the ANA proposed that the entry level for professional nursing should be the baccalaureate of science in nursing degree (BSN), and that this would be implemented by 1985. Associate degree nurses (ADNs) would be technical nurses, and those previously licensed will be allowed the right to retain the title RN in the proposed new licensing schema.

In 1984, the ANA revised the timetable for implementation, and to date little success has been attained in this direction. By 1988, 30 state nurses associations had addressed the issue and 28 had adopted resolutions advocating the BSN as the professional entry requirement. The ANA House of Delegates in 1995 reaffirmed this commitment to the BSN as entry level into professional nursing, and voted to assist states in implementing strategies that would make such a goal a reality (ANA, 1995). Since that time, a few states are beginning to endorse possible legislation that would allow a specified time frame, currently 10 years after initial licensure, for associate degree and diploma nurses to achieve a BSN.

Only two states had any success in changing the entry requirements (North Dakota and Maine). Maine had some initial movement toward changing its statutes to conform with a BSN entry requirement, and North Dakota fully implemented this provision in the 1987 legislative session. Schools of nursing in North Dakota offered a BSN degree or higher, and ADN nurses coming into the state were granted provisional licensure, with an 8-year provision for completion of the BSN degree. These provisions were revoked in the 2003 legislative session, and North Dakota now allows all levels of educational preparation for RN licensure (North Dakota Century Code, 2003).

New research studies and professional association publications are supporting the fact that the discipline of nursing should consider reexamining the issue of how education affects patient safety issues. Aiken and her colleagues (2003) were the first researchers to conclude that there was a relationship between nurses' educational levels and patient mortality rates. They concluded that "in hospitals with higher proportions of nurses educated at the baccalaureate level or higher, surgical patients experienced lower mortality and failure-to-rescue rates" (Aiken et al., 2003, p. 1617). The American Association of Colleges of Nursing (AACN) in 2003 reported that the National Advisory Council on Nursing Education and Practice has advised Congress and the U.S. Secretary for Health and Human Services that at least two-thirds of the nursing workforce should be educated at the baccalaureate level or higher by 2010. Currently, approximately 47.2% of the nation's nurses are educated at the baccalaureate level (AACN, 2008).

There is a growing body of research that continues to support the linkage between the educational status of nurses and lower mortality and failure-to-rescue rates. These latest studies include an article by Aiken et al. (2008) revalidating the 2003 findings that there is a positive link between educational levels of RNs and patient outcomes, and an article by Friese et al. (2008) concluding that "moving to a nurse workforce in which a higher proportion of staff nurses have at least a baccalaureate-level education would result in substantially fewer adverse outcomes for patients" (p. 1159). Tourangeau et al. (2007) had previously concluded that a 10% increase in baccalaureate-prepared nurses was associated with 9 fewer deaths for every 1,000 discharged patients.

Licensure Across Jurisdictions

Because each state or territory has its own nurse practice act and because states or territories have mandatory licensure, provisions are included within state nurse practice acts for licensing nurses with valid licenses in other jurisdictions. There are essentially four means of granting licensure across jurisdictions:

1. **Reciprocity** is an agreement by two or more states granting recognition to licensure by other state boards of nursing. For reciprocity, the licensing requirements of the involved states must be equivalent. Such a provision allows licensed nurses to be granted additional licensure merely by application and payment of required fees. The concept of reciprocity also allows states with similar disciplinary actions to revoke a license in a state based solely on revocation in a sister state (*Schoenhair v. Pennsylvania,* 1983).
2. **Endorsement,** a similar concept, allows a state to grant licensure to an already licensed nurse from another state if the two states' qualifications and licensure requirements are comparable. Usually, the state granting endorsement requires that a similar licensure examination exists in both states. This means of granting licensure is distinguished from reciprocity in that no prior agreement existed between the two involved states, and individual nurses must petition for licensure by endorsement. Cases are decided on an individual basis.
3. **Licensure by examination** is required when the petitioned state does not grant licensure by reciprocity or by endorsement. Essentially, licensure by examination means that the individual must meet all of the state requirements and successfully complete a licensing examination before licensure is granted.
4. **Licensure by waiver** is similar to licensure by examination. If the petitioning candidate meets or exceeds some of the requirements for licensure, that portion previously demonstrated may be waived for the candidate, while he or she must demonstrate other requirements. States may choose to waive educational requirements, experience requirements, or examination requirements while requiring that deficiencies be met.

As with any new graduate within the state, a given state may grant a temporary license to out-of-state nurses. **Temporary licenses** allow nurses to practice while permanent licensure is pending or may allow them to practice for a limited period of time. For example, the state may grant temporary licensure for a semester or two while the nurse completes graduation requirements for an advanced nursing degree.

Foreign nursing school graduates desiring to practice nursing in the United States must meet the requirements of the state or territory in which they reside and must pass the licensing examination. Each state nurse practice act specifies requirements for foreign nursing school graduates. States require that graduates of a foreign school apply for an occupational visa, successfully complete a VisaScreen verifying proficiency in English, and earn a certificate from the Commission on Graduates of Foreign Nursing Schools or pass the National Council Licensure Examination for Registered Nurses (NCLEX-RN).

The Committee on Graduates of Foreign Nursing Schools (CGFNS), sponsored independently by the ANA and NLN, administers an examination to foreign-educated nurses that addresses their command of the English language, knowledge of nursing concepts and skills, and ability to pass the licensing examination. Following passage of the CGFNS examination, foreign nurses are allowed to obtain an occupational visa in the United States. The committee also has a Credentials Evaluation Service (CES) to evaluate transcripts and credentials from foreign countries.

In 1998, the U.S. House of Representatives approved legislation that would have allowed additional foreign nurses to practice in the United States in hospitals with a documented nursing shortage. Called the *Health Professional Shortage Area Nursing Relief Act* (1998), the bill was designed to provide an expedited means of allowing foreign nurses to practice in areas of critical need in the United States. Opposed by President Clinton and reluctantly supported by the ANA, the bill was defeated before it reached the U.S. Senate.

Disciplinary Action and Due Process Requirements

To give credence to the state board of nursing's ability to enforce licensure requirements, the board also has the authority for disciplinary action. Various actions may be taken, depending on the severity of the violation. Allowable **disciplinary actions** include:

1. Private reprimand or censure
2. Public reprimand or censure
3. Probation
4. Suspension of licensure
5. Refusal to renew licensure
6. Revocation of licensure
7. Imposition of a fine
8. Other discipline, such as requiring a continuing education course or a specific course that is the basis for the discipline (for example, requiring a licensee to successfully complete a pharmacology course if the licensee was disciplined for medication errors)

Not all of these measures have the same significance. For minor violations, the nurse may receive a warning or reprimand. Continued violations may be cause for probation or temporary suspension of licensure. Major violations are appropriately managed through licensure revocation or refusal to reissue licensure. Some of the possible violations for which disciplinary actions may be instigated include, but are not limited to:

1. Conviction of a felony or crime involving moral turpitude (an action contrary to justice, honesty, modesty, or good moral principles)

2. Use of fraud or deceit in obtaining licensure
3. Violation of the provisions of the nurse practice act
4. Aiding or abetting any unlicensed person with the unauthorized practice of nursing
5. Revocation, suspension, or denial of licensure to practice nursing in another jurisdiction
6. Habitual use of, or addiction to, alcohol or drugs
7. Unprofessional conduct that is likely to deceive, defraud, or injure the public or patients
8. Lack of fitness by reason of physical or mental health that could result in injury to the public or individual patients

During licensure suspension or probation, the board of nursing has the authority to impose conditions such as:

1. Obtaining substance abuse rehabilitation and counseling
2. Obtaining special counseling
3. Requiring supervision for specific techniques or procedures to validate competency
4. Requiring satisfactory completion of educational programs

For example, in *Thornton v. Alabama Board of Nursing* (2007), a nurse's license was suspended pending successful completion of a substance abuse program. The nurse appealed this decision to the Court of Civil Appeals of Alabama. The court ruled that an arrest for one driving under the influence (DUI) charge does not prove that the nurse has a substance abuse problem, reduced the charge to a reckless driving offense, and found that this lesser charge did not create grounds upon which to revoke a nurse's license. However, because the nurse failed to report this incident on her license renewal form, the board could discipline her for false statements.

Disciplinary actions may arise in one of several ways, depending on applicable state law. Generally, a written complaint is filed with the state board of nursing by an individual, a health care agency, or a professional organization. This single complaint triggers action on part of the board. The complaint may be initiated directly by the state board of nursing in some states. The complaint is screened and an investigation is initiated, if appropriate. A board hearing is then scheduled, and the nurse is entitled to a clear statement of the charges, the right to question and produce witnesses, the right to an attorney, and the right to a fair determination based on the evidence presented. The board may also request that the nurse provide a written response to the board regarding the allegations. This process is outlined in Table 11.1.

During the investigation phase, the board will contact any and all witnesses for information and statements about the complaint. The board may subpoena patient records and obtain copies of the health care institution's policies and procedures. The board may also retain an independent nurse consultant to review nursing notes and actions taken by the nurse being investigated for appropriateness. In cases in which diversion of drugs is suspected, the Drug Enforcement Agency (DEA) may also become involved. The DEA usually conducts its own investigation and may use undercover agents to monitor the nurse at work. The DEA's evidence will later be used by the board at the hearing.

Because state boards of nursing are agencies of state administrative law, the nurse is constitutionally allowed due process rights. Common due process rights of nurses include the following:

1. A clear statement of the allegations
2. A notice of time and place of hearing, disciplinary conference, or other proceeding
3. A right to legal counsel or to consult with legal counsel
4. A presentation of one's own witnesses and evidence
5. A cross-examination of the state's witnesses and challenge of state evidence

TABLE 11.1 Process for Disciplinary Hearings
Filing of the sworn complaint
Individual complaint
Health care agency complaint
Professional organization complaint
Review of the complaint
Notice of hearing to the involved nurse
Hearing before the board of nursing
Evidence presented by board and nurse
Witnesses called by board and nurse
Decision by the board of nursing
Disciplinary action
If found not guilty of misconduct, no action by board of nursing
If found guilty of misconduct, the board of nursing may:
Issue a reprimand, public or private
Place the nurse on probation
Deny the renewal of licensure
Suspend the nurse's license
Revoke the nurse's license
Allow the nurse to enter a diversion program
Court review
Review the board decision and concur with its finding
Order a new trial
Appeal to a higher court

6. A full hearing before an authorized board that functions in a fair manner

7. A written record of the hearing transcript

8. A judicial review, if requested, of the board's decision

Thus, nurses have the right to adequate notice of the alleged misconduct, an opportunity to present information concerning the alleged misconduct, and the right to appeal the board's action. Some states impose stricter rights; for example, not only do nurses have the right to be heard, they also have the right to call witnesses and to be represented by legal counsel. Some states also schedule a conference with their attorney and the nurse before commencing the formal hearing.

Following the announcement of the disciplinary action to be taken (as warranted), the nurse may file a lawsuit to appeal the board's decision. Depending on the jurisdiction, the nurse may file the case in the lowest court of the state or in a special court that handles appeals from state agencies. The appropriate court reviews only the state board of nursing's original decision against the nurse, not the nurse's alleged misconduct. The court's charge is to determine if the board acted properly. Whether the nurse or the state board of nursing prevails, the losing side may further appeal the decision through the court process to the highest court in the given state.

Among the more common reasons for the state board of nursing to investigate a nurse are:

1. Negligent or substandard care provided a patient (*Leahy v. North Carolina Board of Nursing*, 1997; *Kelly v. Guttormsson*, 2007; *Mississippi Board of Nursing v. Hanson*, 1997; *Rowe v. Sisters of the Pallottine Missionary Society*, 2001)
2. Sexual relations with a patient (*Tapp v. Board of Registered Nursing*, 2002)
3. Abusive behavior, either physical or oral (*Hill v. Pennsylvania Department of Health, Division of Nursing Care Facilities*, 1998)
4. Substance abuse and/or diversion of narcotics (*Hurst v. Ball Memorial Hospital, Inc., 2007*; *Kelly v. Guttormsson*, 2007; *Mullarrney v. Board of Review*, 2001; *Primes v. Louisiana State Board*, 2008; *Regester v. Indiana State Board of Nursing*, 1998; *State Board of Nursing v. Berry*, 2000; *The Mercy Hospital, Inc. v. Massachusetts Nurses Association*, 2005)
5. Physical or mental impairment (*Kraft v. State Board of Nursing*, 2001; *Ross v. Indiana State Board of Nursing*, 2003)
6. Fraud, usually committed in the application process (*Thomas v. Department of Health Services*, 2004; *Thompson v. Olsten Kimberly Qualitycare, Inc.*, 1997; *Thornton v. Alabama Board of Nursing*, 2007)

Failure by the state board of nursing to comply with the constitutional rights of due process or of state law may result in the reversal of the board's decision by the judiciary. The court in *Colorado State Board of Nursing v. Hohn* (1954), the landmark case in this area of the law, ordered the nurse's license reinstated, because the hearing was held with less than the full board present and state law mandated a full board hearing.

Typically, state nurse practice acts require that a quorum of the board be present for a disciplinary hearing and for disciplinary decisions. For example, the court in *Stevens v. Blake* (1984) held that a majority of the board of nursing must be in accord for final disciplinary decisions. The court further held that it is not necessary that a majority be present physically for each step involved in the process.

Adequate notice of an alleged misconduct means more than just 10 to 20 days' notice that a hearing will be held by the state board of nursing. Adequate notice encompasses knowledge or reason to have the knowledge that the particular conduct is prohibited by the state nurse practice act. This means that the wording of nurse practice acts may not be too vague or overly broad. This is usually avoided by a standard of conduct that is widely recognized as unprofessional. For example, the court in *Leahy v. North Carolina Board of Nursing* (1997) upheld a 1-year revocation of a nurse's license for what the board ruled were two significant lapses in professional judgment. The nurse appealed the ruling by filing this lawsuit. In both instances that ultimately caused the registered nurse to lose her license, she did not respond to reports from the LPNs under her supervision that there was grave concern for the condition of the patients the LPNs were monitoring. One patient's respirations had dropped from 20 to 8 per minute, and another patient had blood in his urine.

In the case of the patient with decreased respirations, the LPN first notified the RN, then reported the patient's condition to a supervisor. The supervisor immediately assessed the patient, notified the physician, and administered Narcan as ordered. In the second patient's situation, the RN told the LPN not to call the urologist, even though another RN had requested that the physician be notified. The charges filed against the nurse were failing to set her priorities appropriately in determining which patients presented the greatest danger and most needed care, failing to recognize her patients' conditions, failing to supervise appropriately the care given patients by LPNs, and failure to make patient information available to other health care providers, namely the supervisor and the physician.

At the hearing, the board of nursing did not have an expert witness testify to the standards of care owed by this nurse. Instead, the board served as expert witnesses in determining the standard of care owed these patients and in determining the accountability of the nurse. At trial, the Supreme Court of North Carolina agreed with the board that no expert witnesses were necessary because the licensing board may use its own experience and specialized knowledge to evaluate a situation presented before it for a ruling. Thus, the nurse's challenge to revocation of her license failed.

GUIDELINES

Steps in Disciplinary Proceedings for Nursing Misconduct

1. A sworn complaint is filed with the state board of nursing by an individual, a health care agency, or a professional organization, or the complaint may be originated by the board of nursing itself.
2. If there is sufficient evidence, the state board of nursing will hold a formal review of the matter, during which both sides may be represented by legal counsel and witnesses are called. Sometimes, a less formal meeting with the nurse and the state's attorney will occur before the formal board hearing.
3. Depending on the outcome of the hearing, the board may take disciplinary action.
4. The nurse may appeal the board's decision in state court. The court reviews the actions of the board, not the original act of misconduct by the nurse, and either upholds the board's action or grants a new trial.
5. Whichever side loses at trial level may decide to further appeal the court decision to the next highest court in the state. That court may also uphold the lower-court's decision or reverse the decision, and the court may also reinstate the nurse's license if the nurse filed the appeal.

In a 1994 case in Iowa, *Burns v. Matzen,* a provision in state law requiring licensing boards to revoke the licenses of habitually intoxicated health professionals was upheld by the Iowa Supreme Court. The board of nursing placed a registered nurse on probation in accordance with the statute after finding that the nurse was habitually intoxicated. The nurse challenged the decision and the statute. The nurse argued that the law was unconstitutionally vague because licensees could not sufficiently discern what conduct would constitute habitual intoxication and therefore could not avoid violating the statute. The court upheld the statute, ruling that a "person of ordinary intelligence should easily understand what type of conduct is to be avoided" (at 4). The court concluded that the licensing board could determine whether a nurse violated the statute on a case-by-case basis without developing a specific definition. The nurse's probationary status was upheld.

Miller v. Tennessee Board of Nursing (2007) illustrates how courts can rule on the various disciplinary actions a board of nursing imposes. In that case, an LPN was working from 7:00 P.M. to 7:00 A.M. and was assigned to five patients, including a patient for whom an obstetrical consultation was needed. The other four patients were essentially stable. At about 4:30 A.M., the LPN became ill and vomited in the bathroom. She immediately went to the nurses' station and notified the other four nurses who were working with her that she was leaving. The charge nurse instructed her to notify the supervisor before leaving, but the LPN did not communicate with the nursing supervisor before exiting the facility. She gave as her reason for not discussing the situation with the supervisor that she was afraid that the supervisor would send her to the emergency center, and the LPN did not want to be billed for such a visit. She testified that she intended to see her family physician early that same morning.

The facility notified the LPN that it was terminating its contract with her and reported the LPN to the state board of nursing for abandonment. The board of nursing imposed a $1000 penalty for abandoning her patients and suspended her nursing license pending a psychological examination. The court of appeals in this case concurred with the board of nursing that the LPN had wrongfully abandoned her patients and that the fine was appropriate, but refused to uphold the suspension of her license pending a psychological examination. There was no basis, said the court, to suspect that this nurse had a psychological condition that affected her fitness to practice as a nurse.

Courts have also ruled that the board of nursing may not do more than disclose the existence of a pending investigation. In *Neal v. Fields* (2005), a formal complaint was filed against the nurse with the board of nursing. The nurse then experienced difficulty when applying for a new position, and she sued the board of nursing for violation of her constitutional rights. The court ruled that the nurse's rights were not violated so long as no false or unproven allegations against the nurse were communicated to a prospective employer.

Fraudulent conduct may be the basis for disciplinary action. In *Thompson v. Olsten Kimberly Qualitycare, Inc.* (1997), a home health nurse was fired for alleged double billing of patients, for signing documents as an RN when she was really an LPN, for absenteeism, and for being verbally abusive toward co-workers. The grounds for her termination were reported to the state board of nursing, and she sued for defamation.

A person licensed as a professional health care provider must report to the board of nursing personal knowledge of any conduct of a licensed professional nurse believed to be grounds for disciplinary action. This includes conduct that appears incompetent, unprofessional, unethical, fraudulent, or indicative that the nurse is mentally or physically unable to engage safely in the profession of nursing. Any person, facility, or corporation making such a report to the board in good faith is immune from civil liability or criminal prosecution over such a report. The nurse was entitled to her day in court to attempt to prove that her employer was not acting in good faith, however, and the case was remanded to the trial court for decision on this one issue.

Boards of nursing may require licensees to agree to additional examinations and tests in conjunction with their hearing. In *Ross v. Indiana State Board of Nursing* (2003), a hospital staff nurse was alleged to have committed acts of incompetence, including mixing up patients' names on blood samples, not administering medications and then falsifying medication administration records, and removing chest tubes without the necessary qualifications to remove such tubes. The board of nursing required him to undergo a mental health evaluation before commencing the hearing. The nurse agreed to undergo a psychiatric evaluation, but insisted that the board of nursing incur the cost of such tests.

The court agreed with the nurse and said that the board of nursing would be required to bear the costs for such tests. "A citizen has a Constitutional right to maintain professional licensure and to work in a chosen field until proven unfit. Having to pay for a mental health evaluation to keep a professional license, before charges of unfitness have been proven, violates Due Process of Law" was the conclusion of the court (*Ross v. Indiana State Board of Nursing*, 2003, at 120). The court also noted that this ruling did not apply to mental health treatment or evaluation that may be ordered or agreed upon so that a nurse actually proven guilty of misconduct or unfitness can keep or regain a license.

Many of the cases before individual state boards of nursing involve chemical dependency, substance abuse, or narcotics diversion (*Hurst v. Ball Memorial Hospital, Inc.*, 2007; *Kelly v. Guttormsson*, 2007; *Primes v. Louisiana State Board*, 2008; *The Mercy Hospital, Inc. v. Massachusetts Nurses Association*, 2005). Generally, such cases concern the fact that the evidence against the nurse was circumstantial (*Hurst*), that issues with chemical dependency directly resulted in negligent actions and adverse patient outcomes (*Kelly*), or that the nurse was diverting narcotics for his or her own use (*Primes* and *The Mercy Hospital, Inc.*).

An interesting cause of action before the Iowa State Board of Nursing is *Hoffman v. Iowa Board of Nursing* (2006). In that case, a nurse worked for both physicians in a two-physician office practice. When the physicians decided to terminate the partnership, the nurse inherited the chore of photocopying the charts of the physician who was relocating. She decided to complete this chore on a Saturday while the office was closed. She brought her two children, ages 11 and 13, to assist her, and one of the physicians said he would pay the children to photocopy the charts.

When the second physician came in the office and noted what was occurring, he stopped the children from photocopying the charts and filed a complaint with the state board of nursing for violation of patients' medical confidentiality. The board of nursing brought disciplinary action against the nurse and she filed a lawsuit.

The court ruled in the nurse's favor. The children were not allowed to read the charts, merely feed the pages into the copy machine, press the "start" button, and perform manual tasks. Additionally, no confidential material left the physician's office. Thus, there was no breach of any patient's medical confidentiality rights.

GUIDELINES

Nurse Practice Acts

1. Obtain a current copy of your state's nurse practice act. This may be done by writing or contacting the state board of nursing or the local or state office of the state nurses association. Additionally, copies may be obtained via the Internet.
2. Read the act carefully for the following elements, ensuring that you understand what each element means to you as a professional nurse:
   a. Definition of professional nursing
   b. Requirements for licensure
   c. Exemptions
   d. Grounds for disciplinary actions
   e. Criteria for out-of-state licensure
   f. Creation of the state board of nursing
   g. Penalties for practicing without a license
3. Know the state board of nursing rules and regulations regarding professional standards of care and dishonorable conduct. As you read the rules and regulations, know what each enumerated rule and regulation means, and apply each to your individual nursing practice.
4. Know whom to contact and what to do if the nurse practice act is violated by licensed or unlicensed practitioners. Remember that you have an obligation to uphold the state nurse practice act and to see that others likewise uphold the act.

In 1983, the Texas Court of Appeals upheld the suspension of a nurse's license for "unprofessional and dishonorable conduct . . . likely to injure the public" (*Lunsford v. Board of Nurse Examiners,* 1983, at 391) when the nurse failed to adequately assess a potential cardiac patient. The nurse argued that she had acted according to a direct physician order and could not have allowed admission for the patient to the hospital whether or not she had completed the patient assessment. The board, and subsequently the court, ruled that her failure to assess and implement appropriate nursing actions was within the adequate notice provision of the state nurse practice act and was within the specific rule promulgated by the Texas Board of Nurse Examiners.

A newer case that seems to reiterate this same cause of action is *Rowe v. Sisters of the Pallottine Missionary Society* (2001). In *Rowe,* the court stressed the need for nurses to be patient advocates, noting that nurses were to use all levels of the hospital chain of command in assuring that patients receive appropriate and competent medical and nursing care. Specifically, the institution policy in this case called for the RN who believed that appropriate care was not being administered to a patient to discuss his or her concerns with the physician and then alert the clinical manager or patient care coordinator. The patient care coordinator or clinical manager would then discuss the issue with the physician and, if not resolved, alert the nurse administrator. The nursing administrator would then alert the assistant executive of medical affairs, who would in turn notify the chief of the service if the issue could not be resolved. The policy also noted that the nursing administrator could, at any point, request assistance from administration. The court found that although the policy was sound, it was not followed in this instance.

EXERCISE 11.3

A physician was accused of professional misconduct for having his office nurse sign her name to his preprinted prescription forms for medications that the physician prescribed for his patients. The physician did not delegate any medical discretion to the nurse; in fact, it was the physician who determined the type of medication, administration, strength, and other particulars of the prescription the patient was to be given. The state board of nursing charged the nurse with professional misconduct for agreeing to sign these prescriptions.

How should the board of nursing find in such a case? Is the nurse guilty of professional misconduct? Is the physician guilty of professional misconduct? Would your answer about the nurse's misconduct differ if the physician is found to have committed professional misconduct by the board of medicine?

Penalties for Practicing Without a License

Most nurse practice acts allow for a fine or imprisonment for practicing without a license. Fines or confinement represent charges that may be pursued against the illegal practitioner. Generally, fines range from $50 to $500, and the term of confinement does not exceed 60 days.

Civil suits may also be filed against the nonlicensed practitioner. Such suits may be filed prior to, concurrent with, or after criminal charges. The civil suits are brought by those harmed by the nonlicensed practitioner and usually concern standards of care.

DIVERSION PROGRAMS

The nursing profession, through **diversion programs,** is showing a commitment to the rehabilitation of nurses who are psychologically unable to function or addicted to either drugs or alcohol. Rather than disciplining these nurses through the traditional disciplinary process, these nurses are diverted to rehabilitation programs. Diversion programs also allow the state board of nursing to protect the public while complying with the Americans with Disabilities Act of 1990 (ADA). See Chapter 15 for a more complete discussion.

A case that supports this compliance with the ADA is *Scott v. Beverly Enterprises-Kansas, Inc.* (1997). The nurse failed to mention in his interview for a charge nurse position in a nursing home that his license was restricted. He was not allowed access to narcotics or other mind-altering medications. The restriction had been imposed following a long history of trouble with narcotics addiction. When he finally produced and tendered his license to his employer as required by law, shortly after being employed, he was immediately fired. He sued for disability discrimination.

He claimed that he was a successfully rehabilitated drug abuser, having been "clean" and sober for 30 days before he reported to work at this job. The nurse's suit alleged that he was a "qualified individual with a disability," protected from employment discrimination by the ADA. The District Court for Kansas dismissed his lawsuit.

First, the court noted, a nurse with a restricted license who cannot have access to narcotics is not a "qualified individual with a disability" with respect to a nursing position for which the job description requires the ability to administer and/or account for narcotics and other mind-altering drugs on a daily basis. Second, this nurse was not a "successfully rehabilitated drug user," merely because he had been clean and sober for 30 days. He was still a current drug user in the court's opinion. Unfortunately, for employers who must make difficult decisions, and for employees who have successfully overcome addictions, the courts have not clearly defined just how long persons with past problems must be in remission before they get protection from the antidiscrimination laws.

Voluntary alternatives to traditional disciplinary actions, diversion programs sometimes referred to as *peer assistance programs* entail attendance at group sessions such as Alcoholics Anonymous, Narcotics Anonymous, or counseling sessions; voluntary submission of urine samples for substance abuse testing; and special provisions by employers. Facilities that allow diversion program nurses to work within their units must comply with specific guidelines, generally

EXERCISE 11.4

Investigate the existence of a diversion or peer assistance program for substance abuse and/or mental illness within your state. If one exists, find out how it is administered and its success rate. How does the program assist these nurses? If there is no program, what does the state board of nursing do for nurses who have substance abuse or mental illness issues? Are the members of the board of nursing working to implement such a diversion program?

From an ethical perspective, decide which ethical principles such programs foster. Include in your answer ethical principles from both a nurse and patient perspective. What are the ethical responsibilities of nurses who know that a co-worker or peer has a substance abuse problem? Does the mere knowledge of such information increase one's ethical responsibilities to patients who may be cared for by the affected nurse? What are the ethical issues involved from the perspective of the entire profession?

filing quarterly reports with the board of nursing; working on general nursing units rather than emergency centers, intensive care units, and post-anesthesia care units; working no overtime while in the program; and working daytime hours as opposed to night shifts. Some programs also forbid recovering employees from assuming charge positions and from administering narcotics to patients.

In most states, nurses may petition the board for reinstatement of full licensure after 12 to 24 months and must show compliance with the provisions of the program and the ability to perform in the workplace. The advantage of the program is that recovering nurses are allowed to be fully rehabilitated and productive in their chosen career as opposed to being denied licensure to work in the nursing profession. If nurses fail to comply with the provisions of the program, the board of nursing institutes more traditional disciplinary provisions.

ARTICULATION WITH MEDICAL PRACTICE ACTS

Medical practice acts are to physicians what nurse practice acts are to nurses—state laws that allow the individual to practice in a given discipline. Most medical practice acts define medicine as acts of diagnosis, prescription, treatment, and surgery. Some states' acts include only the first three elements. **Articulation of medical practice acts** with nurse practice acts is one way that these professionals work together to ensure quality patient care.

Incorporated into the language or the intent of medical practice acts is broad delegatory language, enabling the physician to delegate to qualified and skilled persons the legal ability to perform certain actions and skills. This broad delegatory language, coupled with standing orders and protocols, has increased the functions of nurses while causing an overlap between nurse practice acts and medical practice acts. For example, nurses in a variety of critical care units may actually perform some medical acts because of valid standing orders and protocols. For example, if the electrocardiogram rhythm strip shows ventricular fibrillation (a medical diagnosis), the nurse may inject lidocaine or perform electric cardioversion (a medical treatment).

Not all jurisdictions recognize and implement **standing orders** in the same manner. Some states allow standing orders to take precedent if the patient fits a particular classification (for example, because the patient is in the coronary care unit, the coronary care standing orders are immediately valid), while other states mandate that the patient be seen by the physician and the standing orders be signed by a physician before they may be implemented. However a particular state approaches standing orders and protocols, they are a means of expanding the scope of nursing practice.

Another way of articulating medical practice acts with nurse practice acts is by passing laws that make some functions common to both professions. For example, some state laws allow both nurses and physicians to diagnose and treat patients as long as the nursing diagnosis does not alter the patient's medical regimen. Other states allow nurses to evaluate and diagnose patients but not to treat them. The more modern nurse practice acts are beginning to allow for the treatment and diagnosis of patients by professional nurses.

A third approach to increase nursing's role is by joint statements between the disciplines of medicine and nursing. **Joint statements** are part of an evolving process and, in fact, are stopgap measures until states are able to develop and implement broader definitions of nursing practice. Joint statements thus serve as the basis for expanded nursing practice. There would be no need for joint statements if nurse practice acts were amended at the same time the joint statements were written.

SCOPE OF PRACTICE ISSUES

In recent years, the courts have attempted to settle scope of practice issues and the articulation of medical practice acts with nurse practice acts. As a general rule, negligence issues have caused scope of practice issues to be considered second rather than first.

Scope of practice issues speak to the actions or duties of a given profession. The phrase *scope of practice* legally refers to permissible boundaries of practice for the health professional, and the scope of practice is defined by statute, rule, or a combination of statute and rule. For example, in a state that statutorily allows nurses to diagnose and treat patients, individual, licensed nurses may diagnose and treat the patients they encounter. In a state that expressly forbids diagnosis and treatment as a nursing function, nurses would be practicing medicine without a license if they undertook to diagnose and treat the patient. In a state in which both nurses and physicians may diagnose and treat patients, the scope of practice issues overlap, and reasonable and customary practice becomes a key issue.

From a legal perspective, scope of practice issues usually arise in one of two instances: (1) Some negligent act was associated with the scope of practice issue, or (2) the standard of care owed the patient is increased because of the medical or nursing action.

A landmark case that illustrates the first instance is *Cooper v. National Motor Bearing Company* (1955). One of the first cases that mandated nurses to be patients' advocates, this case concerned an occupational health nurse who failed to recognize the patient's signs and symptoms as being indicative of cancer and who further failed to refer the patient to his physician for treatment. The court ruled that occupational health nurses should be able to diagnose sufficiently well to know whether to treat the patient or to refer the patient. Thus, diagnosis, which was outside the scope of nursing practice at that time, was allowed in a limited scope. Note that the court failed to question or decide the greater issue of when such diagnoses were outside nursing's scope of practice.

In a case that demonstrates how scope of practice actions can be performed illegally is *Lang v. Department of Health* (2007). In that case, the Court of Appeals of Washington State upheld sanctions imposed on two dentists who routinely allowed "surgical assistants" to start IV lines and administer anesthetic agents through these IV lines. The court used the state's statutory language to define the scope of practice for these nonlicensed health care personnel. First, said the court, there is no designation for a "surgical assistant" in the state law. Second, persons who are surgical technicians are not allowed to start IV lines, nor are they allowed to administer medications through these lines. Ultimately, the court concluded that starting IVs and administering anesthetics through these IV lines are strictly within the scope of nursing and medical practice.

Standards of care issues frequently arise with nurses in expanded roles, such as nurse anesthetists and nurse midwives. In these types of cases, the court usually applies a medical standard of care, reasoning that a greater duty is owed the patient because the nurse is performing actions that physicians typically perform. *Whitney v. Day, M. D., and Hurley Hospital* (1980) held that nurse anesthetists are professionals with expertise in an area of medicine and as such are held to those higher standards. *Mohr v. Jenkins* (1980) reached a similar conclusion.

One possibility for preventing scope of practice issue differences concerns the hospital or institutional policy and procedure manuals. Since nursing and technology are both fluid and dynamic, up-to-date policies and procedures may ensure that the nurse practices within nursing's scope of practice. Policies and procedures accomplish this goal because they tend to be much more narrow in scope than nurse practice acts and give clarity to actions the nurse may or may not perform. For example, the nurse practice act may have a standard that reads "makes judgments and decisions about the nursing care for the client or patient by using assessment data to formulate and implement a plan of goals and objectives." The hospital policy and procedure manual has a procedure that states, in laundry list fashion, how the patient assessment will be done and when it is to be performed, along with specific guidelines for documentation of the patient assessment. The nurses' assessment data may be inclusive of broad hemodynamic measurements, and the hospital policy and procedure manual should also have a procedure for the performance of hemodynamic measurements and monitoring, arterial lines, thermodilution pulmonary artery catheter lines, and central lines.

Policies and procedures specify the allowable scope of practice within the given setting. They may be more narrow than the scope of practice stated within the nurse practice act, but they may not extend the nurse practice act scope of practice. The professional nurse must choose the nurse practice act over the hospital policy if there is a discrepancy. Professional standards and the nurse practice act mandate quality care for all patients. Professional standards and the state board of nursing's rules and regulations were the central themes reinforced in *Lunsford v. Board of Nurse Examiners* (1983).

To be of maximum value to nurses, the policies and procedures must be current. Ideally, they should be developed jointly by medical and nursing committees and updated periodically. The policies and procedures should be reflective of community standards. The committee developing them must be aware of the nursing role within the given community, and policies and procedures should be written to allow nurses to meet and exceed the public standard.

Institutional policies and procedures mandate that nurses remain current in their practice, either through continuing education classes, in-service education classes, or reading current journal articles and publications. Institutional policies and procedures also help nurses prevent potential liability if they can show how individual nursing actions were within the policies and procedures and thus within the allowable scope of practice.

Other means for preventing scope of practice differences include:

1. Listing accepted procedures in the nurse practice act
2. Requesting the attorney general's opinions for clarification on allowed or prohibited procedures
3. Reviewing recent judicial decisions for definition of roles
4. Requesting joint statements from professional organizations clarifying roles and practices
5. Reviewing rules and regulations of the state board of nursing concerning the permitted scope of practice

Scope of practice issues also concern a nurse's right to refuse patient assignments. In 1996, the Joint Commission for the Accreditation of Healthcare Organizations (now known as the Joint Commission [JC]) acknowledged the right of nurses to refuse selected patient assignments by adding a standard to both its hospital and home care accreditation manuals. The standard requires employers to establish policies and mechanisms to address staff requests not to participate in aspects of care that conflict with their cultural values or religious beliefs. The new standard required each facility to:

1. specify aspects of patient care that might conflict with staff members' values and beliefs.
2. have a written policy on how requests to be excused from care are handled and make that policy available to all staff members for review.
3. develop a process for deciding whether staff requests not to participate in care are legitimate and should be granted.
4. ensure the safe delivery of care in instances in which a staff member's request to be excused is granted. (JCAHO, 1996)

Courts have generally upheld the nurse's right to refuse an assignment based on religious beliefs. For example, nurses can refuse to care for and be a party to abortion, if abortion is against their religious tenets. Discrimination in employment on the basis of religion is one of the protected rights under Title VII of the Civil Rights Act of 1964. One of the earlier cases in this area of the law was *Kenney v. Ambulatory Center of Miami* (1981), in which an operating room supervisor was demoted after she objected on religious grounds to assisting in an abortion case. The court ruled that the center had a legal duty to accommodate Kenney's religious beliefs and ordered that she be reinstated to her former position.

A newer case in this area of the law illustrates that nurses may only refuse to assist with procedures that are against religious tenets. In *Larson v. Albany Medical Center* (1998), the nurse refused to participate in an elective abortion because of her religious beliefs. Instead of a simple refusal, the nurse used the request from her supervisor to assist in the abortion as an opportunity to launch into an argument about abortions. This action, said the court, was not protected by the religious beliefs of the nurse and was insubordinate behavior; thus, the nurse could be disciplined by the institution.

States today typically have conscience clauses that provide for more explicit protection. There is also a Federal Conscience Clause (42 U.S.C. 3009.7), which applies to facilities that receive specific types of governmental funding, such as grants under the Public Health Service Act and Community Health Centers Act. As with the state clause, the federal clause protects only nurses who refuse to assist with abortions and sterilizations because of religious or moral beliefs.

GUIDELINES
Refusal of Care Based on Religious and Moral Principles

1. If you have such beliefs, inform your supervisor or nurse manager and request that you not be assigned to such cases. Beliefs normally do not occur in a relatively short time period but are deeply held and should be conveyed to management when you are hired.
2. If you are currently caring for a client and conditions suddenly warrant an aspect of care that you object to, alert your supervisor or nurse manager so that the patient can be reassigned or other arrangements made.
3. Once you have accepted assignment for a patient's care, you are legally responsible for that care until the patient has been reassigned. If an emergency occurs, you must provide for the care as required, regardless of any personal objections you may have.
4. In a nonemergency situation, follow the institution's policy and procedures for refusing assignments. Whether a written policy exists or the institution is in the process of writing such a policy, be clear that your refusal is based on religious or moral grounds.
5. If there is a dispute about the appropriateness of your refusal, work with the nursing team, risk manager, or other appropriate persons to resolve the issue to everyone's satisfaction.

UPDATING NURSE PRACTICE ACTS

There are several ways to update individual nurse practice acts. Updating may call for a simple revision of the original act or a complete rewriting. Because nurse practice acts are legislative enactments, any changes must be channeled through the state legislative body.

Amendments add to the nurse practice act or its regulation, usually giving nurses the needed legal permission to perform actions and functions that have become part of the community standard.

Amendments have the same force of law as does the original act, and many state nurses acts are amended annually by state legislatures.

Redefinitions involve a rewriting of the definition of nursing and as such automatically change the force of the entire act. For example, the definition of nursing may be rewritten to include diagnosis and treatment or to clarify "diagnosis" to mean "nursing diagnosis." The act is thus clarified for the practicing profession, the scope is broadened, and there has been no repeal or piecemeal amendment to the original act.

Application of sunset laws also aids in keeping nurse practice acts current. Such laws call for a review of the act at a fixed time, such as 6 to 10 years after the enactment of the original act. The purpose of sunset laws is to force a periodic review by legislative bodies and thus prevent an act from becoming hopelessly outdated. The practice act affected automatically expires at the designated date. Most acts are updated during the legislative year immediately preceding application of the sunset law.

The dynamic process of nursing may also necessitate some action before the nurse practice act is revised or amended by the appropriate legislative body. Professional organizations, such as the state nurses association and the state board of nursing, may lobby for needed changes in the nurse practice act and thus force redefinition or amendment of the act. Or the state board of nursing may enact new rules and regulations to ensure that the nurse practice act meets the prevailing community standards. Thus, practicing professional nurses must do more than just know the original nurse practice act. They must remain current on newly adopted rules and regulations of the state board of nursing and understand the lobbying efforts of the professional organizations, because both may have great impact on an individual nurse's scope of practice.

CONTINUING EDUCATION FOR PRACTICING NURSES

Many nurse practice acts speak to continuing education for professional nurses. Whether mandatory or voluntary, the concept of **continuing education** involves a means of ensuring that nurses remain current in their practice. With an expanded and ever-increasing scope of practice issues and increased accountability for technical nursing skills and functions, nurses must maintain current and competent practice standards. Although state boards of nursing and professional nursing organizations continue to argue for and against mandatory continuing education, there is no argument that nurses must remain competent to practice in all practice settings.

Today, much of the debate has turned toward developing mechanisms to ensure continuing competency, rather than accrual of continuing education hours. Such validation of continuing competency would more greatly ensure that nurses are competent to care for specialty patients, to perform management roles, or to function as quality nursing educators. Merely attending a continuing education session or completing a short quiz about the content of a journal article does not ensure that the nurse remains competent, nor that any learning actually occurred. In fact, many continuing education programs are designed to explore broader topics such as alternative therapies or newer roles in nursing—issues that the nurse may not be able to readily incorporate into practice arenas. Continuing competency, it is hoped, will be able to better ensure that nurses are lifelong learners and that they remain competent, whatever their role or field in nursing. Nurses may still be able to attend sessions that explore new paths for nurses or revisit the history of nursing, and state boards of nursing will have a better benchmark upon which to renew licenses.

REPORTING PROFESSIONAL VIOLATIONS OF THE NURSE PRACTICE ACT

An important concept for professional nurses concerns the difficulty of knowing how and when to report a co-worker for violations of the state nurse practice act. Mandatory reporting exists to protect the public's health and safety through the discovery of unsafe or substandard nursing practice or conduct. Mandatory reporting to the board of nursing or other appropriate state agency is not a substitute for employer-based disciplinary actions.

Reporting may be for unprofessional conduct, the inability of a nurse to practice with reasonable skill and safety as a result of a mental or physical condition, conduct that reasonably appears to be a contributing factor in the death of a patient or that appears to be a contributing factor in the harm to a patient that requires medical intervention, conduct involving patient abuse, extended scope of practice, and/or substance abuse. Looking the other way may be easier, but all nurse practice acts require the reporting of violations of the act. Failure to report violators becomes grounds for disciplinary action. For example, most nurse practice acts also hold the nonreporting nurse to be in violation of the nurse practice act. Nurses who report in good faith are protected from defamation lawsuits, since they are required to report violations of the nurse practice act.

Unprofessional conduct includes, but is not limited to, failing to report to the board or the appropriate authority in the organization in which the nurse is working, within a reasonable time of the occurrence, any violation or attempted violation of the nurse practice act or duly promulgated rules, regulations, or orders.

The most obvious means of reporting violations is within the organizational structure. Most nurses have a direct chain of command to hospital or institutional administrations, and the staff nurse should report violations of the act to the immediate supervisor, usually a nurse-manager or charge nurse. Reports should be factual and documented in writing. Reports should include as complete a description of the violation as possible, listing other witnesses and giving patient names, as appropriate. The report should be complete so that administrative staff can investigate and gather additional evidence.

Administrative personnel have a duty to act on reported violations. They may insist that the violator receive counseling, attend further education classes, or perform supervised demonstrations to ensure quality nursing actions. The administrative personnel may not allow the violator merely to terminate employment, thus allowing the violator to change places of employment without ever seeking help or changing actions. In such a case, the hospital administrator has a duty to report the violator to the state board of nursing.

Individual staff nurses may also incur the same duty. Suppose a nurse reports a colleague for substance abuse or substandard nursing care to the appropriate supervisor. Later, the reporting nurse learns that the reported nurse has quit her job and is now working for another hospital within the same city (or state). Upon questioning the supervisor, the reporting nurse learns that no action was taken by the hospital administration. The nurse was merely questioned and voluntarily resigned. To date, the second hospital has not asked for a reference concerning the nurse. If there was sufficient evidence to report the nurse to your supervisor in the first place, then there is sufficient evidence to file that same report with the state board of nursing. An affirmative duty to report the nurse to the state board of nursing exists in such a case.

Reporting a violator of the nurse practice act may be done by writing to the state board of nursing, describing the substance abuse or substandard care, and including all pertinent documentation. Sign the letter, because anonymous complaints are summarily disregarded by most boards of nursing and administrators, and the nurse has not fulfilled the affirmative duty to safeguard nursing practice by an anonymous letter. Most state boards of nursing will preserve confidentiality. This last step usually proves unnecessary. Once the nurse is reported through the proper hospital channels, administrative staff will aid the nurse with necessary counseling, education, or rehabilitation.

NATIONAL PRACTITIONER DATA BANK

The **National Practitioner Data Bank (NPDB)** was created by the Health Care Quality Improvement Act of 1986 and became operational on September 1, 1990. Although primarily aimed at affecting the practice of medicine, the NPDB also affects the professional practice of nursing. The NPDB records three types of data:

1. Information relating to medical malpractice payments on behalf of health care practitioners
2. Information relating to adverse actions taken against clinical privileges of physicians, osteopaths, and dentists
3. Information concerning actions by professional societies that adversely affect membership

The information is then available to health care facilities needing the information to verify credentialing of potential practitioners. Failure to report results in fines and penalties if mandatory reporting is identified.

The NPDB affects nursing primarily from the perspective of advanced nursing practice because nurse practitioners, nurse midwives, clinical nurse specialists, and nurse anesthetists are subject to credentialing procedures similar to those named in the act as well as the quality of care at facilities that employ nurses. Although far from a perfect system, the NPDB remains an effective means on a nationwide scale to track and identify professionals found liable of malpractice or who have had professional memberships or professional privileges revoked.

CERTIFICATION

Certification is a form of credentialing that has both legal and professional implications. Certification indicates a level of competence above minimum criteria for licensure and verifies that an individual has met certain standards of preparation and performance.

Certification of individuals awards the person so certified with the right to use the title conferred by the certificate. Certification affirms the special qualifications that the individual has achieved in a defined area of clinical practice.

Many specialty nursing organizations offer certification to professional nurses. Some organizations mandate advanced degrees in nursing as prerequisites for certification, whereas others do not add this prerequisite. The ANA through the American Nurses Credential Center offers a wide variety of certifications, as do other professional organizations. For example, the Emergency Nurses Organization, the American Association of Critical-Care Nurses, and the Association of Operating Room Nurses offer specialty certification in those areas of clinical practice.

EXERCISE 11.5

Interview personnel within your facility to see what certificates are required to hold various nursing positions within the facility. Is there a pay differential for certification? How are staff nurses (e.g., critical care nurses or emergency center nurses) urged to attain certification? Do these certifications assist in enhancing the quality of nursing care delivered within the facility?

COMPLEMENTARY AND ALTERNATIVE MEDICINE

Complementary and alternative medicine (CAM), sometimes referred to as integrative medicine, are modalities not generally used by health care providers to treat illnesses such as therapeutic touch, biofeedback, guided imagery, acupuncture, and massage therapy. Because CAM embraces wellness or a health maintenance model, it is becoming more popular in the United States as patients are beginning to understand and value its effectiveness. Washington State was the first in the country to pass legislation in this area (Rabkin, 1999). This early legislation addressed insurance benefits.

In 1992, the National Institutes of Health established the Office of Alternative Medicine to promote the unbiased study of nonconventional therapies. Many medical and nursing schools now offer such coursework, usually as elective courses rather than required courses for a given degree program. A 2002 survey by the National Center for Complementary and Alternative Medicine (NCCAM) found that 74.6% of participants used some form of CAM for conditions ranging from insomnia to back pain and that more than 62% of the participants had used some form of CAM in the past 12 months. The most common CAM therapies in the United States were prayer, herbalism, breathing meditation, meditation, yoga, diet-based therapy, progressive relaxation, mega-vitamin therapy, and visualization.

Although the popularity for CAM is increasing, there is still a dearth of uniform standards of practice to provide guidance to nurses and physicians who regularly use such therapies. Some states explicitly outlaw certain alternative therapies, whereas others require licensure or certain standards of education before performing these therapies. In Nevada, for example, the nurse may employ CAM if the nurse has the documented competence, knowledge, skill, and ability in application of the therapy and the patient has granted informed consent. In Arkansas, state licensure laws regulate therapies such as massage, acupuncture, and physical therapy. In New York, professional nurses can apply CAM if they have the appropriate education, clinical experience, and supervision required in order to maintain competency.

Nurses must also know their state law before performing such therapies. For example, in a state that does not recognize a certain therapy, the nurse who practices the therapy could be charged with practicing a therapy that is not legally authorized. If the state requires licensure in order to perform a specific therapy, such as massage, and the nurse does not have a license, the charge against the nurse will be practicing without a license. Sometimes, the practice is permitted, but institutional policy forbids its use. Thus, nurses must know and follow state law and individual institution policy.

Before considering the use of alternative therapies, remember a few basic issues. Patients should be fully informed about the alternative therapy before its use, including information about the value and projected outcomes. In some states, certain therapies are still considered experimental, so that signed informed consent form similar to that used for any research subject is required. After using the therapy, ensure that it is fully documented in the patient record. Finally, answer fully any questions about alternative therapies.

The landmark case concerning alternative therapies in nursing remains *Tuma v. Board of Nursing of the State of Idaho* (1979). In that case, Ms. Tuma, a nursing instructor who was in the hospital for the sole purpose of supervising nursing students, was asked by a patient about other therapies for cancer, including natural products such as laetrile and chaparral. At the patient's urging, Tuma agreed to return to the hospital later in the evening so that she could explain the alternative therapies to the patient's family.

The patient's daughter-in-law told the physician about the meeting, and he ordered the chemotherapy discontinued because he felt that the patient no longer wanted the chemotherapy treatments. After talking with Tuma, the family resumed the chemotherapy treatments, and the patient died shortly thereafter.

The physician reported the incident to the director of nursing, and the hospital subsequently filed a complaint with the state board of nursing, alleging that Tuma had interfered with the physician–patient relationship. The board suspended her license for 6 months, and Tuma appealed. The Supreme Court of Idaho held that Tuma's actions did not fall within the board's legislative language of "unprofessional conduct" and reinstated her license.

It is hoped that, given the climate of informed patients and patient empowerment, such a case would never be filed today. But the case does give some direction. Ensure that patients are referred to the physician for questions they might have about their conventional therapy and the alternative therapy. Remember, if the patient or a family member asks about alternative practitioners, some states continue to prevent physicians from making these referrals. If they do, they can be charged with "aiding and abetting the unlicensed practice of medicine."

MEDICINAL USE OF CANNABIS (MARIJUANA)

An issue that is similar to the use of CAM is the medicinal use of cannabis (marijuana). Though 34 states have had some type of legislation recognizing marijuana's medical value, only 12 states have current legislative guidelines for the legal possession of **medical cannabis**— Alaska, California, Colorado, Hawaii, Maine, Montana, Nevada, New Mexico, Oregon, Rhode Island, Vermont, and Washington—though any possession of marijuana remains illegal under federal law. Other states, including Arizona and Maryland, are contemplating such formal legislative action and may soon have such guidelines. Michigan placed the measure on the November 2008 ballot and it passed, with 63% of the population voting for it. California, one of the first states to pass such guidelines, essentially created an exemption from criminal penalties for the medical use of this plant. Basically, the legislation did not legalize marijuana, but merely changed the way medical patients and their primary caregivers would be treated by the state court system. If charged with marijuana possession, patients can claim entitlement to an exemption from the law. The burden of proof is on the patient to show his or her medical need for marijuana use and to show that the drug was used on the recommendation of a prescribing physician.

Researchers face similar challenges in obtaining medical cannabis for use in research trials. Though the United States Federal Drug Agency (FDA) recently approved a number of trials for cannabis research, the FDA has not granted licenses to the researchers in these same studies.

The majority of the patients for whom this medication is approved suffer from cancer, AIDS, or glaucoma. Positive effects of marijuana in these patients include reduction in nausea, increased appetite, reduced eye pressure, and control of muscle spasms. Note, though, that merely having one of these illnesses is not sufficient; a physician must recommend the use of marijuana for these patients. There is also a pill form of the chemical available under the trade name Marinol. Currently, Marinol is used only for patients with severe nausea and vomiting caused by cancer chemotherapies. The use of this drug is restricted by its continuing high cost and the number and seriousness of side effects.

Issues for nurses in this arena are numerous. Nurses are patient advocates, working to assist patients toward as healthy a state as is possible for the individual patient. Nurses are also educators, helping patients to understand the positive and negative effects of medications so that they can make an informed decision about using the medications. With marijuana, this is even more important, as patients must realize that the consumption of marijuana violates federal law at present. Nurses must be true to themselves and their own ethical principles and decide for themselves how to best advocate for patients.

MULTISTATE LICENSURE AND MUTUAL RECOGNITION COMPACTS

Advances in the health care delivery system have resulted in a variety of changes. One of the changes includes the increasing use of new telecommunication technologies. The new technologies are raising questions related to the regulation of health care.

Historically, regulation of health professionals has been a state-based function whereby each state or territory regulates the health care workforce within its geographic boundaries. Thus, all health care professionals practicing within a state or territory are required to be licensed by the jurisdiction in which they practice. However, with recent technologies, including telehealth consultation, telephone triage, and air-transport nursing, to name but a few, practice is no longer limited by geographic boundaries.

The ANA (1998) described *telehealth* as the removal of time and distance barriers for the delivery of health care services and related health care activities. Communication technologies provide a means for health care professionals to practice across state lines. In many instances, this may mean providing services in states in which the professional does not hold current license. Some telehealth employers and nurses may not consider the provision of telehealth services as "practicing," or may consider it unnecessary to obtain licenses in all jurisdictions in which patients who receive their services reside. Yet this provision of service in various states has posed a potential problem of widespread unlicensed practice and presents challenges for boards of nursing in states where patients receive services from nurses located in different states.

One of the solutions to the issue of providing care and/or medical advice is through mutual recognition and the nurse licensure compact. **Mutual recognition** allows the nurse to have a valid nursing license in his or her state of residency and be able to practice in reciprocal states, subject to each state's laws and regulations, through the **nurse licensure compact.** First implemented in Utah in 2000, the nurse licensure compact is now law in 23 states.

The mechanism to implement this mutual recognition of nurse licensure is the interstate compact. Interstate compacts are not a new concept, and were in existence in the early 1900s. Essentially, an interstate compact is an agreement between two or more states, entered into for the purpose of addressing a problem that transcends state lines. The compact must be initiated and voted on by the state legislative bodies to be enforceable. Like any other contract, modification of the compact is possible only by the unanimous consent of all party states. In addition, because the compact is law, it is subject to the traditional principles of statutory interpretation. An interstate compact gains its forcefulness because of its dual-contract nature.

The compact ensures that the nurse is properly licensed in the state of residence or "home state." The nurse must meet that state's licensure requirements and abide by the nurse practice act and other applicable laws within this home state. Other states where the compact is in effect and where the nurse practices but does not live are called *remote states*. These remote states grant the nurse the privilege to practice in their state as a provision of the interstate compact. The nurse practicing in the remote state is expected to practice within the scope of practice and according to the standards of the remote state.

Both the state of residence and remote state boards of nursing must be able to take disciplinary action to protect the citizens, regardless of where the nurse or the patient is located. Both the state of residence and the remote state may take action to limit or stop the practice of an incompetent or unethical nurse in their state. The state of residence acts against the license per se, using probation, suspension, or revocation as its mechanisms of action, and the remote state acts against the practice privilege granted by the compact by limiting or stopping the practice with a cease-and-desist order. Both processes include due process of law, and the effects of both processes are essentially the same.

Perhaps this area remains the most problematic. Opponents of the compact continue to argue that nurses, working within the compact language, could find themselves subject to multiple investigations and disciplinary proceedings arising from one incident. All party states, home and remote, are granted broad powers regarding discipline, including the power to issue subpoenas. Thus, nurses could be required to bear the cost of investigation and disciplinary proceedings in all states involved with the incident.

The compact includes a Coordinated Licensure Information System (CLIS), which is an essential component of the interstate compact giving the compact state boards of nursing timely licensure and discipline information on each nurse. The compact provides for reporting and maintenance of licensure and discipline information. The CLIS is primarily for use by the compact state boards of nursing, but with levels of limited access to comply with providing public information to employers and consumers as exists under the current regulatory system.

Though not fully implemented at the current time, two states in 2002 adopted a model nurse licensure compact for recognition of advanced practice nurses. Some of the reasons that the compact is not fully implemented for nurse practitioners, clinical nurse specialists, and nurse midwives is that there is less conformity among the states on the definitions and standards that apply to these advanced practice nurses. Though the 1999 Institute of Medicine report entitled *To Err Is Human* recommended that there is a need to more uniformly regulate the practice and standards of advanced practice nurses, this has not yet become a reality.

SOME ETHICAL CONCERNS

Issues arise from an ethical perspective when working with complementary and alternative medicines (CAM). Often patients are afraid to reveal that they are using such therapies or may not realize the consequences that the use of such therapies exposes them to when used in combination with more standard therapies. For example, the use of herbal remedies can either potentiate or decrease the effectiveness of a variety of prescribed medications. When patients reveal to the nursing staff their use of over-the-counter medications or other alternative modalities, nurses need to help the patients understand why knowledge of such use is needed to ensure their optimal health care.

Other ethical concerns in the area of CAM concern patient safety issues, a critical value in the *Code of Ethics for Nurses* (ANA, 2001). Safety issues arise because the Food and Drug Administration (FDA) does not regulate vitamins and herbals as carefully as it does medications and foods. Additionally, there are no regulations regarding names and advertising; thus consumers may believe that they are using therapies that target a specific disease or ailment when such is not the case. Nor is there any standardization regarding mega-dosages of vitamins, and it is possible that consumers are being harmed when they consume these mega-dosages.

Finally, the use of CAM can cause a clash in health care values between the health care provider and the patient. For example, how do health care providers respond to requests for nontraditional health care measures, such as the administration of some herbal remedy, in place of more traditional health care measures, such as medications that have been FDA approved for their specific condition or disease? Ethical concerns can also surface when nurses care for patients using medical cannabis. Though a state may approve the drug for medical reasons, federal law does not.

A second ethical issue that continues to affect nurses in clinical practice settings concerns a nurse's right to refuse to give care to specific patients. Though some rights to refuse care exist on religious grounds and for some limited medical reasons and the *Code of Ethics for Nurses* (ANA, 2001) mandates that nurses provide optimal patient care, there are concerns for the safety of the nurse and potentially his or her family members should a major influenza epidemic arise. Much of these same concerns were voiced with the outbreak of the severe acute respiratory syndrome (SARS) virus, the bird flu, and now the H1N1 influenza strain.

SUMMARY

- Credentials are proof of qualifications, usually in written form, stating that an individual or an organization has met specific standards.
- Professional licensure is the legal process by which an authorized authority grants permission to a qualified individual or entity to perform designated skills and services in a jurisdiction in which such practice would be illegal without a license.
- Each state, the District of Columbia, and territories of the United States have individual nurse practice acts, and the means of ensuring enforcement of nurse practice acts is through the state board of nursing or the state board of nurse examiners.
- The board's authority arises from various sources of law, including: legislative, through the promulgation of rules and regulations; quasi-judicial, through hearings; or administrative, through licensure control.
- Mandatory licensure, required by all states, the District of Columbia, and the U.S. territories, requires that all persons who are compensated as a professional member in nursing hold valid licensure as a registered nurse.
- Nurse practice acts, which originated to protect the public at large, define the practice of nursing, give guidance within the scope of practice issues, and set standards for the nursing profession.
- Elements of nurse practice acts include: the definition of professional nursing, requirements for licensure, exemptions from licensure, means of ensuring licensure across jurisdictions, disciplinary actions and due process requirements, and penalties for practicing without a license.
- Diversion programs allow the state boards of nursing to protect the public while complying with the Americans with Disabilities Act of 1990; rehabilitation rather than a more disciplinary program is provided for nurses with substance abuse issues.
- Multiple means, including standing orders, joint statements, and protocols, exist so that nurse practice acts articulate with medical practice acts.
- Scope of practice issues address the actions or duties of a given profession and are defined by statute, rule, or a combination of statute and rule.
- Nurse practice acts may be updated through amendments, redefinitions, application of sunset laws, or total revision of the act.
- Mandatory reporting of violations of the nurse practice act exists to protect the public's health and safety through the discovery of unsafe or substandard nursing practice or conduct and is an expectation of all professional nurses.
- The National Practitioner Data Bank, established in 1986, serves as a clearinghouse for the reporting of adverse actions taken against the clinical privileges of physicians, osteopaths, dentists, and primary health care professionals.
- Certification indicates a level of competence above minimum criteria for licensure and verifies that an individual has met certain standards of preparation and performance.
- Complementary and alternative medicine (CAM), sometimes referred to as integrative medicine, are modalities not generally used by health care providers to treat illnesses such as therapeutic touch, biofeedback, guided imagery, acupuncture, massage therapy, and the medical use of cannabis.
- Mutual recognition (multistate licensure) allows the nurse to have a valid nursing

license in his or her state of residency and be able to practice in reciprocal states, subject to each state's laws and regulations, through the nurse licensure compact.

• There are multiple and varied ethical concerns involved in the professional practice of nursing.

APPLY YOUR LEGAL KNOWLEDGE

1. How do nurse practice acts provide for consumer protection and for nursing advancement?
2. Does the state board of nursing have the authority to change the practice of professional nursing?
3. What are the main differences between licensure and credentialing? Is that difference crucial to consumer protection?

4. Are mutual recognition compacts needed in the professional practice of nursing?

YOU BE THE JUDGE

A nurse had been working in a critical care unit for more than 25 years, gaining respect for her competence and dedication, before suspicions began to gather that she was diverting narcotics for her own use. The acute care hospital had recently installed a "computerized medicine cabinet" for enhanced distribution and better monitoring of narcotics. The cabinet recorded the nurse's personal keypad code and the patient's data before it could be unlocked and narcotics dispensed. The nurses were also required to document the narcotic usage by hand-writing the patient's name, medication, time, route, and dosage on a more traditional paper medication administration record (MAR).

Discrepancies were noted between this nurse's patient electronic data for narcotic administration and the handwritten notations made on the paper record. The nurse was first questioned by her supervisors and then she was suspended, as they did not find her explanations credible. Her grievance was upheld by the arbitrator assigned to the case and the hospital appealed.

At trial, other nurses from the same unit testified that they frequently completed their paper record documentation during their breaks or at the end of the shift, often when they could not remember exactly what medications or dosages they had administered to patients. There was additional information that the nurses would electronically sign for narcotics and prepare IV drip bags in advance of when they were needed and then discard these same IV bags when they were no longer required or the physicians had changed the medication orders. Additionally, these nurses testified that they often deviated from the physician's order for an IM injection, electing to give the medication by an IV route. Finally, there was testimony that the hospital had no formal policy for which nurse was to document narcotics in the paper record when two nurses, such as a preceptor and a mentee, both had responsibility for the patient. The nurse who was suspended testified that she, too, frequently entered data into the paper record long after she had administered the medication and, in some rare instances, entered the data on the following day.

QUESTIONS

1. Did the facility have sufficient evidence to suspend the nurse from employment?
2. How should the testimony of the other nurses in the unit affect the outcome of this case?
3. What additional questions should the institution address before the court rules in this case?
4. How would you have ruled in this case?

REFERENCES

Aiken, L. H., Clarke, S. P., Cheung, R. B., Sloane, D. M., & Silber, J. H. (2003). Educational levels of hospital nurses and surgical patient mortality. *Journal of the American Medical Association, 290*(12), 1617–1623.

Aiken, L. H., Clarke, S. P., Sloane, D. M., Lake, E. T., & Cheney, T. (2008). Effects of hospital care environment on patient mortality and nurse outcomes. *Journal of Nursing Administration, 38*(5), 223–229.

American Association of Colleges of Nursing. (2003). *Fact sheet: The impact of education on nursing practice.* Washington, DC: Author.

American Association of Colleges of Nursing. (2008). *Fact sheet: Creating a more highly qualified nursing workforce.* Washington, DC: Author.

American Nurses Association. (1990). *Suggested state legislation: Nursing practice act.* Washington, DC: Author.

American Nurses Association. (1995). *Report of the House of Delegates: 1995.* Washington, DC: Author.

American Nurses Association. (1998). *Competencies for telehealth technology in nursing.* Washington, DC: Author.

American Nurses Association. (2001). *Code for nurses with interpretive statements.* Washington, DC: Author.

American Nurses Association approves a definition of nursing practice. (1955). *American Journal of Nursing, 55*(12), 1474.

Burns v. Matzen, #93–100 (Iowa, 1994). *Hospital Law Manual, 2*(11), 4.

Civil Rights Act of 1964, Public Law 82-352, 78 *Statutes* 241, July 2, 1964.

Colorado State Board of Nursing v. Hohn, 129 Colo. 195, 268 P.2d 401 (Colorado, 1954).

Cooper v. National Motor Bearing Company, 136 Cal. App.2d 229, 288 P.2d 581 (California, 1955).

Federal Conscience Clause, 42 U.S.C. 3009.7, December 19, 2008.

Friese, C. R., Lake, E. T., Aiken, L. H., Silber, J. H., & Sochalski, J. (2008). Hospital nurse practice environments and outcomes for surgical oncology patients. *Health Services Research, 43*(4), 1145–1163.

Health Care Quality Improvement Act of 1986, Pulbic Law 99–660, November 14, 1986, amended 42 *United States Code,* Section 11101, January 26, 1998.

Health Professional Shortage Area Nursing Relief Act, H.R. 2759 (1998).

Hill v. Pennsylvania Department of Health, Division of Nursing Care Facilities, 711 A.2d 1068 (Pa. Cmmwlth., 1998).

Hoffman v. Iowa Board of Nursing, 2006 WL 2421643 (Iowa App., August 23, 2006).

Hurst v. Ball Memorial Hospital, Inc., 2007 WL 1655794 (S. D. Ind., June 1, 2007).

Institute of Medicine. (1999). *To err is human: Building a safer health system.* Washington, DC: National Academy Press.

Joint Commission for the Accreditation of Healthcare Organizations. (1996). *1996 accreditation manual for hospitals: Volume 1, standards.* Oakbrook Terrace, IL: Author.

Kelly v. Guttormsson, 2007 WL 2245085 (Minn. App., August 7, 2007).

Kenney v. Ambulatory Center of Miami, 400 So.2d 1262 (Fla. App., 1981).

Kraft v. State Board of Nursing, 631 N.W.2d 572 (North Dakota, 2001).

Lang v. Department of Health, 2007 WL 1218011 (Wash. App., April 26, 2007).

Larson v. Albany Medical Center, 676 N.Y.S.2d 293 (N.Y. App., 1998).

Leahy v. North Carolina Board of Nursing, 488 S.E.2d 245 (North Carolina, 1997).

Lunsford v. Board of Nurse Examiners, 648 S.W.2d 391 (Tex. Civ. App., Austin 1983).

Miller v. Tennessee Board of Nursing, 2007 WL 2827526 (Tenn. App., September 26, 2007).

Mississippi Board of Nursing v. Hanson, 703 So.2d 239 (Mississippi, 1997).

Mohr v. Jenkins, 393 So.2d 245 (La. Ct. App., 1980).

Mullarrney v. Board of Review, 778 A.2d 1114 (N.J. App., 2001).

National Center for Complimentary and Alternative Medicine. (2002). *National health interview survey.* Washington, DC: National Institutes of Health.

National Council of State Boards of Nursing. (2006). *Model nursing practice act and model nursing administrative rules.* Chicago: Author.

Neal v. Fields, 2005 WL 3208664 (8th Cir., December 1, 2005).

North Dakota Century Code. (2003). Chapter 43-12-1-09-3.

People v. Stults, 683 N.E.2d 521 (Ill. App., 1997).

Primes v. Louisiana State Board, 2008 WL 2877751 (La. App., July 23, 2008).

Rabkin, R. (1999). Mind/body news: A first: All alternative care covered. *Healthy Living, 4*(6), 18.

Regester v. Indiana State Board of Nursing, 703 N.E.2d 147 (Indiana, 1998).

Ross v. Indiana State Board of Nursing, 790 N.E.2d 110 (Ind. App., 2003).

Rowe v. Sisters of the Pallottine Missionary Society, 560 S.E.2d 491 (West Virginia, 2001).

Schoenhair v. Pennsylvania, 459 A.2d 877 (Pennsylvania, 1983).

Scott v. Beverly Enterprises-Kansas, Inc., 968 F. Supp. 1430 (D. Kan., 1997).

State Board of Nursing v. Berry, 32 S.W.3d 638 (Mo. App., 2000).

Stevens v. Blake, 456 So.2d 795 (Ala. Civ. App., 1984).

Tapp v. Board of Registered Nursing, 2002 WL 31820206 (Cal. App., 2002).

Thomas v. Department of Health Services, 2004 WL 24066 (Cal. App., 2004).

Thompson v. Olsten Kimberly Qualitycare, Inc., 980 F. Supp. 1035 (D. Minn., 1997).

Thornton v. Alabama Board of Nursing, 2007 WL 1519052 (Ala. App., May 25, 2007).

Tourangeau, A. E., Doran, D. M., McGillis-Hall, L., O'Brien-Pallas, L., Pringle, D., Tu, J. V., & Cranley, L. A. (2007). Impact of hospital nursing care on 30-day mortality for acute medical patients. *Journal of Advanced Nursing, 57*(1), 32–41.

The Mercy Hospital, Inc. v. Massachusetts Nurses Association, 429 F. 3rd 338 (1st Cir., 2005).

Tuma v. Board of Nursing of the State of Idaho, 100 Idaho 74, 593 P.2d 711 (Idaho, 1979).

Whitney v. Day, M. D., and Hurley Hospital, 100 Mich. App. 707, 300 N.W.2d 380 (Mich. Ct. App., 1980).

CHAPTER 12

Advanced Nursing Practice Roles

PREVIEW

Advanced nursing practice roles have expanded within the past few years so that there are six currently recognized advanced practice roles: nurse anesthetist, nurse midwife, advanced nurse practitioner, clinical nurse specialist, clinical nursing leader, and doctorate of nursing practice. As these roles continue to evolve and expand, there is improvement of the quality of health care in a nation that is cost-conscious, yet demanding of access and quality care.

Nurses who work within these roles face multiple legal issues, especially in a world that is more technologically advanced and complex. This chapter explores advanced practice roles, accompanying legal aspects related to the roles, and challenges that confront practitioners within the roles.

LEARNING OUTCOMES
After completing this chapter, you should be able to

12.1 Outline the roles of advanced practice nurses, including nurse anesthetists, nurse midwives, advanced nurse practitioners, clinical nurse specialists, clinical nurse leaders, and doctorate of nursing practice.

12.2 Describe some of the legal constraints to advanced professional practice encountered by nurses educationally and clinically competent to perform these roles, including:

scope of practice issues
reimbursement issues
malpractice issues
standards of care
prescriptive authority
hospital or admitting privileges

12.3 Analyze means to overcome these legal constraints.

12.4 Compare and contrast the current status of advanced nursing practice with that role in the future.

12.5 Analyze selected ethical issues that may arise with advanced practice roles.

KEY TERMS

admitting privileges

advanced nurse practitioner

advanced practice roles

antitrust issues

clinical nurse leader

clinical nurse specialist

direct access

doctorate of nursing practice

nurse anesthetist

nurse midwifery

prescriptive authority

reimbursement

scope of practice

standard of care

HISTORICAL OVERVIEW OF ADVANCED NURSING PRACTICE ROLES

Early in America's history, women were fulfilling the role of autonomous nursing practitioners and midwives (Reverby, 1987). During the late 1800s, physicians usurped the autonomous health care deliverer status that prevails today. This was accomplished through state medical practice acts and the strong organizational structure of the American Medical Association (Stevens, 1971). The modern **advanced practice roles** originated in the late 1960s and early 1970s when the shortage of primary physicians led to new initiatives to meet America's health care needs.

Today, advanced nursing practice encompasses six distinct practice roles, though there may be some movement that will reduce that number to fewer roles in the not-too-distant future. The hallmark of the majority of these roles is that nurses have the ability to combine the caring role of the nurse with the more traditional curing role of the physician. Interestingly, the roles that nurses performed generally became their occupational titles. While a specialized body of knowledge and academic degree rather than a title distinction is required for these roles, for the most part advanced practice nurses are still known by these occupational titles.

Nurse Anesthetist

Perhaps the oldest of the expanded roles in nursing is that of the **nurse anesthetist.** In 1878, Sister Mary Bernard was administering anesthesia at St. Vincent's Hospital in Erie, Pennsylvania. Agatha C. Hodgins served as a nurse anesthetist in Cleveland, Ohio, at the turn of the century and was as well known for her ability to administer anesthesia as she was for teaching doctors and nurses her techniques (Mannino, 1982).

The two world wars, as well as the Korean and Vietnam wars, increased the need for nurses proficient in administering anesthesia. Both at home and at the war front, nurses were needed to expand the numbers of medical personnel giving anesthesia. The physician shortage of the early 1960s continued to support the need for this expanded nursing role, and additional schools of nurse anesthesia quickly opened. Nurse anesthetists are registered nurses who have completed a formal program of clinical education in planning anesthesia care, administering anesthetic agents, and monitoring the anesthetized patient. Nurse anesthesia was the first expanded role in nursing to seek recognition via certification and education. All states require current certification through the American Association of Nurse Anesthetists for individuals to practice as certified registered nurse anesthetists (CRNA); to be allowed to write the certificate examination, applicants must have completed a master's program. Depending on the particular program, the CRNA earns a master's degree in nursing, allied health, or the biological and clinical sciences (American Association of Nurse Anesthetists, 2003).

The first legal challenges to this role arose in the mid-1930s. In what has become a landmark decision, the California Supreme Court held that the giving of anesthesia by nurses was not "diagnosing nor prescribing by nurses within the meaning of the California Medical Practice Act" (*Chalmers-Francis v. Nelson*, 1936, at 402). This holding allowed nurses to administer anesthesia within the scope of nursing practice.

Nurse Midwifery

The practice of **nurse midwifery** also has its origins in the late 1800s and early 1900s. At that time, midwifery was becoming a regulated, legally recognized profession through state legislative enactments. Prior to such state enactments, the art of midwifery was a lay art, practiced by women who learned about childbirth either by their own experiences or through others trained in the art. After the state enactments, the art of midwifery became more common among nurses. The first nurse midwifery educational program was opened in 1952 by the Maternity Association of New York City.

Although nurse midwifery practice is legal in all 50 states and the District of Columbia, the practice of nurse midwifery still has some legal uncertainties. Authorization of nurse midwifery may be found in nurse practice acts, medical practice acts, rules and regulations specific to nurse midwives, allied health laws, public health laws, or a combination of any of these. Some states, depending on the jurisdiction, also regulate nurse midwifery through state agencies.

The practice of nurse midwifery involves the independent management of essentially normal prenatal, intrapartum, postpartum, and gynecological care of women, as well as the care of normal newborns. Certified nurse midwives (CNMs) provide family planning and birth control counseling and normal gynecological services such as physical examinations and preventative health screenings. Working in acute care settings, freestanding clinics, health departments, ambulatory care facilities, and physician offices, CNMs offer holistic, continuous care; education of women through the childbearing period and years; and primary care for women's health needs. CNMs offer an alternative childbearing experience to the low-risk patient.

As with nurse anesthesia, the earliest cases in nurse midwifery addressed the issue of whether the practice constituted the practice of medicine. The case of *People v. Arendt* (1894) held that the midwife in question was guilty of practicing medicine without a license. Since that time, nurse midwives have worked to develop a clear definition of the status of the role of nurse midwife.

Advanced Nurse Practitioners

Known in some states as nurse practitioners, the role is clarified as **advanced nurse practitioners** (ANPs) for states that refer to all registered nurses (RNs) as nurse practitioners. This role began in 1965 when Drs. Loretta Ford and Henry Silver began a program at the University of Colorado that placed nurses in new practice settings and increased their traditional patient care responsibilities. Goals of the ANP movement were to prepare nurses with master's and doctorate degrees for independent expert practice, teaching, and clinical research. The ANP has a client caseload much as a practicing physician carries a client caseload. Long-term goals included increased access to quality health care as well as expanded use of nursing skills in health assessment and maintenance. This increased access to quality health care was mainly seen in rural areas and was used by patients for whom minimal health care was available.

Today, ANPs are nurses who have specialized in one or more practice specialties, including gerontology, women's health, family health, pediatric health, school health, home care, adult health, acute care, psychiatric and mental health, oncology, or emergency care nursing. Most provide primary care to low-risk patients and many serve as the primary health care provider. Practitioners work in acute care settings, ambulatory settings, occupational settings, college and university student health settings, long-term care facilities, assisted living facilities, public health departments, nursing service centers, physician offices, or their own offices. ANPs may work independently, in a peer relationship with physicians, or dependently under the physicians' standing or direct orders. Depending on the state nurse practice act, the ANP may independently diagnose, treat, and prescribe for a given patient or may be limited to managing the care of the patient as a delegated role.

Legal challenges for this role have included scope of practice issues, much like the challenges to nurse anesthetists and nurse midwives. One case upheld the suspension of a nurse's license for treating patients without a physician's supervision (*Hernicz v. State of Florida, Department of Professional Regulation,* 1980). Other cases have upheld the right of the nurse to practice as an advanced nurse practitioner (*Bellegie v. Board of Nurse Examiners,* 1985; *Sermchief v. Gonzales,* 1983). Idaho was the first state to enact specific legislation defining and promoting the independent role of the advanced nurse practitioner in 1971.

Clinical Nurse Specialist

Although the major development of the **clinical nurse specialist** role occurred during the 1960s and 1970s as changes in nursing science and practice were rapidly developing, the first program was started by Rutgers University in 1954. The concept of a master's level nurse prepared as a specialist in a clinical area was a departure from the then-traditional functional preparation in teaching, administration, and supervision. Clinical nurse specialists were developed for the purpose of improving the quality of nursing care provided to patients and their families during the 1960s when significant advances in technology paralleled advances in specialty medicine, primarily cardiovascular and pulmonary surgical specialties.

This role evolved in response to needs expressed by both patients and nurses. Traditionally, as nurses advanced in education and experience, they moved away from the bedside and entered either administrative or educational roles. Nurses with advanced nursing knowledge and skills who attempted to remain in staff positions in institutions usually failed due to the economics of the hospital because it was more cost-efficient to have staff nurses and licensed practical nurses give direct patient care.

Several schools of nursing began to offer curricula that would allow nurses to obtain an advanced nursing degree and to specialize in clinical nursing so that they could continue to work directly with patients, family members, and staff. The specialization also allowed the nurse to be proficient in teaching, research methodology, and consultation. This allowed the clinical nurse specialist (CNS) not only to be directly involved with patient care, but to be indirectly involved with increasing the quality of nursing care throughout the institution.

CNSs are expert clinicians in a specialized area of nursing practice, with CNS practice occurring in settings across the health care delivery continuum. This specialty may be defined in terms of a population (pediatrics, gerontology), a setting (critical care, home health care), a disease or medical subspeciality (diabetes, oncology), a type of care (rehabilitative, psychiatric and mental health), or a type of problem (pain, wound care). In addition to providing direct patient care, the CNS influences care outcomes by providing expert consultation for nursing staff and by implementing improvements in health care delivery systems. In 1974, at the American Nurses Association (ANA) Congress for Nursing Practice, the role was defined as requiring a master's degree in nursing. Certification for CNSs is afforded by a number of certification corporations, including the American Nurses Credentialing Center, the Oncology Nursing Certification Corporation, the Rehabilitation Nursing Certification Board, and the American Association of Critical-Care Nurses Certification Corporation.

Traditionally, subroles of the CNS are divided into two broad categories: (1) direct care functions, which include expert practitioner, role model, and patient advocate; and (2) indirect care functions, which include change agent, consultant or resource person, clinical teacher, researcher, liaison, and innovator. Today, the CNS's roles include those of case manager, coach, systems coordinator, and gatekeeper. In these newer subroles, the CNS can contribute to improved quality and cost-effective services during the transition of health care delivery from the acute care setting to community, integrated, seamless health care. The involvement of the CNS in these roles is predictable given the clinical nurse specialist's history as change agent. All of the roles may be independent, collaborative, or supervised, depending on the state nurse practice act.

The roles of the ANP and the CNS are beginning to blend, so that it is often difficult to distinguish the two roles. Like nurse practitioners, CNSs work in a variety of practice settings, including acute care settings, mental health settings, long-term care facilities, home health settings, public health departments, college and university student health settings, hospice settings, physicians' offices, and their own offices. CNSs may have independent prescriptive authority, provide primary or secondary care, and have admitting privileges. A trend is toward using a more general title to include both CNSs and ANPs, as their roles are so similar in practice settings today.

Clinical Nurse Leader

The **clinical nurse leader** (CNL) evolved as a direct result of the continuing nursing shortage, increasing numbers of identified errors in health care delivery, and fragmentation of care, primarily in acute care facilities. Beginning in 2000, the American Association of Colleges of Nursing (AACN) began convening taskforces to identify means to improve the quality of patient care and to determine how best to prepare nurses for skills and competencies that were needed to competently care for patients in an ever more complex health care delivery system (Tornabeni & Miller, 2008). This new role was envisioned by the AACN to be a person who: "designs, implements, and evaluates client care by coordinating, delegating, and supervising the care provided by the health care team, including licensed nurses, technicians, and other health professionals" (AACN, 2005, paragraph 2). Further, the AACN challenged the nursing profession to produce quality graduates who:

- Are prepared for clinical leadership in all health care settings;
- Are prepared to implement outcomes-based practice and quality improvement strategies;
- Will remain in and contribute to the professions, practicing at their full scope of education and ability; and
- Will create and manage microsystems of care that will be responsive to the health care needs of individuals and families. (AACN, 2007, p. 5)

Today, the CNL, educated at the master's degree level, is an individual prepared as an advanced generalist. CNLs have a unique set of competencies that are applicable to any health care setting. These competencies include patient and caregiver advocate, team manager, information manager, systems manager/risk anticipator, clinician, outcomes manager, and educator. Inherent in the role is the ability of the CNL to coordinate and facilitate the multiples services and disciplines that impact the patient and the quality of his or her care as well as ensuring the delivery of evidence-based care. Communications, patient and interdisciplinary, are critical for quality patient care. The role of the CNL "focuses on understanding the interdependency of all disciplines providing care and the needed to utilize the expertise of the team in order to effectively capitalize on the intellectual capital that exists within a highly educated workforce" (Tornabeni & Miller, 2008, p. 611).

Doctorate of Nursing Practice

The **doctorate of nursing practice** (DNP) degree is a practice-focused doctoral program designed to prepare experts in specialized advanced nursing practice. DNP programs focus on practice that is innovative and evidence-based, reflecting the application of research findings to clinical practice. Though the degree program varies according to educational institution, the program generally includes an advanced practice role as a nurse practitioner, nurse anesthetist, nurse midwife, or clinical nurse specialist; leadership; and application of clinical research. Some institutions have expanded the program to include nurses who specialize as nursing educators and health administrators.

The DNP has evolved since the advent of the first professional nursing doctorate program, the doctor of nursing (ND), was initiated by Francis Payne Bolton School of Nursing at Case Western Reserve University in 1979. Benefits of the DNP program include:

- Development of needed advanced competencies for increasingly complex practice, faculty, and leadership roles;
- Enhanced knowledge to improve nursing practice and patient outcomes;
- Enhanced leadership skills to strengthen practice and health care delivery;
- Better match of program requirements, credits, and time with the credential earned;
- Provision of an advanced educational credential for those who require advanced practice knowledge but do not need or want a strong research focus;
- Enhanced ability to attract individuals to nursing from non-nursing backgrounds; and
- Increased supply of faculty for practice instruction. (AACN, 2004, p. 4).

The purpose of transitioning advanced practice programs from the graduate level to the doctoral level is:

> in response to changes in health care delivery and emerging health care needs, additional knowledge or content areas have been identified by practicing nurses. In addition, the knowledge required to provide leadership in the discipline of nursing is so complex and rapidly changing that additional or doctoral level education is needed. (AACN, 2004, p. 7)

Additionally, transitioning advanced practice nursing to the doctoral level makes it similar to other professional practice doctorates such as are awarded graduates in medicine, pharmacy, dentistry, physical therapy, and psychology. With the development of DNP programs, it is envisioned that the master's degree entry for specialized advanced nursing practice will fade and that the DNP will be the preferred preparation for specialty practice.

EXERCISE 12.1

Investigate the use of advanced practice nurses within your area. What are the state requirements concerning these roles? What types of educational requirements exist for these roles? How do these nurses function in the community and hospital health care delivery systems? Are the state nurses associations and/or other professional organizations working to expand the role of these nurses?

LEGAL LIABILITY OF EXPANDED NURSING ROLES

In some ways, professionals practicing in expanded nursing roles have dual legal liabilities. One, they are licensed to practice by the state board of nursing and are accountable for its rules and regulations. Two, these same professionals have acquired advanced standing under the delegatory language of the state medical practice act or have acquired advanced standing under the state nurse practice act, public health laws, or other state laws, and are accountable for this independent or interdependent role.

Several questions arise from a legal perspective regarding the potential liability of the practitioner in an expanded role. Most of the questions come under the overall classification of standards of care and scope of practice issues.

SCOPE OF PRACTICE ISSUES

A major legal issue is the permissible **scope of practice,** which refers to the permissible boundaries of practice for a health professional, as defined by statute, rule, or a combination of statute and rule, and which defines the actions and duties of nurses in these roles. Physicians were the first professionals in virtually all states to define their scope of practice and, by the 1800s, had defined medicine to include curing, diagnosing, treating, and prescribing. Physicians also ensured against interference in their practice by incorporating provisions that made it illegal for anyone not licensed as a physician to perform acts included in their definition.

Nurses gained legal control of their profession in the early 1900s. By 1930, all states had passed nurse practice acts. Autonomous practice was defined as supervision of patients, observation of symptoms and reactions of patients, and accurate recording of patient information. The remainder of the nursing scope of practice was defined as complementary (interdependent) or dependent on the physician. With the advent of advanced nursing practice, it became apparent that such a definition of scope of practice would prevent independent practice, and several courses of action were undertaken to remedy the situation.

One means of increasing the scope of practice was by amending or totally altering state nurse practice acts. States began to accomplish this by promulgating rules and regulations to expand the scope of practice. In 1971, Idaho became the first state to broaden its definition of nursing to statutorily include diagnosis and treatment as part of the scope of practice of the ANP. Although the intent of the statute was clear, the statute required that acts of diagnosis and treatment be authorized by rules and regulations jointly developed by the boards of nursing and medicine, and that all institutions employing ANPs develop policies and guidelines for their practice. This latter requirement resulted in constraints in the ANP's practice.

Currently, all states and the District of Columbia have enacted legislation regarding the ANP's scope of practice. All 50 states plus the District of Columbia have ANP title protection. In 24 states and the District of Columbia, the board of nursing has sole authority for ANP scope of practice and there are no statutory or regulatory requirements for physician supervision, collaboration, or direction. Another 16 states give the sole authority to the state board of nursing for scope of practice issues, but have a requirement for physician collaboration. Five states (California, Florida, Georgia, Massachusetts, and South Carolina) require physician supervision, though the board of nursing has sole authority for scope of practice issues. The final five states (Alabama, Mississippi, North Carolina, South Dakota, and Virginia) mandate that both the board of nursing and the board of medicine have authority for the ANP's scope of practice.

A second means of expanding the legal scope of practice is through court decisions that define the nature of the advanced nurse practitioner's role. Two significant decisions have been made in this area, and they remain the landmark cases today. *Sermchief v. Gonzales,* a 1983 Missouri Supreme Court decision, held that the Missouri legislature, when it enacted the nurse practice act, had intended to avoid statutory constraints on the evolution of new nursing roles and thereby gave ANPs practice authority through the broad wording of professional nursing. In actuality, the court found that professional nurses in that jurisdiction had the right to practice within the limits of their education and experience.

In *Sermchief,* a group of advanced nurse practitioners routinely provided gynecological care, including routine Pap smears, pregnancy testing, and birth control measures, pursuant to protocols jointly developed by nursing and supervising physicians. The Missouri Nurse Practice Act did not require direct physician supervision, but defined professional nursing in more general terms, according to specialized education, judgment, and skill. A group of physicians, predominantly those whose practice had declined because of the advent of the ANPs' practice, brought suit claiming that the nurses, rather than practicing nursing, were instead engaged in the illegal practice of medicine. In a lengthy decision, the court held that the advanced nurse practitioners were indeed practicing within the scope of their education and skills and within the scope of nursing as the Missouri legislature had intended.

Sermchief was a significant decision for nursing. A second significant decision was *Bellegie v. Board of Nurse Examiners* (1985). In that case, the Texas Medical Association and the Texas Hospital Association challenged the authority of the Texas Board of Nurse Examiners to promulgate rules and regulations regarding advanced nursing practice within the state. In finding for the Board of Nurse Examiners, the court held that the Board's regulatory authority was not limited to regulating titles, but extended to regulating the activities and education of nursing within its jurisdiction.

These two decisions clearly began the establishment of nursing's legal status as a full-fledged, independent profession. If nursing is to continue to expand as a truly autonomous professional role, then nurses must work at state and national levels to promote the most effective use of advanced practice nurses.

A third means of expanding the advanced practice nurse's scope of practice is through federal enactments. In 2001, the Centers for Medicare and Medicaid Services published a notice that it intended to drop the current physician supervision requirement for CRNAs from its conditions of participation for hospitals and ambulatory centers. The requirement remains in effect in individual states until the governor of the state where the facility is located sends a formal letter to federal authorities attesting that the governor, in consultation with the state boards of medicine and nursing about issues of access to and quality of anesthesia services, has determined it is in the state's best interest to opt out of the current supervision. Currently there are 14 states that have opted out of this requirement: Alaska, Idaho, Iowa, Kansas, Minnesota, Montana, Nebraska, New Hampshire, New Mexico, North Dakota, Oregon, South Dakota, Washington, and Wisconsin.

Reimbursement Issues

At the federal level, scope of practice issues are also tied to **reimbursement** issues. One of the most significant pieces of legislation for advanced practice nursing was the passage of Medicare reform in the 1997 Balanced Budget Act. That piece of legislation included Medicare reimbursement for both ANPs and CNSs, regardless of geographic setting. Effective January 1, 1998, services are reimbursable by Medicare, if the same services are eligible for reimbursement if provided by a physician and the services are within the scope of practice of the ANP and the CNS. The true significance of the decision was to disavow the payment for services only if they were in "rural settings," narrowly defined to mean a nonmetropolitan statistical area or county. Also significant was that the ANP or CNS may function in a variety of clinical settings, including nursing homes, which had previously been a restricted area for reimbursement. Finally, the legislation was significant in that "collaborative practice" referred to "collaborative" as defined by state nurse practice acts, rather than the more restrictive language of the federal government (Rules and Regulations, 1998).

One limitation in the legislation was the reimbursement for ANPs and CNSs at 85% of the physician reimbursement for the same service. While this was basically the same payment provision that existed under the current insurance codes for reimbursement in states that allowed such reimbursement, it continued to devalue the services of nurses providing identical services as their physician counterparts (Balanced Budget Act, 1997).

Interestingly, the passage of the Medicare Reimbursement Reform Bill as part of the Balanced Budget Act of 1997 addressed (though not necessarily satisfactorily) the three main issues that ANPs have continually included in their lobbying efforts:

1. Elimination of restrictions that allow nurses to practice only in certain geographic settings (for example, rural and underserved areas)
2. Elimination of requirements that make nurses dependent on physician supervision or collaboration
3. Establishment of requirements that same services should result in same payments by insurers and third-party payers, regardless of the specialty or profession of the provider

Though reimbursement remains a central factor in independent practice, the majority of ANPs continue to bill using a physician's name for reimbursement rather than directly billing for third-party reimbursement. Reasons cited for billing using the physicians' names included insufficient information regarding billing codes, the practice's desire to be fully compensated for ANP services, failure of the ANPs to apply for a provider number, and lack of ANP knowledge about changes in the reimbursement policy (Weiland, 2008).

Malpractice Issues

Areas in which advanced practice nurses have incurred liability include:

1. Unlicensed practice of medicine (*Weyandt v. State,* 2001)
2. Conduct exceeding the scope of expertise that causes harm (*Rivera v. County of Suffolk,* 2002); failure to refer appropriately (*Ehteman v. Kaiser Permanente,* 2008)
3. Conduct exceeding physician-delegated authority that results in harm (*Tatro v. State of Texas,* 1983)
4. Negligence in the delivery of health care (*Coleman v. Martinez,* 2007; *Creviston v. St. Mary Medical Center,* 2007; *Oram v. de Cholnoky,* 2008; *Renaissance Surgical Centers v. Jimenez,* 2008)
5. Failure to adequately diagnose (*Jenkins v. Payne,* 1996; *Kim v. Priebe,* 2007)

Lawsuits involving advanced nurse practitioners raise inevitable questions about whether the nurse involved was performing an activity that was:

1. Generic to nursing and thus within the nursing scope of practice
2. A medical activity that is permitted by law as germane to the advanced practice nurse's scope of practice
3. A medical activity not within the scope of practice of the advanced practice nurse
4. A nursing activity that overlaps with a medical activity

Additional questions center on the elements of malpractice, such as the duty owed the patient, breach of that duty as owed, foreseeability, causation, and damages.

If the activity involved in the lawsuit was purely nursing function, then nurses will serve as expert witnesses in determining the standard of care owed the patient. If the activity was a medical function not allowed within the nurse scope of practice, the expert witness will testify to medical standards of care. As the next section illustrates, the courts and nursing are still struggling with standards of care when the activity involved is a nursing function that overlaps with a medical function as opposed to an activity allowable within the scope of the advanced practice nurse.

Some of the more recent cases filed naming advanced practice nursing include ANPs, CRNAs, and CNMs. As one would expect, given the newness of the roles, lawsuits naming CNLs or DNPs have yet to be decided, though they may already be filed in individual states. Reviewing the current cases naming other advanced practice nurses will assist CNLs and DNPs in beginning to appreciate their potential legal liability.

Recent cases naming CNMs have generally centered on the following causes of action: failure to obtain a complete history (*Avila v. New York Health and Hospitals Corporation*, 2007); delay in referring the patient for a timely cesarean section (*Coleman v. Martinez*, 2007; *Ehtemam v. Kaiser Permanente*, 2008; *Oram v. de Cholnoky*, 2008); failure to follow the American College of Obstetrics and Gynecology standards (*Fitzhugh v. St. Luke's South Hospital*, 2007); and failure to monitor a patient receiving Pitocin (*Tremain v. United States*, 2007).

ANPs have seen the numbers and severity of malpractice claims rise in the past few years, most notably due to the increased numbers of ANPs and the expanding scope of their practice (Burroughs, Dmytrow, & Lewis, 2007). Recent cases naming ANPs have also involved issues surrounding obstetrical care (*Infant v. Hospital*, 2007), apparent abuse of an infant (*Chapa v. United States*, 2006), and failure to adequately screen patients (*Hilliard v. McIntyre*, 2007; *In re Nicholas*, 2005).

A recent case involving a CRNA was *Renaissance Surgical Centers v. Jimenez* (2008). In that case, a 49-year-old patient was dismissed by the CRNA from the surgical center in the evening after having surgery for an umbilical hernia repair, abdominoplasty, and liposuction. He suffered a fat embolism that same night and died at home. The family sued the surgeon, the CRNA, two staff nurses, and the facility. Ultimately, all but the CRNA and the facility were dismissed from the lawsuit.

In holding the CRNA liable, the court noted that he had failed to follow the established standard of care for a patient receiving an epidural administration of Duramorph, a preservative-free morphine sulfate. The manufacturer's standard package insert warnings specifically state for epidural use of Duramorph that 24-hour post-operative skilled monitoring of the patient is required, which meant that this patient should have been kept in an inpatient setting so that he could have been observed for complications.

STANDARDS OF CARE

The question that arises frequently in negligence cases is what legal **standard of care,** or duty of care, is to be applied to nurses in expanded roles. Nurses who perform functions and actions traditionally recognized as medical should be familiar with court decisions concerning standards of professional care. Earlier cases mainly held that nurses in expanded roles are held to the medical standard of care (*Harris v. State through Huey P. Long Hospital*, 1979; *Hendry v. United States*, 1969). *Whitney v. Day, M.D., and Hurley Hospital* (1980) held that nurse anesthetists are professionals who have expertise in an area akin to the practice of medicine. Some courts of law continue to hold that "nurses performing medical services are subject to the same standards of care and legal responsibilities as physicians" (*Hypolite v. Columbia Dauterive Hospital*, 2007).

Because ANPs' responsibilities lie in an area of medical expertise, the standard of care is to be based on the skill and care normally expected of those with like education and expertise. This fact was first elaborated in a 1925 case *(Olson v. Bolstad),* which disallowed any liability on the part of the physician involved and found that the nurse midwife was solely negligent. While that court also set the medical standard as the standard of care for the midwife, it specifically stated that the physician incurred no liability in relying on the midwife to perform her duties properly.

Fein v. Permanente Medical Group (1985) was one of the first cases to disagree with this line of holdings. In *Fein,* the court set the standard of care for the ANP. In that case, a patient was misdiagnosed by an ANP and, subsequently, by a physician as having muscle spasms rather than a myocardial infarction. After examining the patient and obtaining a history, the nurse diagnosed muscle spasms and gave the patient a prescription for Valium. The court labored to find that the ANP was held to the standard of a nurse practitioner performing diagnosis and treatment, not to the standard of a physician performing diagnosis and treatment. Specifically, the court held that "the examination or diagnosis cannot be said—as a matter of law—to be a function reserved to physicians rather than to registered nurses or nurse practitioners" (at 140). Therefore, a physician working with ANPs or an ANP functioning in a similar setting would be qualified to establish the standard of care.

Recent court cases continue to debate the topic of standards of care for ANPs. Some courts uphold a separate standard of care for ANPs (*Ali v. Community Health Care Plan, Inc.,* 2002; *Cox v. Board of Hospital Managers,* 2002), while other courts hold the ANP to the same standard of care as primary care physicians (*Hypolite v. Columbia Dauterive Hospital,* 2007; *Judy v. Grant County Health Department,* 2001). In *Ali,* the court rejected the longstanding common law rule and decided that advanced nursing practice is legally distinct from the practice of medicine, and held that a nurse midwife was not to be judged by the standard of care for obstetrical/gynecology physicians: "When the clinical judgment and actions of a nurse with advanced standings are called into question in a civil malpractice lawsuit, the nurse is to be judged by the acceptable standards for nurses with comparable standing in the nurse's specific field of clinical expertise, not by the standards for physicians practicing in the field" (*Ali v. Community Health Care Plan, Inc.,* 2002, at 147).

Similarly, the court in *Cox* noted that physicians are judged by different standards of care depending on whether they are general practitioners or specialists. Nurses are not judged by the standard of care of physicians. However, there is a comparable distinction between nurses with basic general skills and nurse specialists with advanced practice standing. The court noted that the standard of care for a neonatal nurse practitioner is the level of skill and care ordinarily possessed and exercised by practitioners in the same specialty practicing in the same or similar practice settings. This finding contrasted with a finding the previous year in *Judy.* The earlier case had held that ANPs working in primary care were held to the same standard of care as physicians performing the same tasks and diagnoses. "There is only one standard of care for primary care providers" (*Judy v. Grant County Health Department,* 2001, at 346). *Hypolite* (2007) reverts to this earlier point of view. The lesson is that this continues to be an evolving issue, and ANPs are cautioned to know and follow prevailing standards of care.

Additionally, court cases may also herald new areas of liability for advanced practice nurses (*Cohen v. State Board of Medicine,* 1996; *Ruggiero v. State Department of Health,* 1996). Though both of these cases involved physicians' licenses, they address issues that could equally affect advanced practice nurses. In *Cohen,* a physician had prescribed controlled substances susceptible to abuse, including narcotics, barbiturates, and benzodiazepines, without seeing the patient and without determining the medical necessity and appropriateness of the medications. One patient, an admitted addict, received prescriptions for Dilaudid for himself, his wife, and his son and daughter. This patient's wife came into the office but was never examined. His children were never seen in the office. Another patient received a prescription for Esgic over the telephone one day and was admitted for detoxification and chemical dependency treatment the next day. The physician's license was revoked for 5 years.

GUIDELINES
Nursing in Expanded Practice Roles

1. The nurse in an expanded practice role must first recognize that along with the role's increased autonomy comes increased accountability and liability. While nurses are always accountable for their actions and omissions, the nurse in an expanded practice role adopts a higher standard of care for the services and actions performed.

2. Function and accept patients and responsibilities within your field of expertise and within your allowable scope of practice. Review carefully the state nurse practice act, medical practice act, pharmacy act, and public health laws for scope of practice issues. Review and understand the rules and regulations promulgated by the state board of nursing for allowable scope of practice.

3. Understand the allowable scope of practice if your state requires that you function under the delegatory language of the state medical practice act. Be sure you do not exceed any physician-delegated responsibilities.

4. Ensure that you have obtained valid informed consent and have obtained such consent from the proper person(s) before proceeding to care for or treat a particular client. As with physician malpractice lawsuits, informed consent is frequently cited in nursing malpractice suits.

5. Be sure the client knows of your status as a nurse in an expanded role and understands that you are not a physician. Impersonation of a physician is fraud and opens you to licensure suspension or revocation as well as to other civil lawsuits. As more nurses obtain doctoral degrees, this area of potential liability will face heightened challenges.

6. Seek assistance from other specialists and physicians when circumstances exceed your scope of knowledge and expertise. Failure to refer the patient to a physician or more qualified advanced nurse practitioner when your skills are exceeded or when complications arise has been the basis of previous lawsuits. The failure to refer in a timely manner may place you in the position of acting beyond the allowable scope of practice for your expanded role.

7. Do not practice independently unless your state recognizes independent practice by the advanced nurse practitioner. Some states require a supervising or collaborating physician, and you may not exceed the bounds of that supervision or collaborative role.

8. Maintain your current skills and continue to broaden your knowledge and skills through continuing education and advanced nursing degrees. Maintain your certification or seek certification through appropriate associations as proof of your qualifications, knowledge base, and skills in a defined functional or clinical area of nursing.

9. Document carefully and accurately any nursing care given. Legible and dependable nursing records are vital if a nurse functioning in an expanded nursing role hopes to successfully defend a future lawsuit.

In *Ruggiero,* the physician's license was revoked for failure to maintain proper patient records and improper infection control practices. Records consisted of a journal in which the physician noted patients he had seen that day. At a later date, he relied on his memory to write entries about the patients into their medical records. Food and medications were improperly stored together in the same refrigerator, the sink designed for handwashing was filthy, and used instruments were left on open trays without disinfectant.

EXERCISE 12.2

A patient was seen by an ANP in a county health care clinic for a skin disorder. The ANP prescribed antibiotics and a topical cream for the skin condition. The patient actually was suffering from pemphigus vulgaris, an uncommon autoimmune skin disorder from which she died 3 months later. What questions would you ask this ANP in determining if there was any liability on the ANP's part? To what standard of care should the ANP be held?

PRESCRIPTIVE AUTHORITY

Prescriptive authority is central to independent practice by advanced practice nurses. Only 50 years ago, most drugs not classified as narcotics were available as over-the-counter medications, and nurses worked independently with physicians in recommending such medications. This was changed by the 1938 Federal Food, Drug, and Cosmetic Act.

Legal issues in this area involve the extent of professional decision making allowed the advanced practice nurse and the range of drugs from which the advanced practice nurse may select. States generally fall into one of three categories in relation to prescriptive authority. The vast majority of states continue to require some degree of physician involvement or delegation in the area of prescriptive authority, whether through direct supervision or through the use of a formulary that dictates allowable drug prescription. Included in the prescriptive authority is the ability to also dispense controlled substances. Thirty-four states require this physician involvement. Thirteen states and the District of Columbia allow independent prescription authority for advanced practice nurses. These states include controlled substances within this prescription authority. The remaining three states require some physician involvement or delegation for prescribing medications and disallow any prescriptive authority of controlled substances.

ADMITTING PRIVILEGES

The lack of admitting or hospital privileges for ANPs is one means of limiting the practice of these nurses. **Admitting privileges** are granted by individual facilities, and the extent of the privilege varies from allowing the practitioner to visit patients to permitting direct admission and entries in the medical record. Admitting privileges are facility controlled, and no state or federal legislation is involved.

Central to admitting privileges in a state that allows independent practice for advanced practice nurses are **antitrust issues.** Such issues arise when health care professionals, seeking access to health care facilities controlled by physicians with whom they compete, are denied these privileges based on the fact that they represent competition for the physicians in the locality. Because most hospital credentialing committees that vote on extending hospital privileges to qualified practitioners are composed exclusively of physicians, this area of the law has become one of great concern for advanced nursing practice.

Antitrust issues arise whenever:

1. There is exclusion of a class from membership on the medical or hospital staff.
2. There are questions about the fair market value of a service.
3. One society or association attempts to restrict its members' use of a second class of practitioners.

The issue that the courts must decide is whether the antitrust laws can eliminate professional group boycotts motivated by anticompetition interests, while preserving legitimate professional self-regulation aimed at maintaining the competence and professional conduct of a profession.

The two leading cases decided to date assisting practice nurses to secure hospital privileges are *Bahn v. NME Hospitals* (1987) and *Wrable v. Community Memorial Hospital* (1987). These issues are better addressed on a local level, rather than a state or federal level. Perhaps the biggest hurdle to overcome is the prevailing practice of allowing advanced practice nurses to admit patients to an institution under the name of a supervising physician. This practice decreases the autonomy of the advanced practice nurse while ensuring that only physicians are credentialed by the institution.

EXERCISE 12.3

Investigate prescriptive authority and admitting privileges for advanced practice nurses within your community and state. How do these two issues affect the overall ability of nurse practitioners to start their own practice? Which of these two issues has the most impact on nurses in your area?

DIRECT ACCESS TO PATIENT POPULATIONS

Physicians have traditionally been the gatekeepers of the health care delivery system. **Direct access** to alternate providers, such as advanced practice nurses, has been curtailed by medicine regulators and accreditors, including state health departments and the Joint Commission. Nurses have only recently taken definitive action for discharge planning, including when the patient is released from the health care facility.

Some of the current proposals for allowing advanced practice nurses direct access to patient populations concern managed care corporations. Today, managed care corporations retain the power of the physician as the gatekeeper, but negotiations for advanced practice nurses in these corporations are advancing in some areas of the country. These negotiations are being undertaken in light of the current research on patient outcomes and who provides more optimal services in relationship to cost containment and patient satisfaction. Such research needs to continue if advanced practice nurses are to be allowed more direct access to patients.

STATUTE OF LIMITATIONS

Statutes of limitations dictate that actions must be heard within a prescribed number of years or be barred from ever being heard. Most states impose a 1- to 2-year limitation on medical malpractice suits. Whatever the jurisdiction, there seems to be the same statute of limitations for all health care providers in the state. Reread Chapter 3 for more information concerning statutes of limitation.

ETHICAL PERSPECTIVES AND ADVANCED NURSING PRACTICE

Ethical judgment, incorporating ethical principles in all aspects of advanced practice nursing, occurs on a daily basis and begins with respecting each person one encounters and supporting the individual's ethical rights. Many of the decisions that advanced practice nurses make require a significant degree of balancing principles, for example, balancing the person's autonomy rights while advocating for specific treatment modalities for a patient who elects no treatment.

Balancing principles may also be seen when the advanced practice nurse advocates for equal use of scarce resources for patients who are underinsured, respecting their right to have adequate and appropriate health care treatment.

Perhaps, as Chase (2007) suggests, one of the greatest challenges from an ethical perspective concerns the allocation of the APN's time. If the advanced practice nurse gives too much of his or her time to an individual patient, then other patients, equally deserving of this scarce resource, are made to wait or have less time with the primary care provider and potentially are not assessed so that accurate diagnoses are made. The converse could also be true; if the advanced practice nurse routinely holds each patient to his or her allotted time, then the patient may be the person for whom an incorrect or incomplete diagnosis is made.

EXERCISE 12.4

Query advanced practice nurses in your area regarding ethical issues in their practice. What are these advanced practice nurses' main ethical issues? Do they relate to ethical principles as opposed to ethical theories? How does understanding their concerns assist you in better understanding and addressing ethical concerns in your own nursing practice?

SUMMARY

- Advanced nursing practice roles first evolved in the late 1800s with the emergence of the certified registered nurse anesthetist and certified nurse midwifery roles.
- Advanced nurse practitioner and clinical nurse specialist roles emerged in the late 1960s and early 1970s as a direct result of a nationwide physician shortage.
- Clinical nurse leaders emerged in 2000 as a direct result of the continuing nursing shortage, increasing numbers of identified errors in the health care delivery system, and fragmentation of nursing care.
- The doctorate of nursing practice focuses on innovative, evidence-based practice that reflects application of research findings to clinical practice.
- Dual legal liability exists for all of the advanced practice roles, as these practitioners are licensed in their individual state as registered nurses and have expanded roles through certification and/or secondary state licensure.

- Scope of practice is the permissible boundaries of practice and may be influenced by amending or altering state nurse practice acts, through court decisions that redefine nursing roles, by federal amendments, and through changes in reimbursement laws.
- Malpractice issues affect nurses in advanced practice roles and directly relate to their dual roles as an RN and as a primary health care provider.
- A standard of care issue that remains is whether the advanced practice nurse functions under a medical standard of care or an advanced practice standard of care.
- Prescriptive authority expands the role, though in the majority of states this remains a supervised or delegated role.
- Admission privileges and direct access to patients are needed to more fully expand the authority of the advanced practice nurse.
- Ethical issues that confront advanced practice nurses center on balancing ethical principles in everyday clinical settings.

APPLY YOUR LEGAL KNOWLEDGE

1. How does the state nurse practice act affect the role of advanced nursing practice within a given state?
2. Are there areas in which advanced nursing practice is making more of an impact than others? Do these correspond with the primary purposes of advanced nursing practice?
3. What must professional nursing do to ensure that advanced nursing practice is fully used by persons most needing these professionals' care?
4. Why is advanced practice nursing vital to the continued growth of the discipline of nursing?

YOU BE THE JUDGE

Certified nurse midwives (CNMs) were employed by an acute care institution as the primary care providers for new mothers. The patient was pregnant with her first child and she presented at the institution at 8:30 A.M. The mother stated labor had started about 2:30 that morning, when she experienced leakage of her amniotic fluid. She continued to labor throughout the day. At 11:35 that evening, the CNM finally notified the obstetrician on call that a cesarean section was indicated, and the infant was born at 12:15 A.M. The infant suffered an intracranial bleed and today is severely retarded.

Expert witnesses who testified for the mother stated that the intracranial bleed was directly related to the mother's extended labor and that the CNM should have consulted the obstetrician much earlier in the day. Expert testimony for the CNM and the institution stated that the CT scan taken shortly after the infant's birth showed an intracranial bleed that was related to thrombi caused by a placental infection and was not the result of the delay in performing the cesarean section. The trial court accepted the testimony of the defendant's expert witnesses and found no liability on the part of the defendants.

QUESTIONS

1. Who should testify as the expert witnesses in this case?
2. What questions would you anticipate were asked of the expert witnesses regarding the standard of care given this mother during the time she was in labor?
3. How might the defense have presented this case so that there was a clearer answer for the judge and jury?
4. Would you overturn the finding of the trial court? Why or why not?

REFERENCES

Ali v. Community Health Care Plan, Inc., 261 Conn. 143, 801 A.2d 775 (Connecticut, 2002).

American Association of Colleges of Nursing. (2004). *AACN position statement on the practice doctorate in nursing.* Washington, DC: Author.

American Association of Colleges of Nursing. (2005). *Working paper on the role of the clinical nurse leader.* Washington, DC: Author.

American Association of Colleges of Nursing. (2007). *White paper on the education and role of the clinical nurse leader.* Washington, DC: Author.

American Association of Nurse Anesthetists. (2003). *Questions and answers: A career in nurse anesthesia* [fact sheet]. Park Ridge, IL: Author.

Avila v. New York Health & Hospitals Corporation, 2007 WL 4234838 (Sup. Ct. New York, October 18, 2007).

Bahn v. NME Hospitals, 669 F. Supp. 998 (E.D. Cal., 1987).

Balanced Budget Act of 1997, Public Law 105-33, 111 *Statutes* 350, August 5, 1997.

Bellegie v. Board of Nurse Examiners, 685 S.W.2d 431 (Tex. Ct. App. Austin, 1985).

Burroughs, R., Dmytrow, B., & Lewis, H. (2007). Trend in nurse practitioner professional liability: An analysis of claims with risk management recommendations. *Journal of Nursing Law, 11*(1), 52–60.

Chalmers-Francis v. Nelson, 6 Cal.2d 402 (1936).

Chapa v. United States, 2006 WL 1763663 (D. Neb., June 23, 2006).

Chase, S. K. (2007). The art of diagnosis and treatment. In L. M. Dunphy, J. E. Winland-Brown, B. O. Porter, & D. J. Thomas (Eds.), *Primary care: The art and science of advanced practice nursing* (2nd ed., pp. 40–57). Philadelphia, PA: F. A. Davis Company.

Cohen v. State Board of Medicine, 676 A.2d 1277 (Pa. Cmwlth., 1996).

Coleman v. Martinez, 2007 WL 5022487 (Cir. Ct. Hillsborough Co., Florida, November 19, 2007).

Cox v. Board of Hospital Managers, 2002 WL 1722063 (Michigan, July 25, 2002).

Creviston v. St. Mary Medical Center, 2007 WL 5171070 (Sup. Ct. Lake Co., Indiana, November 30, 2007).

Ehteman v. Kaiser Permanente, 2008 WL 464886 (Med. Mal. Arbitration, Orange Co., California, January 10, 2008).

Fein v. Permanente Medical Group, 38 Cal.3d 137, 695 P. 2d 665 (California, 1985).

Fitzhugh v. St. Luke's South Hospital, 2007 WL 1224005 (Dist. Ct., Johnson Co., Kansas, February 6, 2007).

Harris v. State through Huey P. Long Hospital, 371 So.2d 1221 (Louisiana, 1979).

Hendry v. United States, 418 F.2d 744 (2nd Cir., 1969).

Hernicz v. State of Florida, Department of Professional Regulation, 390 S.2d 194 (Fla. Dis. Ct. App., 1980).

Hilliard v. McIntyre, 2007 WL 1650357 (Ct. Com. Pl., Wyoming Co., Pennsylvania, March 27, 2007).

Hypolite v. Columbia Dauterive Hospital, 2007 WL 2851006 (La. App., October 3, 2007).

In re Nicholas, 2005 WL 3118683 (N.Y. App., November 23, 2005).

Infant v. Hospital, 2007 WL 1287709 (Sup Ct. San Joaquin Co., California, January 4, 2007).

Jenkins v. Payne, 465 S.E.2d 795 (Virginia, 1996).

Judy v. Grant County Health Department, 557 S.E.2d 340 (West Virginia, 2001).

Kim v. Priebe, 2007 WL 2415592 (Sup. Ct. Peirce Co., Washington, April 30, 2007).

Mannino, M. J. (1982). *The nurse anesthetist and the law.* New York: Grune & Stratton.

Olson v. Bolstad, 161 Minn. 419, 201 N.W. 918 (1925).

Oram v. de Cholnoky, 2008 WL 793692 (sup. Ct., Stamford-Norwalk, Connecticut, February 8, 2008).

People v. Arendt, 60 Ill. App. 89 (1894).

Renaissance Surgical Centers v. Jimenez, 2008 WL 3971096 (Tex. App., August 28, 2008).

Reverby, S. M. (1987). *Ordered to care: The dilemma of American nursing, 1850–1945.* Cambridge, MA: Cambridge University Press.

Rivera v. County of Suffolk, 736 N.Y.S.2d 95 (N.Y. App., 2002).

Ruggiero v. State Department of Health, 643 N.Y.S.2d 698 (N.Y. App., 1996).

Rules and Regulations. (1998). Fed. Reg. 63 (211), 58871–58876.

Sermchief v. Gonzales, 660 S.W.2d 683 (Mo. en banc, 1983).

Stevens, R. (1971). *American medicine and the public interest.* New Haven, CT: Yale University Press.

Tatro v. State of Texas, 703 F.2d 823 (5th Cir., 1983).

Tornabeni, J. & Miller, J. F. (2008). The power of partnership to shape the future of nursing: The evolution of the clinical nurse leader. *Journal of Nursing Management, 16,* 608–613.

Tremain v. United States, 2007 WL 2791795 (S. D. Ill., May 31, 2007).

Weiland, S. A. (2008). Reflections on independence in nurse practitioner practice. *Journal of the American Academy of Nurse Practitioners, 20,* 345–352.

Weyandt v. State, 35 S.W.3d 144 (Tex. App., 2001).

Whitney v. Day, M.D., and Hurley Hospital, 300 N.W.2d 380 (Ct. App. Mich., 1980).

Wrable v. Community Memorial Hospital, 205 J.J. Super 428 (1985), aff'd. 517 A.2d. 470 (October 22, 1986), cert. denied, 526 A.2d 210 (April 28, 1987).

CHAPTER 13

Corporate Liability Issues and Employment Laws

PREVIEW

Whenever a nurse is employed by another, be it a hospital, clinic, or physician, the employing entity accepts varying amounts of potential liability for the nurse-employee. The nurse becomes the employer's representative and, because of special legal status, conveys potential liability to the employer. Never, though, does the nurse convey all liability to the employer. Each individual is ultimately responsible for his or her actions.

This chapter discusses theories of corporate liability, including vicarious liability, respondeat superior, borrowed and dual servant doctrines, ostensible authority, and the role of the independent contractor. A variety of federal and state employment laws that affect corporate liability are discussed in depth, and the chapter concludes with some ethical issues that may arise in this area of the law.

LEARNING OUTCOMES
After completing this chapter, you should be able to:

13.1 Describe the doctrines of respondeat superior, borrowed and dual servant, ostensible authority, corporate negligence, and direct corporate liability.

13.2 Define and discuss the role of the individual contractor in the health care delivery system.

13.3 Describe the impact of indemnification from a corporate perspective.

13.4 Describe selected federal and state employment laws that affect the delivery of health care in the United States.

13.5 Describe the employer's obligation to nurse-employees and the professional nurse's obligations to the employing agency.

13.6 Discuss some ethical issues that arise in this area of the law.

KEY TERMS

affirmative action
Age Discrimination in
    Employment Act of 1967
borrowed servant doctrine
Civil Rights Act of 1964
collective bargaining (labor
    relations)
constructive discharge
contract negotiation
corporate liability
dual servant doctrine
employment-at-will
Equal Employment
    Opportunity Act of 1972

Equal Employment
    Opportunity Commission
    (EEOC)
Equal Pay Act
Family and Medical Leave
    Act of 1993
Federal False Claims Act
    of 1986
Federal Tort Claims Act
    of 1946
indemnification
independent contractor
National Labor Relations Act
    (NLRA)

negligent hiring and retention
Occupational Safety and
    Health Act of 1970
ostensible authority
personal liability
Rehabilitation Act of 1973
respondeat superior
vicarious liability
whistleblower law
workers' compensation laws
wrongful discharge

THEORIES OF VICARIOUS LIABILITY

Vicarious liability, or substituted liability, describes the instance in which one party is responsible for the actions of another. The law allows substituted liability to prevent further injustice to the injured party and to encourage employers to ensure employee competence. If injured parties could sue only the nurse or nurses who harmed them, the injured person might not be able to be fully compensated monetarily, unless, of course, these nurses are independently wealthy. Holding the employer equally liable increases the chances that there will be money available to cover incurred damages. It also encourages the employer to hire and retain safe practitioners.

Vicarious liability is not a shift in liability, but an extension of liability allowing justice to be fairly distributed. Vicarious liability extends liability to include the employer, but never to the extent that personal and individual liability are lost.

Respondeat Superior

Respondeat superior, "let the master respond" or "let the master answer," is the common law principle of substituted liability based on a master–servant relationship. While nurses may disagree with what a master–servant relationship implies, the courts have found similar elements: (1) the employer controls the actions of the employee, and (2) substituted liability applies only to actions within the scope and course of employment. The effect of this doctrine is that the employer is given responsibility and accountability for an employee's negligent actions and that the injured party may recover damages from the employer or employing institution.

The rationale for such recovery lies in a benefit–burden analysis. Employers, standing to reap the benefits of the employees' activities, must also bear the burden of the employees' errors. Employers have an obligation to see that those they hire perform in a safe and competent manner. As the court said in *Hunter v. Allis-Chambers Corporation, Engine Division* (1986): "An employer is directly liable for torts caused by his employees against others. The employer could have prevented these torts by reasonable care in hiring, supervising, and, if necessary, firing the tortfeasor" (at 1419).

The landmark case applying the doctrine of respondeat superior in health care settings is *Duling v. Bluefield Sanitarium, Inc.* (1965). In that case, a 13-year-old was admitted to the hospital with a diagnosis of rheumatic heart disease. At 7:00 P.M. on the evening of her admission,

Nancy Duling was seen by the attending physician, and he told her mother that the child could easily develop heart failure. The physician explained to Mrs. Duling the signs and symptoms of heart failure, and to notify the nursing staff immediately if she observed any of those signs and symptoms in Nancy.

Shortly after the physician left, Nancy began exhibiting signs of heart failure, and Mrs. Duling notified the staff. The nurses did not check Nancy and, in spite of frequent pleas by Mrs. Duling for help and an obvious deterioration in Nancy's condition, the nurses waited more than 6 hours before adequately assessing the patient. By that time, Nancy's condition was so serious that subsequent treatment failed to save her life.

The issue at court was whether the hospital was liable for the negligence of the nursing staff for failure to provide competent nursing care. The court enumerated the hospital's standard of care thusly: "A private hospital, conducted for profit, owes to its patients such reasonable care and attention for their safety as their mental and physical condition, if known, may require. The care exercised should be commensurate with the known inability of the patient to care for himself" (*Duling v. Bluefield Sanitarium, Inc.,* 1965, at 759). Thus, the court found that the hospital was liable for the care provided (or, as in this instance, not provided) by its employees.

This reliance on the doctrine of respondeat superior stems from the nurses' responsibility to uphold standards of care and from the employment relationship with the hospital wherein the nurse provides care that meets legal standards and hospital mandates.

Scope and Course of Employment

Two hurdles the injured party must pass before the principle of respondeat superior is allowed are:

1. The injured party must show that the employer had control over the employee.
2. The negligent act must have occurred within the course and scope of the employee's employment.

The first element is fairly straightforward and is usually shown in courts of law by proving employment status. The second element is more difficult, because the injured party must show that the actions were those for which the nurse was hired and that these same actions occurred during the course of the nurse's work.

Courts tend to decide scope and course of business on a case-by-case basis. The first factor that courts of law consistently determine is foreseeability of the action. Should the employer have been able to foresee that an employee could perform a certain action as he or she did? Various case decisions indicate that most activities undertaken by employees will be held foreseeable for the purpose of finding employer liability. For example, the court in *Robertson v. Bethlehem Steel Corporation* (1990) held that if employees acted within the scope of their employment and their actions were in connection with the employer's business, the plaintiff could recover. *Biconi v. Pay 'N Pak Stores, Inc.* (1990) extended the scope and course of employment to intentional torts as well as negligent torts.

Some of the other factors consistently analyzed by courts include:

1. Usual place of employment
2. Whether the act's purpose, in whole or in part, was in furtherance of the employer's business
3. The extent to which the act was similar to or different from authorized acts of the employer
4. The extent to which the act was a departure from the employer's customary methods
5. The extent to which the employer should have expected such an act to occur (American Jurisprudence, 1992)

Two examples may help illustrate these points. Nurse A allows Mr. Jones to fall as she is assisting him back to bed. Mr. Jones is a patient in the intensive care unit who had hip surgery 2 days prior to this incident. Liability would extend to the hospital, as the hospital policy and procedure manual mandates that she properly assess the patient and obtain adequate help before assisting the patient either to or from his bed. Note, however, that if Nurse A failed to assist Mr. Jones in the manner prescribed by hospital policy, the hospital would have cause to argue that this action was not performed according to hospital policy.

In a second example, Nurse A is in the hospital for the sole purpose of collecting her paycheck. Nurse B, a co-worker in the intensive care unit, asks Nurse A to put Mr. Jones back to bed so that Nurse B can finish required documentation and join Nurse A for lunch. Mr. Jones subsequently falls. Nurse A would be solely accountable for her actions, as she was not within the course and scope of her employment at the time of Mr. Jones's fall. The hospital may still be held accountable, however, through the actions of Nurse B, who is also a hospital employee.

Actions that are generally considered to be outside the course and scope of employment include the rendering of voluntary health services, either at the scene of an accident or as part of a community health drive, and the giving of health-related advice on a voluntary basis. Additionally, performing actions that are reserved for physicians or advanced practice nurses is not considered within the scope of employment for staff nurses, unless a true emergency condition prevails.

Health care facilities may also incur liability for actions performed by nurses who function in supervisory roles. These nursing supervisors, similar to the nurses and ancillary personnel they oversee, are employees of the institution. While the nursing supervisor may be liable if there is a negligent act by a hospital employee, the supervisor's liability is more frequently incurred because of a failure to perform supervisory functions in a competent manner, as a reasonably prudent nursing supervisor would.

The doctrine of respondeat superior applies equally to acts of omission as well as commission. In the landmark decision of *Darling v. Charleston Community Memorial Hospital* (1965), the nurses and thus the hospital were found liable for their failure to notify the medical staff or the chief of the medical service when the attending physician failed to deliver proper medical care to James Darling.

In *Darling,* the patient had undergone a cast procedure to set a broken leg. The nurses assigned to care for Mr. Darling subsequent to the cast application assessed his recovery accurately: The circulation to his casted extremity was sluggish, he continued to require ever-increasing amounts of pain medications, and there was a foul odor coming from the cast site. Numerous nurses charted their observations and continued to apprise the attending physician of the symptoms. The attending physician responded to their assessments by ordering increased amounts of pain medications and increasing the antibiotic therapy for Mr. Darling. Ultimately, James Darling was transferred to a second hospital, and, despite aggressive therapy, the physicians were unable to save the leg.

The court, in finding against the nurses and the hospital, stated that it is not sufficient to merely apprise the attending physician of the continuing deterioration in this patient's condition. Hospital staff members have a further responsibility to inform those in authority positions so that the patient may receive competent care. In the case described, the chief of staff or the hospital medical committee could have intervened had they known of James Darling's substandard medical care.

In *Hunt v. Tender Loving Care Home Care Agency, Inc.* (2002), a home health aide who cared for a single patient was involved in an automobile accident and filed claims for workers' compensation. In finding against this health care worker's claim, the court noted that the worker would be within the course of employment if she was injured while transporting patients, completing errands for patients, or traveling between patients' homes. In this case, the health care worker cared for a single client, and travel between the patient's home and the health care worker's home was not in the course of employment.

Contrast this case with the finding in *Glander v. Marshall Hospital* (2003). In *Glander,* a nurse had worked a 12-hour shift and then was required by the hospital to stay and attend a 2-hour required annual in-service update session. On her way home after the in-service session, the nurse caused a motor vehicle collision that killed two people. Apparently, she fell asleep while driving. In finding the hospital 25% liable for the subsequent injury, the court held that the nurse was on a "special errand" for her employer, which meant that she was within the course and scope of her duties when the accident occurred. The rationale used by the court was that this was not the usual commute for the nurse.

The court was explicit in *N. X. v. Cabrini Medical Center* (2002) regarding the duty of hospital staff members in the area of respondeat superior. In that case, a female patient had surgery for removal of genital warts. While in the post-anesthesia recovery area she was sexually assaulted by a male surgical resident. The recovery area where the assault occurred was small and consisted of four beds that were spaced closely together and separated only by cloth curtains. At the time of the assault, several nurses and the unit supervisor were in the area. All of the nurses were aware that this particular resident had entered the patient's curtained area, but none of the nurses paid any particular attention to why he was there or what he was doing.

The resident was not listed on the patient's chart as having any involvement in the patient's case. Only as the resident was leaving did the nursing supervisor speak to him. Soon afterward, the patient complained that he had sexually assaulted her. The patient subsequently filed suit against the resident and the hospital for the assault.

In finding for the patient and against the hospital, the court noted that nurses are not gatekeepers who stop and question physicians, ascertain the reasons for their presence, or stand guard and monitor physicians' interactions with patients. However, when a nurse observes something that common sense would indicate is potentially harmful to a patient, a legal duty is triggered to investigate and ensure the protection of the patient. In this case, the plaintiff's cause of action was further supported by the fact that there was an institution policy that a female staff member was to be present when a male physician examined a patient. The most important message from this case is that the hospital incurred liability not because of the resident's misconduct, which was ruled outside the course and scope of his employment, but because of the nurses' failure to prevent what occurred.

When a lawsuit is filed asserting the respondeat superior doctrine, both the hospital and the nurse are sued. Often, the hospital will attempt to claim that the nurse was acting outside the scope of his or her employment to avoid liability. Thus, nurses must first show that they were within the course and scope of their employment at the time of the incident.

EXERCISE 13.1

Judy Jones, an employee of Doctor Ybarra, and Beth Smith, an employee of Doctor Hunter, were friends, with both of their offices located in the same building. One day, as the nurses were leaving the building for lunch, they noticed an elderly lady in obvious respiratory distress. Judy recognized the individual as a patient of Doctor Ybarra and immediately went back to the office to get the doctor. Meanwhile, Beth Smith, in attempting to help the patient, caused the individual to be injured. Following the patient's untimely death, her estate sued Doctor Ybarra and Doctor Hunter, claiming negligence on the part of Beth Smith. Are either of the physicians negligent under the doctrine of respondeat superior? Is anyone at fault? Should the family be able to recover damages?

Borrowed Servant and Dual Servant Doctrines

The **borrowed servant doctrine,** a term seldom used today though the application can be encountered, is a special application of the doctrine of respondeat superior. A borrowed servant is one who, while in the general employment of another, is subject to the right to direct and control the details of the individual's particular activities. This right to direct and control must be more than a mere cooperation with the suggestions of an authority figure. The borrowed servant doctrine applies when one employer lends completely the services or skills of an employee to another employer, and the key to this doctrine is the right and manner of control.

The borrowed servant doctrine's usual application in nursing occurs when the nurse-employee comes under the direct supervision and control of a physician. Thus, the employer-hospital would not be liable for negligent or intentional torts of the nurse while the nurse is under the direct control and supervision of the directing physician. The directing physician becomes liable under the doctrine of respondeat superior if the injured party can prove exclusive control and course and scope of employment. The right to control, said the court in *Harris v. Miller* (1994), is not presumed because the surgeon is in charge during the operation, but must be proven during the course of the trial.

Traditionally, the borrowed servant doctrine applies to situations within the operating arena or to cardiopulmonary resuscitation. Once referred to as the *captain of the ship doctrine,* the trend in national case law is away from this doctrine. This is reflected by the landmark decision made by the Texas Supreme Court in *Sparger v. Worley Hospital, Inc.* (1977), which concluded that the captain of the ship doctrine is a false application of a specific rule of agency and that one must first determine if the nurses are borrowed servants in deciding liability. More recently the court in *Ruiz v. Adlanka* (2007) concluded that members of the operating room team are all accountable for their own errors and omissions in negligently accounting for sponges and surgical instruments, not merely the primary surgeon.

The **dual servant doctrine** describes the outcome in *Ruiz*, as this doctrine allows for vicarious liability to flow to both the employer-hospital and to the physician. A dual servant is one who can be shown to be serving both entities at the same time. For example, circulating nurses in the operating room remain hospital employees, yet strictly follow the orders of the surgeon in charge. In *Ruiz*, the injured plaintiff had to show that the operating nurses were negligent and that they were following the surgeon's directions during the surgical procedure; thus the surgeon did have control at the time of the incident. They were also employees of the institution and responsible for following the policies and procedures of the institution. As with all vicarious liability situations, the nurse who does not act in a reasonably prudent manner may be held individually negligent along with the employer.

CORPORATE LIABILITY

Corporate liability is the doctrine that evolved as hospitals became more profitable and competitive that holds the institution liable for its responsibilities to patients. The *Darling* case is the landmark case for corporate liability, placing certain nondelegable duties regarding patient care directly on the hospital corporation. Prior to the *Darling* ruling, hospitals bore no liability for the provision of health care, as liability for untoward outcomes had been imputed solely to the health care providers.

Under this doctrine, corporations have a direct duty to the public they serve, ensuring that competent and qualified practitioners deliver quality health care to consumers. A later court case interpreted *Darling* to include the duty to make a reasonable effort to monitor and oversee the treatment that is prescribed and administered by physicians and nurses practicing within the institution (*Bost v. Riley,* 1990).

All of the hospital's corporate duties have a direct impact on the provision of patient care. The emphasis on the hospital's responsibility for adequate care is apparent. Most of the early case law dealt with the hospital's responsibility to select and delineate clinical privileges of physicians. The hospital, however, has duties to the patient outside of clinical privileges, which include adequate staffing, supervision for education and training of staff members, maintaining the premises in a reasonably safe manner, provision of properly functioning and reasonably updated equipment, reasonable care in the selection and retention of employees, and the duty to meet a national standard of care.

A case that illustrates corporate liability is *Carter v. Hucks-Folliss* (1998). In this case, the issue was whether a hospital could be sued for granting clinical privileges to a physician without considering the physician's board status. The court held that while Joint Commission (JC) standards do not require a physician to be board certified in order to obtain clinical privileges, the JC does require the hospital to consider the physician's board status.

In *Carter,* the hospital did not consider the physician's board status before granting clinical privileges. The patient was then injured and brought a lawsuit against the hospital for liability under a corporate liability standard. In holding for the injured patient, the court concluded that legal precedents have established that if a patient suffers harm in an instance in which an accredited health care facility deviates from the standards of its accrediting body, the patient can use that deviation as proof of negligence in a subsequent lawsuit against the hospital. *Wellstar Health Systems, Inc. v. Green* (2002) held that a hospital was liable to the injured patient for the negligent credentialing of a nurse practitioner.

Negligent Hiring and Retention

The doctrine of **negligent hiring and retention** of employees is often used by injured parties when respondeat superior cannot be applied to the specific fact situation. For example, negligent hiring and firing may be applied in situations in which nurses were not acting within the course and scope of employment or in which they were acting solely for personal reasons. This doctrine essentially means that the employer can still be held liable if the injured party can show that the employee was incompetent or unsafe for the position and that the employer knew or should have known that the employee was incompetent or unsafe.

Like respondeat superior, negligent hiring and retention is based on the master–servant relationship. An employer is under a duty to exercise reasonable care so as to control employees while acting outside the scope of his employment and to prevent the employee from intentionally harming others. Hospitals are under an affirmative duty to provide adequate numbers of staff as well as adequately educated and skilled staff members.

The hospital's obligation under this doctrine is to monitor or supervise all personnel within the facility, ensuring quality care to patients within the facility. The institution would be liable for substandard care or injury incurred by patients if personnel fail to perform in accordance with acceptable standards of care. Institutions must also periodically review staff competency (*Park North General Hospital v. Hickman,* 1990). A second obligation that institutions have under this doctrine is to investigate physicians' and advanced practice nurses' credentials before allowing them admitting privileges. Most important, the doctrine requires that the hospital terminate unqualified practitioners or make available to these practitioners the education and skills needed to competently deliver quality health care to patients. This concept was upheld in *Wellstar Health Systems, Inc. v. Green* (2002). In *Wellstar,* a patient died from complications of a myocardial infarction after an improperly credentialed nurse practitioner sent her home with a prescription for antibiotics for an ear infection.

OSTENSIBLE AUTHORITY

Ostensible authority is an application of agency law that allows a principal to be liable for acts and omissions by independent contractors working within the principal's place of business or at the direction of the principal when a third party misinterprets the relationship as employer–employee. In health care law, hospitals have been held responsible for actions by independent contractors in lawsuits in which reasonable patients argued that they could not distinguish hospital employees from independent contractors.

Ostensible authority is also known as *agency by estoppel*, and, while there is no true agency authority and no agency has been created in respect to an unknowing third party, the court will allow the principal to be held liable to the injured third party (Corpus Juris Secundum, 2000). The courts employ four criteria to establish ostensible authority: (1) subjectivism, (2) inherent function, (3) reliance, and (4) control.

Subjectivism

This criterion refers to the extent that third parties view the person as a hospital employee, and it is subject to the third parties' interpretation of the relationship. In institutions in which the emergency center or urgent care provider is an independent contractor working in the hospital facility, the court looks to the subjective interpretation of a patient in perceiving that the physician is indeed a hospital employee.

Inherent Function

For this element, the courts determine whether the independent contractor is furthering the primary function of the corporation or if the individual's role can easily be seen as distinguishable from the corporation's primary function. For example, emergency center providers are contracted to serve the primary function of the hospital in that they are contracted to provide emergency and needed treatment to persons in a recognizable hospital setting. This is easily distinguished from a contracted food vendor that the hospital contracts to provide food while the hospital cafeteria is renovated.

Reliance

Reliance, perhaps the most subjective criterion, actually involves the faith that the patient places in the hospital's judgment. If the hospital contracted with a specific emergency center provider, then the patient assumes that the provider's credentials and skills have been investigated and that this provider is competent to perform the role of an emergency center physician.

Control

To determine who had the greater control, the independent contractor or the hospital will ascertain the following factors:

1. To what extent the employer determines the details of the work and work setting
2. Whether the work is supervised by the employer or the independent contractor is free to perform the work in the manner he or she sees fit
3. Who supplies the instruments, equipment, and supplies needed to perform the work
4. Where the work is performed
5. What method of payment is used (Corpus Juris Secundum, 2000)

The more control the corporation has in determining these factors, the more likely it is that the court will find ostensible authority.

THEORIES OF INDEPENDENT LIABILITY

Several legal theories and doctrines refer specifically to one's personal responsibilities and liabilities. Such theories serve to make one continually accountable for one's own actions.

Independent Contractor Status

An **independent contractor** is one who arranges with another to perform a service for him or her but who is not under the control or right to control of the second person. In nursing, independent contractor status usually applies to private-duty nurses and to selected advanced practitioner roles. As with ostensible authority, the key issue is control, and neither party may terminate the contract at will. Termination should be a provision of the expressed contract, as should length of contract, dispute resolution, relationship of the parties, duties and responsibilities of the independent contractor, payment schedule, and professional liability insurance.

In theory, the classification of this status makes the nurse solely liable for negligent or intentional torts and should relieve the hospital or employer of liability. In application, however, many hospitals have been assessed liability by courts under the doctrine of corporate liability or nondelegable duty. In one such case, *Zakbartchenko v. Weinberger* (1993), a rabbi was held negligent in the performance of a bris. The court ruled that the hospital would be held liable if the child's parents established that it had relied on the availability of the hospital's facility and personnel in deciding to perform the bris at the hospital. Because they could establish reliance, the hospital was also liable to the parents. This was because the hospital owes certain legal duties to the patient that are completely independent of any derivative liability, such as liability for (1) inadequate facilities, (2) inadequate institutional policies, or (3) improper enforcement of rules and regulations of the JC and other licensing and accrediting bodies.

Personal Liability

Stated simply, the doctrine of **personal liability** makes each individual responsible for his or her own actions. The law does not impose liability on a third party or entity or permit the person primarily at fault to avoid responsibility and accountability. One cannot negate one's responsibility merely because a second or third party also has responsibility.

Neither will the law impose liability on the competent practitioner. The mere fact that a second or third party has liability does not necessarily convey the liability back to the first individual. For example, a team leader assigns a new staff member to care for an uncomplicated patient. The staff member draws a blood sample from the patient in a negligent manner or fails to monitor the patient's vital signs accurately. The new staff member should be capable of performing both tasks competently. The court will find the staff member negligent and therefore liable if a subsequent lawsuit is filed. The team leader would not share in the liability even though he or she was the person who directly assigned the particular patient's care to this nurse. As a team leader, one has a right to expect that staff members are capable of performing functions normally assigned to them. The example changes, however, if the staff member expressed, at the time of the assignment, an inability to competently perform the tasks. Then both the team leader and the assigned nurse could incur liability.

Indemnification

Closely akin to personal liability is the principle of **indemnification,** which allows the employer to recover from the individual personally responsible any damages paid under the doctrine of respondeat superior for the negligent act. Nurses' personal liability for negligent actions makes them subject to this principle after the hospital, via respondeat superior, has paid damages to the injured party. The key to applying this principle is twofold:

1. The employer is at fault in a liability suit only because of the employee's negligence.
2. The employer incurs monetary damages because of the employee's negligence.

The employer can then institute a lawsuit against the negligent employee and recover the amount of damages that the employer paid to the injured party.

EXERCISE 13.2

Jose, an 8-year-old boy, was injured while playing basketball with his friends. It was a pleasant summer evening about 10:00 P.M. when he fell, dislocating his shoulder. He was admitted to your hospital, in extreme pain, and seen by the emergency center physician. After what seemed like forever, an x-ray was done and the physician told Jose's parents that surgery would be "done the first thing in the morning" as there was no anesthetist on call, but that the anesthetist would arrive about 8:00 A.M. Jose was sedated and spent a long and painful night at the hospital. Following surgery, he developed a permanent disability of his shoulder and arm due to the delayed surgery. His parents bring suit against the hospital, the emergency center physician, and the anesthetist. What are their grounds for liability, and who, if anyone, should be found liable for Jose's injury?

EMPLOYMENT LAWS

The federal and individual state governments have enacted a cadre of laws regulating employment. To be effective and legally correct, nurses must be familiar with these laws and how individual laws affect the institution and labor relations. Many nurses have come to fear the legal system because of personal experience or the experiences of colleagues. However, much of this concern may be directly attributable to uncertainty with the law or partial knowledge of the law. By understanding and correctly following federal employment laws, nurse-managers may actually lessen their potential liability because they have complied with both federal and state laws. Table 13.1 gives an overview of key federal employment laws that pertain to the health care sector. The table is not an exhaustive list of labor laws, but presents those most pertinent for nurse managers to know. One law, the Health Insurance Portability and Accountability Act of 1996, was previously covered in Chapter 9 and is not repeated in this chapter.

EQUAL EMPLOYMENT OPPORTUNITY LAWS

Employment discrimination laws seek to prevent discrimination based on gender, age, race, religion, handicap or physical disability, pregnancy, and national origin. In addition, there is a growing body of law preventing or occasionally justifying employment discrimination based on sexual orientation. Discrimination practices include bias in hiring, promotion, job assignment, termination, compensation, and various types of harassment. The main body of employment

TABLE 13.1 Selected Federal Labor Legislation

- Wagner Act; National Labor Act of 1935: established multiple rights concerning unionization and created the National Labor Relations Board
- Fair Labor Standards Act of 1938: established minimum wages and maximum hours of employment
- Federal Tort Claims Act of 1946: permitted the U.S. government to be sued by its employees
- Taft-Hartley Act of 1947: established a more equal balance of power between unions and management
- Executive Order 10988 (1062): allowed public employees to join unions
- Equal Pay Act of 1963: made it illegal to pay lower wages to employees based solely on gender
- Civil Rights Act of 1964: protected against discrimination due to age, race, color, gender, or national origin
- Age Discrimination Act of 1967: made it illegal for employers to discriminate against older men and women in employment practices
- Occupational Safety and Health Act of 1970: established the development and enforcement of standards for occupational health and safety
- Rehabilitation Act of 1973: afforded protection to handicapped employees
- Wagner Amendments (1974): allowed nonprofit organizations to join unions and allowed collective bargaining in nursing
- Federal False Claims Act of 1986: granted protection for whistleblowers on the federal level
- Americans with Disabilities Act of 1990: prevented discrimination against disabled individuals in the workplace (these laws are discussed in depth in Chapter 16)
- Civil Rights Act of 1991: addressed sexual harrassment in the workplace and overrode and/or modified previous legislation in this area
- Family and Medical Leave Act of 1993: allowed men and women medical leave from their employment to care for a child, spouse, or parent with a serious medical condition, and for the birth or adoption of a child

discrimination laws is composed of federal and state statutes. Additionally, the U.S. Constitution and some state constitutions provide protection when an employer is a governmental body or the government has taken significant steps to foster the discriminatory practice of the employer. Employment discrimination laws are enforced by the **Equal Employment Opportunity Commission (EEOC)**. Additionally, states have enacted statutes that address employment opportunities, and the nurse-manager should consider both when hiring and assigning nursing employees.

The most significant legislation affecting equal employment opportunities today is the amended **Civil Rights Act of 1964** (43 Federal Register, 1978), part of the Nineteenth Century Civil Rights Act. Section 703(a) of Title VII makes it illegal for an employer "to refuse to hire, discharge an individual, or otherwise to discriminate against an individual, with respect to his compensation, terms, conditions, or privileges of employment because of the individual's race, color, religion, sex, or national origin." Title VII was also amended by the **Equal Employment Opportunity Act of 1972** so that it applies to private institutions with 15 or more employees, state and local governments, labor unions, and employment agencies.

In 1991, the amended Civil Rights Act was signed into law. This act further broadened the issue of sexual harassment in the workplace and supersedes many of the sections of Title VII. Sections of the new law define sexual harassment, its elements, and the employer's responsibilities for harassment in the workplace, especially prevention and corrective action.

The Civil Rights Act is enforced by the EEOC as created in the 1964 act; its powers were broadened in the Equal Employment Opportunity Act of 1972. The primary activity of the EEOC is processing complaints of employment discrimination. There are three phases: investigation, conciliation, and litigation. Investigation focuses on determining whether on not Title VII has been violated by the employer. If the EEOC finds "probable cause," an attempt is made to reach an agreement or conciliation between the EEOC, the complainant, and the employer. If conciliation fails, the EEOC may file suit against the employer in federal court or issue to the complainant the right to sue for discrimination.

The EEOC also promulgated written rules and regulations that reflect its interpretation of the laws under its auspices. Included in these written rules and regulations are those relating to staffing practices and to sexual harassment in the workplace. The EEOC defines sexual harassment broadly, which has generally been upheld in the courts. Nurse-managers must realize it is the duty of employers (management) to prevent employees from sexually harassing other employees. The EEOC issues policies and practices for employers to implement to both sensitize employees to this problem and to prevent its occurrence; nurse-managers should be aware of these policies and practices and seek guidance in implementing them if sexual harassment occurs in their units. Additional information regarding this cause of action may be found in Chapter 16.

Cases filed alleging gender discrimination include *Auston v. Schubnell* (1997), *Bair v. Colonial Plaza* (2008), *Harwood v. Avalon Care Center* (2006), *Memisevich v. St. Elizabeth's Medical Center* (2006), and *Robertson v. Total Renal Care* (2003). In *Auston,* the court found that a male nurse could file a gender discrimination lawsuit, because male nurses are members of a protected class of persons. To succeed with a discrimination case, a male nurse must show that similarly situated female nurses were treated more favorably than he was. Even if differential treatment of a member of a protected class can be shown, the employer still has the option to try to convince the court that there is a legitimate nondiscriminatory reason for the employer's actions. In this case, 53 female nurses and this 1 male nurse lost their weekend "Baylor" positions when the hospital decided to phase out the "Baylor" positions as part of a cost-containment measure. "Baylor" positions allowed nurses to work 24 hours every weekend and receive full-time benefits.

In *Bair,* the court upheld the male nurse's gender discrimination lawsuit. This male nursing aide was hired for the night shift in a nursing home; during the day he worked as a waiter. He was abruptly reassigned to the day shift, told to quit his work as a waiter, and his salary was reduced because of reassignment to days. He was also informed that he could not work in the nursing home during the evening and night shifts because the facility had initiated a new policy that prohibited male nurses working either the evening or night shifts. The rationale for this policy was a potential fear of sexual assaults to female patients by male caregivers during the late hours.

The nursing assistant worked the day shift for a short period of time and then quit. He filed suit against the facility for gender discrimination and the court agreed. The nursing home's policy was discriminatory on its face, casting male caregivers as potential sexual predators based solely on their gender. This discrimination created a hostile work environment and the former nursing aide was entitled to damages.

Contrast this last case with the cases of *Robertson* and *Harwood.* In *Robertson,* a male nurse was dismissed after disputing with his employer about the on-call schedule for a renal dialysis unit. Restating that he could sue as a member of a minority class under civil rights laws, the court concluded that he had acted in an unprofessional manner as compared to his female co-workers when notified of on-call assignments he did not want. Robertson was prone to calling in the day before he was scheduled to be on call, sometimes leaving the facility with no on-call nurse. Other nurses in the unit complained when the on-call schedules were first posted, found a replacement, or consented to be on call even when they did not want to be on call. In *Harwood,* the court noted that merely stating discrimination is not sufficient. The alleged victim must show that detailed particulars of a nonminority's infraction were identical to his in all essential respects and that different outcomes occurred, or there is no valid basis for comparison of the outcomes.

Finally, in *Memisivech*, a Bosnian male nurse alleged that he was dismissed from his current nursing position because of his gender and nationality. Though the court agreed that he could file a discrimination lawsuit, he also had the burden of showing how these two factors influenced his dismissal. Like any other alleged victim, said the court, he must show that he was qualified for the position he held. In this case, the nurse had seven documented patient care errors against him during his probationary period, including two errors that posed serious patient safety issues that would justify terminating any nurse. Based on his performance record, the court determined that he was not qualified for this nursing position and thus was not eligible to sue for discrimination.

Lawsuits may be filed alleging race or national origin discrimination. Courts have held that to prevail in this type of discrimination suit the minority employee must be able to show that he or she has somehow been treated differently than a nonminority employee was treated, resulting in less harsh disciplinary action on the part of the nonminority employee (*Chambers v. Principi*, 2006; *Cone v. Health Management Association, Inc.*, 2007; *D'Cunha v. New York Hospital Medical Center of Queens*, 2006; *Dickinson v. Springhill Hospitals, Inc.*, 2006; *Hatchett v. Health Care and Retirement Corporation*, 2006; *Johnson v. Bryson*, 2007; *Williams v. Bala Retirement and Nursing Center*, 2007). For example, in *Johnson*, an African American aide was not able to show the court that she was meeting the employer's legitimate expectations. Her disciplinary write-ups were basically the same during the time she was working on a unit with an African American supervisor as when she worked on a unit with a Caucasian supervisor. Additionally, the aide could not point to a specific nonminority employee who, having been counseled for the same disciplinary offenses, received more favorable treatment than this aide had received.

Cone appears to begin to impose a slightly different standard in these cases. This case involved an African American nurse who applied for a transfer from a unit on which she worked as a staff nurse on the night shift to a unit where she would be working as a case manager on the day shift. The day-shift position was awarded to a Caucasian nurse who was less qualified and had 2 years less nursing experience than did Cone. In its defense, the hospital noted that the position was given to the nurse who demonstrated the most interest and enthusiasm for the position and whose interview showed more confidence and authority.

In its finding, the court noted that part of its responsibility is to decide if the legitimate, nondiscriminatory reason the employer has offered is really legitimate and nondiscriminatory or merely a pretext for discrimination. This court appears to be one of the first to acknowledge that it does not second-guess the employer's reasoning process, but instead looks to see if the reason the employer has proposed is "unworthy of credence." Only if the employer's explanation is inherently unbelievable will the court dismiss that reasoning and find that discrimination has occurred.

Two additional cases are worthy of note. In *D'Cunha*, two nurses were disciplined when a laporatomy sponge was inadvertently left in a patient, requiring a second surgery for its removal. The registered nurse of Asian Indian descent was dismissed by the facility and the Caucasian nurse was reprimanded, but not dismissed. In its defense, the facility noted that the minority nurse refused to take any responsibility for the occurrence and had three prior operating room errors that involved the safety of a patient. The Caucasian nurse willingly took responsibility for her involvement in the error and had no prior infractions. Thus, the facility acknowledged that they were treated differently, but not because of their race.

Hatchett concerned the issue of equality of pay for a minority nurse. An African American nurse who worked as the night-shift nursing manager earned $2 less per hour than did her

Caucasian, day-shift counterpart. Both nurses had approximately the same educational backgrounds and years of experience. They had the same job title and, at least on paper, the same responsibilities and authority. However, the day-shift manager had a much larger staff to supervise, addressed customer-service issues, admitted and discharged patients, and was required to serve on a variety of committees, including quality assurance committees and patient care conferences. Her counterpart supervised a much smaller staff and completed a patient-census form. Thus, the court held that the pay differential could be justified on nondiscriminatory grounds.

Lawrence v. University of Texas Medical Branch at Galveston (1999) and *Piskorek v. Department of Human Services* (2003) both present examples of reverse discrimination lawsuits. In *Lawrence,* two candidates applied for the same position, and the facility awarded the position to the minority candidate. While conceding that Caucasian nurses may sue for reverse discrimination, the facts of the case did not support such a conclusion. The minority candidate hired for the position had superior qualification for the position and thus was the better candidate.

In *Piskorek,* a racially biased remark was made by an African American nurse that caused Piskorek to believe that the nursing supervisor was prejudiced against her and that, because of this prejudice, Piskorek was not reinstated following a medical leave. However, the court noted that to show racial discrimination, the remark must have been made by someone who is an employment decision maker. In this case, the individual making the remark could not and did not decide about the nurse's reinstatement. That decision was made by the director of human resources and was based solely on Piskorek's physician's written statement.

An area of the law that is emerging concerns discrimination involving the mandating of specific languages that may or may not be spoken in health care settings. For example, in *Equal Employment Opportunity Commission v. William O. Benson Rehabilitation Pavilion* (2007), the EEOC obtained a combined settlement of $900,000 for a case filed on behalf of a group of Jamaican nursing home employees who were not permitted to speak their native Creole language in the facility. Other national minorities who worked in this facility were allowed to converse among themselves in their own national language.

There may be circumstances that mandate the use of a given language in health care settings. For example, the court in *Montes v. Vail Clinic, Inc.* (2007) ruled that clear and precise communication was essential in the operating room environment between nurses, who primarily did not speak Spanish, and the housekeeping staff, who primarily spoke Spanish as their first language. Maintaining sanitary conditions in this arena was of paramount importance to the hospital's operations and to the health and safety of patients. Quick and efficient cleaning and turnaround of the operating suites are legitimate business considerations for a surgical facility. Thus, the court noted it was not discrimination to mandate English only in the surgical department and only for job-related discussions. Spanish-speaking employees were allowed to speak in Spanish during their breaks and while conversing on the job about non-job-related topics. The ruling in *Barber v. Lovelace Sandia Health Systems* (2005) was similar. It is discriminatory and unlawful for employers to prevent minority members from speaking to one another in their native national language if they so choose unless the employees are notified in advance of their employers' legitimate expectations for use of English in job-related conversations.

Individuals have brought suit for religious discrimination (*El-Sioufi v. St. Peter's University Hospital,* 2005; *Howard v. Life Care Centers,* 2007; *Morrissette-Brown v. Mobile Infirmary Medical Center,* 2007; *Nead v. Eastern Illinois University,* 2006; *Praigrod v. St. Mary's Medical Center,* 2007). In

El-Sioufi, an Islamic nurse sued because of an anti-Islamic comment made by a nursing supervisor. The Islamic nurse also objected to working on Christmas, claiming that it was discrimination to force a non-Christian to work on a religious holiday so that a Christian would not have to work that day.

In addressing these issues, the court noted that the following four questions must be answered with a "yes" for a legitimate discriminatory lawsuit to go forward:

1. Does the employee belong to a minority group?
2. Was the employee performing the job at a level that met the employer's legitimate expectations?
3. Did the employee suffer an adverse employment action?
4. Did other employees, nonmembers of the same minority group, not suffer similar adverse employment action? (*El-Sioufi v. St. Peter's Hospital,* 2005, at 1178)

In this case, the court noted that the supervisor had apologized when confronted by the Islamic nurse. Additionally, the court ruled that it is not religious discrimination to expect an employee to work on a day that has religious significance to others but does not have significance to the employee in question.

Howard and *Morrissette-Brown* concerned individuals whose religion precluded their working on Saturdays. In both cases, the health care facilities offered reasonable accommodations to working on Saturdays, including allowing the individual to trade shifts with other workers, using seniority to request a Saturday as the scheduled day off, and offering to re-train an employee so that she could be part of the flex-CNA system. Both courts noted that the employers' obligations were to offer reasonable accommodation, communicate with the employee to discover exactly what the employee is requesting, and offer a solution that is reasonable to both sides of the controversy. Both courts also held that the law does not subordinate one employee's desire to have weekends off for whatever reason to another employee's desire to adhere to his or her religious beliefs and practices.

In *Praigrod,* a nurse was excluded from consideration for a nursing position because she did not have relevant clinical experience, while other non-Jewish nurses who also lacked relevant clinical nursing experience were hired for the same types of nursing positions. The court held that if a person who qualifies as a minority is treated differently than others, the employer must be prepared to explain why or discrimination is presumed.

The issue in *Nead* concerned a nurse's belief that life begins at conception and that she could not distribute emergency contraception ("morning-after pills") to students in a university health care center. She was thus bypassed for possible promotion and sued, alleging religious discrimination. The court in this case noted that to avoid liability for religious discrimination the employer would need to show that accommodating the employee's religious beliefs would impose an undue hardship on the employer, noting that such undue hardship usually occurs with employee's requests to be absent for nontraditional religious days and observances. The court upheld Nead's discrimination lawsuit, as there was no evidence presented that the employer would suffer hardships if this nurse did not have to dispense emergency contraception. Other personnel in the facility could dispense the emergency contraception as needed.

Discrimination suits can center on veterans' rights. *Tarin v. County of Los Angeles* (1997) involved a lawsuit brought by a nurse who had been called up for active duty during Desert Storm. She was then restored to her former civilian nursing position as required by the Veterans Reemployment Rights Act. The nurse later filed an application for promotion to a more desirable nursing position. Following an unfairly low performance rating on the required evaluation for the promotion, the nurse brought suit claiming discrimination. At trial, she was able to show that the supervisor completing the evaluation gave the low scores because she was angry about the nurse's being absent during her military service and thus gave no credit for her performance while in the military. The court held that this nurse had a valid discrimination suit.

A final potential source of discrimination occurs with the pregnant worker. In *Center for Behavioral Health, Rhode Island, Inc. v. Barros* (1998), the court held that it is unlawful for an employer to discriminate against an employee on the basis of gender and that basis of gender includes pregnancy, childbirth, and other related medical conditions. In this case, the nurse's progressive disciplinary process changed drastically after she informed her supervisor she was pregnant. The court concluded that the abrupt change in how these matters were handled after she became pregnant could support only one conclusion: She was a victim of discrimination. This right to be free from unequal treatment was also supported by the court in *Duncan v. Children's National Medical Center* (1997). The burden of proof, though, remains on the individual bringing the lawsuit to show that the motive for discriminating against a pregnant worker is due to the pregnancy and not to any other legitimate factors (*Brittain v. Family Care Services, Inc.* 2001; *Wallace v. Methodist Hospital System,* 2001).

Employers may seek exceptions to Title VII on a number of bases. For example, it is lawful to make employment decisions on the basis of national origin, religion, and gender (never race or color) if such decisions are necessary for the normal operation of the business, though the courts have viewed this exception very narrowly. The U.S. District Court for the Southern District of Florida upheld the right of a hospital to create a "women-friendly" environment in the obstetrical/gynecological unit without inferring that the hospital discriminates against male nurses (*Wheatley v. Baptist Hospital of Miami, Inc.,* 1998). Promotions and layoffs based on bona fide seniority or merit systems are also permissible (*Firefighters Local 1784 v. Scotts,* 1984), as are exceptions based on business necessity (*Herrero v. St. Louis University Hospital,* 1997).

In *Herrero,* a 63-year-old woman of Filipino origin was terminated due to the elimination of her position. She sued for employment discrimination, but the court could find no evidence that her termination was based on race, nationality, age, or gender discrimination. Rather, the court said, this was a bona fide reduction of force, based on economic necessity and guided by business judgment. The layoffs were based strictly on job classification, employment status, prior job experience, seniority, and licensure and/or certification.

A final option for persons who have endured intolerable conditions at work caused by illegal acts of discrimination is to resign. Once the individual has resigned, he or she may file a claim of **constructive discharge.** To claim constructive discharge, the employee must show that the employer deliberately created intolerable working conditions with the intention of forcing the employee to quit. Courts do not give the benefit of the doubt to employees who are unreasonably sensitive to their working conditions. Constructive discharge occurs only when a reasonable employee would find the conditions intolerable. An employee who is scrutinized and reprimanded more than others does not have unreasonable working conditions, merely because the job is less enjoyable and the employee experiences added stress (*French v. Eagle Nursing Home, Inc.,* 1997).

Note, though, that being offered a night shift rather than the day shift on returning to work after an approved leave could open the door for a constructive discharge cause of action (*Hunt v. Rapides Healthcare System, LLC,* 2001). In that case, the nurse returned after a 12-week leave, which was allowed by the Family and Medical Leave Act. Explicit in that law is the fact that the employee returning from leave is entitled to return to the same position that he or she enjoyed prior to taking the leave. This court specifically noted that a night-shift position is not equivalent to a day-shift position.

Courts allow suits under a constructive discharge cause of action very judiciously. In *Yearous v. Niobrara County Memorial Hospital* (1997), the court defined intolerable conditions as working conditions that, when viewed objectively, are so difficult a reasonable person would feel compelled to resign. In other words, the employee must have absolutely no other choice but to quit. In this case, the court found that the hospital had used questionable judgment in hiring a new director, but that the nurses had also exercised questionable judgment by taking an inflexible "either she goes or we go" stance. When the nurses resigned, there was still the option of whether or not to leave the employment position; the hospital board was requesting that they rescind their resignations, pledging that the board would try to resolve the problems within internal channels. Thus, they were not constructively discharged.

EXERCISE 13.3

A Caucasian female of Russian descent was terminated from her employment as a staff nurse in an acute care hospital. She filed a discrimination lawsuit stating that she had frequently been harassed and discriminated against by her supervisor, a Caucasian nurse of Norwegian descent. The nurse alleged that this supervisor had announced during a staff meeting that there were too many Russian-speaking patients and nurses and that this would "have to change." Eventually all the Russian-speaking nurses in the unit were replaced by nurses who did not speak Russian.

How do you think the court would rule in such a case? If this is a successful discrimination lawsuit by the terminated nurse, is this a natural-origin discrimination suit or one that more correctly relates to race and color? Is the distinction important? Is it important that both the nurse claiming discrimination and the nurse who allegedly committed the discrimination were both Caucasian?

FEDERAL TORTS CLAIMS ACT OF 1946

The **Federal Tort Claims Act of 1946** was enacted to allow patients and persons with claims against federal workers to be able to sue the U.S. government. Prior to that time, the government was immune, even if negligent actions of its employees caused injury or loss of property to non-governmental individuals. Based on this law, the government is substituted as the defendant in civil actions filed to recover damages against federal employees, and the Federal Tort Claims Act is the sole remedy available to a patient injured by a federal employee providing health care.

Under this act, the court first establishes whether the individual was an employee or an independent contractor with the government. This is done because greater liability exposure occurs with employees than with independent contractors. For example, in *Broussard v. United States* (1993), the court held that no negligence had occurred on the part of the defendant because the physician was an independent contractor at the time of the injury. There was a contract between the government facility and the physicians that the physicians would assume full responsibility and accountability for their own actions. In *Bird v. United States* (1991), the ruling had been just the opposite, and a nurse anesthetist was considered a government employee because the nurse was under the same control and supervision as a regularly employed governmental employee.

AGE DISCRIMINATION IN EMPLOYMENT ACT OF 1967

The outcome of the **Age Discrimination in Employment Act of 1967** was that it became illegal for employers, unions, and employment agencies to discriminate against older men and women. The prohibited practices are nearly identical to those outlined in Title VII of the Civil Rights Act. The Age Discrimination in Employment Act of 1967, in a 1986 amendment, prohibits discrimination against individuals over the age of 40. The practical outcome of this act has been that mandatory retirement is no longer seen in the American workplace.

Some of the practices prohibited under the Age Discrimination in Employment Act include placing older nurses in positions that are being phased out merely as a means of easing the worker out of a job and forcing older workers to waive their rights as part of a termination program. Termination programs include early retirement and reduction-in-force efforts. Waivers were part of the amendments to the Age Discrimination in Employment Act. Known as the Older Workers Benefit Protection Act, this act mandates that waivers must be written in such a manner that employees understand their options and that employees are given 21 days to decide whether to sign the waiver or decline.

As with Title VII, there are some exceptions to this act. Reasonable factors, other than age, may be used when terminations become necessary. Such reasonable factors could be a performance evaluation system and some limited occupational qualifications, such as tedious physical demands of a specific job. Reasonable factors could also entail negative comments that a worker expresses in an exit interview (*Weigel v. Baptist Hospital,* 2002). In that case, a 56-year-old nurse complained about preferential treatment for younger nurses in shift assignments and leave requests. She subsequently resigned and, on the exit interview form, voiced multiple complaints about her dissatisfaction with her working conditions. Later she reapplied at the same facility and was denied a position as a per-diem nurse. The court ruled that her negative exit comments were a valid, nondiscriminatory basis for the hospital's failure to rehire her.

As the nursing community ages (the current average age of the employed registered nurse in the United States is 46.8 years [Health Resources and Services Administration, 2007]), the number of age discrimination cases may well rise. This is especially true as the health care industry continues to downsize and employ more cost-cutting measures. A case example in this area of the law is *Scanlon v. Jeanes Hospital* (2007). In that case a registered nurse with an exemplary record of service had been employed at the same hospital for 37 years. She was abruptly fired over a written complaint filed by a nursing assistant, stating that the nurse had mistreated an obstetrical patient who had a miscarriage. Sixty-one years of age at the time of her dismissal, the nurse sued her formed employer for age discrimination.

Evidence that was discovered during the trial showed that the hospital had made no investigation of the complaint and that the aide's report was taken at face value even though this same aide had previously reported others rather than taking accountability for her own errors and omissions. No other nurses were questioned or interviewed and, contrary to the hospital's policy, the nurse was not given the opportunity for a hearing in which she was entitled to legal representation. The court entered a $256,800 judgment for the nurse, noting that arbitrary action against a person in the 40- to 70-year-old age category is assumed to be discriminatory unless the employer can show that the substance and process were fair. The court further noted that, given the lack of supporting evidence, the only rational explanation for the nurse's dismissal was age discrimination.

In cases that support an employer's actions, the court will uphold the employer's right to terminate or alter a job classification of an employee who is 40 to 70 years of age. Two recent cases exemplify this concept. In *Stephens v. Kettering Adventist Healthcare* (2006), a 60-year-old nurse was mistreating patients in a neonatal unit. The nurse manager and the human resources representative obtained the written statements of six nurses in the unit who had witnessed the abuse. The nurse in question was informed that there was an investigation underway and that she could name any witness to dispute the allegations being made. Unable to produce witnesses supporting her innocence, she was fired, and two part-time nurses, both in their 20s and 30s were hired. The court upheld the dismissal, noting that the nurse's incidents of patient abuse had been fully investigated and well documented and that she had only met three of the four criteria for a successful age discrimination lawsuit:

1. Be 40 to 70 years old.
2. Perform job responsibilities according the employer's expectations.
3. Be discharged.
4. Be replaced by a substantially younger person.

A second case example, *Robinson v. CARES Surgicenter* (2008), concerned an older surgical nurse who requested a transfer to a desk job from her current job, which required a considerable amount of standing during the day. The request was granted, but with a $5.95 per hour pay reduction, based on the facility's standard pay rate for pre-admission testing versus perioperative nurses. The nurse filed a lawsuit for age discrimination.

The court ruled in favor of the facility, noting that the crux of any discrimination suit is to examine comparisons between the alleged victim and other employees in similar situations or as similar as can be found. Upon examination of the pay scales and seniority of the nurses within the facility, the court determined that the nurse in question was still earning more than other comparable nurses in the facility.

REHABILITATION ACT OF 1973

The purpose of the **Rehabilitation Act of 1973** is "to promote and expand employment opportunities in the public and private sectors for handicapped individuals," through affirmative action programs and the elimination of discrimination. Employers covered by the act include agencies of the federal government and employers receiving federal contracts in excess of $2,500 or federal financial assistance. The Department of Labor enforces Section 793 of the act, which refers to employment under federal contracts, and the Department of Justice enforces Section 794 of the act, which refers to organizations receiving federal assistance. The EEOC enforces the act against federal employees, and individual federal agencies promulgate regulations pertaining to the employment of the disabled.

AFFIRMATIVE ACTION

The policy of **affirmative action** (AA) differs from the policy of equal employment opportunity (EEO). Centers for affirmative action enhance employment opportunities of protected groups of people, whereas EEO is concerned with using employment practices that do not discriminate against or impair the employment opportunities of protected groups. Thus, AA can be seen in conjunction with several federal employment laws. For example, in conjunction with the Vietnam Era Veteran's Readjustment Act of 1974, AA requires that employers with government contracts take steps to enhance the employment opportunities of disabled veterans and other veterans of the Vietnam era.

The United States Fair Labor Standards Act of 1938, better known as the FLSA (FLSA, 1938), was one of the first laws established to govern national minimum wage, provide time-and-a-half for overtime in certain job classifications, and prohibit child labor abuse. The **Equal Pay Act** of 1963, an outgrowth of the original 1938 law, makes it illegal to pay lower wages to employees of one gender when the jobs:

1. Require equal skill in experience, training, education, and ability.
2. Require equal effort in mental or physical exertion.

3. Are of equal responsibility and accountability.

4. Are performed under similar working conditions (at 56).

Courts have held that unequal pay may be legal if based on seniority, merit, incentive systems, and a factor other than gender. Though the primary cases filed under this law in the area of nursing have been by nonprofessionals, a newer case involves the equal pay of nurse practitioners and physicians assistants in *Beck-Wilson v. Principi* (2006). Though not yet a definitive ruling for nurse practitioners, the case has been remanded back to the trial level on the finding that the federal district court judge was wrong in granting a summary judgment without giving the nurse practitioners a chance to plead their full case. The question in the case concerned the unequal pay between the predominately male physician assistants and the predominately female nurse practitioners.

Cases that concern nurses filed under FLSA generally involve issues regarding the qualification of nurses for overtime pay and the classification of nurses who are eligible for overtime pay. For example, *Belt v. EmCare, Inc.* (2006) concerned the overtime pay of hourly nurse practitioners, and this court ruled that because these nurse practitioners were not "practicing medicine," they were entitled to overtime pay. *Rawls v. Augustine Home Health Care, Inc.* (2007) and *Bergman v. Private Care, Inc.* (2008) concerned whether employees in domestic service who provided companionship services for individuals who were unable to care for themselves were also eligible for overtime pay. Noting that the act provides an exception for such services performed in clients' private homes, the court remanded the case back to the trial level to address specifically the levels of care provided by this corporation and to determine where progressive levels of assisted living cease to be private dwellings and become more of an institutional setting. *Barfield v. New York City Health and Hospitals Corporation* (2006) extended the right for overtime pay to agency nurses.

OCCUPATIONAL SAFETY AND HEALTH ACT

The **Occupational Safety and Health Act of 1970 (OSHA)** was enacted to assure that healthful and safe working conditions would exist in the workplace. Among other provisions, the law requires isolation procedures, the placarding of areas containing ionizing radiation, proper grounding of electrical equipment, protective storage of flammable and combustible liquids, and now the gloving of all personnel when handling bodily fluids. The statute provides that if no federal standard has been established, state statutes prevail. Nurse-managers should know the relevant OSHA laws for the institution and their specific area. Frequent review of new additions to the law must also be undertaken. Newer updates are occurring in the areas of Methicillin-resistant *Staphylococcus aureas* (MRSA), personal protective equipment, latex allergy, sonography, combustible dust, and occupational exposure to chlorinated solvents. Sonography identifies ergonomic factors, offering a variety of possible solutions for the safer movement and positioning of patients.

Violence in the workplace is an issue that OSHA continues to address in its rules. Violence is perhaps the greatest hidden health and safety threat in the workplace today, and nurses, as the largest group of health care professionals, are most at risk of assault at work. In 1996, the Occupational Safety and Health Administration developed voluntary guidelines to protect health care workers and consumers; these voluntary guidelines are still in effect today. Twenty-four states, Puerto Rico, and the Virgin Islands have now adopted their own standards and enforcement policies, with the majority of these standards and policies being identical to the federal guidelines.

The OSHA laws guarantee all workers the right to a "safe and healthful workplace." This may be accomplished through the use of written policies, employee education and training, proper staffing levels, and follow-up of incident reports. Employers may be penalized if they fail to reduce the potential for workplace violence. Measures that nurses may take in this area include the following:

1. Participate in or initiate regular workplace assessments, identifying unsafe areas and potential hazards. Factors that are known to contribute to assaultive behavior include inadequate staffing, invasion of personal space, seclusion or restraint activities, and lack of experienced staff members.
2. Work with management to make necessary changes, monitor incidents, and determine if control measures are effective. Possible actions include scheduling experienced clinicians on each shift, educating staff to deal with escalating violence, enforcing wearing of proper identification by staff members, and developing a buddy system when working with patients/family members who are known to react violently.
3. Be alert for potential violence and suspicious behavior and report it immediately.
4. Assess patients for their potential for violence, especially if they have known histories of violent behavior.
5. Be supportive of colleagues who encounter workplace violence. Ensure that they report all incidents and receive necessary treatment, including counseling.
6. Encourage co-workers to address violence in their personal lives and conflict in the workplace.

An issue that OSHA has not yet addressed, but that nursing is now addressing in depth, is the issue of safe patient handling, preventing injury to health care workers while ensuring that patients are protected as they are transferred/moved in health care settings. The American Nurse Association's (ANA) data show that more than 52% of nurses complain of chronic back pain, 12% leave the profession while citing chronic back pain as the determining factor for their leaving, and 20% transfer to a different unit, out of direct patient care or other employment settings, because of back pain, neck, and shoulder injuries (McPeck, 2006). Given these data and recognizing that there simply is no safe manual patient lifting, the ANA promotes legislation that would require hospitals and other health care institutions to develop programs to prevent work-related musculoskeletal disorders and eliminate manual patient lifting. Toward this end, 10 states have now passed legislation and an additional 8 states have introduced legislation that mandates health care facilities provide the needed equipment and education for a total no-lift policy. It is hoped that the momentum now in place will lead to federal laws that would require mechanical lifting equipment and friction-reducing devices for all health care workers, patients, and residents across all health care settings.

EMPLOYMENT-AT-WILL AND WRONGFUL DISCHARGE

Historically, the employment relationship has been considered as a "free will" relationship. Employees are free to take or not take a job at will, and employers are free to hire, retain, or discharge employees for any reason. Recent case examples in which courts have upheld the termination of employees include *Davis v. Department of Veterans Affairs* (2006), *Odie v. Department of Employment Security* (2007), and *White v. Fort Sanders-Park West Medical Center* (2007). In each of these cases, termination for cause was ruled justifiable when the employee violated a work rule or employer policy.

Over the past several decades, there has been a growing trend toward a restricted application of the at-will employment rule. Many laws, some federal but predominantly state, have been slowly eroding this at-will employment. Evolving case law provides at least three exceptions to the broad doctrine of **employment-at-will.**

These three exceptions are:

1. The public policy exception
2. Implied contracts and the concept of wrongful discharge
3. The "good faith and fair dealing" exception

The first exception is a public policy exception. Public policy favors the exposure of crime, and the cooperation of citizens who possess direct knowledge of those crimes is essential in the effective implementation of that policy. This exception involves cases in which an employee is discharged in direct conflict with established public policy. Examples of such discharge include discharging an employee for serving on a jury, for reporting an employer's illegal actions (better known as *whistleblowing*), and for filing a workers' compensation claim.

Several cases attest to the number of terminations for retaliation causes of action against health care employees. Often called *whistleblowing cases,* the health care workers are terminated for speaking out about unsafe practices and violations of federal laws and for filing lawsuits against employers. Whistleblowing may be defined as the act of someone, believing that public interest overrides the interest of the organization he or she serves, who publicly exposes the organization for its involvement in corrupt, illegal, fraudulent, or harmful activity (Annotations, 1999). The term *whistleblower* actually derives from the practice of English bobbies (policemen), who would blow their whistle when they noticed the commission of a crime.

Essentially, a **whistleblower law** states that no employer can discharge, threaten, or discriminate against any employee regarding compensation, terms, conditions, location, or privileges of employment because the employee in good faith reported or caused to be reported, verbally or in writing, what the employee had a reasonable cause to believe was a violation of a law, rule, or regulation of state or federal law. Most whistleblowers are internal—that is, they report misconduct to a fellow employee or supervisor within the agency. External whistleblowers are those who report misconduct to outside persons or entities. The employee does not have to cite a reference to any specific law in reporting what is or is believed to be illegal conduct. The whistleblower law extends to an employee who supports another employee who reports illegal conduct, because retaliation against a whistleblower is in itself an illegal action (*Appeal of Linn,* 2000). Individuals who are contemplating reporting violations of laws under a whistleblower law should be aware that although there is a federal whistleblower law, additional protections and regulations vary by state. Federally, individuals are protected under the United States **False Claims Act of 1986** (Federal False Claims Act, 1986), and 23 states currently have False Claim Acts. Consult an attorney, the nurse's union representative, or other knowledgeable source before taking action.

The court outlined the elements that must be shown in order to prevail in a successful whistleblower retaliation case. In *Taylor v. Memorial Health Systems, Inc.* (2000), the following criteria were outlined:

1. The whistleblower must disclose or threaten to disclose an allegation in writing and under oath to the appropriate state or federal agency.
2. The allegation must be about an activity, policy, or practice of the employer that is or was a violation of a state or federal law, rule, or regulation.
3. The employee must have given the employer written notification and a reasonable time to correct the problem/issue.
4. The employee must have suffered retaliation in the form of some actual harm (*Taylor v. Memorial Health System, Inc.,* 2000, at 757).

The nurse in *Taylor* had complained to hospital administration and then to state authorities that a male physician was fondling female patients in the examination rooms of the facility's emergency center and was examining female patients alone without a third person being present, as was the facility's written policy. Before reporting the sexual abuse of these patients to the state department, the nurse had first complained verbally and then in writing to all levels of the facility's administrative staff, including the supervisor in the emergency center. In retaliation, the facility reassigned the nurse to a different department, and reduced her from a full-time to a part-time employee so that she was not eligible for benefits and was unable to earn the money she needed to pay her bills.

Multiple whistleblower suits continue to be filed annually, including *Arends v. Extendicare Homes* (2008), *Berde v. North Shore* (2008), *Rohrbrough v. University of Colorado Hospital* (2007), *Salonga v. D & R RCH Corporation* (2008), *Skare v. Extendicare Health Services* (2008), *Stroli v. Board of Review* (2008), *Taylor v. Alterra Healthcare* (2007), *Thompson v. Merriman CCRC, Inc.* (2006), *Vanhook v. Britthaven* (2007), *Wendeln v. Beatrice Manor, Inc.* (2006), *Yonker v. Centers for Long Term Care* (2006), and *Young v. Trinity Hill Care Center* (2006). Some of the cases have supported the whistleblower's retaliation claims. For example, in *Wendeln,* the issue concerned the improper handling of vulnerable adults by paid caregivers. An aide had previously informed the nursing director and the administrator of a nursing home that another aide was not following the agency's rules regarding the safe transfer of elderly patients. Specifically, the other aide was transferring residents by herself, without the use of a gait belt or other safety device. She again reported this information to the staffing coordinator, who investigated the matter and reported the aide in question to the state department of health and human services.

Within the week after reporting the aide in question, the staff coordinator came in to find that the locks has been changed on her office and that she was to resign. The Supreme Court in Nebraska upheld her right to sue and endorsed a $79,000 verdict in her favor, holding that improper handling of vulnerable adults constitutes abuse and that nurses, physicians, and other health care workers have a duty to report such abuse. In reporting such abuse, they are protected by law from employer retaliation for performing their legal duty.

Arends supports the need to formally complain about actions that violate state or public laws prior to filing a cause of action for employer retaliation. In that case, the licensed practical nurse (LPN) was requested to complete patient care plans, as a possible state survey was to be conducted the following day. She was subsequently fired for alleged absenteeism, medication errors, and not completing the care plans as requested. When she was hired at another facility, the LPN learned that state nursing regulations in Minnesota mandated the responsibility for patient care plans to registered nurses, and the LPN filed a retaliation lawsuit against her former employer. The suit was dismissed, as the LPN had never complained to her supervisors about her assignment on the grounds that it was an illegal action.

Stroli reinforces the criterion that the whistleblower must take reasonable steps to resolve safety issues prior to resigning a position with the agency. In this case, a registered nurse worked for 20 years at a community blood bank as the trainer for phlebotomists and apheresis technicians. The nurse complained to her supervisor about safety conditions in the facility, specifically the increased number of trainees for whom she was responsible. At the time of her resignation, there were several complaints pending before the agency's quality assurance committee. Additionally, the court noted that the nurse never followed through in an effort to work out her grievances, nor had she voiced her discontent about the process for handling grievances with her supervisors. Finally, the safety issues she raised were incompliance with current state and federal regulations. The case reinforces the final criterion of *Taylor* (2000) in that the employee must suffer retaliation and not voluntarily resign.

Skare limits whistleblower retaliation protection if the whistleblower is employed in a position that requires him or her to expose unlawful behavior internally. In this case a nursing director of an extended care facility discouraged the admitting of a 900-pound patient, as the nursing director believed that the facility could not adequately care for such a patient. Later, she repeatedly reported regulatory and legal compliance problems to the management at her facility and she was requested to resign from the facility. The court ruled that she was not entitled to whistleblower protection, as her very job was to work with and report compliance issues internally.

Whistleblowers are not protected if complaints are made to other than the proper authorities and agencies. An aide in *Thompson* (2006) was dismissed after he was observed reading pornographic magazines at a nursing home. Shortly afterward, one of the female residents began clamping her legs together when bathed, a sign that other staff members took to indicate that she may have been sexually abused by the aide before his dismissal. An investigation was initiated and several of the night staff were issued corrective notices for failing to report signs of possible patient abuse to administrative personnel.

Shortly after this investigation, a family member of the suspected victim asked about the investigation and its outcome. The night charge nurse informed the family member that the policies and practices of the agency were wholly inadequate to deal with issues of patient abuse. The family member, understandably distressed, complained to management about these allegations.

The night nurse was dismissed and her dismissal was upheld by the Court of Appeals of Ohio, noting that the laws protecting whistleblowers are drafted expressly to protect good-faith reports of abuse to proper authorities and only to proper authorities. Disparaging comments to others about possible abuse are not protected by the law.

The court in *Rohrbough* appears to be beginning to restrict the rights of the whistleblower while giving greater latitude to employers. A prior 2006 United States Supreme Court ruling restricted the right of a public employee to claim free-speech protection under the First Amendment for speaking out on a subject of public concern that falls within the scope of the public employee's duties as a public employee. In *Rohrbrough,* the nurse claimed she was terminated for complaints to her superiors and for allegations she raised in occurrence reports and a report to an organ procurement agency related to inadequate staffing and various mix-ups in the transplant unit where she worked. The court determined that this nurse was speaking out not as a private citizen, but as an

EXERCISE 13.4

The director of nursing in a brain injury rehabilitation center heard complaints from her staff members that patients were not being released upon attainment of their treatment goals or upon the patients' requests for early discharge. After she spoke with management about these concerns, a directive came from the director of marketing and admissions that patients were to be kept in the facility for the entire 4-year period during which Medicare funding existed. The director was concerned that this was a violation of the law and could constitute Medicare fraud.

While attending a conference, the director spoke with the state director of the traumatic brain injury program. He confirmed her understanding that such patients should be released. She gave this information to her superiors when she returned from the conference and was dismissed within the month. In their defense, the facility stated it had dismissed the director for violating patient confidentiality by speaking to the state director rather than reporting her concerns to the state authorities.

How would you expect the court to rule in this case? Do the facts of this case constitute a valid whistleblower case? Why or why not? What are the nurse's ethical obligations in such a case? How do these obligations complement the nurse's legal responsibilities?

employee of the University of Colorado Hospital, a public institution. Thus her freedom of self-expression was limited because part of her duty as a public employee is to raise legitimate issues of public concern. Though other cases have not yet followed this line of reasoning, it would seem that at least one court is attempting to expand the advocacy role of professionals in the health care arena.

The second exception involves situations in which there is an implied contract and the concept of **wrongful discharge.** The courts have generally treated employee handbooks, company policies, and oral statements made at the time of employment as "framing the employment relationship" (*Toussaint v. Blue Cross and Blue Shield,* 1980). In that case, the court held that a statement in the company's policy handbook that stated an employee would be discharged only for "good cause" provided an enforceable contract between the employer and employee.

Courts will uphold the rights of employees who are discharged in violation of the hospital's policy. In *Chicarello v. Employment Security Division, Department of Labor* (1996), the court held that an employee has the right to expect an employer to follow its own employment policies for progressive discipline procedures. For example, the court pointed out, if an employee is to be warned for two unexcused absences and fired only after two warnings, the employee cannot be terminated any sooner than that time period for excessive absenteeism. Employees have the right to have the employer's job performance expectations known to them, the right to have unsatisfactory job performance pointed out, and the right to make necessary corrections before being subject to discipline. Then, and only then, can the employer terminate the employee. A similar finding occurred in *Mealand v. Eastern New Mexico Medical Center* (2001). In *Mealand,* the court held that disclaimers in handbooks stating that the handbook is not the basis for an employment contract will generally be disregarded by the courts.

Note, however, that the courts also enforce the policies presented in employee handbooks. In *Watkins v. Unemployment Compensation Board of Review* (1997), an employee was terminated for refusing to attend a counseling session. Under the guidelines in the employee handbook, an employee's attendance at such a session was mandatory. The employee walked out before his supervisor was finished speaking with him and was terminated. The court ruled that the firing was justified on grounds of willful insubordination.

Another case in this area of the law has an entirely different holding than *Toussaint,* though it does not appear to be changing this employment exception. In *Pavilascak v. Bridgeport Hospital* (1998), a licensed practical nurse accepted employment with the defendant hospital and received a copy of the employee handbook, acknowledging in writing that she had received the handbook. She worked in various units at the hospital over the next 5 years, with her final position as a scrub nurse in the operating area of the obstetrical unit. During her time at the facility, she received favorable performance evaluations, merit raises, and bonuses.

She was terminated in 1991 after two significant events. The first occurred when a laparotomy sponge was left inside a patient after a cesarean section. Both she and the circulating nurse received written warnings. The second event occurred when the nurse left the sterile environment of a cesarean section to prepare for another operation scheduled to take place shortly after the first operation. This, according to the nurse, was standard procedure for the hospital. She had been instructed to remain in the first operating area, but left to set up the second sterile field. She was then ordered to return to the first operating room, but, by the time she returned, the operation had been completed.

Three days after the second event, she received a written notice that she had breached accepted standards by leaving the first operation. According to the nurse, this written notice resulted from a personality conflict with her supervisor. She left on vacation and, when she returned, was notified that she had been terminated, effective immediately.

The licensed practical nurse sued the hospital, claiming breach of an express contract, breach of an implied contract, and negligent infliction of emotional distress. She also made a claim of promissory estoppel, claiming that she had been promised that she could not be discharged without cause, and that she had reasonably relied on that promise to her detriment, even though the hospital did not have a written contract with her. At trial level, the nurse prevailed on the grounds of promissory estoppel and negligent infliction of emotional distress. The hospital prevailed on the issue of alleged breach of an implied and expressed contract. Both sides appealed the ruling.

The appellate court ruled in favor of the hospital on all counts, rejecting the nurse's causes of action. The appellate court rejected the finding that the hospital had made a promise to the nurse upon which she reasonably relied. Since the hospital's manual permitted the hospital to discharge employees "with or without cause, at any time," it was illogical to infer that the hospital had made a "clear and definite promise that the nurse would have employment as long as she adequately or satisfactorily performed her job" (*Pavilascak v. Bridgeport Hospital*, 1998, at 585). A similar result occurred in *Tremlett v. Aurora Health Care, Inc.* (2002). Having a signed employment contract might have altered the outcome of these two cases. Contracts are discussed in greater detail in Chapter 14.

The third exception is a "good faith and fair dealing" exception. The purpose of this exception, which courts use sparingly, is to prevent unfair or malicious terminations. In *Fortune v. National Cash Register Company* (1977), an employee was discharged just before a final contract was signed between his employer and another company, for which the employee would have received a large commission. The court held that he was discharged, in bad faith, solely to prevent the paying of his commission by National Cash Register.

Nurses are urged to know their respective state law concerning this growing area of the law. Mid-level management nurses and those in higher management positions should also review institution documents, especially employee handbooks and recruiting brochures, for unwanted statements implying job security or other unintentional promises. Managers are also cautioned not to say anything during the preemployment negations and interviews that might be construed as implying job security or other unintentional promises to the potential employee.

EXERCISE 13.5

A nursing aide had worked in a skilled care facility for 17 years prior to be terminated by the facility. On the day she was terminated, she was working with approximately 25 residents in the day room, providing assistance as needed. Earlier that day, the aide had taken extra-strength Tylenol for a toothache. She would later testify that she believed it was this medication that made her drowsy and caused her to fall asleep while taking care of the residents. She fell asleep for approximately 10 to 20 minutes between the hours of 4 and 5 P.M.

A visitor woke her because a resident was screaming for help. The aide's reply was that that resident did that all the time, and the aide reassured the visitor that the resident's cries were nothing about which to worry, as it was the resident's habit to shout for help when nothing was wrong. The remark to the visitor was taken to mean that the aide thought it was all right for her to sleep while in the job, even if a resident needed assistance.

Following her termination, the aide sued for wrongful discharge. How would you expect the court to rule in the subsequent lawsuit? Do any of the exceptions to dismissal for cause apply to this case? If none of the exceptions apply, how would the circumstances need to be altered in order for the court to find that the aide was unlawfully discharged?

One of the best ways to reduce potential liability for wrongful discharge is to develop appropriate guidelines prior to hiring new employees. Avoiding pitfalls and implementing effective hiring practices are means of avoiding such lawsuits. The accompanying guidelines outline potential strategies for avoiding these pitfalls.

GUIDELINES

Effective Hiring Practices

1. Develop clear policies and procedures regarding the hiring, disciplining, and termination of employees. These policies and procedures should be readily available to all concerned parties. Ensure that individuals in management positions adhere to the policies and procedures.

2. Include in the policies and procedures the organization's right to add, delete, or revise the policies and procedures as outlined.

3. Review each applicant's background, work references, and verification of current licensure carefully before offering employment to the individual. Do not offer employment before these aspects are thoroughly considered.

4. Develop a two-tiered interview system for screening applicants. The first interview should be conducted by a member of the human resources department and the second interview by the supervisor of the department to which the applicant is applying.

5. Define clear personnel policies and procedures in an employee handbook and have each employee sign that he or she has received a copy of the handbook. Indicate on the signed form that the employee has received, read, and understood the employee handbook and individual job description.

6. Develop constructive performance evaluations that ensure continuation of desirable behaviors and provide instruction on areas requiring improvement. These performance evaluations should include a written statement regarding the employee's performance and be signed by the person doing the evaluation as well as the employee receiving the evaluation.

7. Develop and implement a progressive disciplinary action policy.

8. Provide in-service education programs for supervisors regarding employee interviews, evaluation, and discipline. If such programs are not available, ask the facility's administration to develop such programs.

COLLECTIVE BARGAINING

Collective bargaining, also called **labor relations,** regulated by the Collective Bargaining Act of 1974, is the joining together of employees for the purpose of increasing their ability to influence the employer and improve working conditions. Usually, the employer is referred to as *management,* and the employees, even professionals, are referred to as *labor.* Those persons involved in the hiring, firing, scheduling, disciplining, or evaluating of employees are considered management and may not be included in a collective bargaining unit. Those in management could form their own group but are not protected under these laws. Nurse-managers may or may not be part of management; if they have hiring and firing authority, then they are part of management.

Collective bargaining was also defined and protected by the 1935 **National Labor Relations Act (NLRA)** and its amendments. The National Labor Relations Board (NLRB) oversees the act and those who come under its auspices. The NLRB ensures that employees can choose freely whether they want to be represented by a particular bargaining unit, and it serves to prevent or remedy any violation of the labor laws.

Collective bargaining became a reality for nurses with enactment of the Employee-Management Cooperation in the Federal Service Executive Order (10988) in 1962 and the 1974 amendments to the Wagner Act. These two enactments made it possible for public employees and for nonprofit health care organizations to join collective bargaining units, respectively. The American Nurses Association has long supported the right of nurses to bargain collectively. Since 1946, the American Nurses Association, through its state constituent associations, has collectively represented the interests of nurses within the individual states. Two of the main reasons proposed for this support were:

1. Collective bargaining allows for achieving the basic elements of professional status.
2. Collective bargaining allows a mechanism for nurses to resolve conflicts within the workplace setting, thereby enhancing quality of care to patients.

Collective bargaining is a power strategy based on the premise of increased power in numbers. Collective bargaining assists in the following areas:

1. Basic economic issues as salary, shift differentials, overtime pay, length of the work day, vacation time, sick leave, lunch breaks, health insurance, and severance pay
2. Unfair or arbitrary treatment in scheduling, staffing, rotating shifts, on-call assignments, transfers, seniority rights, and posting of job openings
3. Maintenance and promotion of professional practice as acceptable standards of care, other quality of care issues, and adequate staffing ratios

Three issues against collective bargaining by professionals include the following: (a) charges of unprofessionalism, (b) unethical behavior especially when faced with a divisive strike situation, and (c) imperiled job security because of the concept of a closed shop in which everyone must join the union. Most health care unions are open shops, allowing nurses to either join the union or not. All of these issues have many sides that can be argued; many nurses now acknowledge that they have progressed because of collective bargaining and unionization.

GUIDELINES

Timetable for Calling a Strike

1. Make sure you are following the most recent federal guidelines; check the current status of the law before proceeding, and be sure to comply with all procedural requirements of the act.
2. The party wishing to end or modify a contract must notify the opposition 90 days prior to the contract expiration date.
3. If within 30 days of notification the two sides cannot agree, notification of the dispute must be given to the Federal Mediation and Conciliation Service and its corresponding state agency.
4. This federal agency will appoint a mediator within 30 days and, if needed, an inquiry board.

5. The mediator or inquiry board makes its recommendations within 15 days after appointment.
6. Fifteen days after the preceding recommendations, if the parties still cannot agree, the employees may plan to strike, and a strike vote by union members is conducted.
7. With the majority of employees voting to strike, the union must give 10 days' notice of the scheduled strike, giving to management the exact day, time, and place of the strike. (Note: No strike may be scheduled before the contract actually expires.)
8. In many states, public-sector employees are prohibited from striking. Binding arbitration is required to settle differences.

The process of unionization is a complex one. Table 13.2 highlights some of the terms used in unionization and collective bargaining. In the first phase, organizing, a labor organization called an *organizing council* is formed. During this pre-union organization, employers are not permitted to ban discussion about unions or to retaliate against a worker who is trying to organize a union. Generally, the worker has the right to talk about unions, to distribute union membership cards, and to pass out brochures, so long as this distribution is done on a worker's own time and in non-work areas such as the cafeteria, locker room, or parking lot. Employers have an obligation to provide the union with the names and addresses of workers who may be eligible to join the

TABLE 13.2	**Collective Bargaining Terms**
Arbitration	The terminal step in the grievance process during which an impartial third party attempts to come to a reasonable solution, taking into consideration both management and labor issues; may be either a voluntary or a government-enforced compulsory process; the third party has the final power of decision making in the dispute.
Closed shop	Synonymous with *union shop*; all employees must belong to the union and pay dues.
Collective bargaining	The relations between employers and labor; employers act through their management representatives, and labor acts through its union representatives.
Conciliation and mediation	These are synonymous terms describing the activity of a third party to assist the disputants in reaching an acceptable agreement; this individual has no final power of decision making, as does the arbitrator.
Free speech	Under Public Law 101, Section 8, the "expression of any views, argument, or dissemination thereof, whether in written, printed, graphic, or visual form, shall not constitute or be evident of unfair labor practice under any provision of this Act, if such expression contains no threat of reprisal or force or promise of benefit."
Grievance	Process undertaken when the perception exists on the part of a union member that management has failed in some way to meet the terms of the labor agreement.
Lockout	Consists of closing of a place of business by management in the course of a labor dispute for the purpose of forcing employees to accept management terms.

TABLE 13.2 Collective Bargaining Terms *Continued*	
National Labor Relations Board	Formed to implement the Wagner Act and serves to (1) determine the official bargaining unit when a new unit is formed and who should be in the unit and (2) adjudicate unfair labor changes.
Open shop	Also known as an agency shop; employees are not required to join a union, although they may if they so desire and one exists within the workplace.
Professionals	Have the right to be represented by a labor union; cannot belong to a union that also represents nonprofessionals, unless a majority of the professionals vote for inclusion into the nonprofessional unit.
Strike	A concerted withholding of labor supply in order to bring economic pressure upon management and force management to grant employee demands.
Supervisors	Those having the authority to hire, fire, transfer, and promote employees; supervisors are excluded from protection under the Taft-Hartley Act and cannot be represented by a union.
Union shop	Also known as a closed shop; all employees are required to join the union and to pay dues.

union. Additionally, members of the union have the right to enter the workplace if the workplace is open to other members of the public. Finally, there can be no threats or intimidation of workers, nor can the employer bribe employees with such things as pay raises or other special benefits in order to discourage unionization.

In *Washington State Nurses Association v. National Labor Relations Board* (2008), the court reinforced the concept that during negotiations for unionization or to extend a new collective bargaining agreement, management can ban the wearing of union insignia in direct patient-care areas, but cannot ban the wearing of union insignia in other areas of the health care facility, including the cafeteria, gift shop, and the first-floor lobby. In this case, the RNs were banned from wearing buttons that stated "RNs Demand Safe Staffing."

In *Highland Hospital v. National Labor Relations Board* (2007), a group of nurses began a decertification campaign in a hospital that had a valid nurses union. They circulated a petition that the union would no longer be recognized as the nurses' representative in the hospital. Hospital management took the position that the petition proved a majority of the hospital's nurses' wishes to no longer be represented by a union and announced that they were not recognizing the union. The hospital then announced a pay raise for all of the nursing staff without consulting the union.

The court found that the hospital was liable for unfair labor practices. The nurses' decertification petition was ambiguous as to whether those signing it wanted no union or desired an alternate union to represent them. Additionally, there was no confirmation that a majority of the nurses would vote for decertification; thus the pay raise was seen as a bribe to discourage continued unionization of the nursing staff.

There must be demonstrated evidence that that a labor organization has support for the creation of a union. This is usually done through "authorization cards" that are signed by workers who wish to join a union. At this stage, the employer may voluntarily agree to unionization or refuse to voluntarily recognize the labor organization. If 30% of the workforce has signed authorization cards, an election with the regional office of the NLRB is called. This election period is normally tense, and both management and union officials attempt to influence the vote in their favor.

The NLRB works to ensure a fair election. There are multiple rules for both sides and, if either side violates the election rules, it is grounds to question the validity of the election process. The election itself is done by secret ballot and workers are given the choice between one or more unions or no union. If no choice receives a majority of the votes, a run-off election may be held. If the election is unsuccessful, a second election may take place a minimum of 12 months after the first election. If the NLRB discovers that the employer engaged in objectionable conduct, a rerun election will be ordered without the waiting period. If over 50% of the workers vote for a particular union, the organization is "certified" and the employer is required to bargain with the organization. This is termed a **contract negotiation** period. Even if the union wins, there may be another election 12 months after the first election, with any worker or employee group requesting the second election. During the contract negotiation period, each side appoints a spokesperson, and good-faith bargaining is mandated by law for both sides. This includes the duty to meet and confer, the duty to bargain in good faith, and the duty to cover certain subjects in the negotiations. Employers must, upon request, supply the union with relevant information such as the cost of wage and benefits packages and the statistics regarding the employment of women and minorities, if relevant. Mandatory subjects of bargaining include wages and fringe benefits, grievance procedures, health and safety, nondiscrimination clauses, no-strike clauses, length of contract, management rights, discipline, seniority, and union security.

During this phase, there may be stalemates, mediation, and binding arbitration. An arbitrator is a neutral party whose purpose is to be fair to both sides; the arbitrator's solution and recommendations are binding to both sides, so often the two sides are more likely to negotiate for small favors.

If the two sides cannot agree and are unwilling to call for arbitration, work stoppages by employees and lockouts by management can occur. With 10 days' notice, the union can then proceed to a strike. Usually, ratification of the agreement is reached because no side wants a strike, and negotiations take on added fervor during work stoppages and lockouts.

Once ratified, collective bargaining does not end but enters the enforcement stage. Grievances can be brought by either management or employees if there are disputes and complaints. Grievances typically can be solved without further steps being taken, but there are specific provisions in the contract negotiations for resolution, including arbitration.

From a management position, nurse-managers and upper-level management can do several things to prevent unionization. Since most unions form because of real or perceived disagreement with management, a well-rounded, high-quality, effective leadership team is needed to prevent dissatisfaction from becoming rampant. Some suggestions for management include:

1. Provide opportunity for participation in organizational decision making; a participative approach may extend to unit self-governance.
2. Maintain salaries in relationship with the education required and the responsibility given.
3. Treat professionals as true professionals; this entails affording respect, trust, and value to all professionals in the organization.
4. Develop, implement, and refine a grievance procedure. This ensures that staff members have direction when they feel dissatisfied and prevents dissatisfaction from becoming so overwhelming that unionization is the only foreseeable answer.
5. Conduct timely and regular surveys and meetings to allow staff an opportunity to express their feelings and views. Open channels of communications are crucial in maintaining positive working relationships.

Once the contract has been accepted and nurse-managers are managing and leading within a union framework, they must know and remember some issues. First, know and understand the contract provisions. A thorough understanding and following of the contract can prevent most grievances. Second, treat all persons being supervised with equal respect and consideration, both union and nonunion members. This will prevent a charge of discrimination and serves to maintain morale. Third, should an issue arise, perform as a professional, be nondefensive, and do not crumble under the pressure. Admit wrong statements or decisions and negotiate a better solution to the problem, assuring that the institutional mission and goals will be upheld. If necessary, seek assistance from upper management, especially if the conflict cannot be immediately resolved. And, fifth, continue to expand personal knowledge of management principles through either formal education or continuing education, and practice those principles.

CASE LAW AND THE NATIONAL LABOR RELATIONS ACT

On March 10, 1993, the Sixth Circuit Court held that staff nurses, including licensed practice nurses (LPNs) at a nursing home facility, were supervisors under the definition of the NLRA and therefore were not entitled to the act's protections (*National Labor Relations Board v. Health Care and Retirement Corporation of America*, 1993). The case was granted review by the Supreme Court to determine whether the duties of nurses in directing the activities of lesser-skilled employees qualify the nurses as supervisors.

The facts of the case were relatively uncomplicated. The LPNs had brought action, alleging that they were disciplined by the nursing home for engaging in protected conduct for the purpose of collective bargaining. The four LPNs involved in the initial action were staff nurses whose primary responsibilities involved monitoring the work of nurse's aides, evaluating the aides' performances, and resolving grievances brought by the nurse's aides. Based on the LPNs' job description, the corporation asserted that these nurses were supervisors and therefore not within the protection of the NLRB because employers cannot be compelled to negotiate with representatives of supervisors. The act defines *supervisor* as

> any individual having authority, in the interest of the employer, to hire, transfer, suspend, lay off, recall, promote, discharge, assign, reward, or discipline other employees, or responsibility to direct them, or to adjust their grievances, or effectively to recommend such action, if in connection with the foregoing the exercise of such authority is not of a merely routine or clerical nature, but requires the use of independent judgment. (29 USCA, Section 152[11], 1935)

The nurses (through the NLRB) argued that since the primary focus of staff nurses is to exercise their own professional skills to care for patients, the staff nurse does not operate in the interest of the employer's interests. They further argued that the direction of the nursing assistants' work by staff nurses is given routinely in connection with the treatment of patients to ensure that quality care is provided to all patients within their care units. There is no evidence that the staff nurses' direction of employees' work goes into personal authority, which more directly promotes the interests of the employer and is not motivated by patient care needs. The administrative law judge who heard the case initially agreed with this statutory argument and held that the protective provisions of the act did cover staff nurses.

But the Supreme Court, on May 23, 1994, disagreed. Justice Kennedy, writing for the court, criticized the NLRB's insistence on the interest of the employer as the test for determining whether staff nurses are supervisors. He concluded that when staff nurses exercise professional responsibilities by caring for a patient, they act in the interest of the nursing home, whose business is patient care.

The NLRB further argued that the health care profession should be treated differently from other professions because the concern over divided loyalty between supervisors and subordinate employees plays no role in health care professions. Nurses, the Board argued, would not divide loyalty between subordinates and the employer, but nurses would place their professional responsibility to care for patients above any loyalty. The court also rejected this argument.

The court's decision is most important in treating the health care profession as other professions. Interns, residents, salaried physicians, and nurses can be classified as supervisors in the future, overturning the longstanding precedents of the NLRB, which held that health professionals were covered by the NLRA. Any professional who uses independent judgment and is employed by an employer subject to the NLRA could be exempted from the protections of the act because of their supervisory status.

Ultimately, the court concluded that it was "up to Congress to carve out an exception for the health care providers, including nurses, should Congress not wish for such nurses to be considered supervisors" *(National Labor Relations Board v. Health Care and Retirement Corporation of America,* 1993, at 1556). Indeed, the court further stated, Congress had made no attempt to carve nurses or health care professionals out of the NLRA's definition of supervisor in the 1974 amendments. Perhaps Congress did not specify this action because it was satisfied with the NLRB's careful avoidance of applying the definition to health care professionals whose activities were directed at quality patient care. If nurses and other health care professionals wish to change this current status, new legislation will need to be enacted in Congress.

The sole attempt to date to enact such legislation occurred in 2007 when the Re-Empowerment of Skilled and Professional Employees and Construction Tradeworkers (RESPECT) Act was introduced into federal legislation. If passed, this act would have dramatically changed the definition of "supervisor" under the NLRA. The proposed legislation would have removed from the definition of supervisor the assignment and responsibility for directing other employees and mandated that the supervisor spend a majority of his or her work time in such activities as the hiring, transferring, suspending, recalling, promoting, rewarding, and disciplining of other employees. Seen by many as a proposal that would essentially eliminate supervisors and drastically change the balance between management and employees, the proposed legislation was soundly defeated.

Court cases continue to confuse the issue regarding the status of nurses as supervisors or non-supervisors. The decision reached in *Providence Alaska Medical Center v. National Labor Relations Board* (1996) recognized that the judgment used by registered nurses in monitoring and assessing patients is part of the professional role, rather than part of any statutory supervision as defined by the National Labor Relations Act. This decision paved the way for the nurses of Providence Hospital to organize and to be represented by the Alaska Nurses Association as the bargaining agent.

Two newer cases, *Extendicare v. Health Services, Inc.* (2006) and *Jochims v. National Labor Relations Board* (2007), extended the uncertainty in this area of the law. In *Extendicare,* nursing home registered nurses (RNs) and licensed practical nurses (LPNs) were determined to be supervisors, using their independent judgment to direct and discipline other employees. The court in that case concluded that although the director of nursing and the administrator made the final decisions about termination, the RNs' and LPNs' actions in disciplining and directing other nursing home personnel made them supervisors. This contrasts with the holding in *Jochims,* where the court held that a charge nurse in a long-term care facility was not a supervisor because she did not have authority to make decisions about whether to reprimand, suspend, dismiss, or otherwise discipline personnel. She did, however, use independent judgment in determining patient care and in evaluating personnel with whom she worked.

Other examples of case law concerning nursing and collective bargaining have centered on fair labor practices (*National Labor Relations Board v. Promedica Health Systems, Inc.*, 2006; *St. Margaret Mercy Healthcare v. National Labor Relations Board*, 2008; *Sunrise Senior Living, Inc. v. National Labor Relations Board*, 2006), upholding an arbitrator's final opinion (*Virginia Mason Hospital v. Washington State Nurses Association*, 2007), and the issue of union dues in closed shops (*St. John's Mercy Health System v. National Labor Relations Board*, 2006; *United Food and Commercial Workers v. St. John's Mercy Health Systems*, 2006). The first cases concerned the rights of nurses to join a union and to engage in concerted activities for the purpose of mutual aid or protection. Employers are not permitted to interfere with union activities by threats, intimidation, or retaliation. Nor can employers enforce no-solicitation rules against union organizers and then allow other non-union solicitation to occur. For example, if the agency permits nurses to collect for the March of Dimes, sell Girl Scout cookies, sell hygiene and cosmetics in direct patient-care areas, information regarding unions can also be viewed in direct patient-care areas. *Virginia Mason Hospital* concerned the ability of management to mandate flu vaccinations, which an arbiter had ruled was outside the management's "prerogative clause." Such a clause only gives the employer rights to generic operational issues and not the right to impose policies such as mandatory immunizations and vaccinations. The court in this case ultimately upheld the arbitrator's ruling.

The last two companion cases concerned the issue of requiring mandatory dues collections in institutions that are closed shops. In *St. John's Mercy Health System* and *United Food and Commercial Workers*, the hospital had argued that state law required the hospitals to maintain an adequate level of nursing staffing and that dismissing non-union nurses in the time of a nursing shortage prevented the institutions from observing the state law. The courts rejected the nursing shortage argument, noting that the hospital in question had previously dealt with a nurses' strike in the past by hiring temporary replacement workers and by closing some hospital units.

Finally, in *McKenzie v. Kadlec Medical Center* (2007), the court ruled that when an employer takes an action not authorized by the collective bargaining agreement in place, the employee's right to file a civil lawsuit is not circumvented. In this case, the nurse was accused of stealing narcotics from the hospital. She was confronted by her co-workers and forcibly prevented from leaving the premises for a period of time in which she was strip-searched and forced to give a urine sample and take a Breathalyzer test. The holding was that the employer in this case was strictly bound by the collective bargaining agreement and that the employer could be liable for civil assault and battery, false imprisonment, invasion of privacy, and defamation in a civil lawsuit.

EXERCISE 13.6

A nursing assistant reported for work smelling of alcohol. His nurse manager sent him for an evaluation by the nursed practitioner in the employee health office. The nurse practitioner saw the assistant, suspected he was impaired, and requested that he be seen by the medical director. At this point, the nursing assistant called his union representative, who advised him to refuse any further testing. He was terminated and brought a lawsuit for unjust termination.

What further evidence should the court require in order to find for the institution and against the nursing assistant in this case? Does the fact that there was a union in place affect the outcome of this case? Would any previous history concerning the relationship between the institution and the nursing assistant affect the outcome of this case?

FAMILY AND MEDICAL LEAVE ACT OF 1993

The **Family and Medical Leave Act of 1993** was signed into law in February 1993 and became effective upon its enactment. The law was passed due to the large number of single-parent and two-parent households in which the single parent or both parents are employed full-time, placing job security and parenting at odds. The law was also passed due to the aging population of the United States and the demands that aging parents place on their working children. The act attempts to balance the demands of the workplace with the demands of the family, allowing employed individuals to take leaves for medical reasons. Such medical reasons include the birth or adoption of a child and the care of a child, spouse, or parent who has a serious health problem. Essentially, the act provides job security for unpaid leave while the employee is caring for a new infant or other family health care needs. The act is gender-neutral and allows both men and women the same leave provisions.

To be eligible under this law, the facility must employ at least 50 persons within a 75-mile radius for each working day during each of 20 or more calendar days in the current or preceding year. *La Monica v. Naph-Care, Inc.* (2007) illustrates the importance of this 50-person employment record. In *La Monica,* a licensed practical nurse was refused coverage under the FMLA law because the local healthcare agency where she worked only employed 33 persons within the 75-mile radius of the location where she was employed. Additionally, the employee must have worked for at least 12 months and worked at least 1,250 hours during the preceding 12-month period. *Mutchler v. Dunlap Memorial Hospital* (2007) clarifies this aspect of the law regarding actual hours worked during the previous 12-month period. In this case, nurses who agreed to work two 12-hour shifts on weekends were given "bonus" hours; that is, they were credited with working 68 hours each 2-week period rather than the actual time that they worked. When the nurse in this case requested leave under the FMLA, she was denied, as she had worked less than the required 1,250 hours. The court in its holding did note that the employer cannot rescind a previously approved FMLA leave if the employer later discovers that the employee has not worked the number of hours as required by the law.

Although its title suggests otherwise, the act does not distinguish between family leave and medical leave per se. The act merely speaks of leave. Family leave is available due to an addition in the household, whether through the birth of a natural child or the placement of a child through adoption or foster care. The leave must be taken within 12 months of the birth or placement. Intermittent leave may be taken, if agreeable to both the employer and employee. The employee may take up to 12 weeks of leave, which is unpaid. The act allows the employee to elect, or the employer to require, that the employee use all or part of any paid vacation, personal leave, or family leave as part of the 12 work weeks of family leave provided under the act. The employee who plans to use leave under the act must give the employer 30 days' notice prior to the date that the leave begins or such notice as is practical.

Medical leave may be taken to care for a spouse, son, daughter, or parent of the employee when that person has a serious medical condition. Employees are also permitted to use medical leave for their own serious health condition. The amount of medical leave is 12 weeks during any 12-month period. Medical leave may be taken intermittently or on a reduced-leave schedule when medically necessary. An employee can elect or an employer may require that the employee use vacation, personal, medical, or sick leave as part of the 12 weeks of leave available. Sick leave may be used for medical leave, but not as part of family leave available under the act. The 30 days requirement for notification also applies to medical leave, unless it is impractical to do so. In such an instance, the employee must give as much notice as is practical.

De la Rama v. Illinois Department of Human Services (2007) illustrates this last point. Here the court held that the individual must timely inform supervisors of the reason for an absence from work. The nurse in this case called in sick every day for a month before she was asked to supply a doctor's validation for her absences. Although she had been diagnosed with fibromyalgia, the physician's validation only described her condition as a generalized muscular neck and lower back pain and stated that she needed an additional week off from work. Three months after her first absences, the employer was finally notified of her fibromyalgia and the human resources department retroactively granted her request for FMLA leave eligibility. When the nurse attempted to return to work after yet another 3-month absence, she was terminated.

The court ruled that merely calling in "sick" does not fulfill the requirements of the employee's obligations that are prerequisite for legal protection under the FMLA. The employee must expressly communicate that he or she had a serious medical condition, expressly say what that condition is, and expressly state that he or she needs to take FMLA leave for a specified period of time, as best that the employee can foresee the required time period. *Silcox v. Via Christi Regional Medical Center* (2006) illustrates the importance of a serious medical condition. In that case, merely being treated by a chiropractor for back pain did not qualify as a serious medical condition.

In a case filed under the Family and Medical Leave Act, the court redefined one purpose of the act (*Jeremy v. Northwest Ohio Development Center,* 1999). The court stated that a substance abuse disorder fits the legal definition of a serious health condition and that employees can use their right under the Family and Medical Leave Act to pursue treatment for a substance abuse disorder under the care of a health care provider. Absences from work caused by abuse of alcohol or other substances, apart from ongoing treatment, are not protected by the Family and Medical Leave Act.

Individuals who take advantage of the Family and Medical Leave Act are entitled to reinstatement of the same or an equivalent position when they return in a timely manner (*Greenlee v. Christus Spohn Health Systems,* 2007). An employee can be denied reinstatement if the employee would have lost his or her position during the leave period even if he or she had been working. That is, if the employee's position would have been legitimately reduced or eliminated if the employee was working, the Family and Medical Leave Act does not require reinstatement. In fairness, though, the burden of proof is on the employer to show that the position would have been eliminated regardless of whether the employee was on leave or not (*Campbell v. Gambro Healthcare, Inc.,* 2007).

Individuals must also return to work at the end of the 12-week period. The court ruled in *Santos v. Shields Health Group* (1998) that when the employee extends leave under the Family and Medical Leave Act beyond the 12-week limit, the facility can terminate the employee. The court in this case ruled that the employee did have a serious medical condition and was entitled to leave under the act. However, at the end of the 12 weeks, the employee must be ready and able to return to work. Similarly in *Kleinmark v. CHS-Lake Erie* (2008), the court found that a hospital has no duty to extend an employee's leave beyond the 12-week period. Any extension of a FMLA leave must be granted fairly and evenhandedly or the hospital opens itself to charges of discrimination.

On January 28, 2008, then President George W. Bush signed an amended act, which became effective January 16, 2009. The amendments permit a spouse, son, daughter, parent, or next of kin to take up to 26 work weeks of leave to care for a member of the armed forces, including a member of the National Guard or Reserves, who is undergoing medical treatment, recuperation, or therapy, is otherwise in outpatient status, or is otherwise on the temporary disability retired list, for a serious injury or illness. Additionally, the act permits an employee to take leave for any qualifying exigency arising out of the fact that the spouse, or a son, daughter, or parent of the employee, is on active duty (or has been notified of an impending call or order to active duty) in the armed forces in support of a contingency operation.

WORKERS' COMPENSATION LAWS

Workers' compensation is a form of insurance that provides compensation for medical care when employees are injured during the course and scope of their employment. In exchange, the employee forfeits the right to sue his or her employer for negligence. The laws were enacted to reduce the need for litigation and to mitigate the requirement that injured workers prove that the injury was their employer's "fault." The first state **workers' compensation law** was passed in Maryland in 1902, and the first law covering federal employees was passed in 1906. By 1949, all states had passed some kind of state workers' compensation law. In most states today, coverage under the law is provided by private insurance companies.

Case law that arises in this area most often concerns health care providers who work outside formal institutional settings (*Hollin v. Johnston County Council on Aging*, 2007; *Jamison v. Workers' Compensation Appeal Board*, 2008; *Janicki v. Kforce.com*, 2006; *Murphy v. Mt. Sinai Hospital*, 2007), injuries sustained while caring for patients (*Coosa Valley Health Care v. Johnson*, 2007; *Huffaker v. St. Mary's Health System*, 2006; *Nurses 4 You, Inc. v. Ferris*, 2007), and mental health of workers (*Jones v. Washington University*, 2006). Generally, nurses who work outside the formal institutional setting are entitled to workers' compensation if they are involved in motor vehicle accidents going to and from clients' homes (*Hollin*, *Janicki*, and *Jamison*). *Murphy* extended this coverage to a nurse practitioner who was attending a continuing education nursing conference, as the institution had paid for him to attend the conference.

Huffaker concerned the rights of a nurse for workers' compensation when she developed an allergy when exposed to latex gloves. The court noted that a nurse is entitled to workers' compensation when the worker first misses work due to the physical complications of the occupational disease. *Nurses 4 You Inc.* and *Coosa Valley Health Care* concerned injuries that the nurses had sustained during the course of their employment. The courts in both cases noted that when the injury occurs during the work day and in the course of completing work-related activities, the worker is entitled to workers' compensation benefits.

The court in *Jones* addressed the issue of whether mental stress can be the basis for a successful workers' compensation claim. Mental stress caused over a period of time by the hours, duties, and responsibilities of employment and other work-related factors is not covered, but mental stress from a specific traumatic incident, such as a physical assault on the job, even if not accompanied by a physical injury, is covered under workers' compensation. In this case, the nurse was administering dialysis treatment to a male patient who suddenly reached inside her scrub top and grabbed her breast. Immediately prior to this action, the Caucasian patient had made crude racial remarks to the nurse, who was African American. The nurse broke down emotionally after leaving the work setting.

EXERCISE 13.7

Four days after starting her employment at a medical center, a laboratory assistant's hair, mouth, eyes, and clothing were splashed with blood from a patient who was positive for hepatitis C. The assistant was sent to the laboratory for blood tests, which confirmed that she was positive for hepatitis C. These tests were repeated 6 months later with the same results.

Some time later, the assistant was unable to work and ultimately resigned her position with the hospital. Contending that she had an occupational disease and that this was the first time she was unable to work, she filed for workers' compensation. Should this assistant be able to collect workers' compensation for her occupational disease? Why or why not?

She was already scheduled for a few days of vacation and then began seeing a psychiatrist, who determined that she was suffering from depression and post-traumatic stress disorder from the incident.

DUTY OWED THE EMPLOYER

Professional nurses owe the employer and themselves the highest standards or qualities of the profession. These include:

1. Maintaining the standards of their state nurse practice act
2. Continuously upgrading their skills and education through mandatory or voluntary continuing education
3. Being a patient care advocate as needed to ensure quality care to all patients
4. Recognizing and applying legal principles as they apply to all areas of patient care

ETHICAL CONCERNS IN THIS AREA OF THE LAW

Ethical concerns that emerge in this area of the law are multiple and varied. One of the issues involves the procedures for restraining and testing employees suspected of substance abuse. As noted by the facts in *McKenzie v. Kadlec Medical Center* (2007), forcibly detaining an employee so that she could be strip-searched and forced to give a urine sample and take a Breathalyzer test supports the need for ethical behavior and humanistic approaches to all employees, regardless of their suspected behaviors or actions. All employees are deserving of ethical consideration, including respect, justice, and fair play.

The multiple forms of discrimination that may be seen in health care settings are not only legally actionable, but also address ethics. The federal government made a major commitment to placing ethics into law with the passage of the Civil Rights Act of 1964, but case law evidences the fact that issues with discrimination persist today. Perhaps one way to approach these types of issues is through in-depth diversity education that promotes ethical behavior. Benefits of educational programs in this area may include promotion of intercultural relationships, improvement of teamwork and the ability to more effectively meet patient needs and achieve positive outcomes, recognition of different thinking styles that promote creative decision making and problem solving, and acceptance of others.

A third issue is the concept of employment-at-will and the ability of employers to dismiss employees for cause or for no cause, perhaps including the aspect that a given supervisor may not like the individual or that the employer may want to bring into the institution individuals to whom he or she owes favors. In the current economy, with the ever-increasing numbers of individuals unemployed, it is not unreasonable to anticipate that some workers may be dismissed for these types of frivolous reasons. In most industrialized countries, employers can only dismiss with cause, such as for incompetent work performance or disregard of patient safety issues. Perhaps this is the most ethical approach, as dismissal is predicated on the employee's actions or nonactions, rather than a more arbitrary system.

A fourth issue concerns patients' dependency on nurses, which hinders the patients' freedom and autonomy. Being required to move at the nurses' convenience or being confined to a specific place may not be in the patients' well-being or may cause the patient to feel undignified. From a nursing perspective, nurses may give preference to patients who are lighter and thus easier to move or are less physically restricted. Patients may not be moved in as timely a manner if the nurse perceives the movement as a personal risk to his or her well-being, a time burden, or less of a priority. Balancing these needs of patients and nurses may pose ethical challenges in multiple clinical settings.

SUMMARY

- Vicarious or substituted liability describes the instance in which one party becomes responsible for the actions of another party.
- Respondeat superior, meaning "let the master respond," is predicated on the fact that the employee for whom another party becomes partially responsible is acting within the course and scope of his or her employment.
- The borrowed servant and dual servant doctrines describe how a health care provider may be serving two masters at the same time, the employer and someone who has direct control over the health care provider's actions.
- Corporate liability is the doctrine that holds the health care institution liable for its direct responsibilities to patients, such as appropriate hiring and retention practices and the provision of safe working environments.
- Ostensible authority allows the health care institution to also be liable for independent contractors if the four criteria of subjectivism, inherent function, reliance, and control are satisfied.
- Personal liability makes each person responsible for his or her own conduct and can never be totally negated merely because a second or third party also has responsibility.
- Indemnification allows an employer to recover from an individual personally responsible any damages paid under the doctrine of respondeat superior for negligent actions.
- Employment laws, enacted by either federal or state legislatures, serve to guide nurses in all health care settings.
- Ethical concerns in this area of the law concern procedures for restraining and testing employees suspected of substance abuse, forms of discrimination in health care settings, employment-at-will dismissals, and ethical challenges related to the lifting and movement of patients.

APPLY YOUR LEGAL KNOWLEDGE

1. How are hospitals liable for acts of individual nurses, even if no lawsuit is brought against the individual nurse?
2. Can an institution be held liable for the actions of independent contractors?
3. How does the doctrine of indemnification further the concept that individuals are ultimately responsible for their own actions?

YOU BE THE JUDGE

Mrs. Dolan has worked at Happy Valley Retirement Home for a number of years; she is currently the home's director of nursing. The home recently developed and implemented a no-contact policy requiring that nurses, from the director of nurses to the nurse's aide, are to refrain from contacting any patient's family member or members without first obtaining permission from the home's administrator. The rationale behind this policy was not explained, though several of the nursing staff did request such information.

Mrs. Dolan believes that the policy is abusive and a direct violation of the state's nursing home residents' bill of rights law. Specifically, she is concerned that the no-contact policy prevents her from working directly with the resident's family members and assuring them about the condition of their loved ones. Mrs. Dolan has made her feelings about this issue known to the administrator of Happy Valley. She has also contacted a senior-citizens advocacy group and the state department of health about her concerns. When the administrator of

Happy Valley discovered that Mrs. Dolan had spoken with the state department of health, he terminated her. She has now filed a lawsuit claiming retaliation for her whistleblower activities.

QUESTIONS

1. Did Mrs. Dolan follow the correct procedure for voicing her concerns about this no-contact policy?

2. Does the no-contact policy meet the definition of a violation of public policy significant enough to be reportable?
3. Did the home terminate Mrs. Dolan in retaliation for her action, or was the action appropriate given her public voicing of her disapproval of the new policy?
4. How would you decide this case?

REFERENCES

Age Discrimination in Employment Act of 1967, Public Law 90-202, 81 *Statutes* 602 (December 15, 1967).

American Jurisprudence. (1992). 4A Agency.

Annotations. (1999). 99 A.L.R. Fed. 775.

Appeal of Linn, 761 A. 2d 502 (New Hampshire, 2000).

Arends v. Extendicare Homes, 2008 WL 1734205 (D. Minn., April 10, 2008).

Auston v. Schubnell, 116 F.3d 251 (7th Cir., 1997).

Bair v. Colonial Plaza, 2008 31546686 (W. D. Okla., August 1, 2008).

Barber v. Lovelace Sandia Health Systems, 2005 WL 3664323 (D. N. M., December 31, 2005).

Barfield v. New York City Health and Hospitals Corporation, 2006 WL 1462269 (S. D. N. Y., May 30, 2006).

Beck-Wilson v. Principi, 441 F. 3d (6th Cir., March 17, 2006).

Belt v. EmCare, Inc., 2006 WL 758277 (5th Cir., March 24, 2006).

Berde v. North Shore, 2008 WL 1748333 (N.Y. App., April 15, 2008).

Bergman v. Private Care, Inc., 2008 WL 517606 (S. D. Fla., January 30, 2008).

Biconi v. Pay 'N Pak Stores, Inc., 746 F. Supp. 1 (D. Oregon, 1990).

Bird v. United States, 949 F.2d 1079 (10th Cir., 1991).

Bost v. Riley, 262 S.E.2d 391 (N.C. App. 1980), 51 ALR 4th 235 (1990).

Brittain v. Family Care Services, Inc., 801 So.2d 457 (La. App., 2001).

Broussard v. United States, 989 F.2d 171 (Texas, 1993).

Campbell v. Gambro Healthcare Inc., 2007 WL 706934 (10th Cir., March 9, 2007).

Carter v. Hucks-Folliss, 505 S.E.2d 177 (N.C. App., 1998).

Center for Behavioral Health, Rhode Island, Inc. v. Barros, 710 A.2d 680 (Rhode Island, 1998).

Chambers v. Principi, 2006 WL 2255261 (S. D. Miss., August 7, 2006).

Chicarello v. Employment Security Division, Department of Labor, 930 P.2d 170 (New Mexico, 1996).

Civil Rights Act of 1964, Public Law 82-352, 43 Federal Register 19807 (amended, October 31, 1978).

Collective Bargaining Act of 1974, Public Law 93-360, Section 2(5) 88 Stat. 395 (July 26, 1974).

Cone v. Health Management Association, Inc., 2007 WL 1702867 (D. Ga., June 11, 2007).

Coosa Valley Health Care v. Johnson, 2007 WL 80506 (Ala. Civ. App., January 12, 2007).

Corpus Juris Secundum. (2000). 2A Agency, Sections 1–59.

Darling v. Charleston Community Memorial Hospital, 211 N.E.2d 253 (Illinois, 1965), cert. den'd, 383 U.S. 946 (1966).

Davis v. Department of Veterans Affairs, 2006 WL 3251733 (Fed. Cir., November 9, 2006).

D'Cunha v. New York Hospital Medical Center of Queens, 2006 WL 544470 (E. D. N.Y., March 6, 2006).

De la Rama v. Illinois Department of Human Services, 2007 WL 54060 (N. D. Ill., January 5, 2007).

Dickinson v. Springhill Hospitals, Inc., 2006 WL 1785295 (11th Cir., June 29, 2006).

Duling v. Bluefield Sanitarium, Inc., 142 S.E.2d 754 (West Virginia, 1965).

Duncan v. Children's National Medical Center, 702 A.2d 207 (D.C. App., 1997).

El-Sioufi v. St. Peter's University Hospital, 887 A. 2d 1170 (N. J. App., December 29, 2005).

Employee-Management Cooperation in the Federal Service, Executive Order 10988 (January 17, 1962).

Equal Employment Opportunity Act of 1972, 78 *Statutes* 253; 42 U.S.C. 2000e (March 24, 1972).

Equal Employment Opportunity Commission v. William O. Benson Rehabilitation Pavilion, 2007 WL 1516479 (E. D. N.Y., April 20, 2007).

Equal Pay Act of 1963, Public Law 88-38, 77 *Statutes* 56 (June 10, 1963).

Extendicare v. Health Services, Inc., 2006 WL 1307474 (6th Cir., May 9, 2006).

Fair Labor and Standards Act of 1938, chapter 676, 52 *Statutes* 1069 (June 25, 1938).

Family and Medical Leave Act of 1993, Public Law 103-3 (February 5, 1993).

Family and Medical Leave Amended Act of 2008, Public Law 110-181 (January 28, 2008).

Federal False Claims Act of 1986, Public Law 99-562, 100 *Statutes* 3153, 31 USC sections 3730 et seq. (October 27, 1986).

Federal Torts Claims Act of 1946, 60 *Statutes* 842 (August 2, 1946).

Firefighters Local 1784 v. Scotts, 467 U.S. 561, 34 FEP Cases 1702 (1984).

Fortune v. National Cash Register Company, 272 Mass. 96, 264 N.E.2d 1251 (1977), 42 U.S.C. Section 12101 *et seq.* (1990).

French v. Eagle Nursing Home, Inc., 973 F. Supp. 870 (D. Minn., 1997).

Glander v. Marshall Hospital, 2003 WL 649127 (Cal. App., February 28, 2003).

Greenlee v. Christus Spohn Health Systems, 2007 WL 38284 (S.D. Tex., January 4, 2007).

Harris v. Miller, No. 345A91, 1994 N.C. LEXIS 16 (January 28, 1994).

Harwood v. Avalon Care Center, 2006 WL 234906 (D. Ariz., August 10, 2006).

Hatchett v. Health Care and Retirement Corporation, 2006 WL 1525688 (6th Cir., June 1, 2006).

Health Resources and Services Administration. (2007). *The registered nurse population: Findings from the 2004 National Sample Survey of Registered Nurses.* Washington, DC: Author.

Herrero v. St. Louis University Hospital, 109 F.3d 481 (8th Cir., 1997).

Highland Hospital v. National Labor Relations Board, 2007 WL 4208324 (D.C. Cir., November 30, 2007).

Hollin v. Johnston County Council on Aging, 2007 WL 3515 (N.C. App., January 2, 2007).

Howard v. Life Care Centers, 2007 WL 4964716 (M. D. Fla., October 29, 2007).

Huffaker v. St. Mary's Health System, 2006 WL 2522141 (Tenn. Work Comp., September 1, 2006).

Hunt v. Rapides Healthcare System, LLC., 277 F.3d 757 (5th Cir., 2001).

Hunt v. Tender Loving Care Home Care Agency, Inc., 2002 WL 31162401 (N.C. App., October 1, 2002).

Hunter v. Allis-Chambers Corporation, Engine Division, 797 F.2d 1417 (Cir. App., 1986).

Jamison v. Workers' Comp. Appeal Board, 2008 WL 3834955 (Pa. Cmwlth., August 19, 2008).

Janicki v. Kforce.com, 2006 WL 1793244 (Ohio App., June 30, 2006).

Jeremy v. Northwest Ohio Development Center, 33 F. Supp.2d 635 (N.D. Ohio, 1999).

Jochims v. National Labor Relations Board, 480 F. 3d 1161 (D.C. Cir., March 23, 2007).

Johnson v. Bryson, 2007 WL 3290455 (E. D. Ark., November 5, 2007).

Jones v. Washington University, 2006 WL 1735324 (Mo. App., June 27, 2006).

Kleinmark v. CHS-Lake Erie, 2008 WL 2740817 (N.D. Ohio, July 10, 2008).

La Monica v. Naph-Care, Inc., 2007 WL 81851 (N.D. Ohio, January 8, 2007).

Lawrence v. University of Texas Medical Branch at Galveston, 163 F.3d 309 (5th Cir., 1999).

McKenzie v. Kadlec Medical Center, 2007 WL 433088 (E.D. Wash., February 5, 2007).

McPeck, P. (2006). Watching our back: RNs get a lift from "no lift" policies. Available online at http://www2.nurseweek.com/Articles/article.cfm?AID=22078

Mealand v. Eastern New Mexico Medical Center, 33 P.3d 258 (N.M. App., 2001).

Memisevich v. St. Elizabeth's Medical Center, 2006 WL 2277964 (W. D. N.Y., August 9, 2006).

Montes v. Vail Clinic, Inc., 2007 WL 2309766 (10th Cir., August 14, 2007).

Morrissette-Brown v. Mobile Infirmary Medical Center, 2007 WL 3274898 (11th Cir., November 7, 2007).

Murphy v. Mt. Sinai Hospital, 2007 WL 414277 (N.Y. App., February 8, 2007).

Mutchler v. Dunlap Memorial Hospital, 2007 WL 1263968 (6th Cir., May 2, 2007).

National Labor Relations Act, Ch. 372, 49 *Statutes* 449 (1935).

National Labor Relations Board v. Health Care and Retirement Corporation of America, 987 F.2d 1256 (6th Cir. 1993), cert. granted 62 U.S.L.W. 3244 (U.S. Oct. 5, 1993), 114 S.Ct. 1178 (1994).

National Labor Relations Board v. Promedica Health Systems, Inc., 2006 WL 2860771 (6th Cir., October 5, 2006).

Nead v. Eastern Illinois University, 2006 WL 1582454 (C.D. Ill., June 6, 2006).

Nurses 4 You, Inc. v. Ferris, 2007 WL 505799 (Va. App., February 20, 2007).

N. X. v. Cabrini Medical Center, 739 N.Y.S.2d 348 (N.Y. App., 2002).

Occupational Safety and Health Act of 1970, Public Law 91-595, 84 *Statutes* 1590 (December 29, 1970).

Odie v. Department of Employment Security, 2007 WL 4233453 (Ill. App., November 30, 2007).

Park North General Hospital v. Hickman, 703 S.W.2d 262 (1985), 51 ALR 4th 235 (1990).

Pavilascak v. Bridgeport Hospital, 48 Conn. App. 580 (1998).

Piskorek v. Department of Human Services, 2003 WL 21212583 (N.D. Ill., May 22, 2003).

Praigrod v. St. Mary's Medical Center, 2007 WL 178627 (S.D. Ind., January 19, 2007).

Providence Alaska Medical Center v. National Labor Relations Board, 121 F.3d 548 (9th Cir., 1996).

Rawls v. Augustine Home Health Care, Inc., 2007 WL 1952988 (D. Md., July 5, 2007).

Re-Empowerment of Skilled and Professional Employees and Construction Tradeworkers Act, H. R. 1644/S.B. 969 (2007).

Rehabilitation Act of 1973, Public Law 93-112 (September 26, 1973).

Robertson v. Bethlehem Steel Corporation, 912 F.2d 184 (Cir. App., 1990).

Robertson v. Total Renal Care, 2003 WL 22326579 (N.D. Ill., October 10, 2003).

Robinson v. CARES Surgicenter, 2008 WL 1744410 (N.J. App., April 17, 2008).

Rohrbrough v. University of Colorado Hospital, 2007 WL 3024449 (D. Colo., October 16, 2007).

Ruiz v. Adlanka, 2007 WL 2640633 (Sup. Ct. Lake Co., Indiana, June 8, 2007).

Salonga v. D & R RCH Corporation, 2008 WL 2101429 (Sup. Ct. Alameda Co., California, February 8, 2008).

Santos v. Shields Health Group, 996 F. Supp. 87 (D. Mass., 1998).

Scanlon v. Jeanes Hospital, 2007 WL 2972558 (E. D. Pa., October 10, 2007).

Silcox v. Via Christi Regional Medical Center, 2006 WL 2536602 (10th Cir., September 5, 2006).

Skare v. Extendicare Health Services, 2008 WL 341464 (8th Cir., February 8, 2008).

Sparger v. Worley Hospital, Inc., 547 S.W.2d 582 (Texas, 1977).

St. John's Mercy Health System v. National Labor Relations Board, 2006 WL 229912 (8th Cir., February 1, 2006).

St. Margaret Mercy Healthcare v. National Labor Relations Board, 2008 WL 638059 (7th Cir., March 11, 2008).

Stephens v. Kettering Adventist Healthcare, 2006 WL 1307476 (6th Cir., May 9, 2006).

Stroli v. Board of Review, 2008 WL 2122336 (N.J. App., May 20, 2008).

Sunrise Senior Living, Inc v. National Labor Relations Board, 2006 WL 1526122 (4th Cir., May 31, 2006).

Tarin v. County of Los Angeles, 123 F.3d 1259 (9th Cir., 1997).

Taylor v. Alterra Healthcare, 2007 WL 2571978 (E. D. Mich, September 4, 2007).

Taylor v. Memorial Health Systems, Inc., 770 So.2d 752 (Fla. App., 2000).

Thompson v. Merriman CCRC, Inc., 2006 3302508 (Ohio App., November 15, 2006).

Toussaint v. Blue Cross and Blue Shield, 408 Mich. 579, 292 N.W.2d 880 (1980).

Tremlett v. Aurora Health Care, Inc., 2002 WL 1424224 (Wis. App., July 2, 2002).

United Food and Commercial Workers v. St. John's Mercy Health Systems, 2006 WL 1409416 (8th Cir., May 24, 2006).

Vanhook v. Britthaven, 2007 WL 2142691 (Ky. App., July 27, 2007).

Vietnam Era Readjustment Act of 1974, 38 *United States Code* 4212 (1974).

Virginia Mason Hospital v. Washington State Nurses Association, 2007 WL 4463924 (9th Cir., December 21, 2007).

Wallace v. Methodist Hospital System, 271 F. 3d 212 (5th Cir., 2001).

Washington State Nurses Association v. National Labor Relations Board, 2008 WL 2096970 (9th Cir., May 20, 2008).

Watkins v. Unemployment Compensation Board of Review, 689 A.2d 1019 (Pa. Cmwlth., 1997).

Weigel v. Baptist Hospital, 2002 WL 1489616, 89 BNA Fair Employment Practice Case. 718 (6th Cir., July 15, 2002).

Wellstar Health Systems, Inc. v. Green, 2002 WL 31324127 (Ga. App., October 18, 2002).

Wendeln v. Beatrice Manor, Inc., 2006 WL 903598 (Neb., April 7, 2006).

Wheatley v. Baptist Hospital of Miami, Inc., 16 F. Supp.2d 1356 (S. D. Fla., 1998).

White v. Fort Sanders-Park West Medical Center, 2007 WL 241024 (Tenn. App., January 29, 2007).

Williams v. Bala Retirement and Nursing Center, 2007 WL 2571526 (E. D. Pa., August 31, 2007).

Yearous v. Niobrara County Memorial Hospital, 128 F.3d 1351 (10th Cir., 1997).

Yonker v. Centers for Long Term Care, 2006 WL 516851 (D. Kan., March 2, 2006).

Young v. Trinity Hill Care Center, 2006 WL 1461166 (Conn. Super., May 11, 2006).

Zakbartchenko v. Weinberger, 605 N.Y.S. 205 (New York, 1993).

CHAPTER 14

Nursing Management and the Nurse-Manager

PREVIEW

As the role of the professional nurse expands to include increased expertise, specialization, autonomy, and accountability, nurses in management roles must develop additional understanding of a changing legal climate. This chapter explains key concepts underlying nursing management, including corporate liability issues, supervision of others, the temporary reassignment of nurses to units other than those with which they have primary expertise, and the role of agency nurses within health care settings. Additionally, nurses may undertake to practice in more independent settings and in independent roles. As nurses undertake employment opportunities that are more independent of hospital settings, understanding and knowing aspects of contract law become more imperative. Thus, this chapter also explores contract law, defining the various aspects of formal and informal contracts, and the chapter concludes with a discussion of the legal issues involved in contract law.

LEARNING OUTCOMES
After completing this chapter, you should be able to:

14.1 Analyze the concept of corporate liability, including the nurse-manager's role in preventing such liability.

14.2 Define three separate issues concerning staffing from the aspect of the nurse-manager's legal liability.

14.3 Describe the goals of risk management.

14.4 Define and describe principles and terms used in contract law.

14.5 Describe the four elements of a valid contract.

14.6 Define the statute of frauds and its relationship to contract law.

14.7 Define types of contracts and give examples of when each type would be used.

14.8 Identify and analyze three remedies for breach of contract law.

14.9 Describe the purpose of alternative dispute resolution and give four means by which resolution may be performed.

14.10 Describe how contracts may arise after employment.

14.11 Identify some of the ethical concerns in this area of the law.

KEY TERMS

abandonment
adequate staffing
agency personnel
alternative dispute resolution
arbitration
breach of contract
contract
contract termination
corporate liability
corporate negligence
duty to orient, educate, and evaluate

expressed contract
fact finding
failure to warn
float staff
formal contract
hiring practices
implied contracts
injunction
mediation
monetary damages
oral contract

ostensible authority (apparent agency)
personal liability
policies and procedures
specific performance
statute of frauds
summary jury trial
vicarious or substituted liability

LIABILITY

The issues of liability from the perspective of the nurse-manager involve concepts such as **personal liability, vicarious liability,** and the continually evolving aspect of **corporate liability.** The first two of these concepts were covered in the preceding chapter. Corporate liability involves several aspects, and many of its facets have evolved through case law.

A case that well illustrates the principal of corporate liability is *Roach v. Kelly Health Care et al.* (1997). In *Roach,* the agency used certified nursing assistants rather than home health aides to provide care to the clients it served. The certified nursing assistants received 60 hours of training that emphasized caring for patients in institutionalized settings under direct supervision. Home health aides received not only the 60 hours of training but also an additional 60 hours that emphasized home care of individuals.

One of the clients the agency served was an 87-year-old widow who was confused and had fallen at home. Care was provided on a 24-hour basis by the home health service. The aide caring for her had not checked on the client for a 5-hour period and found the widow on the floor with her face against a baseboard heater. The widow sustained severe head, face, and neck burns. Although the agency argued that their staff members were qualified to care for this patient, the court held that home health aides were required in caring for such a complex client. The court noted in its holding that the agency had not complied with regulations mandating conferences every second week, nor had they complied with weekly telephone conferences as mandated. The court also held that the nursing supervisor did not have direct supervisory responsibility as she was totally unaware that there were any problems arising from the care of this client.

A similar cause of action occurred in *Ponce v. Ashford Presbyterian Community Hospital* (2001). The hospital failed to provide qualified labor and delivery nursing staff, resulting in permanent injury to the newborn as the physician had to wait for a second nurse to assist in the delivery. The court ruled that the hospital was 50% at fault for not providing an adequate nursing staff. In *Greenwood v. Paracelsus Health Care Corporation* (2001), the opposite result occurred because the hospital was able to show it had provided qualified staff, but the surgeon used only his private-duty surgical nurse as his assistant.

Courts have also applied a corporate doctrine in instances where nurses failed to serve as patient advocates. Citing what is now known as **corporate negligence,** the court in *Whittington v. Episcopal Hospital* (2001) held that when a hospital, through its administrative officers and staff, knows there is a serious problem with patient care issues and allows the patient care problems to continue and escalate without intervening, the hospital will be held accountable. In this particular case, an obstetrical patient who had severe pregnancy-induced hypertension expired during a cesarean section. The patient, who had presented to the emergency center with an elevated blood pressure, excessive weight gain, proteinuria, and post-term pregnancy, was allowed to return to her home rather than remain in the hospital for observation, evaluation, and therapy. At trial, the nurses testified they knew the patient required additional care and observation, and they had allowed her to be discharged rather than using internal mechanisms of communication to prevent the discharge, such as notifying their supervisor, the administrator on call, or the chief of staff.

Gess v. United States (1996) illustrates the need for the facility to be accountable when staff members exhibit suspicious behavior and to take necessary action to safeguard patients. In that case, a medical technician, who had a history of psychiatric hospitalizations and reports of domestic violent behavior, was tried for injecting newborn infants with lidocaine. He was in a position to care for infants in the newborn nursery, and he was always the first on the unit to initiate the process of resuscitation, albeit unsuccessfully in some cases. The subsequent criminal investigation revealed that he had injected one new mother and 11 newborns with lidocaine or similar medications.

The court held that there was an obvious pattern to these adverse patient care incidents that should have alerted the hospital that the incidents were neither random nor isolated. The court emphasized that health care institutions have a responsibility to discover and eliminate the cause of such incidents before significant damage has been done. Quality assurance, through the follow-up to incident reports, is one mechanism to alert institutions about suspicious patterns and persons in adverse patient care situations, such as this pattern of ongoing intentional criminal misconduct.

Courts also impose corporate liability on institutions for failing to act when a physician is incompetent or impaired. A Pennsylvania anesthesiologist was sentenced to 10 years in prison for stealing narcotics from patients who had surgical procedures performed. During the 3 months he worked at the hospital, several patients complained of unbearable pain, including full sensation at the beginning of surgical procedures. The institution noted that this one physician requested more narcotics than did other anesthesiologists, and that he could not fully account for some of the medications he received for patients under his care. The hospital knew the anesthesiologist had abused drugs in the past and had successfully completed a drug rehabilitation program.

Acting on reasonable suspicion based on these patient complaints, the laboratory analyzed blood samples from two preoperative patients and found that they had only trace amounts of narcotics in their blood. A urine sample was obtained from the anesthesiologist, which tested positive for narcotics. He was suspended and later arrested when he reentered the institution using a retained key. He confessed and admitted that he had previously been arrested in California, New York, Ohio, and Massachusetts for various crimes, including drug possession, kidnapping, and assaulting a police officer. The court held the institution responsible under a corporate liability cause of action for not having done a criminal background check on this physician, especially given his history of drug abuse. The hospital claimed that a criminal background check was not part of its credentialing policy and thus none was requested ("Theft of Drugs," 1997).

Nurse-managers play a key role in assisting the institution to avoid corporate liability. For example, nurse-managers are normally delegated the responsibility to ensure that staff remain competent and qualified; that personnel within their supervision have current licensure; that corporate management be alerted if staffing levels are dangerously low or there is an incorrect mix of staff for the acuity of the patients requiring care; and that incompetent, illegal, or unethical practices are reported to the proper persons or agencies. Whether the nurse-manager reports these data in writing or verbally depends on the agency policies and the type of reporting that must be done.

CAUSES OF MALPRACTICE FOR NURSE-MANAGERS

Nursing managers are charged with maintaining a standard of competent nursing care within the institution. Several potential sources of liability for malpractice among nurse-managers may be identified. These causes of action include negligent hiring, negligent retention of incompetent or impaired employees, inappropriate assigning of staff, failure to supervise and educate staff, and failure to warn employees of potential problems with previously employed staff. Once identified, guidelines to prevent or avoid these pitfalls can then be developed.

Duty to Orient, Educate, and Evaluate

Most health care facilities have continuing education departments whose function it is to orient nurses new to the institution, and to supply in-service education for new equipment, procedures, and interventions. Nonetheless, nurse-managers have a **duty to orient, educate, and evaluate.** These individuals are responsible for the daily evaluation of whether nurses are performing competent care. The key to meeting this expectation is reasonableness. Nurse-managers should ensure that they respond promptly to all allegations, whether by patients, staff, or other health care personnel, of incompetent or questionable nursing care. Nurse-managers should thoroughly investigate, recommend alternatives for correcting the situation, and include follow-up evaluations in nurses' records, showing that the nurses are competent to care for patients within clinical settings.

A Texas case, *St. Paul Medical Center v. Cecil* (1992), concerned allegations that the hospital was negligent in retaining, supervising, and assigning a nurse. In that case, a term obstetrical patient presented at St. Paul Medical Center, stating that her "water had broken." The nurse checked the patient by means of a pelvic examination and assessed the patient's vital signs, fetal heart tones, and contractions.

An hour later, the patient was again assessed, this time by a resident, and he determined that the membranes had ruptured and that meconium was present. Another hour passed, and the nurse attached an external fetal monitor and recorded the printout. During the third hour after admission, the resident attached an internal fetal monitor, whose printout showed severe fetal hypoxia, bradycardia, and more meconium. Though the resident told the nurse to alert the attending physician of the need for an immediate cesarean section, there was still an hour delay before a severely brain-damaged infant was delivered.

One issue that arose in the defense of the nurse-defendant concerned evaluations that had been written about the nurse's performance 3 months before this incident arose. At that time, the nurse had been rated as an unsatisfactory employee who sometimes fell asleep while on duty, had difficulty in using electronic fetal monitors, and was reluctant to seek the supervisor's advice or consult with the supervisor when problems arose concerning labor and delivery issues. No subsequent evaluations could be found to support that any of these problems had been addressed or that any had been resolved. The court found the hospital and the nurse both liable to the patient. Liability was averted on the part of the physician, as he settled out of court prior to the start of the trial.

One of the many lessons to be learned from this case is the importance of following through on incompetent staff members with reassignment to less critical areas of the institution, retraining so that the nurse can safely perform staff nursing skills and intervene in an appropriate and timely manner, or discharge. The second lesson is the importance of reevaluation and ensuring that current evaluations show the improved competency of the nurse in question.

Additional case examples in this area of the law include *Bunn-Penn v. Southern Regional Medical Corporation* (1997), *Healthcare Trust v. Cantrell* (1997), *Jackson v. Harper Hospital* (2006), and *Shelly v. Bethshan* (2007). In *Healthcare Trust,* a surgical technician was involved. At the time of the incident in question, surgical technicians were not subject to mandatory licensing or certification under state law. The court, however, looked for guidance from the then-current version of *Standards and Recommended Practices for Perioperative Nursing,* published by the American Organization of Operating Room Nurses (AORN). This publication was accepted by the court as evidence of the legal standard of care. The court believed that the publication established a necessity for surgical personnel to have specific training in the tasks and procedures they were asked to perform.

Specifically, the surgical technician should not have been allowed to hold retractors in a pediatric hip arthroplasty. Never having been educated for that task with pediatric patients, the technician was not aware of the risk to the sciatic nerve that could result from even the slightest deviation from the surgeon's manual positioning of the retractor. Assignments of surgical personnel to specific tasks and specific procedures in the operating area must be based on individual qualifications, said the court. The court concluded that it was negligence for a surgical facility to permit a surgical technician to perform tasks for which the technician does not have specific training. It was also negligence for a surgical facility to assign a surgical technician to a procedure with which the technician is unfamiliar. Training and familiarity with procedures performed on adults is not directly transferable to pediatric situations. Surgical technicians must be cleared, and their competence and training for the specific tasks and procedures in question must be documented.

The courts in *Jackson* and *Shelly* similarly concluded that the hospital had a responsibility to train health care providers to be alert for complications that could arise and how to properly use equipment so that patients are not injured. In *Jackson,* this training included the need to correctly position elderly patients securely with pillows, wedges, rolls, and/or restraints in order to prevent the patients from possibly becoming entangled in the bed side rails in positions from which they cannot remove themselves.

Bunn-Penn illustrates what must be done to prevent liability on the part of the nurse-manager. In that case, a male emergency center technician was accused of sexually assaulting a female patient in the emergency center. Nurses had complained to the nurse-manager that the male technician seemed too eager to assist female patients who were undressing and that he stayed too long with female patients while they were undressing. The nurse-manager herself noted that he seemed eager to assist female patients on and off bedpans. The hospital's practice was that a male caregiver was to help a female patient with this latter task only when extra assistance was needed due to the size of a particular patient.

The nurse-manager spoke to the technician about these issues. She indicated that how he had acted was not appropriate caregiving and told him what he needed to do in the future about such issues. She continued to monitor his actions and noted no further evidence of inappropriate care involving female patients until the incident occurred that was the foundation for this lawsuit.

The court ruled that the nurse-manager was the supervisor at the hospital who was directly responsible for the technician's conduct on the job. She fulfilled her duty, held the court, by counseling the technician, informing him of appropriate care measures, and monitoring him to ascertain that his inappropriate actions had ceased. She had also acted promptly when complaints by other staff members surfaced. The nurse-manager was justified in believing that all of her and the other staff nurses' concerns over this employee's inappropriate behavior had been resolved.

Failure to Warn

A newer area of potential liability for nurse-managers is the area of **failure to warn** potential employers of staff incompetence or impairment. Information about suspected addictions, violent behavior, and incompetency of staff members is of vital importance to subsequent employers. If the institution has sufficient information and suspicion on which to discharge an employee or force a letter of resignation, then subsequent employers should be aware of those issues.

One means that courts have used to address this issue is through a qualified privilege to certain communications. As a general rule, qualified privilege concerns communications made in good faith between persons or entities with a need to know. Most states now recognize this qualified privilege and allow previous employees to give factual, objective information to subsequent employers. Chapter 7 should be reviewed for more information on this defense.

Hiring Practices

Nurse-managers participate in the hiring of new employees. To avoid potential liability in this area, the nurse-manager must be conversant with effective **hiring practices** and careful of potential pitfalls. One such pitfall is representations made about the position during the interview that may later lead to a breach of express or implied contract claims. Such representations usually occur in prehiring interviews, contract negotiations, letters offering the position to an individual, or employee handbooks. Representations may be made about future wages, benefit increases, terms of employment, or cause-for-termination standards.

Employee handbooks frequently create enforceable rights about specific disciplinary procedures. In *Daldulav v. St. Mary Nazareth Hospital Center* (1987), the court ruled that an employee handbook or other policy statement creates enforceable contractual rights if the traditional requirements for contract formation are presented. These elements include a policy statement containing a promise clear enough for the employee to reasonably believe it to be an offer, with acceptance of the employee's beginning or continuing to work after learning of its existence. In a later case, *Karnes v. Doctor's Hospital* (1990), the court disagreed with this ruling, stating that the employee handbook did not create an express or implied contract. Note, though, that the facts of this latter case are quite different. In *Karnes,* the employee stated that she was aware of the at-will employment and had not read the handbook. The lesson seems to be ensuring that language in the handbook does not constitute expressed conditions or the court will treat it as contractual. A second lesson may be requiring newly hired staff members to sign a form indicating that they have read and understand the content of the handbook. These signed forms should be retained in the personnel department with other employee documents and forms.

Oral comments made during the interview may also be seen as binding on the employer, particularly those promising continued employment. Thus, during oral negotiations, the nurse-manager should:

1. Avoid making promises about career opportunities.
2. Use words such as "possible," "potential," and "maybe" when describing career opportunities.

3. Refrain from predicting future pay raises or benefits, and refer to past pay raises as merely a guide.
4. Use words such as "now" and "presently" when referring to benefits.
5. Note that all employee benefit plans are subject to change.

EXERCISE 14.1

Review your institution's employee handbook, given either to new employees or to all employees during a calendar year. Do the handbooks contain specific terms that you would argue create a duty on the part of the institution? For example, "the employee will be given three disciplinary warnings before termination" could be seen as creating such a duty. Are there other examples? How would you initiate change in the handbook so that language creating a duty is completely eliminated?

STAFFING ISSUES

Three different issues arise under the general term *staffing:*

1. Adequate numbers of staff members in a time of advancing patient acuity and limited resources
2. Floating staff from one unit to another
3. Using temporary or "agency" staff to augment hospital staffing

Adequate Numbers of Staff

Accreditation standards, namely the Joint Commission (JC) and the Community Health Accreditation Program (CHAP), as well as other state and federal standards, mandate that health care institutions must provide **adequate staffing** with qualified personnel. This includes not only numbers of staff, but also the legal status of the staff members and the staffing mix. For instance, some areas of the institution must have greater percentages of registered nurses (RNs) than licensed practical nurses/licensed vocational nurses (LPNs/LVNs), such as critical care areas, post-anesthesia care areas, and emergency centers, whereas other areas may have equal or lower percentages of RNs to LPN/LVNs or nursing assistants, such as the general floor areas and some long-term care areas. Whether short staffing or understaffing exists in a given situation depends on a careful, objective analysis of the number of patients, patient acuity, amount of care required by each patient, and the number and classification/type of staff members. Unless the state has enacted legislation-mandated staff-to-patient ratios, courts generally determine whether under-staffing indeed exists on a case-to-case basis.

To address the issues associated with adequate staffing, the American Nurses Association (ANA) in 1997 convened a panel of nurses to begin to develop an understanding of the factors that contribute to the working conditions of nurses. The panel's discussion included:

- Feasibility of identifying minimum safe staffing levels
- Levels and variability of patient acuity
- Individualized nurse factors such as experience and education
- Organizational resources and support available to the patient care unit
- Issues related to the work environment (ANA, 2005, p. 4)

The panel concluded that there were three different models that could begin to address this issue. The first approach was to implement nurse staffing plans, with input from direct care nurses, assuring that nurse-to-patient ratios were based on patient need and other relevant factors. A second approach was for legislators to mandate specific ratios. The third approach was to require health care institutions to disclose staffing ratios to the public or a regulatory body (ANA, 2009).

California was the first state to adopt legislation that mandated fixed nurse-to-patient ratios, passing this historic legislation in 1999. Although an additional 15 states have introduced similar legislation since that time, California remains the only state that has set requirements for every patient care unit in every hospital in the state (ANA, 2009). These types of ratios require set nurse-to-patient ratios based solely on numbers of patients within given nursing care areas and do not take into account issues such as patient acuity, level of staff preparation, or environmental factors. Though mandating such ratios is a first step toward beginning to assure adequate numbers of nurses, many states are now moving toward the concept of safe staffing rather than specific nurse-to-patient ratios.

Adequate and safe nurse staffing is critical to ensuring the delivery of quality patient care, and changes in staffing levels, including changes in the overall number and/or mix of nursing staff, should be based on a comprehensive and inclusive evaluation of multiple nursing-sensitive indicators. Adequate staffing should be based on the consideration of three critical factors: the maintenance of the quality of patient care, the quality of the organizational outcomes, and the quality of nurses' work life (ANA, 2005). If these are accomplished, adequate and safe staffing issues will be assured.

Thirteen states plus the District of Columbia have now enacted legislation or adopted regulations to address staffing issues. Most of these states have passed safe staffing measures rather than mandating ratios. Generally, these safe staffing measures call for a committee to develop, oversee, and evaluate a plan for each specific nursing unit and shift based on patient care needs, appropriate skill mix of RNs and other nursing personnel, the physical layout of the unit, and national standards or recommendations regarding nursing staffing. Washington State's plan also includes a provision that the staffing information is posted in a public area of the nursing unit, updated at least once per shift, and that the information is available to patients and visitors upon request (Safe Nurse Staffing Legislation, 2008). A federal Safe Nurse Staffing Act was defeated in 2007.

Although the institution is ultimately accountable for staffing issues, nurse-managers may also incur some potential liability because they directly oversee numbers of personnel assigned to a unit on a given shift. Courts have traditionally looked to the constant exercise of professional judgment, rather than a reliance on concrete rules, in times of short staffing. This means that using judgment to ensure patient safety and quality care is more important than ensuring that each unit has the exact nurse-to-patient ratio. For nurse-manager liability to occur, it must be shown that a resultant patient injury was directly due to the "short staffing" and not due to the inappropriate or incompetent actions of an individual staff member. Remember, staffing problems never cancel the institution's obligation to maintain a reasonable standard of care.

An older case had set the stage for such an upholding. In a 1990 Georgia case, a hospital was sued for negligence to provide adequate staffing. The case concerned the ability of emergency center staff members to adequately diagnose and intervene appropriately with a patient who suffered a myocardial infarction. The court concluded that the hospital was required to provide staff competent to exercise a reasonable degree of care and skill when delivering health care to patients (*Harrell v. Louis Smith Memorial Hospital*, 1990).

Guidelines for nurse-managers in short-staffing issues include alerting hospital administrators and upper-level managers of concerns. First, though, nurse-managers must have done whatever was under their control to have alleviated the circumstances, such as approving overtime for adequate coverage, reassigning personnel among those areas they supervise, and restricting new admissions to the area. This includes listening to staff members about their competencies, knowing which patients require special expertise and unique care, and knowing what is reasonable to ensure the continuing safety of patients. This may also involve soliciting such information from staff members because some staff members may be reticent to volunteer the needed information.

Second, remember that nurse-managers have a legal duty to notify the chief operating officer, either directly or indirectly, when understaffing endangers patient welfare. One way of notifying the chief operating officer is through formal nursing channels, for example, by notifying the nurse-manager's direct supervisor. Higher administration must then decide how to alleviate the short staffing, either on a short-term or long-term basis. Appropriate measures could be closing a certain unit or units, restricting elective surgeries, procuring additional temporary staff, or hiring new staff members. Once nurse-managers can show they acted appropriately, used sound judgment given the circumstances, and alerted their supervisors of the seriousness of the situation, then the institution becomes potentially solely liable for staffing issues.

If the hospital has no collective bargaining contracts, the employment is considered to be at-will employment. The hospital is free to set the terms and conditions of employment, including numbers of hours worked and when the hours will be worked. The federal Fair Labor Standards Act, which governs employment conditions, and most state labor laws do not restrict the number of hours that nurses can work in a given pay period or week. Additionally, under employment-at-will, workers can be terminated at any time and for any reason, including failure to follow a direct order, such as mandatory overtime.

One means that nurse-managers in employment-at-will states use is insisting that nurses work mandatory overtime as a means of alleviating short staffing. A New York licensure case illustrates what can happen when such mandatory overtime is requested. In *Husbert v. Commissioner of Education* (1992), a nurse was notified by the supervisor that one of the day-shift nurses would be required to work an extra shift due to staff shortage. Under the hospital's mandatory overtime policy, the nurse with the least seniority was required to stay. The RN told the supervisor she would stay, but she left after an hour, informing no one she was leaving. Twenty-nine patients were left with no RN supervision, though there were nurse's aides and orderlies who remained to give direct care to the patients. Many of the patients were elderly, suffering from multiple illnesses and requiring multiple intravenous injections. Three of the patients were intubated and ventilator-dependent.

The case was brought before the hearing panel, which found that the policy was appropriate, that the nurse was aware of the policy, and that a true emergency understaffing issue existed on the day of the occurrence. The panel found that the nurse had abandoned the patients, and her license was suspended for 1 year. Because there had been no reasonable notice given to the nursing supervisor, the supervisor had no opportunity to find a replacement nurse. When she left the floor, the RN had informed the staff that she was going to see the supervisor and that she should be paged if an emergency arose.

The case illustrates nurses' responsibility to the hospital for assisting in times of short staffing by providing reasonable patient care in as safe a manner as possible. For a variety of reasons, management did not resort to continuous use of mandatory overtime until fairly recently, mainly because it is demoralizing to staff and can lead to increased absenteeism, burnout, and staff turnover. More important, mandatory overtime is frequently dangerous from a patient perspective, because mistakes and oversights occur more often when one is overworked and tired.

Fifteen states now prohibit the use of mandatory overtime by nurses, 12 through enacted legislation and 3 via provisions in the nursing regulations. Generally these laws state that the health care facility may not require an employee to work in excess of agreed to, predetermined, and regularly scheduled daily work shifts unless there is an unforeseeable declared national, state, or municipal emergency or catastrophic event that is unpredicted or unavoidable and that substantially affects or increases the need for health care services. Additionally, many of these laws define "normal work schedule" as 12 or fewer hours, and employees are protected from disciplinary action or retribution for refusing to work overtime; monetary penalties can result from the employer's failure to adhere to the law. Some states also mandate that health care facilities are required to have a process for complaints related to patient safety. Note that nothing in these laws negates voluntary overtime.

Nurse-managers must work to ensure that competent care remains the standard of the institution and work to ensure that mandatory overtime is not a concept used within their institutions if they work in states that have no restrictions on mandatory overtime. Nurse-managers in states where statutes preventing mandatory overtime have been enacted should ensure that these statutes are followed and that no retaliation or disciplinary action ensues if nurses elect not to work overtime.

Staff nurses also have some responsibilities to ensure that understaffing does not persist. First, nurses should discuss the issues and concerns with the nurse-manager, either individually or collectively. Nurses may also fill out Assignment Under Protest forms, which are available at some hospitals or state nursing associations, or which they themselves have created. Document specific problems related to the understaffing, such as not being able to timely administer medications, failure to adequately teach patients about their home instructions, or failure to perform ordered treatments. Document in a factual manner, citing numbers of patients, acuity levels, numbers and mix of staff, and specific examples of what actually occurred, not what could have occurred. Also, list positive actions that can be implemented to alleviate the shortage, both short term and long term, as applicable. Work together with management in a constructive and positive manner to resolve chronic understaffing issues.

Float Staff

Float staff, staff members who are rotated from unit to unit, is the second issue that concerns overall staffing. Institutions have a duty to ensure that all areas of the institution are adequately staffed. Units temporarily overstaffed either due to low patient census or a lower patient acuity ratio usually float staff to units less well staffed. Floating nurses to areas with which they have less familiarity and expertise can increase potential liability for the nurse-manager, but to leave another area understaffed can also increase potential liability. Floating nurses from one area to another can also create problems for the nurse who is floated. Accepting the float assignment places the nurse in jeopardy of caring for patients for which one is not fully qualified, and rejecting the assignment places one at risk of disciplinary actions.

Winkelman v. Beloit Memorial Hospital (1992) illustrates this point. Ms. Winkelman sued the hospital for wrongful discharge after she was terminated for refusing to float to the hospital's post-operative and geriatric care area. For 16 years, she had worked exclusively in the newborn nursery, an arrangement that the hospital had approved when she was hired and had honored all the years she worked in the nursery. The hospital, however, also had a policy that nurses would be floated as needed to maintain quality nursing care in all units of the hospital.

When asked to float to an adult unit, Winkelman immediately contacted her supervisor and explained the working arrangement that she had with the institution. She explained that she had never been floated before, that she was unqualified to float to an adult unit, and that floating would place patients, her license, and the hospital at risk.

According to Winkelman, she was given three options: float as requested; find a replacement nurse to float; or take an unexcused absence from the institution and go home. She chose the latter option. The supervisor maintained at trial that only the first two options were made available to Winkelman, and that there was no option to take an unexcused absence. Later, based on these actions, the hospital insisted that Winkelman had voluntarily resigned and, despite her objections, refused to reinstate her.

She sued and eventually recovered $40,000 in lost wages. The court found that she had been terminated for refusing to float, noting that in this instance the refusal to float was an appropriate action based on her education and experience. The court noted in the ruling that "the sick should be given care only by those who are in fact qualified to do so. . . . licensure does not itself confer a particular qualification" (at 215). Similarly, the court in *Whittier v. Kaiser Foundation Hospitals* (2007) found that the nurse had acted appropriately in not acting on an assignment that would have required her to work in an area of the hospital where she was not qualified and where patient safety could have been an issue.

Before floating staff from one area to another, the nurse-manager should consider staff expertise, patient care delivery systems, and patient care requirements. Nurses should be floated to units as comparable to their own unit as possible. From a legal perspective, the nursing care delivered by the float staff need not be perfect, but it must be consistent with that provided by a reasonably prudent nurse with similar skills and expertise under similar circumstances. This requires the nurse-manager to match the nurse's home unit and float unit as closely as possible or to consider negotiating with another nurse-manager to cross-float the nurse. For example, a manager might float a critical care nurse to an intermediate care unit and float an intermediate care unit nurse to the floor unit. Or the manager might consider floating the general floor nurse to the postpartum floor and floating a postpartum floor nurse to labor and delivery.

Staff nurses need to be aware that patient **abandonment** could become an issue. If the staff nurse accepts the float assignment, reports to the unit in which he or she will assist, is assigned responsibility for patient care, and then decides not to fulfill that responsibility, he or she could be charged with patient abandonment. The nurse who is to be floated must negotiate before accepting the float assignment. Once accepted, the nurse must fulfill this assignment.

A recent case that illustrates patient abandonment is *Miller v. Tennessee Board of Nursing* (2007). In that case, a licensed practical nurse (LPN) was assigned to care for five patients on the night (7:00 P.M. to 7:00 A.M.) shift. She became ill during the shift and informed the other nurses that she needed to leave. The charge nurse instructed her to speak with the nursing supervisor before leaving, which the LPN did not do. Instead, she merely left the premises. The hospital terminated her employment contract and reported her to the state board of nursing. The court upheld this finding, noting that the nurse had wrongfully abandoned her patients when she left the hospital premises without assuring that the patients assigned to her care would receive nursing care for the remainder of the shift.

Reasons that a nurse should consider in refusing an assignment include lack of a specific skill or competency and the lack of proper orientation so that patient safety is compromised. Open communications regarding staff limitations and concerns as well as creative solutions for staffing can alleviate some of the potential liability involved and create better morale among the float nurses. A newer option is to cross-train nurses within the institution so that nurses are familiar with two or three areas and can competently float to areas in which they have been cross-trained.

Staff nurses have a responsibility to the employer to float to other units in times of need or overstaffing on their primary unit. This includes taking advantage of the opportunity to orient to other units in the institution so that when floated to that unit, the nurse will already know unit policies and procedures and be more apt to give quality nursing care. An older New Mexico case reiterates the employee's responsibility. In *David W. Francis v. Memorial General Hospital* (1986), an intensive care nurse refused to float to an orthopedic unit because he did not feel qualified to act as charge nurse on that unit. The hospital offered to orient him, but he declined and was later terminated at the institution. The court sided with the employer, noting that the employee's unwillingness to orient or even try working with hospital administration undermined his case.

GUIDELINES

Float Nurses

The responsibilities of a nurse temporarily assigned to another unit include:

1. Before accepting a patient assignment, state any hesitancy you might have about it to appropriate persons (direct supervisor, nurse-manager, or team leader). Make your objections clear and specific. Follow your verbal hesitancies with a written memo to your supervisor, and make a photocopy of the memo for your records. In the written memo, state ways in which you would feel more comfortable in the reassignment, such as with a formal orientation period or more specific knowledge of the nursing routine for the new unit.

2. State your qualifications and skills concerning assessment skills, performance of routine procedures, and the like to the appropriate charge person. Thoroughly understand the patient assignment before accepting it, because once accepted, you are legally accountable for the nursing care of the patients and could be charged with abandonment if you choose to leave before the next shift of nurses arrives.

3. Identify your immediate resource person, and ask any questions you might have about the assignment, orders, routine procedures, and the like. Resource persons might be the charge nurse, a physician, a team member, or an interdisciplinary staff person.

4. Recognize and give yourself credit for your strengths as well as enumerating your weaknesses. Ask for help only if truly needed, remembering that you are capable of routine nursing procedures and assessments.

5. Remember that much of the case law involving float nurses concerns the broad area of medications. Double-check references, call the pharmacist, or contact your direct supervisor prior to administering any medication about which you are unsure. If numerous unfamiliar medications are to be given to several patients, arrange to perform more routine nursing procedures for the patients while another nurse who is familiar with the medications, unit, and patients administers all the medications.

The responsibilities of the charge nurse to whose unit a nurse is temporarily reassigned include:

1. Thoroughly assess the qualifications of the reassigned nurse. Ask specific questions so that you may competently make patient assignments. Offer to orient the assigned nurse to the unit, and start with the more critical policies and procedures first.

2. Make the patient assignments carefully. Refrain from taking advantage of the float nurse by overloading the float nurse or by assigning difficult patients merely because this nurse is

not a permanent member of your staff. The float nurse may later decide to ask for permanent assignment to your unit based on your fairness and management style.

3. Continue to reassess the reassigned nurse. Offer assistance as needed, and follow behind the float nurse as much as possible to reassure yourself that competent patient care is being delivered.

4. Keep your immediate supervisor apprised of changes within the unit or in patient status. Whether additional help is available or not, you may escape potential liability as you correctly assess the situation and ask for help when it is needed.

5. Reassign patients as dictated by changes in their status or in the number of patients because of admissions to the unit.

6. Run interference as much as possible to assure all the nurses on the unit that you are continually balancing the needs of the patients with the individual demands and needs of the nursing staff.

7. Be aware that much of the case law in this area involves medication errors. Be constantly available as a resource person, and ask questions to ascertain that the float person understands proper dosages, administration routes, and potential side effects. Alternately, give the medications yourself, and allow the float nurse to assume other responsibilities of direct and indirect patient care.

8. Nurses who feel appreciated may perform to higher expectations. Remember to reassure the float nurse that he or she is performing well and is appreciated.

9. Listen carefully to the float nurse's concerns and comments and act accordingly, so that potential liability may be averted.

Agency Personnel

The use of temporary or **agency personnel** has created increased liability concerns among nurse-managers. Until recently, most jurisdictions held that such personnel were considered to be independent contractors and that the institution was not liable for their actions, although their primary employment agency did retain potential liability. Some jurisdictions still follow this principle. Other courts have begun to hold the institution liable under the principle of apparent agency or ostensible authority.

Ostensible authority (or **apparent agency**) refers to the doctrine whereby a principal becomes accountable for the actions of his or her agent. Apparent agency is created when a person (agent) holds himself or herself out as acting on behalf of the principal. In issues concerning agency nurses, the patient is unable to ascertain if the nurse works directly for the hospital (has a valid employment contract) or is working for a different employer. At law, lack of actual authority is no defense.

The principle of apparent agency applies when it can be shown that the reasonable patient believed that the health care worker was an employee of the institution. If it appears to the reasonable patient that this worker is an employee of the institution, then the law will consider the worker as an employee for the purposes of corporate and vicarious liability.

The borrowed servant doctrine may also be employed by courts in deciding cases involving agency staff. With this doctrine, the special master or hospital must have complete control and direction of the servant (nurse), and the general master (employment agency) must have the exclusive right to discharge the employee. Usually, the hospital can be shown to have complete supervisory control over agency nurses while they are in the hospital setting, including assigning them to specific units, assigning patients to their direct care, and making them accountable for following hospital policies and procedures. The agency retains accountability for paying the nurse's wages, furnishing unemployment benefits, and requiring the nurse to maintain validation forms regarding clinical skills.

Whether the agency providing the nurse shares in the liability should patients be injured depends, in large part, on the nature of the relationship with the hospital and agency and the language and words used in their written agreement. In *Hansen v. Caring Professional, Inc.* (1997), a patient had a jugular venous catheter. The catheter became dislodged, presumably while the agency nurse was assisting the patient to sit up in bed, and air entered into her brain. The patient suffered permanent brain injury caused by the bolus of air. Although the nursing staffing agency had provided the temporary nurse to the hospital, the court said that the agency had no right to control the manner of the nurse's work, nor the time, place, or scope of her practice.

The contract between the nurse and the agency described her as an "independent contractor." Indeed, the nurse was responsible for all of her own expenses, none of her income was withheld by the agency, and she was exclusively supervised by the hospital. Part of the evidence produced at trial clearly showed that she had received a Form 1099 to document her earning as an independent contractor from her agency, and not a W-2 form as an employee. Therefore, the court ruled that the agency could not be held accountable for the nurse's alleged malpractice, because no employer–employee relationship had been established.

The court in *Ruelas v. Staff Builders Personnel Services, Inc.* (2001) reached a similar conclusion, though for an entirely different reason. The court concluded that the agency has no practical or even theoretical right to control how its nurses perform their clinical responsibilities. The agency must ensure that its nurses are licensed and must ensure that the nurse's education, experience, and certifications are valid and correct. But the agency is not legally responsible for wrongful conduct of the nurses on the job, when the hospital has full control over how the agency nurses perform their jobs.

A different outcome occurred in *Gallegos v. Presbyterian Healthcare Services, Inc., Lloyd's Professional Healthcare Services, Inc., and Speller* (1995). A New Mexico court returned a $166,323 verdict against the hospital, a nurse's aide, and the aide's employment agency after an elderly patient fell and broke her hip. While being cared for by the nurse's aide, who had no prior hospital experience, the patient fell. Her hip was surgically repaired and the patient underwent 2 weeks of rehabilitation. The patient died 2 months after the fall, either from consequences of the fall or her underlying pathology.

The family filed suit, alleging negligence, wrongful death, and reckless hiring and retention of the aide, who had no previous training as an aide. The trial judge dismissed the wrongful death claim since it could not be determined to what degree the fall had hastened her death. A nurse testifying for the family stated that the fall would not have occurred if the aide had been trained properly and had experience working as an aide. The jury allocated 45% of the liability to the hospital that supervised the aide at the time of the fall, 50% of the liability to the aide's employment agency for its failure to verify her training or lack of training as an aide, and 5% of the liability to the aide herself.

This newer trend of the law makes it imperative that the nurse-manager consider temporary workers' skills, competencies, and knowledge when delegating tasks and supervising their actions. If there is reason to suspect that the temporary worker is incompetent, the nurse-manager must convey this fact to the agency. The nurse-manager must also either send the temporary worker home or reassign the worker to other duties and areas. Screening procedures, the same as those used with new institution employees, should also be performed with temporary workers.

Additional areas that nurse-managers should stress when using agency or temporary personnel include ensuring that the temporary staff member is given a brief but thorough orientation to institution policies and procedures, is made aware of resource materials within the institution, and is made aware of documentation procedures. It is also advisable that nurse-managers assign a resource person to the temporary staff member. This resource person serves in the role of mentor for the agency nurse and serves to prevent potential problems that could arise merely because the agency staff member does not know the institutional routine or is unaware of where to turn for assistance. This resource person also serves as a mentor for critical decision making for the agency nurse.

GUIDELINES

Staffing Issues

1. When you first realize that a unit will be understaffed, try to get qualified help immediately. Options include asking nurses to work overtime or come in on a day off, floating nurses from other units, and employing temporary agency nurses.

2. Keep a record of all requests for additional staffing in a log or journal. This ensures an accurate record of what transpired should litigation develop as a result of staffing. While such a record may not prevent some liability, it will show what steps were taken and how you attempted to address the problem.

3. Make frequent visits to the understaffed unit, assessing the situation and working with the charge nurse to set priorities. Transferring patients to other units may be a viable option, depending on the specialty of the understaffed unit and staffing in other units.

4. If you use an agency nurse, assign him or her to fully staffed units and float one of that unit's staff to the understaffed unit. The staff RN will probably be more help for the understaffed unit, particularly since he or she knows the hospital policies and procedures and needs to ask fewer questions. If possible, float a staff RN who has been cross-trained to the understaffed unit.

5. Pitch in and help as you can. This includes nursing as well as clerical tasks. Reassign ancillary personnel to also assist with clerical and non-nursing tasks, further freeing nursing staff to meet high-priority tasks.

6. Plan ahead for potential understaffing. When hiring new personnel, ascertain if they can assist with additional work time. Even 4 hours would be an assistance in times of short staffing, and nurses may be willing to help if they are not required to work a full 8- or 12-hour shift. Orient new employees to at least two units, so that you have more leverage in times of short staffing on one unit.

7. Talk to management about establishing a nursing resource pool or per diem nursing staff. These nurses would be knowledgeable about the hospital's policies and procedures, could be oriented to a variety of units, and are then available for staffing emergencies.

EXERCISE 14.2

Terry Sanchez, an agency nurse, floated to labor and delivery and was informed that a 38-weeks-pregnant patient of Dr. Kwan was on her way to the hospital. Dr. Kwan had a standing order that all of his patients were to have fetal monitors. Terry, after placing the monitor on the patient, failed to note that the patient's monitor indicated a pattern consistent with fetal distress. Dr. Kwan, arriving 45 minutes later, looked at the monitor and ordered an immediate cesarean section, but the child was born severely brain damaged. In the subsequent suit against the hospital, Dr. Kwan, and Terry Sanchez, who would be found liable and why? Which of the defendants could show absence of liability and why?

Are there factors that the nursing supervisor should have considered before assigning Terry to this unit? Would this have averted liability on the part of the supervisor, should you conclude there was liability?

POLICIES AND PROCEDURES

Risk management is a process that identifies, analyzes, and treats potential hazards within a given setting. Although the terminology is somewhat different, the steps of the risk management and nursing processes are similar: assess, plan, intervene, and evaluate. The object of risk management is to identify potential hazards and to eliminate them before anyone is harmed or disabled. *Gess v. United States* (1996), cited earlier in this chapter, illustrates this vital role of health care agencies in preventing harm. In *Gess,* the court noted that the actions of Gess should have leaped from the incident reports had anyone been closely monitoring the reports. His was the name that was common on all the reports; in fact, he was the very first person to begin resuscitation efforts in the majority of the patients involved. The court concluded that he was the only commonality to all the reports, and the hospital should have noted this immediately. The purpose of quality assurance, held that court, is to be alert for suspicious patterns in adverse patient situations and to take corrective actions. A good starting point is to match personnel on duty with the incidents, consider what is known about their backgrounds, and monitor their actions.

Written **policies and procedures** fall within the scope of risk management activities and are a requirement of the Joint Commission. Individual institutions may also have protocols and critical pathways that fall within the scope of risk management. Such documents set standards of care for the institution and direct practice. Factors that shape a successful risk management program include the visibility and accessibility of the risk management department staff, as well as risk management guidelines that are clearly stated, address multiple issues that may arise within a given institution, and can be implemented, as appropriate, by various levels of staff, and are based on evidence-based practice. Nurse-managers should review the policies and procedures frequently for compliance and timeliness. If policies are outdated or absent, request that the appropriate person or committee either update or initiate the policy.

CONTRACT PRINCIPLES

A **contract** is a legally binding agreement made between two or more persons to do or to refrain from doing certain actions. Every contract, to be enforceable by law, must have four essential features:

1. Promises or agreements must be made between two or more persons or entities for the performance of an action or restraint from certain actions. Most nursing contracts specify the conditions and performances the nurse will undertake, but contracts may also be made to prevent certain actions.

2. All parties to the contract must have a mutual understanding of the terms and meaning of the contract.
3. Compensation in the form of something of value in exchange for the action or inaction must be expressed by the contract terms. Usually, this compensation is in monetary terms such as a specified salary or dollar amount per hour earned wage, but other items of value may be seen as compensation.
4. The contract must fulfill a lawful purpose. There can be no enforceable contract for illegal acts or fraud.

Contracts serve to provide one or more parties with a legal remedy if another party does not perform its obligations pursuant to the terms of the contract. Contracts, especially those in writing, serve to minimize misunderstandings and offer a means for parties of the contract to resolve any disputes that may arise.

Legal Elements of a Contract

Legally, contracts have four elements:

1. *Offer:* The person or the entity (a hospital or home health care agency) extends an offer to someone to be hired or with whom the person or entity will have a contractual relationship. The person extending the offer is the offeror, and the person to whom the contract is extended is the offeree.
2. *Acceptance:* The actual acceptance of or agreeing to the terms and conditions of the contract creates the contract. Acceptance may be in written form or verbal. Contracts may also be accepted by the beginning performance of the offeree, for example, when the nurse shows up promptly on the first day of work in a new position.
   Exceptions to verbal acceptance have been created by the law. The **statute of frauds** is the legal principle that a contract does not need to be written to be enforceable. Exceptions to this statute include agreements involving marriage, the sale of land or interests in land, the sale of goods over a certain dollar figure, suretyship (agreements to pay or perform actions in the event that the principal is unable to meet his or her obligations), and agreements that cannot be performed within a 12-month period.
3. *Consideration:* This element concerns the economic costs of an agreement. Consideration is what is negotiated between offeror and offeree. Often, consideration is seen as the salary figure or dollar figure per hour worked, but consideration may also include a set fee per unit of work or other objects of value.
4. *Consent (sometimes referred to as mutuality of agreement and obligation):* This element involves the mutual assent to the agreement, or actions that lead the parties to the contract to reasonably believe that an agreement has been reached. As with acceptance, the beginning performance by the offeree would indicate to both parties consent to the contract.

Consent also involves the competency of the parties to the contract to enter into a valid contract. Issues that courts of law evaluate in determining competency include the age of the parties (adults versus those under the age of majority) and the mental capacity to understand the terms and meanings of the contract.

Additional issues that may be considered include the legality or lawful purpose of the contract. Courts of laws will not enforce contracts made for other-than-lawful purposes. Contracts that provide for criminal or tortuous actions or actions opposed to public policy will not be enforced. Thus, the entire range of criminal and tort law is incorporated into this element.

TYPES OF CONTRACTS

A **formal contract** is required by law to be in writing. To prevent fraudulent practices, all states have statutes of fraud requiring certain contracts to be in written form. Some formal contracts also require that they be written under seal, stamped with an official seal, or written on a special imprinted paper. All other contracts are considered simple contracts, whether written or oral.

An **oral contract** is equally binding as a written contract, though the terms of the contract may be more difficult to prove in courts of law. The terms of the contract are subject to memory and interpretation, and often there may be a change in personnel during the term of the contract, causing new interpretations. For these reasons, most contracts are written and include language that the contract survives the employment of the original signors.

An **expressed contract** concerns terms and conditions that were specifically negotiated or discussed during the creation of the contract. These expressed terms may be either oral or written, and both parties to the contract have an opportunity to either question or renegotiate the expressed terms at the time of entering the contract. **Implied contracts** concern terms or conditions of the contract that each side anticipated were a part of the contract but that were never actually expressed or discussed. Most expressed contracts have some implied provisions as well. For example, the nurse is expected to perform quality, safe nursing care and to follow the policies and procedures of the hospital even though such expectations were not explicitly written or verbalized, and the employer is expected to provide a safe work site for the employee and to have the necessary supplies and equipment to ensure competent nursing care.

GUIDELINES

Negotiating an Individual Employment Contract

Before accepting a contract with a potential employer:

1. Address employment practices and ensure that you are aware of the following:
   a. Exact work hours and schedules
   b. Time off, including individual days off, vacation time, and sick leave
   c. Float policies
   d. Mandatory or requested days off without pay
   e. Accruement of vacation and sick time
   f. Periodic evaluations, including purpose and by whom
   g. Style of nursing care, such as primary or team nursing
   h. Philosophy of nursing
   i. Status of the institution as a collective bargaining unit or employment-at-will institution
   j. Classification of nurses such as Staff Nurse I, II, or III, and how to advance from one level to the next
   k. Orientation time and educational expectations
   l. Number of required hours of continuing education per year
   m. Leaves of absence such as bereavement, medical, jury duty, and personal leaves
   n. Seniority and how it is accrued, how it affects temporary and permanent work reductions, and how it is lost
   o. Grievance procedures

    p. Existence of clinical ladder programs, qualifications, and employee eligibility to apply for such programs

    q. Use of private car for transportation, as applicable

2. Understand the payment scale in the following areas:

    a. Base salary

    b. Differentials for evening and night-shift work; charge nurse responsibilities; working specific units such as intensive or intermediate care; weekend shift work; holiday pay; and salary differences for degrees, certification, and/or years of experience

    c. Raises, either as cost of living or merit

    d. Number of paid holidays per year and restrictions on when they may be taken

    e. Change in base scale for clinical ladder positions

    f. Reimbursement for use of private car as applicable

3. Ask about benefits and who pays the cost of such benefits for the following:

    a. Group hospitalization, vision, and dental plans

    b. Term life insurance policies

    c. Retirement plan

    d. Parking

    e. Savings programs and employer-sponsored credit union

    f. Conversion of accrued sick leave and vacation time to terminal pay

    g. Professional liability insurance

    h. Child care facilities

    i. Housing

    j. Formal education reimbursement programs

    k. Insurance for private car as needed to see patients in home settings

Individual contracts are negotiated between a single individual and the offeror, whereas collective contracts are those negotiated by collective bargaining units for the benefit of the unit. Most individual contracts are informally offered and accepted, whereas collective contracts are negotiated formally, specifying all particulars of the contract, and accepted in writing.

EXERCISE 14.3

Obtain a copy of the contract used in your health care facility, if one exists. What terms are expressed, and which terms affecting nursing practice are silent? How would you negotiate the contract differently, or try to negotiate differently, if you were the professional nurse who was to sign the contract? If no contract exists, what conditions and terms would you negotiate for if you were applying for a position in the health care facility?

TERMINATION OF A CONTRACT

Contract termination signifies that the terms of the contract have been fulfilled or that the parties to the contract agree to the contract's end. Sometimes the term *released from a contract* is used to indicate the ending point of the contract. A release implies that the contract has not been completely fulfilled, but that there has been no breach of the contract. In individual employment contracts with health care agencies, the offeree traditionally writes a letter of resignation and the employer-offeror releases the employee from any further obligations under the terms of the contract.

A second means of terminating a contract is by **breach of contract,** which is essentially the failure of one or both of the parties to abide by the agreement and to meet the contract obligations. For example, if an employee agrees to work at a health care facility for a period of no less than 12 months in return for a sign-on bonus and leaves the institution after 8 months, the employee has breached the contract. Remedies for breach of a contract include monetary damages, injunctions, and specific performance.

A recent case illustrates the importance of contract provisions when working with agency nurses. In *Dunina v. Lifecare Hospitals* (2006), hospital personnel noted that narcotics were missing whenever a certain agency nurse worked in the facility. Administrative staff chose to solve the issue by telling the agency that this particular nurse could no longer work in the acute care hospital. The agency offered the nurse work assignments at other facilities in the city, but she declined the offer and sued Lifecare Hospitals and the staffing agency.

The court found that although there was no formal contract between the agency nurse and the hospital, there was a formal contract between the agency and the hospital. The contract gave the hospital the right to dismiss the agency nurse at the hospital's discretion, with or without cause. The agency nurse's contract with the agency stated that she agreed to be treated as an at-will employee, meaning that the agency had no obligation to provide her with employment or to try to continue an assignment terminated by a client facility. The agency met its obligations by offering her assignments at other facilities. There was no obligation on the part of the agency to get the nurse reinstated at the facility where she wanted to work. The court also noted that had the facility dismissed the agency nurse on the basis of her gender, national origin, age, race, or other protected entity, then the agency would be bound by antidiscrimination laws, just as the hospital was bound by these laws.

Monetary damages are the usual remedy for breach of contractual obligations. Because the underlying goal in breach of contract suits is to place damaged or injured parties in as good a position as they would have been if the provisions of the contract had been fulfilled, the court allows injured parties to be compensated monetarily. In the preceding example, the nurse may be required to pay back the entire sign-on bonus previously received or a prorated portion of it.

If the employer is the person breaching the terms of the contract, the employee wrongfully discharged may bring suit for lost salary and other economic benefits that had been agreed upon by the terms of the contract. The injured employee may also ask for reinstatement as well as monetary damages.

The injured party may request an **injunction,** which is a court order requiring a person to refrain from doing a specific act. The hospital in the preceding example may ask the court to issue an injunction against the nurse, preventing him or her from working at another health care facility for the remainder of the contract term. Although injunctions are not often requested, injured parties may seek injunctive relief, particularly if the business concerns a specialty trade or craft. Injunctions may also be obtained to prevent a former employee from contacting individuals served by the business. In a company that has spent years building an established clientele, the company may seek an injunction preventing the former employee from contacting, either directly or indirectly, any of the persons doing business with the previous employer.

A Louisiana case illustrates this concept (*Nursing Enterprises, Inc. v. Marr,* 1998). In that case, a nurse worked for a nursing staffing agency developing new business relationships with client hospitals and other providers. She also recruited staff nurses, attempting to match their backgrounds and career goals with the clients' needs.

A dispute with her employer over a promotion resulted in her tendering her resignation. After tendering her resignation, but before it became effective, she, her husband, and a nurse-partner leased office space, set up new phone lines, and had an attorney draw up and file articles of incorporation for a new nursing staffing agency. The new agency was successful from the start. The former employer sued and won injunctive relief and an award of compensation for lost business from the trial court.

At the appellate level, the court held that it is not unfair competition for a former employee to enter into competition with a former employer. It is unfair competition, and grounds for a successful lawsuit, for an employee to copy or remove confidential information that belongs to the employer. Files and records are the employer's personal property and the information in the files and records is protected as trade secrets.

However, an employee is free to use the general knowledge of the employer's business practices the employee carries away in his or her mind. The employee is also free to go to phone books and directories for potential client information, even if that yields essentially the same client names as the former employer's client base. According to the court, the law strongly favors business competition.

Similarly, in *Mercury Staffing, Inc. v. Newark Extended Care Facility, Inc.* (2007), the contract between the nursing agency and the nursing facility prohibited the facility from directly hiring any of the nurses sent to the facility by the agency unless the agency was willing to pay the agency a finder's fee of 25% of the nurse's first annual salary. When the facility directly hired seven nurses who had been referred to work at the facility by the nursing staffing agency, the extended care facility was charged $94,622.50 for the breach of contract.

Specific performance is enforcement by the court to comply with the terms of the contract. The court could force the breaching employee to work the remainder of the 4 months of his or her contract, having already received the sign-on bonus. Again, this is seldom sought as a remedy by the injured party because morale and work performance become problematic when workers are forced to stay in jobs or positions after they have either left or announced their decision to leave.

ALTERNATIVE DISPUTE RESOLUTION

Nurses are frequently reluctant to challenge contract disputes in courts of law because of perceived harm to their reputation and the time that such suits take from their personal and professional lives. Because of such concerns, there are now alternative means of resolving contract disputes. The contract as signed should have a provision that **alternative dispute resolution** processes will be used as needed.

Mediation

Mediation allows the disputing parties to resolve differences while maintaining a professional relationship. Mediators are neutral third parties who facilitate disputes by assisting both parties to identify their specific needs and concerns and work toward an agreeable solution. Costs of using mediators are usually shared by the parties, and several consultants offer this service.

Arbitration

Arbitration involves the selection of a neutral third-party arbitrator who is knowledgeable in the area of contention and who renders a decision and award. Often used in employment contract disputes, this neutral third party is knowledgeable about working conditions, terms of employment contracts, and factors leading to such disputes. He or she is empowered to make a final decision, and that decision is usually binding to both sides of the dispute, although the parties can agree in advance that the decision will not be binding. Arbitration is used with collective bargaining disputes, and both sides must realize that the arbitrator's decision, unlike the mediator's decision, becomes binding on both sides of the dispute.

Fact Finding

The **fact-finding** alternative dispute resolution process is normally reserved for complex multistate and multiparty disputes. Again, a neutral party is employed to sort out the various facts of the dispute and to assist the parties in knowing all the facts of the dispute, from the perspective of all the parties to the dispute.

Summary Jury Trial

A **summary jury trial** is an abbreviated, privately held trial that may be used to give both sides of the dispute an indication of the strengths and weaknesses of their case and the potential outcome should they decide to seek trial resolution.

NURSES AND CONTRACTS

Understanding contracts may not significantly alter one's nursing care, but such an understanding can aid nurses in their decision to accept a position and can increase job security and satisfaction by giving nurses some control within the work setting. Remember, however, that nurses must be satisfied with all the terms of the contract before accepting it. Nurses' bargaining power is in knowing exactly what they want in the work setting and in negotiating for it before the contract is accepted. There is no negotiating power once the contract is accepted. Contract negotiation is therefore an important skill for nurses.

Nurses may also contract with other agencies during the course of operating a privately owned business. For example, a nurse or group of nurses may decide to open a home health care agency. They will need contracts for employees hired as direct patient caregivers, for clerical workers, for space rentals for the agency, for other agencies that deal with the home health care agency such as durable medical suppliers, and for clients served by the agency. The terms, both expressed and implied, must be understood, and the home health care agency must ensure that all provisions are expressly contracted. Nurses entering such formal, multiparty contracts are encouraged to seek legal representation for all contract negotiations, particularly as state laws vary. A variety of nursing consultants specialize in this area of the law, and a variety of law firms offer this expertise.

EXERCISE 14.4

You are the supervisor in a hospital that has collective bargaining for its professional staff. A staff member requests vacation for the next two weekends. There is a family wedding out of state the first weekend. Her mother is having surgery on the Friday of the second week, and she has promised to help take care of her mother that weekend. Do you schedule the staff member for the vacation? What types of contract questions would you ask before deciding how to best answer this question? Would your answer be different if the employment contract is silent regarding weekends that registered nurses are required to work in this hospital?

CONTRACTS THAT ARISE AFTER EMPLOYMENT

Courts have held that contracts may arise after employment, even in states with employment-at-will doctrines and absence of collective bargaining units. Statements in employee manuals or handbooks may serve to create a valid contract and prevent the discharge of an employee, just as oral statements made to entice a person to take the position may create contract language.

In *Sides v. Duke* (1985), a nurse moved from Michigan to North Carolina, accepting a position from which she was told she could be discharged only for cause, and incompetency was specified as the sole cause for discharge. While at the health care setting, she refused to administer a medication she believed would injure a patient and, indeed, the patient was injured after another nurse gave the medication. During that patient's malpractice suit against the hospital and physician, Ms. Sides was told not to tell the whole truth by the defendants and their counsel. When Ms. Sides testified to the true matter, she was discharged by the hospital.

In her suit for wrongful discharge, she argued two theories of law: contract and tort. She successfully convinced the jury that the move from Michigan to North Carolina in addition to the statement that she could be discharged only for incompetency created an employment contract. Her expectations, based on the employer's statements, changed an at-will employment to a contractual employment.

Employee handbooks can constitute a contract, giving enforceable rights to the employee. For this to happen, the following elements must be present:

1. The handbook must be expressed in language that clearly sets forth a promise the employee can constitute as an offer.
2. The handbook must be distributed to the employee, making him or her fully aware of it as an offer.
3. After the employee learns of the offer, he or she must begin to work or continue to work.

ETHICAL ISSUES

The issue of mandatory overtime, which remains a viable option in the majority of states, raises ethical issues about the safety of patients and safety concerns for the nurse. Ethical nursing practice mandates that nurses not engage in practice that can compromise patient outcomes. The American Nurses Association's (ANA) *Code of Ethics for Nurses* (2001) addresses these ethical issues in the following sections: Provision 3 "The nurse promotes, advocates for, and strives to protect the health, safety, and rights of the patient," and Provision 4 "The nurse is responsible and accountable for individual nursing practice and determines the appropriate delegation of tasks consistent with the nurse's obligation to provide optimal patient care" (ANA, 2001, p. 4). Though several states have now outlawed the practice of mandatory overtime through regulations, nurses may continue to volunteer for overtime work assignments. Nurse-managers and those staff members with whom these nurses work need to continue to be vigilant concerning the safety of the patients and the nurse herself or himself when voluntary overtime occurs.

A second ethical issue concerns how nurse-managers and nursing staff work with management regarding corporate liability. With the court's proclamation that failing to serve as a patient advocate may be considered corporate negligence, nurses have a responsibility to see that patient care is not compromised and thus does not become a potential area of liability. How one approaches unsafe practice issues involves respecting the patient and the staff member and reinforcing beneficence and justice while ensuring that any unsafe practice does not continue.

As the nursing shortage continues and becomes more complex, issues surrounding adequate and safe staffing are also emerging. Determining if adequate numbers and mix of staff are present to assure safe patient care can be very subjective, and nurse-managers are challenged to ensure that staffing ratios are appropriate while also observing cost measures. Balancing these two concerns involves the ethical issues of justice, beneficence, nonmalifience, and respect for all persons involved. Similarly, ensuring that the most capable and efficient person floats to a short-staffed area also incorporates these ethical principles.

SUMMARY

- Liability in health care settings is generally viewed as personal, vicarious, or corporate liability.
- Corporate negligence has been determined by the courts to occur when nurses fail to serve as patient advocates and the health care institution, through its administrative officers and staff, knows that there is a serious risk to patient safety and allows the patient care problems to continue and escalate without intervening.
- Causes of malpractice for nurse-managers include negligent hiring, negligent retention of incompetent or impaired staff, inappropriate assigning of staff, failure to supervise and educate staff, and failure to warn employees of potential problems with previously employed staff.
- Staffing issues include adequate numbers of staff, floating staff from one unit to another unit, and the use of temporary or agency staff members.
- Mandatory overtime has now been prohibited in 15 states.

- Patient abandonment occurs when a nurse accepts a patient assignment and fails to fulfill the patient assignment without first ensuring that another qualified nurse has accepted the patient assignment.
- Risk management is a process that identifies, analyzes, and treats potential hazards within a given setting.
- A contract is a legally binding agreement made between two or more persons to do or refrain from doing certain actions.
- Legal elements of a contract are offer, acceptance, consideration, and consent (frequently known as agreement and obligation).
- There are four types of contracts: formal, oral, expressed, and implied.
- If the provisions of the contract are breached, remedies include monetary damages, injunction, or specific performance.
- Alternate means of resolving contract disputes are by means of mediation, arbitration, fact finding, and summary jury trial.

APPLY YOUR LEGAL KNOWLEDGE

1. What are the most common potential legal liabilities for nurse administration and nurse-managers in health care settings?
2. How can these areas of potential liability be minimized or avoided?
3. What measures should a nurse-manager take to ensure that agency personnel working in the institution meet standards of care?
4. What provision of a nursing contract is the most important, and how does one ensure that nurses understand the importance of contracts within their profession?
5. Why should nurses be concerned about learning contract law? How does such knowledge assist in their future employment?

YOU BE THE JUDGE

A few days after a patient's spinal disc surgery, the surgeon discovered that he had used pediatric rather than adult pedicle screws during the spinal fusion surgery. He promptly informed the patient of the error, urging the patient to have the surgery redone because the screws used were inappropriate for a person of her height and weight. She was, he said, at risk for the screws to fail, causing potential new injuries. The patient and her husband sued the surgeon, the physician who assisted the surgeon, and the hospital.

In the case, the plaintiffs noted that the sales representative for the company that had manufactured and supplied the hardware and screws necessary for the procedure had brought complete sets to the central supply area. Someone in the central supply area had sent the correct hardware, but the incorrect size of screws, to the operating room for the patient's surgery. The circulating nurse and the surgical assistant had merely passed the incorrect screws to the surgeon when he asked for those pieces of equipment. No one in the operating area caught the error at the time of the surgery.

Along with a malpractice claim against the two surgeons involved in the case, the patient is alleging a corporate liability claim. Her contention is that the hospital has a legal responsibility for proper selection of supplies, instruments, and equipment used in treating patients who enter the hospital.

QUESTIONS

1. Under the principle of corporate liability, is there a valid claim in this case?
2. Is the corporate liability of the hospital contingent on a finding that the surgeons were liable for the error in using smaller screws than were indicated for an adult patient?
3. Is there liability on the part of the nurses in this instance?
4. Do contract principles apply in this case, in that the hospital had a contract with the company that supplied the equipment/hardware?
5. How would you decide this case?

REFERENCES

American Nurses Association. (2001). *Code for nurses with interpretive statements.* Washington, DC: Author.

American Nurses Association (2005). *Utilization guide for the ANA principles of nurse staffing.* Washington, DC: Author.

American Nurses Association. (2009). *Nurse staffing plans and ratios.* Washington, DC: Author. Available at http://www.nursingworld.org/mainmenucategories/ANA-PoliticalPower/State/StateLegislature/

Bunn-Penn v. Southern Regional Medical Corporation, 488 S.E.2d 747 (Ga. App., 1997).

Daldulav v. St. Mary Nazareth Hospital Center, Docket No. 62737 (Illinois, 1987).

David W. Francis v. Memorial General Hospital, 726 P.2d 852 (N.M., 1986).

Dunina v. Lifecare Hospitals, 2006 WL 1529475 (Ohio App., June 2, 2006).

Gallegos v. Presbyterian Healthcare Services, Inc., Lloyd's Professional Healthcare Services, Inc., and Speller,

Bernalillo County District Court, Case #CV 95-228 (N.M. D.C., 1995).

Gess v. United States, 952 F. Supp. 1529 (M.D. Ala., 1996).

Greenwood v. Paracelsus Health Care Corporation, 622 N. W. 2d 195 (North Dakota, 2001).

Hansen v. Caring Professionals, Inc., 676 N.E.2d 1349 (Ill. App., 1997).

Harrell v. Louis Smith Memorial Hospital, 397 S.E.2d 746 (Georgia, 1990).

Healthcare Trust v. Cantrell, 689 So.2d 822 (Alabama, 1997).

Husbert v. Commissioner of Education, 591 N.Y.S. 99 (New York, 1992).

Jackson v. Harper Hospital, 2006 WL 2613599 (Mich. App., September 12, 2006).

Karnes v. Doctor's Hospital, 555 N.E.2d 280 (Ohio, 1990).

Mercury Staffing, Inc. v. Newark Extended Care Facility, Inc., 2007 WL 2963225 (N. J. App., October 12, 2007).

Miller v. Tennessee Board of Nursing, 2007 WL 2827526 (Tenn. App., September 26, 2007).

Nursing Enterprises, Inc. v. Marr, 719 So. 2d 524 (La. App., 1998).

Ponce v. Ashford Presbyterian Community Hospital, 238 F.20 (1st Cir., 2001).

Roach v. Kelly Health Care et al., 742 P.2d 1190 (Oregon, 1997).

Ruelas v. Staff Builders Personnel Services, Inc., 18 P.3d 138 (Ariz. App., 2001).

Safe Nurse Staffing Legislation, Washington State HB 3123 (March, 2008).

Shelly v. Bethshan, 2007 WL 4374509 (Cir. Ct. Cook Co., Illinois, October 18, 2007).

Sides v. Duke, 74 N. C. App. 3d 331, 328 S. E. 2d 818 (North Carolina, 1985).

St. Paul Medical Center v. Cecil, 842 S.W.2d 809 (Texas, 1992).

Theft of drugs is serious problem, putting patients and hospitals at risk. (1997). *Health Risk Management, 19*(4), 41.

Whittier v. Kaiser Foundation Hospitals, 2007 LEXIS 22492 (California, 2007).

Whittington v. Episcopal Hospital, 768 A.2d 1144 (Pa. Super., 2001).

Winkelman v. Beloit Memorial Hospital, 168 Wisc.2d 12, 484 N.W.2d 211 (Wisconsin, 1992).

CHAPTER 15

Delegation and Supervision

PREVIEW

Delegation, used throughout all of nursing history, has evolved into a complex, work-enhancing strategy that has the potential for greatly increasing the individual nurse's legal liability. Prior to the early 1970s, nurses used delegation to direct the multiple tasks performed by the various levels of staff members in a team nursing model. Subsequently, the concept of primary nursing became the desirable nursing model in acute care settings, with the focus on an all-professional staff, requiring little delegation. By the mid-1990s, a nursing shortage had again shifted the nursing model to a multilevel staff, with a return of the need for delegation and supervision. This chapter explores the concepts of delegation and supervision and the legal liabilities that can ensue.

LEARNING OUTCOMES

After completing this chapter, you should be able to:

15.1 Differentiate delegation from assignment.

15.2 Discuss the concept of supervision in effective delegation and distinguish between direct and indirect supervision.

15.3 Discuss the role of effective discipline in delegation and supervision.

15.4 Define and evaluate the role of unlicensed assistive personnel in relation to professional accountability.

KEY TERMS

assignment
delegatee
delegation
delegator

direct supervision
effective discipline
indirect supervision

supervision
unlicensed assistive
    personnel

DELEGATION, ASSIGNMENT, AND SUPERVISION

Delegation has been defined in a number of ways, with some consistencies among the definitions. Involved in any delegation are at least two people, a **delegator** and a **delegatee,** with the transfer of authority to perform some type of task or work. A working definition could be that delegation is the transfer of responsibility for the performance of an activity from one individual to another while retaining accountability for the outcome. In other words, delegation involves the transfer of responsibility for the performance of tasks and skills without the transfer of accountability for the ultimate outcome. Examples include the registered nurse (RN) who delegates patients' personal care tasks to certified nursing aides (CNAs) who work in a long-term care setting. In delegating these tasks, the RN retains the ultimate accountability and responsibility for ensuring that the delegated tasks are completed competently.

Typically, delegation involves tasks and procedures assigned to unlicensed assistive personnel, such as certified nurse's aides, orderlies, assistants, attendants, and technicians. Delegation, though, can also occur from licensed staff members to other licensed staff members. For example, if one RN has the accountability for an outcome and asks another RN to perform a specific component of the overall function, that is delegation. This type of delegation typically occurs between professional staff members when one member leaves the unit/work area for a meal break or committee work.

Advantages of delegation include the fact that effective delegation develops a more balanced workload, allowing the delegator the ability to concentrate on and complete other non-delegable tasks. Delegation promotes increased communications between health care providers and provides the opportunity for individuals to develop trust and respect. Finally, delegation also promotes a team environment and potentially leads to greater productivity (Nahavandi, 2006).

Delegation is complex because it involves relationships and communication (Anthony, Standing, & Hertz, 2000). It also involves entrusting others so that they assume responsibility with the delegator for certain tasks and duties. Involved in the delegation process are multiple players, usually with varying degrees of education and experience, who have different scopes of practice. Understanding these variances and communicating effectively to the delegatee involves an understanding of competencies and the ability to communicate with all levels of staff personnel (Potter & Grant, 2004).

The importance of communication was exemplified in *Short v. Plantation Management Corporation* (2000). In that case, the 69-year-old resident of a nursing home had previously had hip replacement surgery. Approximately 4 months after her admission, her right lower leg became swollen and her foot gradually became a darker color. Eventually, the right greater toe turned a purplish color and the resident complained of severe pain. It was only when the resident complained of pain that the professional nursing staff members were made aware of the resident's overall condition. Subsequent surgery was performed to amputate the leg below the knee, and the patient, through her family members, sued for negligent care. At trial, it was noted that the nurse's aides had failed to mention anything about the resident's changing condition to the professional staff and that professional staff never inquired about changes in the resident's condition.

Communication on the part of the individual delegating a specific task is equally important. In *Steele v. Department of Workforce Development* (2006), an aide was terminated from employment at a nursing home for attempting a solo transfer of a patient from her bed to her wheelchair without using a gait belt and without requesting assistance from another person. The aide was terminated, and he appealed when the state denied his unemployment claim. On appeal, the court determined that it was unclear as to whether requirements regarding the patient's care plan were effectively communicated to the aide. Assignment sheets for the patients were kept in a notebook at the nurses' station, but it was unclear if the aide was ever instructed to review the assignment sheets or supervised to ensure that he did review the assignment sheets. Effective communication of what is expected, noted the court, is one of the many basic responsibilities of a supervisor.

Similarly, in *Black v. Department of Social and Health Services* (2007), effective communications may have altered the care of the patient. In *Black*, a resident in a residential treatment center for persons with developmental disabilities was prescribed a helmet that was to be worn at all times so that the patient could not injure himself by hitting himself on the head. The RN in charge delegated the care of the patient to an aide, who stated she did not agree with the order for the helmet, claiming that the helmet interfered with the patient's right of consent. She also stated that she could keep him from hurting himself if the helmet was not worn. The patient was later observed bleeding from a self-inflicted head wound and the aide was discharged from the facility.

At the point when the aide stated she did not agree with the treatment of this patient and that she could keep him from harming himself if the order helmet was not used, the RN responsible for the patient's safety should have changed the aide's patient care tasks. In the alternative, the delegating RN should have supervised more carefully and altered to whom this patient's care was entrusted when the RN first noted that the patient was not wearing the ordered helmet.

Delegation may be distinguished from **assignment,** which is the downward or lateral transfer of both the responsibility and accountability for an activity from one individual to another. Assignment occurs most often in clinical settings between licensed personnel. For example, the team leader/nurse-manager in an acute care setting assigns patients to the licensed staff members working on a given shift. In assigning the care for a specific patient to the staff member, the team leader/nurse-manager also gives the staff member the full responsibility for ensuring that the patient receives competent and timely care.

Involved in both delegation and assignment is the concept of **supervision,** which may be defined as the active process of directing, guiding, and influencing the outcome of an individual's performance of an activity. Supervision may be defined as either direct or indirect supervision. **Direct supervision** is provided when the delegator is actually present, observes, works with, and directs the person who is being supervised. **Indirect supervision** occurs when the delegator is easily contactable, but does not directly oversee the interventions or activities being performed.

The field of nursing involves supervision of a variety of personnel, including professional staff members who directly provide nursing care to patients. The delegator remains personally liable for the reasonable exercise of delegation and supervision activities. The failure to delegate and supervise within acceptable standards of professional nursing practice may be seen as malpractice. Additionally, in a newer trend in the law, failure to delegate and supervise within acceptable standards may extend to direct corporate liability for the institution. For example, in *Fairfax Nursing Home, Inc. v. Department of Health and Human Services* (2003), a nursing home was held to be liable for inadequate practices and procedures in monitoring ventilator-dependent patients. In that case, the professional staff had delegated the task of suctioning a ventilator-dependent patient to a nurse's aide. After suctioning the patient, the aide failed to ensure that the ventilator was reconnected to the patient, and the patient died. The professional staff member did not check to see that the procedure had been done correctly. Review Chapter 13 for a more thorough discussion of corporate liability.

Note, however, that team leaders/nurse-managers are not liable merely because they have a supervisory function. The degree of knowledge concerning the skills and competencies of those one supervises is of paramount importance. The doctrine of "knew or should have known" becomes a legal standard in delegating tasks to licensed or unlicensed individuals whom one supervises. If it can be shown that the team leader/nurse-manager delegated tasks appropriately and had no reason to believe that the individual to whom the task was delegated was anything but competent to perform the task, the delegator will be judged to have no personal liability. But the converse is also true. If it can be shown that the delegator was aware of incompetencies in a given employee or that the assigned task was outside the employee's scope of practice, then the delegator becomes potentially liable for any subsequent injury to a patient.

Team leaders/nurse-managers have a duty to ensure that staff members under their supervision are practicing in a competent manner. The team leader/nurse-manager must be aware of nurses' knowledge, skills, and competencies and that they maintain their competencies. Knowingly allowing a staff member to function below the acceptable standard of care opens both the nurse-manager and the institution to potential liability.

A case example of this concept is *Sparks Regional Medical Center v. Smith* (1998). In that case, the Court of Appeals in Arkansas upheld an $80,000 civil judgment against a hospital in favor of a female medical-surgical patient who was sexually assaulted by a male nurse. The court awarded the monetary damages for extreme psychological trauma, anxiety, distress, and depression.

The court noted in its finding that before this particular incident, the male nurse was seen in the room of two female psychiatric patients having a sexual conversation with them. He was only verbally warned and was not restricted from contact with vulnerable patients, nor was an effort made to monitor his activities more closely. This, said the court, was negligence in supervising an employee to the detriment of a patient's safety. The court also found the hospital liable under the doctrine of vicarious liability.

Some means of ensuring continued competency are continuing education programs and assigning the staff member to work with a second staff member to improve technical skills. Another method is to require the nurse in question to attend additional courses at institutions of higher education. For example, this latter means of increasing nursing proficiency may be used to improve the nurse's knowledge of pharmaceutical agents or to increase the nurse's knowledge and skills in health and physical assessment techniques.

Effective discipline is a vital part of the nurse-manager/supervisor's role in supervision and delegation. Effective supervision assists persons to perform at their best, improving in areas in which their performance requires improvement and ensuring an acceptable level of competent productivity within the unit. The best means for nurse-managers to assist staff in reaching such acceptable levels of output is through setting firm standards for all work and establishing a formal discipline plan to be used when performance fails to meet these preset standards. See the accompanying Guidelines feature for the steps involved in creating an effective discipline plan.

GUIDELINES

Creating an Effective Discipline Plan

1. Set firm work rules and performance standards, communicating them to everyone before any disciplinary action is needed.
2. Design a progressive discipline system that is fair to all concerned and provides an opportunity for employee improvement.
3. Be consistent in applying the disciplinary rules. Once you begin the process, follow the progressive discipline plan exactly.
4. Investigate all facts and circumstances leading to the disciplinary action, making complete and detailed notes.

5. Document carefully and completely all employment actions.
6. Review the employee's work record and all the facts before determining what action must be taken.
7. Give the employee an opportunity to rebut the allegations.
8. Allow the staff member to read the documentation concerning reprimands and other disciplinary actions, and ask the employee to sign the documentation as acknowledgment. If the employee refuses, include a note to that effect in the documentation.

Ultimately, the nurse is responsible and accountable for individual nursing practice and determines the appropriate delegation of tasks consistent with the nurse's obligation to provide optimal patient care (American Nurses Association [ANA], 2008). This obligation is met by the delegation of tasks based on the needs and condition of the patient, the potential for harm, the stability of the patient's condition, the complexity of the task, and the predictability of the outcome (ANA, 2008).

EXERCISE 15.1

Judy Brown is the nurse-manager for an acute care medical-surgical floor. One of the staff members in the unit, Molly Chu, has consistently been absent or tardy in the past month, and Judy has implemented a disciplinary plan with Molly. A provision of this plan is that Molly must notify the nurse in charge if she will be late or absent for a given shift at least 4 hours in advance of the shift. If she fails to follow this plan, Molly knows she will be dismissed from the institution. For the past 2 weeks, Molly has been on time for work and has not needed to call the nurse in charge.

Judy has a planned 1-week vacation, and her responsibilities for the medical-surgical floor will be assumed by Joey Johansen during Judy's vacation. Judy has explained to Joey the need for the disciplinary plan and the terms of the plan that has been negotiated between Molly and Judy. Joey had previously worked with Molly, and he spoke with her about the plan before Judy left for vacation.

On the second day of Judy's vacation, Molly neither called the nurse in charge nor appeared for a scheduled shift. Joey subsequently completed the necessary paperwork for Molly's dismissal. Molly has protested the dismissal, stating that only Judy can fire her, as this type of responsibility is not delegable.

How would you decide this issue? Can this type of action be delegated from one professional staff member to another professional staff member? If you were Joey, would you have handled this issue in another way? From an ethical perspective, was there a better manner for addressing this issue?

PRINCIPLES OF EFFECTIVE DELEGATION

Whether delegating to licensed or unlicensed staff members, there are some general aspects to remember. Perhaps one of the more important issues to remember is that nurses have an obligation in the ANA *Code of Ethics for Nurses* (2001) to delegate tasks appropriately. Provision 4 states "The nurse is responsible and accountable for individual nursing practice and determines the appropriate delegation of tasks consistent with the nurse's obligation to provide optimal patient care" (ANA, 2001, p. 4). Additionally, the ANA *Nursing Scope and Standards of Practice* (2003) mandates that the nurse assigns or delegates tasks based on the individual needs of the patient, the complexity of the task, the predictability of the outcome, and the abilities of the staff person to whom the task is assigned or delegated.

Other issues that must be considered when delegating tasks include the following. One is that the RN who is responsible and accountable for delegation of tasks and procedures retains individual liability for such delegation. A second issue is that only tasks or procedures should be delegated, not the entire nursing process. In other words, the RN retains the accountability and responsibility for determining assessment of the patient's needs, planning what interventions should be enacted, determining whether they are the appropriate interventions, and the ultimate evaluation of the success or failure of the interventions. Delegation thus involves the actual tasks, such as taking vital signs, ambulating the patient for the full length of the hallway, or ensuring that the patient receives at least 1000 cc of fluid in an 8-hour period.

Delegation is not a list of tasks, though, but a responsibility that must be undertaken using critical thinking and professional judgment. Elements essential before delegating to others include understanding the definition of delegation and the need for follow-up. One cannot merely delegate, but must ensure that the delegated tasks were performed and performed correctly. The RN must also understand whether the task is delegable according to the state nurse practice act. Given the individual state, some nursing actions cannot be delegated to unlicensed personnel, such as the required assessment of the patient. Even if the task is delegable, consider if the best course of action might be not to delegate. For example, although feeding a patient could be delegated to another staff member, the RN might decide to do the task herself or himself. One reason for this could be to better assess how well the patient is able to swallow, or it might be the best opportunity the nurse has for effectively teaching the patient about proper nutrition and diet restrictions.

Before delegating, one should also determine the amount of supervision required. Nothing is gained if the amount of supervision needed exceeds the time saved by delegating the task. For example, if the nurse is unsure that the person to whom the task would be delegated can adequately perform the task, then he or she may need to repeat the task. One means of preventing such an occurrence is to use the time needed for the task to educate the delegee or ensure that the delegee receives the proper training before being assigned to the hospital unit.

The National Council of State Boards of Nursing (1997) created a list of the Five Rights of Delegation:

1. Right task
2. Right circumstances
3. Right person
4. Right directions and communication
5. Right supervision and evaluation

Inherent in each of the rights is the concept that merely because one can delegate a task does not mean that the task should be delegated. The more unpredictable the outcome, the less likely it is that a particular task is one that can be safely delegated. The delegator must consider all the aspects of the delegation, including whether delegating the task will ensure the provision of competent and quality nursing care.

UNLICENSED ASSISTIVE PERSONNEL

As management struggles to become more cost-effective and provide for better patient outcomes, the issue of alternative patient care providers has been addressed by health care facilities. Many institutions have now employed **unlicensed assistive personnel** (UAP), persons not authorized under respective nurse practice acts to provide direct patient care. Legal concerns about these UAPs abound.

One of the first areas of legal concern that arises addresses whether these UAPs "practice on the license" of the delegator, as the UAP is not a licensed individual. Remember, only licensed persons are granted that license and only they retain or lose it. A variety of unlicensed personnel have functioned in health care institutions for years without this question arising, including orderlies, nursing aides, and clerical workers. These persons work under the auspices and license of the institution, not the professional nurse. Review the concept of institutional licensure in Chapter 11.

Second, the organization must ensure that there are adequate resources to ensure sufficient staffing so that professional staff members may appropriately delegate patient care tasks. Additionally, the corporation is accountable for documenting competencies for all staff members providing direct patient care and for ensuring that professional staff members have access to this competency information (ANA, 2008).

Third, there should be an institutional mechanism for consistent and adequate orientation and training of UAPs. This is established by nursing administration, taking into consideration how these persons will be used by the institution and where their services are most needed. Patient care responsibilities should be well delineated, and UAPs must be taught when to inform other personnel of patient data (e.g., vital signs) or untoward happenings. Additionally, nurses should know that they have a responsibility to inquire about expected outcomes, such as asking about the blood pressure readings for a patient scheduled to receive potent vasopressor medications or the heart rate in a patient being treated for cardiac palpitations.

Should untoward patient outcomes occur and a lawsuit be filed for malpractice/negligence against the health care providers, issues that will arise include responsible delegation and supervision of UAPs. Professional nurses are responsible for the safe delegation of tasks, including follow-up, to ensure that delegated tasks and procedures were performed and the adequate supervision of UAPs occurred. These are the same issues that professional nurses face daily and are not exclusive to UAPs.

For example, in *Ferry v. State of Oklahoma* (2007), a patient had life-long cognitive deficits related to her cerebral palsy. Her caregivers knew, or were supposed to know, that the patient was not to be left unattended in a bathtub. When she was left unattended by a treatment aide, the patient subsequently drowned. The court found that her death was attributed to the aide who did not know of this treatment restriction, noting that the task was not correctly delegated nor was the aide adequately supervised. Similarly, in *Williams v. West Virginia Board of Examiners* (2004), the 1-year suspension of the license of an RN was upheld by the state nursing board. The basis for this suspension was the inadequate manner in which the nurse carried out her responsibility and accountability for supervising nonlicensed homemakers working in Medicaid clients' homes. Among the many complaints against the individual homemakers were that they were absent when they should have been at the clients' homes, that the homemakers failed to complete required in-service training hours, and that the homemakers did not know what their individual tasks were. Additionally, the nurse falsified records, including that the appropriate nursing care had been given these clients when she herself had no means of knowing what had or had not transpired in the clients' homes.

Finally, in *Ditch v. Waynesboro Hospital* (2007), the court held that a health care facility has the responsibility to ensure that delegated tasks are consistent with safety concerns of a patient. In this case, a patient was seen in the hospital's emergency center following a stroke. When it was decided that she was to be admitted to an acute-care unit, the transfer of the patient was delegated to nonlicensed personnel. During the transfer procedure, the patient fell from the bed, hit her head, and suffered an orbital fracture and a closed head injury. She died due to a subdural hematoma 3 days later.

The court noted that patient safety needs mandate that a professional staff person assess the patient prior to a transfer, accurately assessing the need for the individual patient's safety needs, including the need for restraints during the transfer procedure. This transfer should then be appropriately delegated to personnel who have received adequate instructions regarding the transfer of the patient and are competent to safely transfer a stroke patient from a bed to a stretcher.

Note that at least one court has held that delegation involves more than the physical care of the patient. In *Thurston v. Worker's Compensation Fund* (2003), the court held that the nurse's aides had a responsibility to report both the patient's physical and psychological needs. In this case, nurse's aides were caring for a home health client who had sustained an on-the-job accident that caused serious burns and eventually resulted in the amputation of both the patient's arms. Over time, the patient became more and more depressed, and his alcohol and drug ingestion increased. The home health aides continued to provide quality physical care but failed to mention his worsening depression, and the supervising staff members did not question them about the patient's psychosocial status. The patient subsequently committed suicide. Though the court said it would be speculation to conclude that the patient's death was directly due to less-than-adequate home health care, it did conclude that the duty to supervise delegated tasks extended to more than mere physical tasks.

Supervision is one of the keys to ensuring that proper delegation with UAPs results in positive and competent patient care. Supervision is the "active process of directing, guiding, and influencing the outcome of an individual's performance of a task" (ANA, 2008, p. 3). Supervision is interpersonal and goal directed. It requires that professional nurses understand their own scope of practice, role dimensions, and job descriptions as well as the scope of practice, role dimensions, and job descriptions of UAPs, from legal, ethical, and organizational perspectives. Supervision involves a thorough understanding of the skill sets and contributions that UAPs bring to care delivery in all clinical settings. Finally, supervision involves an appreciation of the division of effort that allows the professional nurse more time to attend to the nursing needs of complex patients and interdisciplinary collaboration.

EXERCISE 15.2

John Jordon, a 62-year-old resident of Happy Dale Nursing Home, weighed more than 300 pounds and was 6 feet tall. He was developmentally disabled and had lost the use of one of his legs due to a series of cerebral vascular events. His plan of care expressly called for two aides to assist him when transferring him from his wheelchair to his shower chair. The care plan also called for him to be transferred to the shower chair in his room because the shower area was too narrow for the two-person assisted transfer to be done there.

Despite the care plan and the direction from the professional nurse in charge, one aide attempted to transfer Mr. Jordon from his wheelchair to the shower chair by propping him against the wall on his good leg. During this maneuver, the resident lost his footing, fell, and injured his good leg.

In the lawsuit that followed, the issues of delegation and supervision were highlighted. Was the professional staff negligent in allowing nurse's aides to transfer this resident? Was this a delegable task? What implication should the court find in the fact that only one aide assisted the resident on this particular day? Is there liability in this case and, if yes, who should be found liable?

Supervision is a means to achieve understood and desired goals. Supervision involves appreciation of teamwork, appropriate assignment of duties, assessment of and provision for ongoing learning needs of UAPs, and oversight of performance with timely feedback to UAPs to ensure quality outcomes.

Effective supervision strategies when working with UAPs include:

1. Know the UAP's role expectations, competencies, strengths, and weaknesses well.
2. Allocate sufficient time for supervision, making rounds, opportunities for the UAP to bring issues and concerns to the staff nurse, and evaluation of the progress of care delivery.
3. Develop and maintain clear channels of communication, including being available to UAPs as needed.
4. Adhere to patient care and work performance standards.
5. Give timely feedback, both positive and negative, and make time for sharing formative information with UAPs.

Professional nurses must also ensure that tasks delegated to UAPs are within a delegable scope of practice and that tasks requiring licensure are not delegated to UAPs. Once delegated, the nurse must ensure that the action was performed and performed correctly.

A case example in which communications would have improved the delegation of the task and ensured a better patient outcome is *A. O. v. Department of Health and Rehabilitation* (1997). An aide was told by the charge nurse to bathe several nursing home patients. He bathed one and then helped a second patient into the shower chair. There were no towels left where he had found them earlier, so he asked the nurse where to find more towels.

The delegating nurse informed him it was his job, not hers, to look for towels. The aide pushed the patient back into her room, still in the shower chair with a belt secured around her waist. He assumed incorrectly that the nurse knew he was looking for towels and would keep an eye on the patient. On his return, he found the patient on the floor of her room, having sustained a fractured wrist. The aide was disciplined by state authority for neglect of a patient.

The District Court of Appeals disagreed with this discipline. Leaving this patient alone for a brief period of time is not neglect as defined by the law, the justices held. Close monitoring of the patient had not been ordered; thus, it was not neglect to leave the patient alone briefly while the aide was searching for bath towels. It could not reasonably be expected before the fact that this patient would suffer harm while being left alone, so the aide cannot be held responsible for her unfortunate injury.

Note that this outcome could have been prevented if communication had been enhanced between the nurse and the aide. The patient would have been more closely watched if the aide had communicated this to the nurse, and perhaps he would have been more inclined to openly communicate if the nurse had not responded so sarcastically to his request concerning the location of additional bath towels.

When deciding to use UAPs in patient care units, nursing management should consider the following factors:

1. The type of UAP support being planned and whether it will be primarily supportive or patient care delivery
2. Previous experience and credentials the UAPs need to be eligible for employment
3. Assignment of responsibility for supervising the UAPs and whether each of these potential supervisors understands both the role and limitations of UAPs
4. The type of staff mix that will be used in the institution
5. Inclusion of professional and nonprofessional staff in work redesign efforts
6. The specific tasks or responsibilities to be delegated
7. The institution's policies, procedures, job descriptions, and performance evaluations and their match with these revised roles and expectations
8. Effective communication of these changes to other health care providers in the institution

9. The types of communications to be available for staff to make their concerns known

10. The types of evaluations to be done to assess the effectiveness of UAPs (Blouin & Brent, 1995)

A case that exemplifies the appropriate use of UAPs is *Hunter v. Bossier Medical Center* (1998). In *Hunter*, the physician's orders to ambulate a post-operative diskectomy and spinal fusion patient were carried out by two nursing aides, because it was Sunday and no physical therapists were on duty. The two aides had 26 years of experience between them.

The patient was assisted in walking to the nurses' station and back up the hall, with one aide assisting him on each side. When he was back in his room, one aide held him against the wall while the other aide changed the bed linens. When he said he felt faint, the aide followed standard protocol and procedure by leaning the patient against her chest and allowing him to slide in a gentle manner to the floor. One aide immediately summoned the nurse for help, and the other aide took his vital signs, asked him if he was all right, and assessed him for external injuries. Then the three of them put him back to bed.

The physician was promptly notified of the patient's fall, and x-rays were done. There was no evidence that the position of the bone graft had slipped. The court ruled that this same technique of assisting a patient to the floor during ambulation is widely taught to licensed and nonlicensed personnel and is a proper method for safely assisting a patient who is about to fall. The court also noted that it was fully documented in the patient's record that this method had been used, apparently successfully averting injury to the patient. Thus, even though the patient continued to suffer back pain, the actions of the nurses were appropriate, and there was no liability found on the part of the nurses or the hospital.

GUIDELINES

Delegation

1. Remember that merely because a task can be delegated does not mean that it should be delegated. Before considering delegating a task, use thoughtful decision making and check to see that:
   a. There is a low potential for harm to the patient;
   b. The delegated task does not entail complex nursing activity or problem solving;
   c. The outcome for the task is highly predictable; and
   d. There is adequate RN supervision and opportunity for interactions with the individual performing the task as well as the patient for whom the task is done.

2. Provide clear and specific directions regarding the task, ensuring that the plan of care has been individualized to the patient's specific needs.

3. Communicate the method of performance to be used, including expected outcomes, and ensure that the task has been adequately performed. If this is the first time the task will be performed, have the delegatee demonstrate the performance of the task.

4. Encourage the individual to whom the task is delegated to ask questions as needed, to always follow the institution's established protocols and guidelines, and to report all observations and activities to the delegator. Remind the delegatee to seek assistance and further direction before proceeding with the delegated task as appropriate.

5. As the delegator, ensure that:
   a. Adequate staffing and other resources needed for safe and effective patient care are provided;

b. Follow-up is provided on any report of concern for safe staffing or safe practice, with needed steps taken to correct any area of concern; and

c. Education concerning delegation is current in the institution.

ETHICAL CONSIDERATIONS IN DELEGATION

Ethical issues that arise with delegation are multiple. A primary issue concerns the differences between delegating versus "dumping" of needed tasks. Delegation has a specific framework, enabling the delegator to delegate tasks while taking into consideration the best possible outcomes from a patient perspective, matching the best person to accomplish the delegated tasks, and continually developing the potential of all members of the team. Dumping generally is seen as the handing off of tasks that the nurse-manager does not want to accomplish or is not interested in completing. Dumping is not a process, nor is it a reciprocated relationship. Ethically, dumping does not allow for respect of the person or justice.

A second ethical issue concerns what might best be described as a fair selection process. This issue concerns to whom tasks are delegated, assuring that nursing care tasks are evenly distributed so that patient outcomes are met while not overburdening any one member of the health care team or treating one more favorably than another. Fair selection involves monitoring the number and quality of delegated tasks so that tasks are fairly shared while challenging and stimulating the growth of each individual employee. Fair selection involves ongoing communications, individual development plans, and accurate and up-to-date performance appraisals. This concept also assures that all members of the health care team share tasks as equally as possible, including the delegation of less favorable tasks and patient assignments.

A third issue concerns the safety and physical needs of patients, ensuring that not only are nursing care tasks fairly distributed, but that the driving force remains the best possible outcome for the patient. This ethical concern acknowledges the importance of viewing ethical concerns from two separate perspectives, patient and health care provider, and balancing these concerns appropriately.

Finally, ethics mandate that an examination of the delegation and supervision processes occurs on a daily basis. Nurse-managers must be cognizant of the fact that delegation and

EXERCISE 15.3

The patient was elderly, had been a resident in a nursing home for some years, and the family had recently questioned the quality of their mother's nursing care. She had fallen several times during the past few months, generally as she attempted to transfer herself from her bed to a wheelchair or from a wheelchair back to her bed. After the resident's last fall, during which she sustained injury to both her hips that ultimately caused her death due to complications, the family filed a lawsuit for negligence.

In the testimony at court, it was discovered that a lack of nursing leadership prevailed throughout the facility. Specifically, this lack of leadership resulted in a disorganization of patient care duties, with no specific aide assigned the care of any resident. This resulted in no one being specifically responsible for ensuring the safety of the resident. Neither were there formal reports by aides at the end of the shift. Also noted was that the facility did not have care protocols for high-fall-risk patients.

How would you begin to remedy the situation at this care facility? What obligations does the corporation have to ensure the appropriate delegation and supervision of care for residents? What obligations does the professional staff have to ensure the appropriate delegation and supervision of care for residents? Are there ethical issues as well as legal concerns that should be considered?

supervision are always ongoing processes and are much more than the mere assignment and follow-up of tasks. The delegator must constantly be aware of the criteria being used to delegate nursing care tasks, ensuring that they are delegated appropriately and fairly, according to agency policy, and allowing for individual development and growth. This reexamination also involves follow-up on providing necessary feedback to employees. Checkpoints should be established to measure progress toward individual goals, and timely performance evaluations should be completed.

SUMMARY

- Delegation is the transfer of responsibility for the performance of an activity from one individual to another while retaining accountability for the outcome.
- Delegation is accomplished through a delegator and a delegatee.
- Assignment is the downward or lateral transfer of both the responsibility and accountability for an activity from one individual to another, generally among licensed staff members.
- In both delegation and assignment, supervision—defined as the active process of directing, guiding, and influencing the outcome of an individual's performance of an activity—is vital.
- Supervisors become potentially liable dependent upon the degree of knowledge one has about another's ability to perform competently.

- Effective discipline, which is a part of the supervisor's role, assists persons to perform at their best, improving in areas in which their performance requires improvement and ensuring an acceptable level of competent productivity.
- When delegating, remember that only tasks and procedures may be delegated, not the entire nursing process.
- Critical thinking, professional judgment, and effective communications are hallmarks of delegation.
- Ethical issues that are considerations in delegation and supervision include fair selection process, delegating versus dumping, meeting the safety and physical needs of patient while developing staff members, and continuously reviewing the delegation and supervision processes.

APPLY YOUR LEGAL KNOWLEDGE

1. How has the role of delegation changed in the time period between the mid-1980s and now?
2. What types of liabilities have surfaced to make the entire concept of delegation and supervision so significant in nursing today?
3. Are there circumstances where a professional nurse both delegates and assigns tasks at the same time?
4. How does the concept of effective discipline assist in preventing potential legal liability?

YOU BE THE JUDGE

A licensed practical nurse (LPN) who worked for a nursing personnel agency worked one evening shift at the Veterans Administration Hospital in a major city. She cared for a patient who had recently undergone hip replacement surgery. Since his surgery, the patient had consistently spiked significant temperatures, and his temperature generally responded well to oral Tylenol, 500 mg, tabs ii, every 4 hours as needed. The charge nurse explained to the LPN that the patient was to continue on vital signs every 4 hours, including temperatures, and that he was to be medicated if his fever was increased, even if only at low-grade levels.

During the evening that she worked, the LPN obtained the patient's temperature at 4 P.M. and again at 8 P.M. He had a low-grade fever at the 4 P.M. hour, and his temperature had risen to 102°F orally at 8 P.M. At both intervals, the LPN administered Tylenol as ordered. The charge nurse did not assess the patient during the evening, nor did she inquire about the patient's condition. The nurse caring for the patient at midnight noted that his temperature was still elevated (102.4°F orally). When notified, the attending physician ordered blood cultures, additional treatment for his ever-increasing fever, and a change in antibiotic therapy.

Despite this aggressive therapy, the patient developed a fatal septicemia, and the patient's family sued for wrongful death. At trial, the court determined that the charge nurse had been derelict in her duty to supervise this patient and assessed partial liability against the LPN and the charge nurse.

QUESTIONS

1. Did the nurse-manager have a responsibility to supervise the care of the patient?
2. Was the care of this patient appropriately assigned to the LPN by the charge nurse, or could the charge nurse have delegated this patient's care more appropriately?
3. If the charge nurse assigned the care of the patient to the LPN, did she retain any supervisory responsibility that would result in her liability in this case?
4. How do the principles associated with delegation and supervision figure into this case?
5. How would you decide this case?

REFERENCES

American Nurses Association. (2001) *Code of ethics for nurses with interpretive statements.* Washington, DC: Author.

American Nurses Association. (2003). *Nursing scope and standards of practice.* Washington, DC: Author.

American Nurses Association. (2008). *Principles for delegation.* Washington, DC: Author.

Anthony, M. K., Standing, T., & Hertz, J. E. (2000). Factors influencing outcomes after delegation to unlicensed assistive personnel. *Journal of Nursing Administration, 30*(10), 474–481.

A. O. v. Department of Health and Rehabilitation, 696 So.2d 1358 (Fla. App., 1997).

Black v. Department of Social and Health Services, 2007 WL 663760 (Wash. App., March 6, 2007).

Blouin, A. S., & Brent, N. J. (1995). Unlicensed assistive personnel: Legal considerations. *Nursing Management, 23*(11), 7–8, 21.

Ditch v. Waynesboro Hospital, 2007 WL 38387 (Pa. Super., January 8, 2007).

Fairfax Nursing Home, Inc. v. Department of Health and Human Services, 123 S.Ct. 901, 71 USLW 3471 (2003).

Ferry v. State of Oklahoma, 2007 WL 632739 (Okla. Dist., January 24, 2007).

Hunter v. Bossier Medical Center, 718 So.2d 636, (La. App., 1998).

Nahavandi, A. (2006). *The art and science of leadership* (4th ed.). Upper Saddle River, NJ: Prentice Hall.

National Council of State Boards of Nursing. (1997). *Five rights of delegation.* Washington, DC: Author.

Potter, P., & Grant, E. (2004). Understanding RN and unlicensed assistive personnel working relationships in designing care delivery strategies. *Journal of Nursing Administration, 34*(1), 19–25.

Short v. Plantation Management Corporation, 781 So.2d 46 (La. App., 2000).

Sparks Regional Medical Center v. Smith, 976 S.W.2d 396 (Ark. App., 1998).

Steele v. Department of Workforce Development, 2006 WL 2521443 (Ind. App., September 1, 2006).

Thurston v. Worker's Compensation Fund, 2003 WL 23011467 (Utah App., December 26, 2003).

Williams v. West Virginia Board of Examiners, 2004 WL 1432298 (W. Va., June 24, 2004).

CHAPTER 16

Federal Laws: The Americans with Disabilities Act of 1990 and the Civil Rights Act of 1991

PREVIEW

The Americans with Disabilities Act (ADA) of 1990 and the Civil Rights Act of 1991 were both signed into legislation during the term of President George H. W. Bush. Both of these acts have significant implications for health care delivery. The ADA affects health care providers as well as consumers, with various sections of the act addressing hiring and retention of providers as well as access to health care. The act was significantly changed in subsequent legislation. The Civil Rights Act of 1991 also affects both health care providers and consumers. This chapter explores these two pieces of federal legislation, defining the purposes of the acts and their application through case law, and concludes with future projections concerning these areas of the law for nurses.

LEARNING OUTCOMES
After completing this chapter, you should be able to:

16.1 Describe the conditions within the United States that caused both the ADA and the Civil Rights Act of 1991 to be written and implemented.

16.2 Describe the various sections, necessary definitions, and intended purposes of the two acts.

16.3 Describe how the acts affect the health care delivery system in terms of consumers and providers.

16.4 Analyze the ever-expanding number of cases filed under both of these acts.

KEY TERMS

Americans with Disabilities
    Act of 1990
Americans with Disabilities
    Amendments Act of
    2008

Civil Rights Act of 1991
disability
essential job functions
hostile work environment
preferential treatment

quid pro quo sexual
    harassment
reasonable accommodations
sexual harassment
undue hardship

THE AMERICANS WITH DISABILITIES ACT OF 1990

Background of the Act

On July 26, 1990, President George H. W. Bush signed the **Americans with Disabilities Act of 1990** (ADA) into law, providing comprehensive protection to Americans with disabilities. The ADA is one of the most significant pieces of legislation since the Civil Rights Act of 1964, and was seen by its sponsors as "the Emancipation Act of disabled persons." The act had been necessitated by the discrimination faced by HIV/AIDS individuals, as those persons identified loopholes not adequately addressed by existing state and federal laws.

In enacting the ADA, Congress was faced with the challenge of combining two legal concepts, disability and equality. The aim was to "provide a clear and comprehensive mandate for the elimination of discrimination against individuals with disabilities" (ADA, 1990, Section 2, [a][1]), thus ensuring equality for the disabled without undue hardships being placed on those regulated by the act.

The act was amended on September 25, 2008, to clarify and reiterate who is covered by the law's civil rights protections. The **ADA Amendments Act of 2008** revises the definition of "disability" to more broadly encompass impairments that substantially limit a major life activity. Essentially, the amended language also states that mitigating measures, including assistive devices, auxiliary aids, accommodations, and medical therapies and supplies (other than eyeglasses and contact lenses) have no bearing in determining whether a disability qualifies under the law. Further changes clarify coverage of impairments that are episodic or in remission that substantially limit a major life activity when active, such as epilepsy or post-traumatic stress disorder. Not altered in the act were record of impairment, reasonable accommodation, and essential job functions. These amendments became effective January 1, 2009, and are discussed in greater depth later in this chapter.

Title I primarily covers employment provisions and is perhaps the best-known portion of the ADA. The act defines a "covered entity" as an employer, employment agency, or labor organization, or joint labor-management committee. While the act was originally restricted to employers of 25 or more employees, it now applies to all employers who have 15 or more employees. The United States, corporations wholly owed by the United States, Indian tribes, and bona fide tax-exempt private membership clubs are not included in the definition of employer. State governments, governmental agencies, and political subdivisions, though not specifically included in the act, were intended by Congress to be part of the ADA. While the ADA does not exclude religious organizations, it does authorize them to give preference in employment to their own members and to require that applicants and employees conform to their religious tenets.

Definitions in the Act

The ADA of 1990 defined **disability** broadly. Individuals were covered if: (1) the disability is a physical or mental impairment that substantially limits one or more of the major life enjoyments of the person; (2) there is a record of such impairment; or (3) the individuals are regarded as having such an impairment. These criteria were amended in the 2008 act to read:

The term *disability* means, with respect to an individual:

(A) a physical or mental impairment that substantially limits one or more major life *activities of such individual;*
(B) A record of such an impairment; or
(C) Being regarded as having such an impairment (ADA Amended Act, 2008, Section 3[1]).

Under the amended act, major life events "include, but are not limited to, caring for oneself, performing manual tasks, seeing, hearing, eating, sleeping, walking, standing, lifting, bending, speaking, breathing, learning, reading, concentrating, thinking, communicating, and working" and "major life activity also includes the operation of a major bodily function, including, but not limited to, functions of the immune system, normal cell growth, digestive, bowel, bladder, neurological, brain, respiratory, circulatory, endocrine, and reproductive functions" (ADA Amended Act, 2008, Section 3[2][A & B]). The act also specifies that an impairment that substantially limits one major life event need not limit other major life events in order to be considered a disability.

The determination of whether an impairment substantially limits a major life event is made without regard to the "ameliorative effects of mitigating measures such as medication, medical supplies, equipment, or appliance, low vision devices (which do not include ordinary eyeglasses or contact lenses), prosthetics including limbs and devices, health aids and cochlear implants or other implantable hearing devices, mobility devices, or oxygen therapy equipment and supplies, use of assistive technology, reasonable accommodations or auxiliary aids or services, or learned behavioral or adaptive neurological modifications" (ADA Amended Act, 2008, Section 3[3][e][I,II,III, and IV]). This section was added to so that the definition of disability was broadened to be as inclusive a possible, while disallowing from the definition of disability impairments that are transitory and minor, noting that a transitory impairment is one with an actual or expected duration of 6 months or less.

Other additions to broaden the definition of disability include clarification that an impairment that is episodic or in remission is a disability if it substantially limits a major life event when not in remission. Finally, the act clarifies the definition for applicants or employees of "regarded as" being disabled if the applicant or employee can show that he or she was subject to an action prohibited by the ADA, such as the failure to hire the person or the termination of the person, based on an impairment that is not transitory and minor. Further, individuals who satisfy the "regarded as" being disabled stipulation are not entitled to reasonable accommodation under the act.

A *record of impairment* refers to someone who has a history of, or has been classified as having, a mental or physical impairment that substantially limits one or more of the major life activities. This provision is intended to ensure that the covered entities do not discriminate against individuals because they have a history of a disability or because they have been misclassified as being disabled. This clause was included because Congress clearly intended to prohibit discrimination against individuals with disabilities based on society's myths and unfounded fears about disabilities.

Reasonable accommodations refer to the employer's responsibilities to provide the necessary structure, reassignment, and equipment modifications or devices; interpreters; or other reasonable needs that would allow the disabled person to perform the job satisfactorily. Employees and potential employees should be prepared to inform the employer of modifications or special needs that will accommodate them. Reasonable accommodations may be as simple as providing amplification devices so that a hearing-impaired person applying for the position of telephone switchboard operator can qualify for the position. Other reasonable accommodations include job restructuring, part-time or modified work, provision of qualified readers or interpreters, or reassignment to another position.

To meet the qualifications of this section, employers must also identify **essential job functions.** These functions are based on the employer's judgment, the job description, and the amount of time performing the given function. The purpose of such a provision is to ensure that if qualified disabled applicants apply for a job, they will not be discriminated against because of nonessential job functions they are not able to perform. However, if there are other, more or equally qualified nondisabled applicants, the employer does not have to hire the disabled person. The issue arises when more qualified disabled applicants are passed over for less qualified, nondisabled applicants.

EXERCISE 16.1

Review all of the components and skills used in staff performance. What are the essential job functions you would want to include when authoring a list of staff nurses' essential job functions? What are their nonessential functions? Give the rationale for your answers. Define what you consider to be essential versus nonessential job functions. Are there areas of overlap? How difficult was it to decide what is essential rather than what is preferred?

Exclusions from the Definition of Disability

There are multiple exclusions from the definition of disability under the ADA. The ADA excludes homosexuality and bisexuality from its coverage. It further excludes transvestism, transsexualism, pedophilia, exhibitionism, voyeurism, gender identity disorders not resulting from physical impairments, and other sexual behavior disorders. The ADA does not protect compulsive gamblers, kleptomaniacs, pyromaniacs, and those who currently use illegal drugs. Moreover, the employer may hold alcoholics to the same qualifications and job performance standards as other employees even if the unsatisfactory behavior or performance is directly related to the alcoholism.

PROVISIONS OF THE ADA

The ADA is closely related to the Civil Rights Act of 1964 and incorporates the antidiscrimination principles established in Section 504 of the Rehabilitation Act of 1973. There are five titles in the act.

Title I

Title I of the ADA prohibits employment discrimination, adopting the remedies and procedures provided by Title VII of the Civil Rights Act of 1964. This title also incorporates the concepts of reasonable accommodation and undue hardship that were established in parts of the Rehabilitation Act.

The purpose of this section is to ensure that people with disabilities are not excluded from job opportunities or adversely affected in any other aspect of employment unless they are not qualified or otherwise unable to perform the job. This protects qualified and disabled individuals in regard to application, salary, promotions, discharge, transfer, and all other aspects of work.

The ADA's prohibition against employment discrimination extends to medical examinations and inquiries on applications. The employer is not allowed to ask about disabilities or about the extent of obvious disabilities. The employer, though, may make inquiries as to the ability of the applicant to fulfill the job requirements. A medical examination may be conducted after a job offer has been extended to the disabled person, provided that all applicants for the position are subjected to the same examinations. Drug testing to determine the illegal use of drugs may be performed, because such screens are not considered medical examinations. Depending on the job, employers may make inquiries about disabilities if the inquiry is job-related and consistent with business necessity. Employers may also conduct voluntary medical examinations that are part of an employee health program made available to all employees at the work site.

Defenses that the employer has to the ADA include **undue hardship.** This provision is available if the accommodation to be made is extremely expensive or difficult to implement. The act provides that the employer must investigate the required accommodations and offer data proving this hardship. Undue hardships are usually based on cost, numbers of employees, and type of business enterprise.

Other possible defenses include the public safety defense and the health and safety defense. Under these two defenses, the employer must prove that reasonable accommodation cannot prevent potential compromised safety and health hazards to others in the workplace. For example, health care institutions have requirements that persons with contagious diseases may not work in the facility during the active phase of the illness.

Though not a true defense, employers with religious affiliations may give preference to individuals of the same religious sect. For example, colleges and universities that are supported by and follow a specific religious affiliation often employ faculty members who ascribe to the same religious affiliation.

Title II

Title II of the ADA prohibits discrimination against disabled individuals by any state or local government entity without regard to the receipt of federal funds and includes comprehensive provisions designed to ensure access to and use of public transportation by disabled persons. Title II incorporates the remedies and procedures set forth by the Rehabilitation Act.

Title III

Title III prohibits discrimination by public accommodations against individuals on the basis of disability in the full and equal enjoyment of the entity's goods, services, facilities, privileges, advantages, or accommodations. Title III mandates the removal of architectural and structural barriers and the provision of auxiliary aids and services in many cases. Public accommodations are required to remove barriers in existing facilities if such removal can be accomplished without substantial difficulty or expense. However, newly constructed facilities and major renovations of existing structures must be designed to be readily accessible to and usable by individuals with disabilities. Title III also includes provisions on discrimination in transportation services provided by private entities. Title III incorporates remedies and procedures from the Civil Rights Act of 1964.

Title IV

Title IV is designed to ensure that individuals with speech and hearing impairments have meaningful access to and use of telephone services. The ADA requires common carriers engaged in intrastate and interstate communications to provide telecommunications relay services to individuals with hearing and speech impairments.

Title V

Title V contains miscellaneous provisions, including some construction clauses. Provisions under this section include the statement that the ADA does not invalidate or limit other federal or state laws, allows insurance carriers to continue classifying risks in the manner consistent with state laws, and prohibits retaliation against persons who file discrimination charges under the act or assist others who file such charges.

LAWSUITS UNDER THE ADA

Disability Discrimination

Since its enactment, the number of cases filed under the ADA continues to be extensive. This is partly due to the flexibility of the act's definitions, which necessitated the amended act of 2008. To prevent the act from being overly narrow, explicit definitions of which individuals are "qualified individuals with a disability will of necessity . . . be done on a case to case method" (ADA, 1990, 42 U.S.C. Section 12101). The protected class is composed of employees or applicants for employment who meet three discrete provisions:

1. The individual must have a disability in the sense that he or she has a "physical or mental impairment."
2. The impairment must be such that it "substantially limits one or more of the major life activities" of the individual.
3. The qualified person must still be able to perform "the essential function of the employment position" sought or in which the individual is currently employed. (ADA, 1990, 42 U.S.C. Section 12111).

Court cases have continued to challenge the definition of a qualified individual with a disability. From the first passage of the act, early challenges to the ADA concerned HIV and AIDS patients, disease states that many saw as the impetus for the act. Early cases presented such issues as mandatory HIV testing, whether the ADA prohibited discrimination against HIV-infected persons, or whether the asymptomatic HIV-infected person was qualified under the ADA. For example, in *Leckelt v. Board of Commissioners* (1990), the court upheld the dismissal of a nurse for refusal to take an HIV antibody test. The court reasoned that the nurse was not otherwise qualified, because he refused to take a test that the court felt was consistent with appropriate infection control procedures. Even though the likelihood that Leckelt would transmit an HIV infection was small, the court found the hospital policy was justifiable given the hospital's need to protect and safeguard patients.

A landmark 1998 Supreme Court decision brought this issue to what appears to be a final determination. The court in *Bragdon v. Abbott* (1998) held that a patient's positive HIV status was a disability under the ADA, even when the HIV-positive person was asymptomatic. A provision in the amended act of 2008 specifically addresses this issue: An impairment that is episodic or in remission is a disability if it would substantially limit a major life activity if active (ADA Amended Act, 2008, Section 3[3][D]).

Courts, though, even with this resolution, have continued to struggle with the definition of disability. In *Sarosdy v. Columbia/HCA Healthcare Corporation* (2003), the court concluded that a person who can work, who can do many jobs in a certain field but not one particular job in that field, is not disabled under disability discrimination law. That case concerned a surgical scrub nurse who has sustained an on-the-job injury to her left hand and was granted a 6-month medical leave. When she failed to return at the end of the leave, she was terminated. No reasonable accommodation was due, said the court, because the nurse was not disabled. This issue appears to have been resolved in the amended act of 2008: An impairment that substantially limits one major life activity need not limit other major life activities in order to be considered a disability (ADA Amended Act, 2008, Section 3[3][C]).

Courts across the country have continue to hold that a variety of conditions do not constitute a disability. Such examples include the finding that a nurse with a lifting disability was not qualified under ADA (*Reible v. Illinois Odd Fellows Home*, 2005; *Squibb v. Memorial Medical Center*, 2007; *Storkamp v. Geren*, 2008); erratic behavior does not give notice to the employer that an employee is suffering from a disabling mental impairment (*Webb v. Mercy Hospital*, 1996); depression and anxiety are not disabling mental conditions (*Rose v. Visiting Nurse Association*, 2007); a nurse's inability to handle the stress of a particular job is not a disability (*Wiggins v. DaVita Tidewater, 2006*); migraine headaches and nonlatex allergies are not disabilities (*Howard v. North Mississippi Medical Center,* 1996); a short-term condition is not a disability (*Doss-Clark v. Babies and Beyond Pediatrics*, 2007; *Garrett v. University of Alabama*, 2007; *Vierra v. Wayne Memorial Hospital,* 2006); and pregnancy is not a disability (*Jessie v. Carter Health Care Center, Inc.,* 1996).

Courts have also examined how individuals with disabilities accommodate their disability. For example, in *Robinson v. St. Mary's Health Care* (2007), a male RN, previously diagnosed with type 2 diabetes, hypertension, sleep apnea, insomnia, and chronic pain from a back injury had prescriptions for Ambien for sleep and an opiate for back pain among other medications for his multiple conditions. While working, he was observed to be leaning against a wall, alternating between appearing to be unresponsive or acting strangely, and, when questioned, was confused and incoherent in his speech. Transferred to the emergency center, his blood glucose levels were within a normal range and his stupor responded quickly to two doses of Narcan. He was subsequently terminated.

In the court case that followed, the court ruled that he did not have a disability despite his multiple diagnoses, as he had been able to competently perform job expectations for a period of 22 years. The court noted that although the sleep apnea, insomnia, and sleep deprivation could be considered disabilities, the effects of the prescription medications directly violated hospital policy, and that health care facilities have a legitimate right to outlaw employee conduct that does or that could threaten patients' safety.

Remember, too, that the perception of a disability is equally important to having a disability from a legal perspective. The courts in *Doss-Clark v. Babies and Beyond Pediatrics* (2007) and *Cusworth V. County of Herkimer* (2006) both concluded that for purposes of disability discrimination, a person falsely perceived by his or her employer to have a disability and who does not in fact have such a disability is protected by the ADA to the same extent as a truly disabled person. Similarly, though chemical dependency is recognized as a disability in the act, the act only protects employees from discrimination who are successfully rehabilitated and are no longer abusing drugs (*Dovenmuehler v. St. Cloud Hospital*, 2007; *Nicholson v. West Penn Allegheny Health System*, 2007).

A nurse cannot refuse to participate in an interactive process that would result in alternative employment and be successful in a disability discrimination lawsuit. For example, in *Webster v. Methodist Occupational Health Centers, Inc.* (1998), a nurse desired to return to work following stroke rehabilitation. Her physician testified that she had a residual decreased ability to sustain attention and concentration at times, as well as mild decreases in visual spatial skills and scanning and occasional impulsivity. He testified that she could probably function effectively, but only in an environment in which she had close supervision and was supported by the resources of other staff members. According to his testimony, it was not appropriate for her to return to a nursing position where she had to be able to work alone.

She could have returned to occupational nursing if the facility were to hire a second nurse to work with her. But hiring a second nurse would effectively amount to paying a double salary for a one-nurse position, and the company refused to accommodate her. There were, however, other positions available through the agency that could accommodate her needs. She refused to consider any other option besides returning to her former job, on the same shift, with an extra second nurse. There were also non-nursing positions available that would use her expertise and accommodate her physical disability. The court ruled that the nurse's refusal to participate in the interactive process between employer and employee rules out her right to sue successfully for disability discrimination after her dismissal from the agency.

Court cases involving disability discrimination in health care settings may be filed by patients or patient families rather than health care providers. In *McElroy v. Nebraska Medical Center* (2007), a patient who had been hospitalized in a psychiatric developmental center for 16 years was denied a kidney transplantation. His assessment for transplant suitability included a comprehensive psychiatric evaluation that supported his diagnoses of delusional disorder, persecutory type, and paranoid schizophrenia. The committee who evaluated this patient concluded that a kidney transplantation was not in the best interest of the patient or the transplant system, because the procedure itself is complex and intrusive and requires long-term adherence to immunosuppressive agents and cooperation with a team of professionals. The court endorsed the committee's finding, noting that it would be highly dubious to expect close cooperation and strict compliance from a person with this patient's psychiatric diagnoses. In *Wood v. Vista Manor Nursing Center* (2006), the family was able to show that the facility had discriminated in denying a patient admission on the basis of the potential patient's positive HIV diagnosis.

Dewitt v. Proctor Hospital (2008) explores an area of the ADA seldom seen in litigation. The ADA contains language prohibiting an employer from discriminating against an employee because of a disability affecting an individual with whom the employee is known to have an association or relationship. In this case, the first known application of the "association discrimination" clause, a nurse was fired from her job over the strain that the spiraling costs (in excess of $180,000) of her husband's cancer treatments were placing on the hospital's self-insured health plan. The hospital's financial situation was well known and the nurse-manager had tried, unsuccessfully, to convince the nurse to drop her husband's costly cancer chemotherapy and radiation treatments and have him admitted to the hospice section of the hospital. When the nurse refused for the fourth time, she was fired. Though the nurse had to prove cause and effect, the court, in finding for the nurse, noted that the only possible reason for the nurse-manager's actions was to stop the cost of expensive treatment for a disabled person with whom the nurse has a relationship.

Reasonable Accommodation

A second area that the courts have addressed concerns reasonable accommodation. This may include but is not limited to job restructuring, part-time or modified work schedules, offering of lower-pay positions for which the individual is qualified, reassignment or transfers to other departments that have vacant positions, acquisition or modification of equipment or devices, educational materials or policies, and the provision of qualified readers or interpreters. What constitutes reasonable accommodation is judged on a case-by-case basis.

Courts have enforced this case-by-case rule. In *Street v. Ingalls Memorial Hospital* (2008), a RN who was a case manager for the hospital fractured her femur and, following her sick leave, was permitted to return to work, with no lifting over 50 pounds and using a cane to walk. The hospital's policy was that no accommodation was necessary as the hospital's policy was that unless an employee could return to work at 100% of capacity and without the assistance of any appliances such as wheelchairs, cane, or walkers, the employee could not work. Additionally, the hospital made no effort to see if the employee was capable of doing her job or if an accommodation could be made.

The court in this case ruled that the hospital's understanding of its legal duties was flawed. Whether her condition was acute or chronic, the nurse was substantially limited in the major life activity of walking. This qualified her as having a disability for the purposes of the ADA. The hospital did not communicate with her to determine what she could do and how she might need assistance in performing her work. There was no way to determine if a reasonable accommodation was needed because the employer failed to initiate any type of communication with her, and the employer, not the employee, bears the legal burden when there is such a failure to communicate.

Failure to offer reasonable accommodation is disability discrimination for which an employee can successfully bring a lawsuit. To file suit alleging that reasonable accommodation has not been made, the employer must first know of the person's disability and be given an opportunity to accommodate the employee. For example, in *Dovenmuehler v. St. Cloud Hospital* (2007), the nurse, who had a history of substance abuse, was terminated in her employment for cause. She then was hired at St. Cloud Hospital without revealing her drug-use history or that she was in a state board of nursing monitoring program. When these facts became known, the hospital decided it did not have the resources to provide the supervision that she required and terminated her employment. She sued for disability discrimination and the case was dismissed. The first test, noted the court, was whether the hiring agency knew of the disability. Here, there was no evidence to support that the hospital, when employing this nurse, had any indication that the nurse had a disability that would require reasonable accommodation.

Often, the court must decide what constitutes reasonable accommodation. In *Feldkamp v. Viau* (2007), a licensed practical nurse (LPN) required knee surgery. When her sick leave and Family and Medical Leave Act leave were exhausted, she was allowed to return to work in the medical records department. This alternate employment continued until a progress report from her physician to the hospital human resources department indicated that the LPN's medical restrictions would be permanent and that she could not return to her previous staff position. The hospital placed her on lay-off status. Notices of alternate job openings were sent to her, but the LPN did not apply for any of these openings. She sued, and the court ruled that a facility that voluntarily supplies a temporary accommodation for a temporary medical condition has no further obligation to continue such an accommodation on a permanent basis. The disabled employee can apply for a different, light-duty job, on the same basis as any other applicant.

A similar finding occurred in *Hosier v. Nicholson* (2006). In that case, the LPN was hired with the understanding that she would be allowed to work in the emergency center or outpatient clinics rather than on patient care floors where the physical requirements were too demanding of her. The nurse suffered from chronic venous insufficiency in her right lower leg, arthritis and degenerative joint disease in her right knee, and lumbar radiculopathy, all of which made it difficult for her to stand or walk for extended periods of time.

During a severe nursing staff shortage, the management was forced to change its policies and all nurses were required to meet the hospital's standards for standing, walking, bending, stretching, lifting, pushing, and pulling. Also, the LPN position in the emergency center was eliminated, forcing this nurse to work on a nursing home care floor. By the end of her first day on this unit, it was obvious that she could not effectively complete patient care assignments. She was discharged and sued for disability discrimination.

The court ruled that a patient care facility has the right to require all of its staff members to meet the legitimate expectations for the physical demands of direct patient care work. A nurse who is unable to meet these demands does not have the right, under the rubric of reasonable accommodation, to have a light-duty position created or continued just to meet the nurse's special circumstances. This, in the court's view, creates an undue hardship for the employer. In *Exarhakis v. Visiting Nurse Service of New York* (2006), the court reached a similar conclusion and further noted that when employers exceed their legal responsibilities, they should not be penalized when circumstances force them to alter extraordinary accommodations.

Neither do employers have an obligation under the ADA to tolerate frequent unpredictable absences as reasonable accommodation. In *Willett v. State of Kansas* (1996), the facility had made reasonable accommodations for a nurse with systemic lupus erythematosus. They had provided a lighter medication cart and assigned her to a portion of the building where walking distances were shorter and there were fewer floor ramps. But the reasonable accommodation standard did not extend to frequent absences because these imposed an undue hardship on the facility, on the clients it served, and on other staff members. An unscheduled absence by a professional nurse required the facility to try to provide quality patient care while short staffed, to call in other staff members who were scheduled time off from work, or to force staff already on duty to stay and work overtime.

The court in *Amato v. St. Luke's Episcopal Hospital* (1997) also addressed the issue of frequent absenteeism on the part of one of its employees. In holding for the hospital and against the employee, the court stated that even if the employee has a genuine disability, a hospital is not required to accommodate sporadic and unpredictable absences. A hospital "having to retain and compensate a surplus employee to be available in the event that another employee fails to report for work is not reasonable accommodation" (at 538).

Note that an employer need not retain a disabled person unless reasonable accommodation may be made. In *Gary v. Department of Human Resources* (2006), a nurse had physical limitations that prevented her from being able to respond to emergency code situations. Since all nurses in the facility were obligated to respond to such emergencies when they occurred, there was no reasonable accommodation and thus disability discrimination was not an issue for the court.

In order to be successful in a case based on reasonable accommodation, the nurse must participate in the interactive process concerning what would constitute reasonable accommodation (*Thornton v. Providence Health System-Oregon*, 2005). In *Thornton*, a nurse suffered from progressively worsening problems with the plantar fascia in his feet. Unsuccessful corrective surgery left him medically restricted from standing or walking for more than 15 minutes at a time. As his condition worsened, he began exploring options that would prevent long periods of standing. He was informed that a telephone triage position was being created, which he refused as it would pay less than his staff position. When the nurse was no longer able to work as a staff nurse, he requested to be considered for the telephone triage position. He was denied this position, as the newly created qualifications for the telephone triage position required previous experience in this capacity.

Though the case is still in the appeals process, the court noted that the legal concept of the interactive process was critical in deciding this case. This concept basically means that the employer has the legal obligation to reach out and communicate as openly as possible with employees who have come forward and asked for assistance to accommodate their disability-related needs. The court further noted that while the employer has no legal obligation to (1) create a new position for such an employee, (2) give a position to a disabled employee for which the employee is not qualified, or (3) train an employee for a position for which an employee is not qualified, the employer does have the responsibility of giving the disabled employee preference over an outside applicant for a position for which the employee is qualified.

Essential Job Functions

The final hurdle for such cases concerns essential job functions. These are defined by the ADA as those functions that a person must be able to perform in order to be qualified for the employment position, not qualifications that would be ideal to possess. Courts have been involved in deciding what constitutes essential job functions. For example, the court in *Feliciano v. State of Rhode Island* (1998) noted that the essential functions for an institutional attendant included the following: performing personal hygiene; transferring and lifting patients; administering minor treatments; bathing, dressing, and grooming patients; cleaning bedpans and other equipment; exercising and walking patients to various locations; and participating in food service to patients at mealtimes. Once persons can perform all the essential functions of a position, then they can be considered qualified individuals with disabilities. Examples of essential job functions include the ability to respond to emergency code situations (*Gary v. Department of Human Resources*, 2006), the ability to input patient data in computerized medical records (*Miller v. Principi*, 2006), and, for nurses working with psychiatric patients, the ability to restrain patients (*Jones v. Kerrville State Hospital*, 1998).

One of the more interesting cases regarding essential job functions remains *Laurin v. Providence Hospital and Massachusetts Nurses Association* (1998). In *Laurin,* the nurse had worked on the maternity unit for 6 years prior to suffering a seizure at home. Her neurologist determined that the seizure was fatigue-related and indicated in a report to the hospital that a daytime position was absolutely necessary for this nurse. The hospital, as part of a collective bargaining agreement, had a policy that stated in part that nurses with less than 15 years of seniority and who worked on 24-hour units must rotate shifts. This meant that the maternity nurses worked about one-third of their shifts at night.

Initially, the hospital did accommodate Laurin by temporarily assigning her to a 6-week, days-only schedule. The hospital expected her to use this period to look for alternative employment, in areas that offered day positions, such as perioperative areas. After she suffered a second seizure, the hospital extended her a day-only position but informed her that her employment would be terminated if she did not return to shift work.

Reasonable accommodation does not mandate that an employer dispense with an essential job function, the court said in its opinion. Thus, the court ruled that availability for night-shift work was an essential job function for a unit that provides care on a 24-hour basis. Other nurses, the court noted, also suffered fatigue from juggling family responsibilities and night-work obligations. Although they might not have been disabled by their fatigue, the court said they had rights that their employer was not compelled to ignore in accommodating a disabled employee.

The court in *Moschke v. Memorial Medical Center of West Michigan* (2003) determined that the ability to take "on-call" work is an essential function of a surgical nurse's job. Such on-call work involved the ability of the surgical nurse to be available when emergency cases or scheduling problems required the staff to work beyond their assigned shifts.

Cases Under Titles III and IV

A case filed under Title III of the ADA, *Parker v. Metropolitan Life Insurance Company* (1997), defined the purpose of the ADA. The court found, in a rather complicated fact scenario, that Title III's prohibitions do not apply to employer-sponsored benefit plans. The court did find that "the purpose of the ADA was to prevent discrimination among nondisabled and disabled persons, not to ensure equal treatment for people with different disabilities" (at 1015).

EXERCISE 16.2

Imagine that a co-worker of yours, also an RN, is HIV positive and works in the emergency center at your hospital. What are the essential job functions of a registered nurse in the emergency department? Do these essential job functions differ from those of nurses in other departments of the hospital? Are there special risks to the nurse and to potential patients? What would be reasonable accommodation for such a registered nurse?

What are the ethical duties owed by nurses who are HIV positive toward potential patients? Should they continue caring for patients in this type of setting, knowing the consequences to themselves and potentially to their families? In what other areas of acute care settings might such nurses be better employed?

A case that directly involves Title IV of the act is *Abernathy v. Valley Medical Center* (2006). Federal regulations for the ADA require hospitals to take reasonable steps to ensure that communications with members of the public with disabilities are as effective as communications with others who do not have disabilities. Additionally, the facility should give primary consideration to the requests of the disabled individual. In this case, a deaf patient checked himself out of the hospital the day after his admission for severe abdominal pain, went to an alternate hospital that had certified in-house sign-language interpreters, and had his surgery at this second hospital. In his lawsuit against the first hospital, he was unable to show that any actual harm had been done to him. He claimed that he felt ignored, frustrated, and unsafe; the hospital staff countered with the fact that he was rude, abrasive, belligerent, challenging, and uncooperative. In their communications with the patient, the hospital used handwritten notes.

The court concluded that exchanging handwritten notes is an ineffective means of communicating with a deaf person during a medical emergency and that informed consent to a life-saving medical intervention such as an open abdominal procedure for an abscess cannot be effectively obtained through exchanging notes. The patient was allowed to recover damages for pain and suffering for the time frame the surgery consult went ahead with hospital personnel refusing to provide the accommodation that the patient requested.

The verdict in *Loeffler v. Staten Island University Hospital* (2007) resulted in an opposite ruling, as the hospital was able to show that it had made a good-faith effort to locate a sign-language interpreter for a deaf patient. When it became apparent that the patient's hearing teenage children could not effectively sign for their father, the hospital's speech and hearing department made a good-faith effort to locate an interpreter. Though the hospital acknowledged that improvements to how the facility accesses interpreters were made after the fact, the hearing-impaired patient can only successfully sue if the hospital has been deliberately indifferent to the patient's need for interpretive services.

Enforcement of the ADA

Enforcement of the ADA is done primarily through the Equal Employment Opportunity Commission. Complaints are filed with this commission and trials by jury may be a second option. The Department of Justice oversees Title III violations. Enforcement ensures one of the primary purposes of the act—that no one, either disabled or abled, will be given a greater advantage in employment opportunities, public services, transportation, and communications.

GUIDELINES

The ADA and Hiring Processes

1. To be a qualified individual with a disability under the ADA definition, the applicant must be able to perform essential job functions. This allows employers to question individuals about their educational and experiential qualifications for the job, plus licensure and required certification if that is a prerequisite of all candidates for the position.

2. Applicants can be questioned about their ability to perform the job safely, with or without accommodation. No accommodations are necessary unless the disabled person requests such accommodations and makes the full extent of his or her disabilities known.

3. No accommodation is required if the needed accommodation would impose an undue hardship on the employer. Such undue hardships include costly or disruptive renovations to the existing facility, or costs disproportionate with the size of the employer, numbers of other employees, and nature of the business place.

4. Applicants may be questioned about their ability to perform essential job functions, and case scenarios can be devised to ascertain qualifications for clinical-based jobs. Questions about disabilities, past medical problems, or previous workers' compensation claims cannot be asked.

5. Employment tests that would screen out disabled workers may not be used unless the test is shown to be job-related and consistent with business necessity. For example, a test for color blindness may be given to applicants for phlebotomy positions if they are required to place blood in different colored tubes. Tests that screen for illegal drug use may be given if required of all applicants for the position, not just disabled job applicants.

6. If preemployment physicals are part of the hiring process, they cannot be done until after the job is offered conditioned on applicants passing the examination. The same medical examination requirements must be made of all persons applying for the position, and all test data must be kept confidential. Only persons with a need to know may be told of the disabled person's medical data following the examination.

7. All applicants should be queried about their qualifications for the position, and policies and procedures of the facility should be explained. Remember, the ADA does not mandate that disabled persons be hired. It mandates that all persons, those disabled and those not disabled, be given the same advantages in job opportunities.

Conclusion

The ADA represents an expansive vision of the capabilities of disabled individuals and rightly regards them as productive members of society. Similarly, the act holds that the societal costs of discrimination against and isolation of disabled individuals far outweigh the economic costs of accommodation. The ADA's scope is vast, and over time the act can be expected to create major changes in the areas of employment, transportation, communications, access to public services and public accommodations, and in all other areas where the disabled have been subject to discrimination, isolation, and segregation. The ADA offers a historic opportunity to fully integrate disabled individuals into the mainstream of American society.

EXERCISE 16.3

Daniel fractured his knee playing sports and requested a medical leave from his staff nursing position. The sports injury aggravated a preexisting knee injury, and his physician ruled him unable to continue in his staff nursing position because of the walking required in the nursing position. Daniel was offered an office position in patient referrals/scheduling with pay and benefits comparable to staff nursing. He refused that assignment.

Daniel then applied for a position in quality assurance and a position as a case manager. Two other individuals were hired into those positions, and Daniel was told that he was not hired for these two positions because the selected individuals were more qualified. He is now filing this lawsuit citing disability discrimination.

How would you decide this case? Does Daniel have a legitimate disability claim? Should he have been hired for either of the two open positions? Does the fact that he refused the office position in patient referrals/scheduling factor into your decision?

CIVIL RIGHTS ACT OF 1991

Background of the Act

Congress, the federal courts, and numerous other courts struggled with issues of sexual discrimination and harassment during the last half of the 20th century. The culminating factor that brought the issue to a final showdown was the Clarence Thomas Supreme Court confirmation hearings in October 1991, heightening awareness and concern about sexual harassment in the workplace. The Thomas hearings pushed sexual harassment to the top of the national agenda, and the **Civil Rights Act of 1991** was signed into law on November 21, 1991.

Definition of Sexual Harassment

The major portion of the act defines **sexual harassment,** identifying two categories of sexual harassment. Overall, sexual harassment is simply "unwelcome sexual conduct that is a term of employment" (29 Code of Federal Regulations, Section 1604.11[a]). The two categories of sexual harassment are discussed separately in this chapter.

Quid Pro Quo Sexual Harassment

Quid pro quo sexual harassment occurs when submission to or rejection of the sexual conduct by an individual is used as a basis for employment decisions affecting the individual. To prove quid pro quo sexual harassment, the individual must show that:

1. The employee was subjected to unwelcome harassment in the form of sexual advances or requests for sexual favors.
2. The harassment complained of was based on sexual advances or requests for sexual favors.
3. The employee's submission to the unwelcome advances was an expressed or implied condition for receiving job benefits, or the employee's refusal to submit to the supervisor's sexual demands resulted in tangible job detriments.
4. The individual is a member of a protected class (an employee in a lower position in the power chain of command).

Additionally, employers are strictly liable for the conduct of supervisory personnel in quid pro quo harassment suits.

Hostile Work Environment

The majority of the cases brought under the act concern **hostile work environment** sexual harassment. In these instances, there are no tangible job benefits or detriments. Here, the employee is subjected to sexual innuendos, remarks, and physical acts so offensive as to "alter the conditions of the employee's employment and create an abusive work environment" (*Meritor Savings Bank v. Vinson*, 1986). Elements that must be shown in this type of case include (1) establishing that the harassment unreasonably interfered with work performance and (2) that the harassment would affect a reasonable person's work environment. The employer is not strictly liable in such a suit, but becomes liable when the individual alleging the harassment files complaints with the employer or when the harassment is so pervasive that knowledge can be inferred.

Because most issues in this area affect women, the court addressed the issue of a "reasonable woman standard." In *Robinson v. Jacksonville Shipyards, Inc.* (1991), the court concluded that

> . . . the cumulative, corrosive effect of their work environment over time affects the psychological well-being measured by the impact of the work environment on a reasonable woman's work performance or more broadly by the impact of the stress inflicted on her by the continuing presence of the harassing behavior. The fact that some female employees did not complain of the work environment or find some behaviors objectionable does not affect this conclusion concerning the objective offensiveness of the work environment as a whole. (at 1492)

The *Robinson* case was the first to carve out the "reasonable woman standard" in dealing with sexual harassment cases, since gender is an issue in this area of perception. *Ellison v. Brady* (1991) had concluded that a complete understanding of the victim's views requires an analysis of the different perspectives between men and women, and what men may consider unobjectionable may offend many women.

In hostile work environment sexual harassment cases, the conduct need not be directed at the individual who files the complaint. It is enough that the behavior or condition was observed or known by the individual and that the behavior affected the psychological well-being of the individual. For example, hostile work environment sexual harassment may be triggered by posting pornography in the office, displaying lewd cartoons labeled with a worker's name, making sexually demeaning comments or jokes, touching or attempting to touch the individual, and making sexual propositions. A hostile work environment can originate from sexually discriminatory verbal intimidation, ridicule, or insults, if "sufficiently severe or pervasive as to alter the conditions of the victim's employment and create an abusive working environment" (*Farpella-Crosby v. Horizon Health Care*, 1996, at 805). The conduct/behavior complained of must be unwelcome, and the victim's perspective is what is relevant.

Conduct akin to that of a quid pro quo sexual harassment case may also exist in this type of suit, but the offending employee has no direct supervision over the individual or there is no corresponding job benefit or detriment connected with the harassment. For example, in *Hamm v. Lakeview Community Hospital* (1996), the U.S. District Court for the Middle District of Alabama ruled that an emergency department nurse's suit for quid pro quo sexual harassment was without merit. Title VII of the Civil Right Act outlaws acts of sexual harassment on the job between an employee and an employer. In this case, the physician was the employee of a separate corporation that had a contract with the hospital (also the nurse's employer) to provide emergency department physician's services, and the court was unwilling to infer that the physician was the hospital's designated agent in supervising the nurse. The nurse more likely would have prevailed if she had brought this suit as a hostile environment suit, since it was conceivable that she could show the hospital knew of the hostile environment and chose to allow the situation to continue.

Employees who feel there is some type of hostile environment sexual harassment should notify superiors or the employer directly, depending on the size of the facility/place of employment and organizational chart. The employer has a duty to investigate the report, document the investigation, maintain confidentiality, and report back to the initiating complainant. The employer should maintain professionalism and speak with the alleged victim and the alleged harasser and other potential witnesses. The employer should consider what action needs to be taken and communicate the results of the investigation back to all parties involved.

Two separate cases serve as examples of the preceding statements. In *Pickett v. Sheridan Health Care Center* (2008), a member of the nursing home's nonlicensed staff sued the nursing home for sexual harassment, citing three separate incidents that involved three different residents. Though the general rule is that an employer may be liable for sexual harassment of its employees by clients or customers, not just supervisors or co-workers, a nursing home caring for elderly dementia and mentally ill patients is a special environment where a certain amount of acting out is expected that would be inappropriate in other contexts.

The court found no basis to sue for sexual harassment for the following reasons. Once the employee reported each incident to her supervisors, prompt and effective action was taken. Resident #1 was counseled about his inappropriate behavior, and the aide was instructed that she was not to enter his room by herself. Resident #2 was counseled and placed on a monitoring program, and the aide was instructed that she would no longer be assigned to his care. The third resident was counseled, monitored, and eventually transferred out of the facility. Thus the aide did not have to care for him. The court in *Equal Employment Opportunity Commission v. Nexion Health* (2006) reached a similar conclusion, noting that health care workers caring for Alzheimer's patients cannot take their racial remarks personally as indicators of a hostile work environment, as these patients are unable to understand or to control what they say and do.

Nicholis-Villalpando v. Life Care Centers of America, Inc. (2007) similarly held that if an employer knows of an incident of sexual harassment, the employer must take appropriate action. In this case, the sexual harassment concerned a co-worker in the facility and the court held that the supervisor must investigate and take action if the harassment is reported or if the supervisor realistically should have known that such action was occurring. The court in *Aden v. Life Care Centers of America* (2007) also held that victims of sexual harassment have the right to use leave and not return to work until the victim of the sexual harassment is assured that management can and will stop the alleged harassment. *Kuhn v. Public Employment Relations Board* (2007) ruled that a supervisor could be terminated for failure to investigate and take action following the report of sexual harassment by an employee. Employers have an affirmative duty under state and federal laws to take derisive action when an employee complains of sexual harassment. *Kampmier v. Emeritus Corporation* (2007) upheld sexual harassment in a case that involved same-sex (lesbian) sexual harassment.

Moss v. Washoe Medical Center, Inc. (2006) outlined the steps that a facility should take when an employee reports alleged sexual harassment. First, temporary steps must be taken to deal with the situation while it is determined whether the complaints are valid. These include protecting the alleged victim from further incidences of harassment and investigating in such a manner that the rights of the alleged harasser are protected. Second, permanent remedial steps must be taken once the investigation is concluded. This may include relocating the victim to another unit or campus of the facility, changing the shifts that either party works, and/or disciplinary, corrective action.

Note that termination of the alleged harasser is not mandatory, and other remedial action may be taken, such as a transfer of the offender to other units or work sites and disciplinary warnings. Generally, courts have held that for serious physical harassment, termination may be required, whereas less serious verbal harassment may justify lesser discipline. Most important, some action must be taken if a potential lawsuit is to be avoided. Courts have concluded that if an employer fails to take corrective action after learning of harassing conduct, the employer is considered to have adopted the offensive conduct and its results as if the offensive conduct had been expressly authorized by the employer's policies.

Finally, in instances where an individual reports a co-worker for alleged sexual harassment, courts have held that retaliation by the employer is not allowed (*Benson v. Carson City Hospital,* 2007). In that case, a female co-worker reported a male nurse for sexual harassment and the male nurse was subsequently terminated. The nurse who brought the charges was then terminated by her nurse-manager, who was a close friend of the male nurse. The important point that the court noted was that retaliation over a complaint of sexual harassment is strictly forbidden, even if the retaliation does not come directly from the perpetrator, but is instigated by a third party.

GUIDELINES

Avoiding Sexual Harassment Claims

1. Try to prevent the harassment from occurring. This is the most effective and cost-effective means to deal with the reality of workplace relationships.
2. Take affirmative action to prevent harassment, such as educational programs to alert persons about how to react to such advances and hostile environments. Express strong disapproval, inform persons of their right to raise sexual harassment issues, and sensitize all concerned. Consider having educational programs as part of the yearly in-service requirements to ensure that all personnel know and understand sexual harassment in the workplace.
3. Develop policies prohibiting either type of sexual harassment. The policy should include strong language prohibiting such actions and stating that such actions will not be tolerated; a procedure for reporting complaints; notice that violators will be subject to stern disciplinary procedures, including discharge; identification of an employee representative to whom complaints should be directed; and a statement that all complaints and investigations will be treated in a confidential manner.
4. Effectively communicate the policy, including placement in policy manuals, bulletin boards, interoffice memoranda, and employee handbooks.
5. Conduct educational programs as needed to ensure that all personnel understand the significance of sexual harassment in the workplace.

Preferential Treatment or Sexual Favoritism

An employer may also be liable for unlawful sexual discrimination when an employee is denied a job opportunity or benefit due to the **preferential treatment** of another employee who submits to the employer's sexual advances. Additionally, there may be liability when employers promote employees who give sexual favors to supervisors rather than promoting other, better-qualified employees.

EXERCISE 16.4

For the following examples, state whether there are grounds for a sexual harassment claim and what type of sexual harassment claim could be brought—quid pro quo or hostile environment.

1. John rejects a homosexual advance by David, a nurse-manager, and is subsequently fired by the unit manager.
2. William, the hospital chief operating officer, asks Judy, the assistant director of nursing, for a date.
3. During a conference sponsored by the institution, Paul makes sexual remarks and behaves in a sexually physical manner with a female co-worker, Judy. Judy immediately complains to her direct supervisor, and 12 hours later, the hospital director of nursing tells her that she needs to stay at the conference, but will no longer be required to work with Paul after the conference.
4. Marilyn and Jeff, both employed by the same institution, are having an affair. They are both upper-level managers, but work in different departments.
5. During a trip, Rita makes sexual innuendos and tells lewd jokes to a male co-worker, Richard. After Richard complains, the company transfers Richard and reprimands Rita.

ETHICAL CONCERNS

The ADA raises some interesting ethical concerns, specifically in the area of justice and fairness. One of the issues concerns how far companies and health care institutions must extend themselves to accommodate employees with special needs. For example, should these disabled workers have an edge over more able-bodied workers? Is it just to expect companies and health care institutions to continue to expend additional revenue to guarantee accommodation in a time of a national recession? Heath care institutions are already burdened with ever-increasing support for those without medical insurance or those underinsured. Should there be a clause that protects the disabled worker but only to the extent economically feasible?

A second issue concerns professionalism and the fact that society should focus on abilities rather than the extent of a person's disabilities. Such a concept challenges everyone to begin to view what is positive rather than merely looking at what a person cannot do or to what extent the person's abilities will limit the institution. Employing individuals with special needs is not charity, but is socially responsible and beneficial for the institution. Differences should be embraced, not feared and excluded. In this era of ever-increasing technology, managers and administrators may be able to craft more creative accommodations and allow for additional employment opportunities for disabled workers.

Finally, respect for others dictates that health care institutions allow equal opportunities for all employees and potential employees. What should be the bottom line is being continually conscious of fairness and equality.

SUMMARY

• The Americans with Disabilities Act of 1990 and the Amended Act of 2008 were enacted to eliminate discrimination against disabled Americans.

• The most noted part of the act concerns Title I, which covers employment provisions and specifies many of the definitions in the act.

- Individuals are considered disabled if they have a physical or mental impairment that substantially limits one or more major life activities, have a record of such impairment, or are regarded as having such an impairment.
- Reasonable accommodations refer to an employer's responsibility to provide the necessary structure, reassignment, and equipment modifications that allow a disabled person to perform the job in a satisfactory manner.
- Essential job functions, based on the employer's judgment, job description, and amount of time performing a specific task, assist in preventing discrimination because of nonessential functions that a disabled person might not be able to perform.

- Lawsuits under the act are numerous and continue to define the definition of disability, reasonable accommodations, and essential job functions.
- The Civil Rights Act of 1991 was enacted to prevent sexual harassment in the workplace.
- Two classifications of sexual harassment were defined: quid pro quo sexual harassment and hostile work environment sexual harassment, with the latter being the most encountered in health care settings.
- Lawsuits in this area of the law have crafted the important steps that employers must take to prevent liability when sexual harassment is reported by employees.
- Ethical concerns center on the principles of justice and respect of others.

APPLY YOUR LEGAL KNOWLEDGE

1. How do staff nurses comply with these two acts in providing competent care to patients?
2. Have these two laws had the effect that their drafters intended? Why or why not?
3. What revisions or redefinitions to the original laws have been created by legal cases filed concerning these two acts? Does the ADA Amended Act of 2008 adequately address these concerns?
4. What would you advise employers to implement or change to prevent further cases from being filed under these two acts?

YOU BE THE JUDGE

As a full-time nurse consultant, Eileen May performed compliance review for her employer's contract with the state department of social and rehabilitative services. She had received favorable performance reviews up until the time that she requested a leave for scleroderma and esophageal dysmobility.

When she returned to work, she attempted to maintain the same working schedule she had performed prior to her medical leave. Unable to maintain this schedule, she requested permission to work at home as a reasonable accommodation under the ADA. Her contention was that this position did not require close supervision and could be performed as solitary unsupervised work. Her request was denied and she was terminated for her inability to perform her current position. She sued for disability discrimination.

QUESTIONS

1. Is Eileen a qualified individual under the provisions of the ADA in that she has a disability as defined by the ADA?
2. Is the request to work at home a reasonable accommodation given the circumstances?
3. What other accommodations could be considered reasonable for this individual?
4. How should this case have been resolved?

REFERENCES

Abernathy v. Valley Medical Center, 2006 WL 3754792 (W. D. Wash., December 18, 2006).

Aden v. Life Care Centers of America, Inc., 2007 WL 29450 (D. Kan., January 3, 2007).

Amato v. St. Luke's Episcopal Hospital, 987 F. Supp. 523 (S.D. Tex., 1997).

Americans with Disabilities Act of 1990, Public Law 101-336, 42 *United States Code,* Sections 12101 *et seq.* (July 26, 1990).

Americans with Disabilities Amended Act of 2008, Public Law 110-325 (September 25, 2008).

Benson v. Carson City Hospital, 2007 WL 2951862 (E. D. Mich., October 9, 2007).

Bragdon v. Abbott, 118 S.Ct. 2196 (1998).

Civil Rights Act of 1991, Public Law 102-166, 29 *Code of Federal Regulations,* Sections 1604 *et seq.* (November 21, 1991).

Cusworth v. County of Herkimer, 2006 WL 1800130 (N. D. N. Y., June 28, 2006).

Dewitt v. Proctor Hospital, 2008 WL 509194 (7th Cir., February 27, 2008).

Doss-Clark v. Babies and Beyond Pediatrics, 2007 WL 1577770 (M. D. Fla., May 31, 2007).

Dovenmuehler v. St. Cloud Hospital, 2007 WL 4233160 (8th Cir., December 4, 2007).

Ellison v. Brady, 924 F.2d 872 (9th Cir., 1991).

Equal Employment Opportunity Commission v. Nexion Health, 2006 WL 2528432 (5th Cir., September 1, 2006).

Exarhakis v. Visiting Nurse Service of New York, 2006 WL 335420 (E. D. N. Y., February 13, 2006).

Farpella-Crosby v. Horizon Health Care, 97 F. 3d 803 (5th Cir., 1996).

Feldkamp v. Viau, 2007 WL 4248283 (Ohio App., December 3, 2007).

Feliciano v. State of Rhode Island, 160 F.3d 780 (1st Cir., 1998).

Garrett v. University of Alabama, 2007 WL 3378398 (11th Cir., November 15, 2007).

Gary v. Department of Human Resources, 2006 WL 2946842 (11th Cir., October 17, 2006).

Hamm v. Lakeview Community Hospital, 950 F. Supp. 330 (M. D. Ala., 1996).

Hosier v. Nicholson, 2006 WL 2816604 (M. D. Pa., September 28, 2006).

Howard v. North Mississippi Medical Center, 939 F. Supp. 505 (N. D. Miss., 1996).

Jessie v. Carter Health Care Center, Inc., 926 F. Supp. 613 (E. D. Ky., 1996).

Jones v. Kerrville State Hospital, 142 F.3d 263 (5th Cir., 1998).

Kampmier v. Emeritus Corporation, 2007 WL 6072 (7th Cir., January 2, 2007).

Kuhn v. Public Employment Relations Board, 2007 WL 4191987 (Iowa App., November 29, 2007).

Laurin v. Providence Hospital and Massachusetts Nurses Association, 150 F.3d 52 (1st Cir., 1998).

Leckelt v. Board of Commissioners, 909 F.2d 820 (5th Cir., 1990).

Loeffler v. Staten Island University Hospital, 2007 WL 805802 (E. D. N. Y., February 27, 2007).

McElroy v. Nebraska Medical Center, 2007 WL 4180695 (D. Neb., November 21, 2007).

Meritor Savings Bank v. Vinson, 477 U.S. 57 (1986).

Miller v. Principi, 2006 WL 2222682 (W. D. Tenn., August 2, 2006).

Moschke v. Memorial Medical Center of West Michigan, 2003 WL 462374 (Mich. App., February 21, 2003).

Moss v. Washoe Medical Center, Inc., 2006 WL 508088 (D. Nev., March 1, 2006).

Nicholis-Villalpando v. Life Care Centers of America, Inc., 2007 WL 28262 (D. Kan., January 3, 2007).

Nicholson v. West Penn Allegheny Health System, 2007 WL 483910 (W. D. Penn., October 23, 2007).

Parker v. Metropolitan Life Insurance Company, 121 F.3d 1006 (6th Cir., 1997).

Pickett v. Sheridan Health Care Center, 2008 WL 719224 (N. D. Ill., March 14, 2008).

Reible v. Illinois Odd Fellows Home, 2005 WL 3358869 (C. D. Ill., December 9, 2005).

Robinson v. Jacksonville Shipyards, Inc., 760 F. Supp. 1486 (M. D. Fla., 1991).

Robinson v. St. Mary's Health Care, 2007 WL 710155 (M. D. Ga., March 6, 2007).

Rose v. Visiting Nurse Association, 2007 WL 1306594 (D. Md., April 26, 2007).

Sarosdy v. Columbia/HCA Healthcare Corporation, 2003 WL 21791358 (Cal. App., August 4, 2003).

Squibb v. Memorial Medical Center, 2007 WL 2325173 (7th Cir., August 16, 2007).

Storkamp v. Geren, 2008 WL 360991 (E. D. N. C., February 8, 2008).

Street v. Ingalls Memorial Hospital, 2008 WL 162761 (N. D. Ill., January 17, 2008).

Thornton v. Providence Health System-Oregon, 2005 WL 3303944 (D. Or., December 5, 2005).

Vierra v. Wayne Memorial Hospital, 2006 WL 288665 (3rd Cir., February 8, 2006).

Webb v. Mercy Hospital, 102 F.3d 958 (8th Cir., 1996).

Webster v. Methodist Occupational Health Centers, Inc., 141 F.3d 1236 (7th Cir., 1998).

Wiggins v. DaVita Tidewater, 2006 WL 2662997 (E. D. Va., September 13, 2006).

Willett v. State of Kansas, 942 F. Supp. 1387 (D. Kan., 1996).

Wood v. Vista Manor Nursing Center, 2006 WL 2850045 (N. D. Cal., October 5, 2006).

PART FIVE

IMPACT OF THE LAW ON NURSING IN SELECTED PRACTICE SETTINGS

CHAPTER 17

Nursing in Acute Care Settings

PREVIEW

This chapter concerns legal issues as they pertain to nurses practicing within acute care settings, performing daily more highly skilled tasks and having responsibility for increasingly more acutely ill patients. No longer are sophisticated machines and technologies seen only in critical care areas, step-down units, or emergency centers. Patients in general medical and surgical units and in clinical settings may have a variety of machines, devices, and other highly technological assists. Thus, employees who work in acute care settings are encountering the need for greater skills and facing potentially more liability. This chapter addresses issues arising within acute care settings, giving guidance on competent, quality health care delivery.

LEARNING OUTCOMES
After completing this chapter, you should be able to:

17.1 Describe the changing health care environment that has created increased responsibility for staff nurses.

17.2 Describe the unique nature of the care of psychiatric and vulnerable patients.

17.3 Differentiate two types of restraints, including the nursing management of the restrained patient.

17.4 Describe the nurse's responsibility in medication errors and five means to avoid such errors.

17.5 Analyze the potential liability for nurses when using technological advances and specialized equipment.

17.6 Compare and contrast the nurse's responsibility for assessing, monitoring, and communicating in clinical settings.

17.7 Discuss selected ethical issues that arise in acute care settings.

KEY TERMS

failure to adequately assess,
   monitor, and
   communicate
medication errors

patient safety
psychiatric and vulnerable
   patients
restraints

suicide prevention
technology and equipment

ACUTE CARE NURSING

The past 30 years have witnessed dramatic changes within the nurse's role in acute care settings. Three decades ago, it was easy to define the practice of medicine and the practice of nursing and to articulate the difference between the two professions. Today, the roles are becoming masked with the advent of:

1. Critical care, intermediate care, and multiple other specialty care units
2. Advanced nursing skills within specialized units such as the operating arena, post-anesthesia care unit, labor and delivery units, and emergency centers
3. Advanced nursing knowledge and skills, physiological as well as psychosocial and cultural skills

Today's nurse must assume responsibility and accountability for patient care that requires knowledge of complex illnesses and use of highly sophisticated machinery.

Nurses can best avoid potential liability by giving safe and competent nursing care, while recognizing potential problems, identifying the risk areas in individual practice, and remaining current in new technology, nursing diagnoses, and the latest institutional policies and procedures. This chapter explores some of the more frequently encountered challenges for nurses working in acute care settings.

PATIENT SAFETY

One of the most important responsibilities of nurses remains that of ensuring **patient safety** needs. The now classic study by the Institute of Medicine (2000) brought the overwhelming significance of patient safety needs to the attention of the nation as well as to members of the health care team, noting that annually more than 7,000 patient deaths occur because of medication errors. This responsibility for patient safety includes protecting patients from falls, protecting patients from injuring themselves or others in the clinical setting, ensuring that medication errors do not occur, and protecting patients from faulty equipment or unsafe conditions. Examples of how nurses ensure such safety measures include inspecting siderails to see that they are functional and used appropriately, foreseeing risks to patient safety (e.g., slick or wet floors), restraining patients as indicated, and responding appropriately to violence in the workplace.

Given the complexities of individuals and society, increasing numbers of nurses are encountering violence in the workplace settings, including greater numbers of hostile and angry patients. Such patients exist in all areas of nursing, though the incidence was once thought to be primarily encountered in the emergency centers of health care institutions (Danesh, Malvey, & Fottler, 2008; Tarzian & Marco, 2008). Patients in this category typically have unrealistic expectations of their treatment plans and may be described as hostile, angry, belligerent, aggressive, or noncompliant. Although nurses have often described these patients as merely "difficult" and "challenging," such patients also present a safety hazard and increase the potential of liability for the nurses who care for them.

Working with these patients is difficult, but there are some interventions that assist in diffusing anger and hostility. Spend additional time, not less time, with such patients, conveying that they are important. Attempt to understand their anger, but do not become part of it by showing hostility in return. Speak calmly and rationally. Respect patients' autonomy, addressing underlying issues and ensuring that these patients are educated about their condition, what to expect from the treatment, and alternatives to treatment. Continue to practice patience.

Know the institution's policy on dealing with violent patients, and diffuse the situation according to the policy. The institution should have a zero tolerance for violence policy in the workplace. Attend seminars on preventing violence in the workplace, and practice techniques for diffusing such situations. Document the patients' complaints or noncompliance and interventions taken to resolve the situation. Consult with colleagues about the best approach to take, and ensure that the entire health care team is reinforcing the approach selected.

Should patients have a serious violent episode, follow these simple rules:

1. Ensure a safe atmosphere by positioning oneself at least four arm lengths away and to the side of patients, so that the nurse's egress is not blocked by the patient. Such positions serve to ensure that the patients do not feel threatened and that the nurse has a means of safely exiting the room if needed.
2. Keep hands in sight and maintain eye contact.
3. Avoid touching, pointing, challenging, or interrupting the patient. Continue to speak calmly, softly, and rationally.
4. Address the patient by name.
5. Request permission to ask questions and listen intently as the patient responds.
6. Acknowledge the patient's feelings, and express understanding without assigning blame.
7. Show empathy and offer solutions that address the patient's concerns.
8. Remain calm and professional. (Bartlett & Rehmar, 1997; Tarizan & Marco, 2008)

PSYCHIATRIC AND VULNERABLE PATIENTS

Patients with serious mental illnesses continue to challenge even the most experienced nurses. Because these patients are not necessarily hospitalized in dedicated psychiatric settings, nurses in all acute care settings must know how to recognize patients with psychiatric or emotional disturbances and how to meet their specific nursing needs. Remember that caring for **psychiatric and vulnerable patients** presents unique issues, and nurses must know what legal risks are involved and how to minimize them while maximizing nursing care.

The law has long recognized psychiatric patients as part of the group of vulnerable persons, along with children, the elderly, the imprisoned, and the mentally challenged. Persons falling within the category of vulnerable do so because they are often unable to recognize their unique circumstances, and, because they are frequently unable to speak for themselves, they cannot assert their rights in health care settings. Several issues arise with these patients.

Suicide Prevention

Nurses have obligations related to **suicide prevention.** Not all self-destructive and depressed patients will be hospitalized in psychiatric units, and some patients, particularly the elderly, the recently anesthetized, and selected postpartum patients, respond to hospitalization with depression and suicidal thoughts. Nurses should listen carefully to comments spoken by patients, because nearly all suicidal patients have some ambivalence and give some warning clues before self-destructive behavior is evident. Once identified as a potential suicidal or self-destructive patient, the duty of care owed the patient increases, as the foreseeable consequences of not meeting the duty of care required are obvious. Identification of such patients offers nurses the opportunity to counsel them, alert psychiatric clinical nurse specialists or psychiatric interveners that these patients are at risk for self-destruction, and implement precautions while they are recovering. Above all, the nurse should treat these patients and their families with concern, consistency, and caring behaviors.

Nurses should have an understanding of which patients are more likely to become self-destructive. The majority of people who commit suicide have a diagnosable mental disorder. Mental disorders that increase suicidal risks include all forms of depression, personality disorders, schizophrenia, alcohol abuse, and organic mental disorders, with major depression and alcohol abuse being the most common psychiatric disorders associated with completed suicide (World Health Organization [WHO], 2006). Physical illness most often associated with suicide include central nervous system disorders, autoimmune disorders, cancer, renal failure patients on dialysis, and patients with peptic ulcers (Maris, Berman, & Silverman, 2000).

Older patients are more likely to commit suicide than younger patients, although younger patients may be more verbal. Women make more suicide attempts, but men, by a two-to-one ratio, are more likely to succeed in their attempts. Most patients who commit suicide have a previous history of suicide attempts or prior hospitalization for self-destruction (WHO, 2006).

Once identified, nurses have a legal responsibility to protect the patient. The court in *Hooper v. County of Cook* (2006) held that a hospital and its staff must exercise reasonable care to protect suicidal patients from self-harm. The patient, admitted to the facility's intensive care unit (ICU), suddenly became combative and uncontrollable at 3:00 on the third day after her admission. A hospital psychiatric nurse examined the patient, and noted that she was having paranoid ideation, which is defined as a belief that people are trying to invade her space and cause her harm. This diagnosis was later changed to ICU psychosis.

The psychiatric nurse phoned the hospital's attending psychiatrist and together they formulated a treatment plan. The patient was to be moved from the ICU to a general medical-surgical unit, where there would be a calmer atmosphere. Haldol would be ordered to control her psychosis, and one-to-one nursing care would be ordered as needed for unpredictable behavior. The patient would be ambulatory and able to get up and walk about as she needed.

That evening following her transfer to the general unit, the patient reported seeing green and purple lights and movement on the ceiling. At 3:55 A.M., she was found by another patient in the bathroom, having hanged herself with her hospital gown. The family sued for wrongful death and the court awarded damages in the amount of $1,212,000, for the failure to implement one-to-one nursing care for a patient at high risk for self-harm.

Reid v. Altieri (2007) reiterates this responsibility of health care providers' duty to protect vulnerable patients. The patient in this case had a longstanding history of outpatient psychiatric care for depression. His wife brought him to the emergency center because she feared he was about to harm himself. While in the emergency center, he informed the triage nurse that he was thinking about hanging himself. A mental health consultant, though, overruled the nurse's decision that the patient should be admitted for observation and treatment. The man's psychiatrist, on the following day, likewise did not admit him, as the hospital failed to include the nurse's notes with the other faxed information from the previous emergency center visit. The patient hung himself later that day and his wife brought this wrongful death lawsuit against the hospital.

The court, in deciding that the hospital was liable for this patient's death, noted that when a patient goes beyond verbalizing thoughts of suicide to an actual plan for suicide, caregivers have an immediate legal responsibility to seek admission of the patient for inpatient psychiatric care.

The court concluded that he should have been admitted, not discharged from the emergency center, and that such admission would have prevented his immediate suicide.

Note that no overt suicidal act is necessary for the nurse to initiate suicide precautions according to the facility policy. In *In re S. B.* (2000), a patient who told a psychiatric nurse that she was not clear if she could be safe or whether or not she was suicidal and who refused to sign a contract for safety had presented sufficient evidence to alert the nursing staff that the patient was at risk for self-destructive behavior. It is only necessary to show that the person has acted in a manner that shows he or she is a clear and present danger to himself or herself.

Courts, though, will also support a finding that the hospital and staff have no liability for a patient's suicide if the facts of the case support a holding that the standards of care were upheld. In *Soderman v. Smith* (2007), a 57-year-old woman had a history of alcohol abuse, depression, and previous suicide attempts. She began drinking heavily, and while intoxicated attempted to take her life with an overdose of Antabuse. When the overdose was not successful, she thought of hanging herself, but instead called 911 for help. She was transported to the hospital by paramedics and admitted on a 72-hour involuntary psychiatric hold.

At the hospital, she was admitted to a locked psychiatric unit and placed on a 15-minute suicide watch until she informed the staff that she was no longer suicidal. The nurse called the psychiatrist for orders to transfer the patient to an adult treatment program, believing that a less restrictive environment would be more beneficial for this patient. While in the adult treatment program, the nursing staff continued to monitor the patient every 30 minutes. The patient went to a group meeting, signed a safety contract, and agreed that she would fully cooperate in her treatment plan. The psychiatric saw her later that same day and she again denied continuing suicidal intent, disclosing the fact that recent family stressors triggered this suicide attempt. The psychiatrist diagnosed major depression and started the patient on antidepressants.

The next day, the patient was withdrawn and anxious. She agreed to remain voluntarily in the hospital and to work through her problems. Her antidepressants were adjusted, and later that evening she said she felt safe and would do nothing to harm herself. Sometime later that night, she was found hanging in the shower, revived, and transferred to an acute care center. Following determination that she was brain-dead, her family decided to discontinue her life support systems.

The court, in finding for the institution, noted that the quality of the care, not the outcome, was the significant factor in this case. There were no errors or omissions that fell below the standard of care, and the fact that the family elected to withdraw life support was not a relevant factor in the court's decision.

Kinchen v. Gateway Community Service Board (2006) concerned a patient who had a violent argument with her boyfriend. When the boyfriend aimed a gun that misfired at her, the patient tried to stab herself, but the boyfriend grabbed the knife and called 911. The police responded to the 911 call, transporting the patient to an acute care hospital. She was seen by the triage nurse, assessed, and denied any suicidal intention or recent suicidal behavior. The nurse consulted with the attending physician and a licensed mental health counselor was called in to see the patient. The counselor arrived at 2:00 A.M., assessed the patient to be low-risk for self-harm, and after consulting with the physician, decided not to initiate an involuntary commitment process.

Two days after her dismissal from the acute care facility, she committed suicide by shooting herself. The court agreed with the psychiatric nursing expert that the standard of care was met, even though there was an unfortunate outcome.

Note, though, that the patient's mental diagnosis also needs to be considered when determining the potential liability for upholding standards of care. *In re Baptist Hospitals of Southeast Texas* (2006) held that a patient who was diagnosed as delusional could not be relied upon to adequately state that she was no longer a danger to herself. Though an effort should be undertaken to ensure that the patient can understand and collaborate with needed medical interventions, close, frequent observation of the patient must be continued. Such patients, concluded the court, should always be considered at risk for self-harm and elopement.

To protect patients who are not able to fully appreciate the need for hospitalization and observation, involuntary commitment may be used. Involuntary commitment in most states is a 72-hour hold. Because such hospitalization is forced on the person, courts have determined that an overt act is needed to show that the patient is a danger to himself or herself. For example, in *Sheliga v. Cumberland River Comprehensive Care* (2007), a man with previous mental health issues became agitated and his speech content was grandiose and delusional while at his employment in a fast-food restaurant. Though he denied any intent to harm himself or anyone else, mental health providers sought to have him involuntarily committed based on his speech and crescendoing agitation. The request for an involuntary hold was denied, as the only legally permissible basis for such a hold is that the patient is a danger to himself or herself or others. This is true, said the court, even if the person has previous mental health diagnoses. The issue of involuntary commitment is covered in greater detail later in this chapter.

Should the nurse identify a patient or potential patient as a suicide risk, several nursing interventions might be initiated. Although not an exhaustive list, some of the more obvious nursing interventions include:

1. Closely supervising the patient by staff and/or family members
2. Removing potentially dangerous objects from the patient's bedside and room
3. Ensuring that the patient takes all medications when given so that there can be no accumulation of medications to be taken all at once
4. Transferring the patient closer to the nurses' station or to another unit as needed for closer observation and frequent checks
5. Transferring a rooming-in infant back to the nursery since postpartum depression may be seen not as self-destruction, but as destructive behaviors aimed at neonates
6. Ensuring that windows in the patient's room cannot be opened or opened only partially (If possible, also ensure that window panes are made of sufficiently heavy glass so that they are not easily broken.)
7. Notifying the physician promptly of changes in the patient's condition and administering medications as needed to prevent further depression or self-destruction
8. Restraining the patient as indicated

EXERCISE 17.1

A patient was transported to the hospital after police were called to a convenience store where the patient was walking about in a confused state. The patient admitted to both the police and the hospital staff that he was thinking about harming himself. The patient was placed in soft restraints pending admission to an acute care psychiatric unit.

Although he was restrained to prevent self-harm, the patient was not provided direct one-to-one patient observation. He slipped out of the restraints, eloped from the facility, went back to the convenience store to retrieve his car, drove another 335 miles, stopped on the interstate highway, and walked in front of an oncoming vehicle. His wife filed a wrongful death suit against the facility and its staff members.

How do you think the court would rule in such a case? Why?

Warning of Intent to Harm

Failure to warn of a patient's dangerous propensities when the victim is identifiable has long been accepted as a liability-producing situation by courts of law (*Tarasoff v. The Regents of the University of California,* 1976). Recent cases have reaffirmed this principle, including *DeJesus v. United States Department of Veterans Affairs* (2007), *Evans v. Benson* (2007), and *Stewart v. North Coast Center* (2006).

Evans reinforces the holding of *Tarasoff* that identifiable victims for potential harm are to be contacted when health care providers know they are at risk for harm. After showing signs of anxiety and verbalizing suicidal thoughts, a manufacturing company employee was referred by his employee assistance program to a psychiatric nurse practitioner. The patient told the nurse practitioner that he was hearing voices, which the nurse categorized as command hallucinations, telling the patient to harm the company's human resources director with whom the patient was having an ongoing conflict regarding his job performance. The patient also revealed to the nurse practitioner that he had access to a gun. The human resources director was a clearly identified potential victim, and the nurse saw it as her legal duty to warn him notwithstanding her legal duty to maintain medical confidentiality.

The patient sued for breach of medical confidentiality. At trial, the patient's psychologist confirmed that the patient was very irritable, having suicidal and homicidal thoughts about the human resources director with whom he was in conflict. The Supreme Court of Iowa dismissed the patient's lawsuit against the human resources director and the company over his termination and the nurse practitioner for breach of medical confidentiality.

In *Stewart,* the family of a murder victim who was killed by a violent psychiatric patient sued the patient's caregivers for the victim's death. The patient, while in treatment, talked about multiple situational problems, including problems with his girlfriend, whom he did not identify, and stated that he desired to work with a therapist on anger management issues. He denied suicidal or homicidal thoughts and that he owned or had access to any weapons.

Three weeks after beginning his treatment, the patient called the nurse stating that he was very angry and was destroying his furniture with a hammer. He also stated that he had built a pipe bomb and was considering using it on himself. Though the patient refused hospitalization, he did consent to new medications, which were immediately started. The following week, he stalked his girlfriend, ran her car off the road, shot and killed her, and then killed himself.

The court ruled that the nurse was not liable for the girl's death as she was not an identifiable victim. The court outlined the two criteria that must be shown for such liability to attach:

1. The caregiver has reason to believe that the patient has the intent and ability to carry out an explicit threat of imminent and serious physical harm to a clearly identifiable victim who is a family member or someone known to the patient.
2. If the threat is verbalized, the mental health caregiver must, if feasible, communicate to a law enforcement agency and, if feasible, communicate to each potential victim the nature of the threat, the identity of the patient or client making the threat, and the identity of each potential victim. (*Stewart v. North Coast Center,* 2006, at 1313098)

DeJesus evidences how important it is that the potential victim or victims be identified by the patient. This case concerned a patient who was transferred from an inpatient psychiatric unit to an intermediate care residence on the hospital campus after some success with achieving control with his intermittent explosive disorder. His discharge came after he had threatened another resident with a knife during an argument while they were working together in the kitchen. The patient's counselor, a registered nurse, was fully aware that the patient had a history of domestic violence, was under a restraining order when he entered the facility for treatment, and had once tried to kill himself. After the kitchen incident and before his discharge, the patient's counselor clearly heard the patient verbalizing thoughts of suicide. He was also giving away all of his personal possessions, including a favorite baseball cap he was never seen not wearing. The counselor attempted to block the patient's transfer to a less restrictive setting to no avail. Following his discharge, he killed his wife, children, two neighbors, and himself.

The court found that it was grossly negligent for the facility to ignore the counselor's warnings and discharge this patient into the community. Given his history, recent actions, and his vocalization that he was suicidal, the facility had a duty to provide additional care, not release him to the community. The court also held that there was no legal duty to warn his family merely because he had an explosive disorder. They were, said the court, not known victims.

Note, though, that there is no legal duty to inform family members of such threats if these family members are already fully aware of the patient's violent tendencies and actions (*Ohlen v. Piskacek,* 2000). In that case, the court refused to hold two mental health workers liable to the wife of a patient. The wife had been assaulted by her husband on previous occasions and was fully aware of his violence toward her.

Failure to Protect from Harm

A variant application of duty to warn involves the failure to protect from harm. This need to protect occurs in instances when patients, because of their vulnerable state and their inability to distinguish potentially harmful situations, must be protected by health care providers.

Lawsuits have also been filed questioning the liability of hospitals when patients are subject to involuntary restraint and administration of medications (*Hanson v. Hospital of Saint Raphael,* 2007; *People v. Simon,* 2007). In *Hanson,* a patient with diagnoses of dissociative identity disorder and substance abuse and a history of self-mutilation was admitted to the hospital following a self-inflicted injury at home. She was placed in four-point restraints so that her wound could be treated and to prevent further self-harm and possible elopement. She was given an injection of Ativan and released from the restraints once she had become more calm and alert. The court found that there were no grounds upon which she could successfully sue the institution.

Similarly, in *People v. Simon* (2007), a patient with a diagnosis of paranoid schizophrenia and a history as a sexually violent predator expressed a death threat toward one of the nurses caring for him. Refusing to take medications, the institution requested permission to involuntarily medicate the patient with the antipsychotic drug Risperdal. Though disagreement with the need to take a prescribed medication does not constitute grounds for involuntary medication of a patient, if the patient completely lacks insight into the illness, such medications may be forced on the patient. In this case, the court found that the patient was in complete denial of his psychiatric condition and, as a result of that denial, refused to even consider treatment with medication. Thus the court allowed the involuntary administration of the medication for this patient.

Courts have also ruled that staff members have a duty to protect patients from harm, especially when vulnerable persons are left in circumstances in which they could be harmed. For example, in *Unnamed Patient v. Unnamed Private Psychiatric Hospital* (2007), a 13-year-old patient with a history of acting out promiscuously with boys her own age was hospitalized with depression and other psychiatric problems that made her vulnerable to sexual manipulation. She repeatedly verbalized that she intended to have sex with a specific male nursing supervisor. No one appeared to take these comments seriously. During her stay at the facility, the patient was accompanied solely by this male supervisor to a remote area of the facility, where they engaged in sexual intercourse in a bathroom. The incident was not reported until

2 weeks after the patient's discharge when she mentioned it to an adult who then called the police. The staff member was arrested, convicted of a lewd act with a minor, and sentenced to 3 years in prison.

In the lawsuit between the facility and the patient's guardian, the facility was found liable to the victim for $900,000 and to the victim's guardian for $350,000 for the guardian's mental anguish and emotional distress. In its finding, the court reiterated the importance of acting when a patient's conduct and/or verbalizations place the staff members on notice of potential patient abuse.

Hospitals have also been held liable for patient elopement. In *Estate of Hollan v. Brookwood Medical Center* (2007), a mental health patient was one of 10 supervised patients who was allowed to be outside on the facility's deck. He managed to scale a 12-foot iron fence, fall 25 feet to the top level of a parking garage, and then crawl to the edge of the garage and fall another 80 feet to his death. The family was awarded $12,000,000 for his wrongful death.

Department of Mental Health v. Hall (2006) also held that the facility was responsible for not preventing a patient's injuries that resulted from the consequences of her own dangerous behavior. A 25-year-old patient with schizophrenia and borderline personality disorder was considered to be a danger to herself and others, having attempted suicide 3 months earlier. She was a patient in a locked unit and had recently been argumentative with multiple staff members.

Believing that she was about to be transferred to a unit where abuse was rumored to occur, she and two other patients attempted to escape by tying bed sheets together to make a rope and climb down from a third-story window. She fell and sustained serious leg injuries in the attempt, resulting in a permanent physical disability. She was awarded $1,000,000 for her injuries.

The court noted that the patient had been crying hysterically about the possible transfer just minutes before the attempted escape, which should have alerted staff members of a possible elopement attempt. The patient was also on every-30-minutes monitoring precautions, and the court accepted the testimony of other patients that the patient care aides were all watching television when the escape attempt occurred. Finally, the court noted that the patient had used a third-floor conference room window for the escape. The conference room had no patient-security window screen or locks as it was not considered a patient-access area, though the door to the room was always unlocked. Additionally, the linen room of this locked psychiatric unit should also have been locked, thus preventing the easy accessibility to the bed sheets used in the escape attempt.

This finding was reconfirmed by the court in *Hofflander v. St. Catherine's Hospital* (2001). That court held that the relationship between psychiatric facilities and psychiatric patients is a special legal relationship. If the facility can foresee that the patient likely will try to elope and fails to take reasonable measures to stop the patient from eloping, the facility is liable for neglect of a vulnerable adult.

Note, though, that courts will not find liability if there was no foreseeable actions to place the staff members on notice that an elopement might occur. *Ball v. Charter Behavioral Health* (2006) concerned a chronic alcoholic patient who was in acute withdrawal when brought to the rehabilitation center. He was convinced to admit himself and was taken to the nurse's station for admission vital signs and medications, specifically Librium. It became apparent by his rising blood pressure that additional medications were needed. The nurse, who believed she had established a rapport with the patient, spoke with him about her need to contact the physician and stepped away to make the phone call. She took about three steps when the patient arose and ran from the facility. As he ran, he fell, hit his head, and subsequently died from the resulting concussion. The case was dismissed, as the court held that there had been no reason to foresee that such a result would happen and that the nurse had acted appropriately.

False Imprisonment/Wrongful Commitment

Psychiatric patients may voluntarily admit themselves for treatment, or, in the case of persons unable to judge what is best for them, the state may involuntarily hospitalize the patient. Case law abounds on the issue of whether the patient should or should not have been detained and whether the patient had the competency to make a rational decision. Some case examples may help clarify these issues.

In *Application of Anthony M. v. Sanchez* (1996), the court concluded that the patient's continued involuntary psychiatric commitment was justified. The court noted that the patient not only suffered from a mental illness, but presented a substantial threat of harm to himself and to others, and was in need of continued treatment and structured care. The patient, while confined to the hospital, threatened a nurse who was carrying a hypodermic needle. He screamed at her that he would take the needle from her and poke out her eyes.

The patient often screamed at the top of his lungs that he was going to kill anyone trying to keep him at the hospital and that, after his release, he was going to come back and "get his revenge." In other outbursts of aggression, the patient hurled verbal expletives at the staff. He also masturbated in front of female staff members.

Additionally, the patient was noncompliant in taking his medication. He was known to try to avoid taking his medications that were being administered to control his anxiety and impulsiveness, while calmly taking other medications without incident. In trying to devise an aftercare plan for the patient, no appropriate caregiver could be found. The only family member willing to take him into her household had significant health problems and had no ability to exert any manner of control on the patient.

The court was also mindful that the patient had a criminal record for rape. Just because the patient could remain stable for a few days in a secure and controlled hospital environment did not mean that his release was appropriate, and the court ruled that the involuntary commitment was justified.

Copeland v. Northwestern Memorial Hospital (1997) held that when a patient comes in voluntarily for mental health reasons, a nurse can and must obtain a full history. The history must include why the person is seeking treatment. If the patient voluntarily discloses that he or she has just committed a crime, the nurse can take appropriate safety measures and notify the police. The nurse and the hospital are not to be held liable in a civil lawsuit for damages if the authorities decide to come to the hospital and arrest the patient for the criminal activity he or she has voluntarily disclosed, while the patient is still choosing to remain voluntarily for assessment and treatment.

The nurse was not engaged in a custodial interrogation and was not in a position to violate the patient's civil or constitutional rights. Custodial interrogation is defined as initiated by law enforcement officials after they have taken the person into police custody or deprived the person of liberty in a significant fashion.

When the nurse in this case questioned the patient about the circumstances leading up to his coming to the hospital and seeking a psychiatric admission, the patient volunteered that he must have just committed an armed robbery during his blackout to get the $1,400 he found he had with him to go on his cocaine binge. At this point, the nurse properly summoned the hospital security guard to sit with the patient, who was still free to go, while she spoke with the physician and called the police. Once voluntarily admitted, the patient was placed in a locked observation room, but was still free to ask to leave and did not have to answer the physician's questions. The court held that the nurse, physicians, and the hospital did not arrest, detain, or interrogate the patient or violate his constitutional rights. Similar conclusions were reached in *S. P. v. City of Takoma Park* (1998).

In *Heater v. Southwood Psychiatric Center* (1996), the court extended the ruling to note that even when there are grounds to hold a person for psychiatric reasons, the law still requires a full court hearing before powerful antipsychotic medication can be given to the person against his or her will. Ativan, ordered only to relieve agitation, can be given without first going to court for authorization. The court in *In re Dorothy W.* (1998) allowed medications for severe paranoid schizophrenia to be given after a court ruling was requested.

An Iowa court (*In the Interest of "J. P.,"* 1998) delineated the criteria for involuntary commitment. They include:

1. A mental illness
2. The lack of sufficient judgment to make responsible decisions with respect to the person's hospitalization or treatment, due to the mental illness
3. The likelihood of inflicting serious physical or emotional harm on self or others, or the inability to satisfy the person's own basic physical needs, if allowed to remain at liberty (at 346)

The court further noted that all three criteria must exist in order to hold a patient involuntarily for psychiatric treatment. "The law is essentially the same in all jurisdictions, due to the United States Supreme Court's nationwide standards for the constitutionality of state mental-health laws" ("Involuntary psychiatric commitment," 1998, p. 4). The court in *In re Adam S.* (2001) reconfirmed that the basic question in involuntary treatment is whether the patient has the mental capacity to make reasoned decisions about the course of treatment.

The court in *State v. Nguyen* (2002) found that a dire and immediate threat to survival is required to hold a patient involuntarily. It is not enough that the patient may have long-term effects of medication noncompliance; the patient must present with evidence of imminent self-harm. In this case, the patient denied having a mental illness and also denied having non-insulin-dependent diabetes. The fact that he might ultimately suffer blindness, limb amputations, and damage to organ systems was not evidence of his imminent self-harm.

Level of Care Required

Courts of law continue to determine the care required for psychiatric patients, as they remain some of the most vulnerable patients. Whether committed voluntarily or involuntarily, they must be afforded the least restrictive environment that is appropriate to meet their needs. The principle of least restrictive environment means that restriction of their civil rights must be no more than is necessary to protect the individual. The court in *In re Turnbough* (2000) also noted that, in close cases, the court must defer to the dignity of the individual rather than taking a strictly paternalistic approach of seeking the utmost security.

In that case, a guardian was appointed for the patient and given the authority to determine where the patient would reside. This patient was a 24-year-old woman with severe cerebral palsy who was also bipolar as evidenced by severe depression, mood swings, hallucinations, and voices telling her to commit suicide. She was unable to care for her physical needs and had deficits in her receptive and expressive language, learning, and self-direction. She needed to take multiple medications during the day, such as mood stabilizers, antidepressants, and antipsychotics. The patient was unable to take these medications by herself or to articulate what, when, and how much of a medication to take.

The patient was prone to outbursts of anger against her caregivers and of rejecting caregivers. Though community volunteers attempted to care for her in a home setting, the patient was frequently noted to display aggression against these volunteers and demand that they leave the house. The court determined that the least restrictive environment for this patient was a nursing home within her community; she did not require inpatient care in a psychiatric facility but did require more care than an assisted living center could provide.

Similar cases found that the least restrictive care environment for mentally ill persons could be ordering involuntary commitment to a psychiatric facility for the involuntary injection of antipsychotic medications (*In re Mental Health of S. C.*, 2000), placement in a transitional setting while awaiting discharge to an adult group home setting (*Angell v. State*, 2000), and placement in a transitional setting while awaiting further legal proceedings (*In re J. S.*, 2001).

Note, though, that patients must be placed in the appropriate setting based on the individual patient's needs. In *Salcido v. Woodbury County* (2000), the court ruled that dementia patients who require mental health treatment have the right to receive such care in mental health facilities rather than merely being placed in extended nursing home settings. The patient in this case was, in the estimation of his psychiatrist, abusive, aggressive, suffering from disinhibited behavior, a poor potential for rehabilitation, and a danger to himself and others. The patient was ultimately committed to a mental health facility.

Confidentiality Right of Mentally Ill Patients

Because of the stigma associated with mental illness, courts have stringently upheld the confidentiality rights of these patients. For example, the court in *Cedars Healthcare Group, Ltd. v. Freeman* (2002) prevented photos to be used that showed other patients who were hospitalized on the same unit as the patient at the time of the alleged occurrence. The policy of strict medical confidentiality, especially with persons receiving mental health treatment, is meant to protect and thereby encourage people who need help to access such help. Even if the other patients' names were deleted from the photos, the mere display of the photo could lead to inadvertent discovery of the patients' identities.

EXERCISE 17.2

Jane Nye was admitted to an acute care psychiatric facility. She was placed on frequent checks for self-harm because Jane had made numerous statements that she was unsure if she was dangerous to herself and did not know if she was suicidal or not. The nurse-manager offered a contract for safety to the patient. In this written agreement signed by the nurse-manager and Jane, the patient agreed to alert the nursing staff if she felt she needed extra support in preventing any self-harm. The contract for safety also assured that Jane would take her medications as prescribed. Jane refused to sign the contract. She also frequently refused to take her medications, to eat her meals, and to perform self-care activities such as bathing and oral hygiene.

The facility has now filed a petition to have Jane committed involuntarily based on these findings. Has the facility presented sufficient evidence that Jane should be committed against her wishes? Why or why not? Does the evidence as presented show an overt act that the court could find as evidence of potential self-harm?

RESTRAINTS

Restraints, both physical and chemical, are used daily in many hospital settings, from the critical care unit to the psychiatric unit. Physical restraints assist in preventing patient falls, discourage patients from disconnecting vital equipment or intravenous and feeding lines, and prevent patients from harming either themselves or others. Chemical restraints also prevent patients from disconnecting vital, life-sustaining equipment; assist in preventing hostile and impaired patients from hurting themselves or others; and allow staff to care for all patients on a given unit.

But restraints are not without serious side effects and harm. Physical restraints can cause skin impairment, impaired respiratory status, strangulation, neurological damage, entrapment, and death. Chemical restraints may result in increased drowsiness, respiratory distress, hemodynamic instability, decreased competency and judgment, and confusion.

All hospitals have policies and procedures outlining when and how restraints are to be used and the nursing care that must be documented on restrained individuals. Because of the inappropriate use of restraints, it is almost universally mandated that hospital staff secure a physician's order before applying restraints, and federal law prohibits chemical restraints in certain nursing home patients. For example, *Eden Park Management, Inc. v. Schrull* (2007) held that drugs causing patients to be restrained cannot be used for convenience or discipline. Such medications are appropriate only if supported by the patient's medical condition. *Wilcox v. Gamble Guest Care Corporation* (2006) used stronger language and held that medications used to restrain a patient solely for the convenience of the staff constituted an illegal use of restraints.

In the past, failing to raise siderails for elderly patients was synonymous with substandard care. However, research is now showing that elderly patients are more likely to fall and suffer injuries when siderails are used. Less intrusive interventions, such as educating patients about the need to call for assistance rather than attempting to move without assistance, keeping night-lights on to reorient the patient to unfamiliar surroundings, using bed monitors that alert staff when a patient is no longer in bed, and placing mattresses on floors to break a possible fall, may be more effective ways of preventing falls in the elderly, especially for the elderly patient whose mind sometimes wanders. Thus, many institutions are reevaluating and rewriting their policies on the use of restraints. The court in *Umbarger v. Hayes Green Beach Memorial Hospital* (2007) ruled that bed rails are a form of physical restraint requiring expert professional judgment.

Sturgill v. Ashe Memorial Hospital (2007) reinforces the need for nurses to use their expert professional judgment regarding when restraints, including raised bed rails, should be used. In that case, a 76-year-old man was assessed as a high fall risk, 8 on a scale of 1 to 10. The nurse elected to initiate the hospital's fall prevention program, meaning that siderails were to be in the raised position and soft restraints could be used without a physician's order. The policy further noted that if the soft restraints were used, the physician was to be notified within the hour of their usage and an order obtained for the continued use. The next day, the nurse removed the soft restraints because she found no order for their continued use. Soon afterward, the patient fell while getting out of bed. An assessment was done, showing that the patient had a low oxygen saturation, abnormal heart rate, and signs of dementia and confusion. The physician refused to order restraints and the patient suffered a closed-head injury when he fell a second time. He subsequently died of complications related to the closed-head injury.

The court noted in its finding of liability that a nurse can and must initiate restraints on an emergency basis if the nurse's assessment indicates that such restraint is necessary for the patient's continued safety. The nurse cannot, though, continue with restraints if the physician does not order their continuation. The nurses were appropriate in placing the restraints, but should have alerted hospital administration and the medical chief of staff when they were unable to secure an order for the continued use of soft restraints or seek other methods of promoting the patient's safety.

Case law consistently has held that siderails on stretchers and gurneys must be in the raised and locked position. Patients using such devices are either in the process of being transported or are under constant supervision. That differs greatly from the patient who is in a hospital room on a general medical or surgical floor.

Examples of patients harmed because they were not properly restrained continue to be prominent in current case law (*Blevins v. Hamilton Medical Center*, 2007; *Estate of Gehrich v. St. Frances Hospital*, 2008; *Estate of Seenandan v. Dependable Ambulette Service*, 2007; *Hogan v. Washington Nursing Facility*, 2007; *Jensen v. Longwood Management Corporation*, 2007; *Paullin v. Oconomowoc Memorial Hospital*, 2007; *Perby v. East Rockaway Progressive Care*, 2008). In each of these cases, the court held that the facility was at fault for failure to use bed rails appropriately, secure patients in wheelchairs, and/or apply restraints as needed.

Facilities have also been held liable for the failure to adequately assess the patient following falls from wheelchairs and beds. For example, in *Jensen v. Longwood Management Corporation* (2007), the court did not fault the facility for the fact that the patient was inadequately restrained as much as it faulted the facility for its failure to assess the patient once he fell from his wheelchair. He was observed for obvious signs of a head injury, but no neurological assessment was done. Had the patient been adequately assessed, the staff members would have found that a stroke caused his initial fall and he could have been timely treated with anticoagulant drugs. In *Brown v. Tift Health Care, Inc.* (2006) and *Cox v. (Name Withheld-Confidential) Nursing Facility* (2007) the results were similar; failure to assess the patient after her fall prevented adequate care for a fractured leg and failure to assess the patient after his fall prevented adequate care for a subdural hematoma, respectively.

Courts have also found no liability for patient falls when standards of care, including the use of restraints, have been appropriately implemented (*Blas v. University of California*, 2007; *Waters v. Andalusia Regional Hospital*, 2007; *Weeks v. Byrd Medical Clinic, Inc.*, 2006). In *Weeks*, it was documented that the patient was observed every 15 minutes as the policy mandated, that the patient had consistently used her call bell to request assistance when she needed to get up and use the bedside commode, and that her mental status had not changed. The court could find no evidence of failure to meet the nursing standard of care when the patient elected to get up by herself and incurred a severe fall. In *Blas*, the court found that a patient's fall was an unexpected accident and no one could be said to be at fault.

A case that outlines the general rule for siderail use is *Pedraza v. Wyckoff Heights Medical Center* (2002). Here the court noted that, as a general rule, a hospital is not liable for negligence for failing to raise the bed rails absent a doctor's expressed medical order to raise the siderails. However, this general rule does not apply in the instance where the hospital establishes a rule that bed rails are to be raised at all times for a particular class of high-risk patients. In *Pedraza*, the hospital's fall/injury prevention protocol for high-risk patients required that nursing staff assess and reassess the patient's mental and physician condition, including medications that could dim the patient's thought process. In addition, the patient was to be assessed every 2 hours, the bed was to be kept in the lowest position, and all bed rails were to be up at all times.

Courts have addressed the issue of use of restraints in emergency conditions. In *Marvel v. County of Erie* (2003), a patient under psychiatric care was brought to the emergency center because of behavior indicating that he was likely to harm himself. On arrival, the nurse assessed the patient as highly intoxicated, exhibiting behavior that was harmful to him, and threatening to leave. The nurse placed the patient in wrist restraints until he could be seen by a physician. This, the court concluded, was appropriate care. However, the court faulted the nurse for not providing continuous, one-to-one supervision of the patient. Such supervision is necessary to prevent further harm.

Interestingly, the court has also addressed the question of what nurses could have done differently when a restrained patient comes to harm because of the use of restraints. In *American Transitional Care Centers of Texas, Inc. v. Palacios* (2001), a patient apparently untied his own wrist and vest restraints, then fell and injured his head while trying to get out of bed by himself. The nurses caring for this patient knew that he could untie the restraints, and they had initiated a system whereby he was checked at least every hour while in restraints. The bed and vest restraints were securely tied, and a nurses' note written 10 minutes before the patient was found on the floor indicated that these devices were securely fastened.

The Supreme Court of Texas concluded by asking what else the nursing staff could have done for this patient. They were aware of his ability to get out of the restraints, they had moved the patient to a room nearest the nursing station, the patient was checked at least every hour, and the family was also aware of the patient's ability to get out of his restraints. The expert witness addressed the issue in general terms, stating that the nurses had breached the duty of care. The court ruled that the expert witness was incorrect to only state that the nursing staff was negligent without answering the more critical question of what additional measures could have been initiated to prevent such a happening.

The court in *Spohn Hospital v. Mayer* (2003) noted that it is below the standard of care for nurses not to respond promptly to a patient's call bell when the patient is confused, disoriented, and in a Posey belt. A nurse cannot assume that such a patient will be kept in bed by restraints, but must anticipate that the patient might try to get out of bed despite the device and become entangled in the device. In this case, the patient's call bell rang several times before the telemetry unit attached to the patient showed a ventricular fibrillation. The patient had gotten out of bed and was strangled by the Posey vest.

The Joint Commission (JC) set forth guidelines in 2003 related to the use of patient restraints. Individual institution policy and procedure manuals should reflect the following:

1. The decision to use physical restraints should be based on the patient's condition at that moment, rather than on a prior history of violent behavior, the fact that he or she had previously discontinued feeding tubes, or what might happen if the patient becomes confused.

2. Whenever possible, attempt alternative, less restrictive approaches first. For example, use a lap tray rather than physical restraints while the patient is sitting in a chair to support and prevent slipping.

3. If restraints are necessary, choose the least restrictive device to restrict the patient. Do not use four restraints if soft wrist restraints are sufficient.

4. Document frequent assessments of the patient, including the removal of restraints for short periods of time. Documentation should include how one assessed circulation and whether the patient was offered food or hydration and assistance with elimination, such as assisting the patient to the bathroom, providing a bed pan, or the fact that the patient had an indwelling catheter. Most institutions have a specialized form to document nursing interventions while a patient is restrained.

5. Obtain an order for the restraints, even if it is after the restraints have been applied. Remember that the patient's safety comes first. Do what is necessary to protect the patient, and then follow institutional policy.

6. The order must include the date and time that restraints were ordered, the type of restraint to be used, the purpose, and a specific short-term time limit, defined as 24 hours or less.

7. For psychiatric patients, the patient may not be restrained for longer than 4 hours for adults, 2 hours for adolescents, and 1 hour for a child under 9 years of age. After this initial period, a licensed practitioner must reassess the patient and continue the restraints as needed, up to 24 hours. If a psychiatric patient requires hospitalization for medical illness and conditions, the parameters change to that of the patient's primary clinical issue.

8. The order for restraints cannot be renewed without reassessment of the patient. Vague orders, such as "restrain until no longer agitated," are not acceptable. If restraints are still required after assessment, a new order must be written (PC 12.00 et seq).

When using restraints, it is vital to follow hospital policy and procedure, documenting adequately why the patient was restrained, how he or she was restrained, how patient safety needs were met during the time restraints were used, and whether restraints were removed or continued. In documentation, record what type of patient behavior necessitated the restraints, including ineffective methods of restraint that may have been used and the exact type of restraint finally applied, such as soft wrist restraints, kerlix hand restraints, or a Posey vest or belt. The date and time of application of restraints should be noted, along with the patient's response to the restraints. Patient safety needs, such as skin integrity, circulation in the restrained extremities, respiratory status, nutrition and elimination needs, and elevation of the patient's head prior to feeding should be noted according to the hospital policy. Also document the need for continued restraint and periodic assessments to ascertain when restraints may be removed.

Perhaps part of the difficulty in complying with patient restraint standards is a basic misunderstanding of what constitutes restraints and how nurses document the use of various devices. Belts, vests, wrist ties, leathers, and siderails may all be restraints, but some can also serve other purposes. For example, a vest restraint may prevent a patient from falling, or its purpose may be to help an elderly patient maintain correct alignment and support while sitting in a chair. Similarly, one could reason that soft wrist restraints are preventative in patients with endotracheal tubes who are ventilator-dependent, as their purpose is to prevent harm and a possible respiratory arrest if the endotracheal tube is removed prematurely. In both instances, documentation of why the device is used is the key to whether the device is a restraint or is being used for some other purpose.

If restraints as applied are not effective, chemical restraints may augment the physical restraints. For example, the ventilator-dependent patient with adult respiratory distress syndrome may be physically restrained to prevent the accidental dislodgment of an endotracheal tube and chemically restrained to allow the ventilator to regulate respiratory rate and tidal volume. Or chemical restraints may be used without physical restraints, as in patients in whom sedation alone is effective.

A newer trend in restraints is to use a bed occupancy monitor (bed alarm) or similar device so that personnel are alerted immediately when a patient is no longer in bed. Although it may not prevent the patient from falling, the device begins to ensure that assistance is provided immediately. Since there are some patients who can successfully free themselves from all restraints, courts will look to how quickly and effectively the patient was treated after falling. Bed occupancy monitors greatly aid in early intervention and assistance.

GUIDELINES
Chemical and Physical Restraints

1. Involve the patient and family in the decision regarding the need for restraints. This allows the nurse to explain the purpose of the restraints, the reasons for their use, and care that will be given while the person is restrained.
2. Document the reason for the restraint, any explanation given to the patient and family, and measures undertaken to ensure the continuing safety of the patient. This includes checking circulation, assisting with range-of-motion exercises, meeting nutritional and hydration needs, and assessing frequently for the continuing need for the restraint.
3. Document a thorough assessment of the extremity to be restrained before applying the restraining devices. This will protect you against allegations that the restraint caused physical harm to the patient if your assessment shows that the skin was bruised or broken prior to applying the restraint.
4. Document your continuing assessment of the restrained extremity according to hospital policy and the removal of restraints for short periods of time, if that is part of your policy.
5. Document the continuing need for restraints and the reasons necessitating the restraints, if possible. For example, if a certain medication is causing the patient confusion, document the discontinuance of the medication.

EXERCISE 17.3

Reread the case of the patient who was harmed because he was able to untie his restraints, fell, and hit his head. From a legal perspective, what more could the nurses have done to prevent his injury? Is there a greater duty to this type of patient from an ethical perspective? What ethical principles must be considered when caring for such a patient?

MEDICATION ERRORS

Medication errors remain the most common source of liability for nurses in all practice settings, and medication errors continue to be the number one cause of mortality and morbidity in hospitalized patients. Though health care providers have long known that medication errors were the most significant cause of liability in health care settings, the now famous Institute of Medicine study (2000) made these statistics known nationally and internationally.

Medication errors are difficult to defend because they are most often easily averted. Schools of nursing most often teach these precautions as the "five rights" of medication administration: right patient, right medication, right dose, right route, and right time. Most medication errors fall into one of the following categories.

Incorrect Patient

Institutional policy and procedure manuals insist that nurses check patient identification bands frequently, even if the nurse is sure of the patient's identification. Such policies exist to prevent giving a medication to other than the patient for whom the medication was intended and to prevent harmful side effects of the medication in the patient. Relatively few lawsuits are filed that specifically address this one issue, and it is presumed that this is because many patients are able to tolerate one dose of an incorrect medication with few significant side effects.

An older case illustrates this concept. In *Demers v. United States* (1990), the plaintiff's husband was admitted to the hospital for the implantation of a pacemaker. Subsequent to the procedure, the patient was administered Cardizem, a medication intended for another patient in the unit, resulting in his premature demise.

Incorrect Dosage, Medication, or Incorrect Route of Administration

More commonly, nurses administer medications in wrong doses or by a route other than that ordered. Such errors can stem from the nurse's lack of knowledge about the medication. For example, in *Schroeder v. Northwest Community Hospital* (2006), a patient, previously diagnosed with complete renal failure for which he was receiving hemodialysis treatments, was admitted for treatment of his rheumatoid arthritis. The physician ordered methotrexate, a medication contraindicated in patients with renal failure. The patient died due to methotrexate toxicity.

In her lawsuit for her husband's wrongful death, the widow alleged that the nurses who administered this medication were negligent for merely following the physicians' orders and for not knowing that this particular medication should have been questioned and that a request for a discontinuing order should have been written. The court agreed with the widow and found liability against the nursing staff and the physicians.

Confidential v. Confidential (2008a) illustrates the importance of clarifying medication orders. The patient, a 33-year-old male, had been admitted for acute appendicitis and routine appendectomy. Demerol, 100 mg IV, was ordered for post-operative pain, and the first dose was given in the post-anesthesia care unit in 25-mg increments. The patient was transferred to a medical-surgical unit with orders for IV Demerol, 75 mg every 3 to 4 hours as needed for pain. The patient began clear liquids on the following day, and 2 days after surgery, his pain medication was changed to Vicodin, two tablets every 4 to 6 hours as needed for pain. Though the new order was written, the physician did not discontinue the order for Demerol. At this point in his recovery, the patient had received a total of 675 mg of Demerol for pain.

The patient continued to experience significant post-operative pain, and the nurses elected to continue giving the Demerol and did not begin the Vicodin. Late on the third post-operative day, the nurse did give one dose of Vicodin, which the patient reported did not relieve his pain. She then gave the Demerol. On the fourth post-operative day, the patient experienced a seizure, became unresponsive, and a code was called. The 55-minute code was not successful. The coroner's report noted that laboratory tests established acute meperidine toxicity as the cause of death, noting that Demerol (meperidine) is metabolized into normeperidine, a chemical substance that remains in the blood and can build to toxic levels. Nurses at the facility had made the decision to continue the Demerol, even though the physician had written orders for oral Vicodin.

Medication errors also occur when medications are given in greater amounts than the amount ordered (*Lakos v. Kaiser Permanente*, 2008; *Morrison v. Mann*, 2007; *Moc v. Children's Hospital*, 2007; *People v. Gutierrez*, 2006). In *Lakos*, a patient was given 80 units of NPH insulin rather than the prescribed 8 units of NPH insulin, which resulted in his premature demise. A nurse applied a 72% acetic acid solution instead of the normal 3% to 5% solution in *Morrison*, causing severe chemical burns. In *Moc*, an infant who was receiving total parenteral nutrition (TPN) was given an overdose of the solution that was approximately 10 times the ordered dosage. The hyperosmolar solution caused permanent neurological brain injuries. An overdose of Heparin (100,000 units rather than the ordered 1,000 units) in *Gutierrez* caused the patient to expire from his stab wounds.

Finally, medications may also be administered using the incorrect route. *Weeks v. Eastern Idaho Health Services* (2007) illustrates this cause of action. In that case, a patient was to receive an IV mixture of dopamine, amiodarone, magnesium sulfate, potassium phosphate, and potassium chloride. The nurse, though, adminsitered 296 cc of this solution into a catheter that had been inserted to drain fluid from the patient's brain hemorrhage, causing an intracranial fluid overload and his ultimate death.

Improper Injection Technique

An older case, *Biggs v. United States* (1987), illustrates this cause of action. In *Biggs*, the patient claimed that the nurse had used incorrect technique in administering an intramuscular injection. The injection, if given 3 to 4 inches above the knee as was claimed, could have resulted in nerve damage and would have been contrary to nursing standards of care. Because the patient exhibited signs and symptoms of nerve damage, the court remanded the case back to trial level on the issue of nursing malpractice.

Incorrect Time of Administration

Giving medications at wrong time intervals may cause patients serious injury. In an older case illustrating this point, a Utah nurse failed to give an antipsychotic medication as ordered, and the patient subsequently jumped from the hospital window and was permanently paralyzed. In finding for the plaintiff, the court stressed the importance of timely given ordered medications and the need to understand the actions and desired effects of such medications so that timely administration would occur (*Farrow v. Health Services et al.*, 1979).

Failure to Note Patient Allergies

When nurses administer medications to which patients have already disclosed an allergy, the court will typically find against the nurse and the hospital. In *Bazel v. Mabee* (1998), Betadine was used as the antiseptic agent on a surgical site following coronary artery bypass surgery. The Betadine was used before and after the procedure to secure venous material for the bypass graft, even though the patient had noted such an allergy on admission. The court found the hospital liable for his subsequent debridement and skin grafts.

Inaccurate Knowledge Regarding the Medication and Its Side Effects

One of the most important aspects of medication administration involves the nurse's full comprehension of the medication's target effects and possible side effects. Standards of care require nurses not only to be able to administer medications correctly, but to understand the pharmaceutical actions of the medications, potential side effects, and contraindications. Nurses must also understand the interactions of medications because most patients receive more than three medications during a 24-hour period, and they must properly question the prescribing physician before administering the medication.

A case that clearly illustrates this aspect is *Hill v. Sacred Heart Medical Center* (2008). The case involved a patient recovering from bilateral knee replacement surgery. The physician ordered subcutaneous injections of Lovenox as a precaution against deep vein thrombosis in the recovery period. These injections were administered over a 9-day period in the patient's left lower quadrant of his abdomen. Over this period of time, the patient developed a rash and bruising in the area where the injections were being administered. The skin was hardened at the injection site, then a large blood blister developed and progressed to a black blister measuring 3 by 8 cm.

Blood tests showed that from day 7 to day 9 post-operatively, his platelet count dropped 70%. On day 9, the patient became pale, confused, drowsy, short of breath, and was eventually very difficult to rouse. Unfractionated heparin was substituted for the Lovenox. Ten hours later, another internist discontinued all anticoagulant medications. The patient then had a stroke, pulmonary embolism, and a deep vein thrombosis, leaving him paralyzed on the right side, all related to heparin-induced thrombocytopenia, an immune reaction to heparin.

The nursing expert who testified in this case acknowledged that the nurses were aware that something was amiss in this patient's reaction to the Lovenox as evidenced by the significant changes at the injection site, but that they failed to advocate for the patient and did not recognize signs and symptoms of a heparin-induced thrombocytopenia. The nurses, testified the expert, should have been aware of the adverse side effects of the medication and should have known that a marked drop in the patient's platelet count indicated that the patient was having an adverse reaction to the Lovenox. Additionally, the nurses should have advocated for the patient when the Lovenox was changed to an unfractionated heparin administration when the patient was already exhibiting major symptoms of an immune reaction to a heparin-based compound.

Kunz v. Little County of Mary Hospital (2007) illustrates the nurse's responsibility for also ensuring that clear and correct information regarding medications is clearly conveyed to all health care providers. In this case, a 75-year-old patient was to be given a very short-term administration of gentamycin, as this drug is contraindicated in patients with known renal insufficiency, but was indicated for a methacillin-resistant *Staph aureas* infection following knee-replacement surgery. The physician elected to give the medication during the time that the patient was in the acute care facility, then planned to discontinue the medication and give IV vancomycin and oral refampin when the patient was discharged to the nursing home. However, the hospital discharge nurse misread the physician's discharge orders and failed to note that the gentamycin was discontinued. In the nursing home, the patient received all three antibiotics, because the nursing staff in the nursing home also failed to clarify the antibiotic orders for this patient. The discharge nurse and the nursing staff in the nursing home shared liability in this case for the patient's irreversible renal failure.

EXERCISE 17.4

You are the medication nurse for a busy medical-surgical unit. After giving a patient her medication, she complains of itching and slight shortness of breath, and you notice obvious signs of an allergic reaction on her skin. Should the patient decide to later file suit and name you in the case, could you be held liable for the allergic response and subsequent harm to the patient? What would be your best defense against liability in such a suit?

PATIENT FALLS

Patient falls remain second to medication errors in untoward events that may happen to patients. Patient falls are among the top incidents that cause or create the potential for serious patient injury or death. Patient falls are also among the most common types of cases that are filed against health care providers.

Remember, though, that merely because a patient falls does not necessarily mean that fault will be assessed against health care providers (*Lewandowski v. Mercy Memorial Hospital Corporation*, 2003). A more recent case example of this principle may be found in *Simon v. Sierra Madre Skilled Nursing* (2007). This case involved a 74-year-old patient admitted to the hospital after suffering a third stroke, which left her completely paralyzed on her right side. At the hospital she made sufficient progress to then be transferred to a skilled nursing facility. The discharge summary from the hospital indicated that restraints were occasionally used, and she was summarized as a low risk for falls.

She fell during the night at the skilled nursing facility. At about 2:00 A.M., an aide heard the patient fall and the charge nurse was immediately informed. The nurse completed a thorough assessment of the patient, noting that the patient had a medium-sized bump on her head. The physician was called and hourly neurological assessments were ordered. These were completed as ordered and at 7:30 A.M. the nurse called the physician because the patient could not be roused. She was sent to the acute care hospital for evaluation, which showed that she had a subdural hematoma that ultimately resulted in her death.

The court noted that restraints, including a Posey vest, had not been ordered, as it was determined that the lowest level of restraint was best for this patient. Siderails were in their raised position and the patient was promptly and completely assessed and observed immediately after the fall. Additionally, the physician was notified in a timely manner of all subsequent occurrences and the patient was timely transferred to the acute care hospital when her condition changed. Thus no liability was held against the facility.

Romaro v. Marks (1996) examined the issue of nurse's responsibilities for preventing falls in patients who are fully able to understand and comply with recommended treatment. The patient was ordered to remain in bed, on strict bedrest, for 24 hours. The patient testified that she was aware of the orders, but she got up to use the bathroom without calling the nursing staff. She fell as she returned to bed from the bathroom. The court dismissed the case, stating that the nursing staff had no obligation for keeping the patient in bed, beyond making sure that she understood the physician's instructions.

Liability will be assessed against the nursing staff if it can be shown that the nurse used poor judgment in preventing a patient's fall. In *McLaughlin v. Firelands Community Hospital* (2006), the patient suffered from Parkinson's disease, scoliosis, osteoporosis, and severe depression. Treatment for her depression included electroconvulsive therapy. Restraints had been ordered because the patient was combative and experienced periods of hallucination. On the night prior to her fall, she could not sleep and continued to hallucinate. Because of her deteriorating mental status, she was transferred to a special care unit, which had a maximum of six patients and a staff of three nurses. The patient was also given additional antidepressant medication and Haldol was added as a new medication. Standard practice on this unit included that patients be monitored every 15 minutes.

The patient slept for most of the next day without her restraints. During the night, a new patient was admitted to the unit. Immediately before this patient arrived in the unit, staff members observed patients already on the unit and found these patients to all be asleep. The three nurses and two aides from the emergency room then entered the new patient's room, leaving the remaining patients unattended. During this time frame, the patient awakened and fell while getting out of bed. The court held that such an event should have been anticipated and found the institution liable for the injury caused by the patient's fall.

Sometimes, allowing a patient to fall is not the only act of negligence or malpractice that is brought in a lawsuit. In *Thomas v. Greenview Hospital, Inc.* (2004), a patient whose right leg had been amputated as the result of her diabetes was allowed to fall while seated in a chair near the nurses' station. Following her fall, she had hip replacement surgery and was placed on bedrest. During the post-operative time frame she developed an infected Stage III decubitus.

The nurses in this case were found at fault for allowing this patient, in a confused state, to be unrestrained while she was sitting in the chair. Additionally, the staff was also at fault for not turning the patient every 2 hours to prevent a decubitus from developing. Finally, the court noted that the air mattress that was ordered when the patient's first signs of skin breakdown became apparent was not started as ordered, but that there was a 2-day delay in placing the mattress on the patient's bed.

When a patient falls, the first duty of care is to the patient. Notify the patient's physician and management personnel after the patient has been fully assessed for injuries. Give the patient's physician a brief description of what happened and a full description of the patient's condition. The emphasis should be on treatment to prevent further injury. Completely document the patient's condition, treatments or tests performed to prevent further injury or done to ascertain the full extent of the injury, who was notified, and when they were notified. Many institutions require that the patient's family also be notified of the fall. In some states, the law requires that patient's families be informed of falls in residential treatment centers and long-term care facilities.

EXERCISE 17.5

Mr. Jones is in the rehabilitation unit of your institution. He is partially paralyzed on his left side as a result of a recent stroke. When caring for him, the nurse assisted him to a bedside commode, then left the room to give Mr. Jones some privacy. Shortly after the nurse left the room, Mr. Jones began to convulse and he fell from the commode, striking his head on the metal bed frame as he fell to the floor.

How do you think the court would decide in such a case? What professional responsibilities did the nurse have to Mr. Jones?

TECHNOLOGY AND EQUIPMENT

Advances in **technology and equipment** have created special problems of liability for nurses. In addition to assessing and monitoring the patient, the nurse must also know the capabilities, limitations, hazards, and safety features of numerous machines and devices. Today, more equipment injuries occur not because of unfamiliarity with the equipment, but because of carelessness or misuse of equipment. Thus, nurses should carefully follow manufacturers' recommendations for use of equipment and refrain from making modifications to the equipment.

Nursing negligence associated with improper use of equipment can arise in a variety of ways. First, after learning the correct use of machinery, the nurse is expected to conform with the manufacturers' recommendations and hospital policy and protocols. For example, in *Espinosa v. Baptist Health Systems* (2006), a patient was injured when the orthopedic trapeze above his bed suddenly came apart as he was using it to lift himself up in bed. His contention at trial was that the nurse and orthopedic technician who assembled the trapeze were negligent in not assembling the device according to the manufacturer's specifications. Though the court noted that the patient would have prevailed in this case, the patient's attorney failed to secure the evidence from an expert witness and the case was dismissed.

Additional cases include *Craig v. Sina* (2007), in which the alarm on a cardiac monitor had been discontinued while the patient used the bedside commode and then not reconnected; the patient suffered irreversible brain damage when the subsequent episode of ventricular fibrillation was not timely treated. In *Bullock v. The Rapides Foundation* (2006), a patient's family member was injured when a stool in the emergency room suddenly rolled backward. In finding liability in this case, the court noted that the medical center had knowledge of the stool's ability to cause potential injury, as there had been eight previous instances where the stool suddenly rolled back when someone sat on it.

Colombini v. Westchester County Healthcare Corporation (2005) exemplifies how dangerous equipment can be and why it is important to be knowledgeable about such equipment. In this case, a 6-year-old boy was sedated and placed in a magnetic resonance imaging (MRI) machine. When the anesthesiologist realized that the boy was not receiving oxygen, he called to the operators of the MRI equipment to attend to the oxygen supply source. Hearing the call for additional oxygen, a nurse who was passing in the hallway outside the imaging room attempted to hand the anesthesiologist an oxygen tank made of ferrous material, which was drawn into the MRI machine by its strong magnetic field. The oxygen tank struck the boy's head, causing his death.

Liability can result from using defective or unsafe equipment, and nurses have a duty to make a reasonable inspection of equipment and refrain from using equipment that is defective or not working properly. In *Christus Health v. Lanham* (2007), the facility was found liable to an elderly patient for a shower chair that collapsed when the patient used it. The court sited JC standards in its finding, noting that the standard of care requires the effective management of the environment of care to control and reduce environmental hazards and risks, prevent accidents and injuries, and maintain safe conditions. The standard of care extends to the employees' responsibility to inspect equipment prior to its use and to remove and report faulty equipment per hospital policy.

Nurses are also expected to give quality, competent care despite equipment failures and faulty equipment. An older case illustrates this point. In *Rose v. Hakim* (1971), an infant who had sustained cardiac arrest during surgery required the use of a hypothermia unit in a pediatric intensive care unit. The continuous-readout thermometer in the hypothermia unit was faulty, and the nurse caring for the child failed to verify the thermometer's accuracy or use ancillary cooling measures such as medications, ice packs, or alcohol sponge baths. The infant suffered a grand mal seizure and respiratory arrest, and was placed on a ventilator for respiratory assistance. When the infant showed signs of poor air exchange on the ventilator, the nurse corrected an obvious kink in the ventilator tubing, but failed to check oxygen concentration and tidal volume delivery. The court held that the infant's subsequent injuries were due primarily to negligent actions and omissions by the nursing personnel, and secondarily to the defective equipment.

Finally, nurses may have a legal duty to assess the equipment's appropriateness. In *Hall v. Arthur* (1998), the surgeon implanted an artificial material during an anterior cervical diskectomy and fusion surgery, rather than bone harvested from the patient's hip or from the tissue bank. Eventually, the patient required a second operation, removing the implant and using the patient's bone. The court ruled that the hospital was also liable because the nurse ordered the synthetic implant without having the unusual request reviewed by the appropriate managers, as was the hospital's policy, and because the product's original package insert specifically contraindicated its use for spinal procedures.

Nurses, through the risk management department, may also have a duty to evaluate whether institutions are following the Safe Medical Devices Act of 1990, amended in 1992. Under this law and its amendments, all adverse incidents related to medical devices must be reported to manufacturers, and in cases of death to the Food and Drug Administration, within 10 working days. The purpose of the law is to investigate and take action the first time an event occurs to prevent reoccurrence and harm to subsequent patients.

FAILURE TO ADEQUATELY ASSESS, MONITOR, AND COMMUNICATE

Nurses are frequently reminded that their most important duty is that of communication, both verbally and through written documentation, to patients, physicians, other staff members, and members of the interdisciplinary health care team. Communication is vital, but one must have something to communicate. Perhaps equally important is the nurse's role in assessing and monitoring patients, then in communicating this information to others.

Failure to adequately assess, monitor, and communicate can occur in all aspects of nursing and in all hospital units. This same failure can occur with all types of nursing procedures and skills, from the simplest to more complex procedures and skills.

Failure to Monitor

Failure to monitor has been found to be the cause of action for liability in multiple recent legal cases, including *Cockerham v. LaSalle Nursing Home, Inc.* (2006); *Confidential v. Confidential* (2007a); *Dutton v. Scott and White Memorial Hospital* (2007); *Frias v. King* (2008); *Harris v. Sumpter Regional Hospital* (2008); *Hughes v. Boyd* (2008); *Johnson v. Methodist Hospital of Dallas* (2007); *Lake Cumberland v. Dishman* (2007); *Lance v. Moores* (2007); *Morton v. Brookhaven Memorial Hospital* (2007); *Page v. Daybreak Venture* (2007); *Reinhardt v. Sunrise* (2008); and *Rodriquez v. Palm Springs General Hospital* (2007), among others. These failure to monitor cases all resulted in significant liability for the health care providers and institutions and comprised a variety of nursing care specialties and skills.

Two of the cases (*Hughes and Rodriquez*) involved the failure to adequately monitor patients during surgical procedures. In Hughes, this failure to monitor resulted in a retained hemostat and a surgical burn, which occurred when a heated IV bag was placed under the armpit of the 62-year-old patient. In *Confidential,* a 32-year-old obstetrical patient's labor was progressing very slowly and it was decided that a cesarean section was required. In preparation for the surgical procedure, a bolus of anesthetic was delivered through the epidural catheter that had been previous placed. The bolus was given at the change of shift and no nurse or physician monitored the patient following its administration. The patient suffered severe respiratory distress, which was not noticed until someone monitoring the fetal monitor read-outs noticed the abnormal reading and alerted other personnel. A crash section was performed and the baby was born basically unaffected by the event, though the mother sustained irreversible brain damage and remains in a persistent vegetative state. The case, primarily because of the cost for skilled nursing care placement for the mother, resulted in a $4,200,000 award.

Inadequate post-operative care may also result from failure to monitor. In *Harris,* a 14-year-old patient fractured his distal femur, which was repaired with a closed reduction and percutanous pinning. At midnight, the patient complained that his leg was numb and that he could not move his toes, at 8:00 A.M. it was noted that there was no pulse in the foot and that the patient was complaining of increased pain, and at 3:00 P.M. an arteriogram showed that there was an absence of blood flow below the knee. The nurses were found liable for the failure to monitor and the failure to understand the significance of ominous signs as well as the failure to report significant findings to the physician in time to save the limb. In *Lance* and *Johnson,* the nursing staff members were faulted for the failure to monitor oxygen level saturations that resulted in significant adverse outcomes for both of these patients.

Three of the cases for failure to monitor concerned medications and/or IV fluid administration. In *Frias,* a newborn infant had a seizure that resulted in permanent neurological injuries when the nurses failed to monitor the infant for fluid overload. *Morton* concerned a patient receiving emergency anticoagulant therapy for a possible myocardial infarction. Though she repeatedly reported to the nurses caring for her that the IV site was painful and swollen, no effort was made to discontinue the IV fluids and restart the IV in another site. *Dutton* concerned a patient who presented with preeclampsia and received Pitocin. The nurses failed to monitor the fetal heart tracings that indicated an emergency cesarean section was indicated. The infant suffered significant neurological deficits at birth related to oxygen deprivation.

Though smoking is banned in most health care institutions today, *Page* concerned what can happen when patients are allowed smoking privileges and are not adequately monitored. The nursing and rehabilitation center where the patient resided had a smoking area that supervised patients could use. The patient had been diagnosed with chronic obstructive lung disease (COLD), used supplemental oxygen, and also used a wheelchair. She wheeled herself, unsupervised, into the facility's smoking area and suffered second and third-degree burns when her supplemental oxygen caused her to become inflamed. The facility was faulted for failure to monitor the patient while smoking as well as failure to keep her cigarettes in a secure place.

Failure to Assess and Notify

Similar to failure to monitor causes of action, causes of action for the failure to assess and notify members of the health care team of adverse findings have resulted in numerous recent court rulings. Some of these cases include *Confidential v. Confidential* (2007b); *De Stasio v. Kocsis* (2007); *Groves v. State* (2007); *John Doe v. Confidential Hospital* (2007); *Lawson v. United States* (2006); *McAllen Hospital v. Muniz* (2007); *McKenna Memorial Hospital v. Quinney* (2006); *Michael v. Medical Staffing Network, Inc.* (2007); *Moeltner v. Rubio* (2007); *Sobti v. Prince William Hospital* (2008); *Vela v. Bay Area Healthcare Group* (2007); *Villarreal v. Rio Grande Regional Hospital* (2008); and *Wert v. (Name Withheld-Confidential) Hospital* (2007), among others.

The failure to assess and notify is perhaps most frequently seen in obstetrical cases. For example, in *Wert*, fetal heart monitoring was initiated immediately upon the mother's arrival. The first tracings were within normal ranges, seemingly indicating that the fetus was healthy and that a normal vaginal delivery was indicated. A few hours later, the tracings showed late decelerations, indicating changes in the fetal heart rate after uterine contractions with diminished long-term variability. No attempt was made to contact the physician, who had left the hospital and was returning to his office.

Twenty minutes later, the fetal heart rate rose to 145 to 150, then abruptly fell to 60 to 100 and remained in that range for some 7 minutes. The mother's uterus became hypertonic, with contractions lasting 5 minutes in duration. Again the physician was not notified and preparations were not made for a possible emergency cesarean section. The physician was finally notified of the adverse findings more than an hour later. An emergency cesarean section was performed and a severely neurologically affected infant was delivered.

Failure to assess and notify was also the holding in *Moeltner*. In this case, the mother was first given 50 micrograms of intravaginal Cytotec by the physician to induce labor, an "off-label" use of the ulcer medication. Four hours later, the nurse began Pitocin as ordered, gradually increasing the dose as ordered. Three hours later, the nurse discontinued the Pitocin and attempted to notify the physician. Two hours after the Pitocin was discontinued, a severely hypoxic and permanently brain-damaged infant was delivered by cesarean section. The nurse was found partially liable for her failure to adequately assess the patient and for failure to timely notify the physician of adverse effects of the Pitocin. The physician was faulted for the use of the drug Cytotec, for ordering Pitocin less than 4 hours after the Cytotec administration, and for delay in starting the cesarean section.

A pediatric case that supports this same cause of action is *Confidential v. Confidential* (2007b). A 31-week-old infant, born to a mother with a history of illegal drug abuse and no previous prenatal care, was assessed by the staff nurses, a neonatal nurse practitioner, and two neonatologists as having a patent anus. A rectal temperature had been taken and charted and the nurse practitioner had charted that the "anus was within normal limits-patent, rectal exam not merited." By the end of his second day of life, the nurses were concerned that the infant had had no bowel movement and that his abdominal circumference has increased by 5 cm, from the original 22 cm to 27 cm. X-rays revealed free air in the bowel, indicating that the bowel had perforated internally and that its contents were now in the peritoneum. Multiple members of the health care team who were associated with the care of this infant were found partially liable for the failure to properly assess this infant.

Two recent lawsuits held that nurses also have the responsibility to do more than assess and notify the physician regarding patient care issues. In *Czarney v. Porter* (2006), a patient was admitted for the treatment of gastrointestional bleeding. The physician ordered the infusion of two units of packed red blood cells, IV fluids, and telemetry monitoring. No infusion rate was given for the blood or the IV fluids, and rather than clarifying the order with the physician, the nurse administered the blood at a rate of 125 cc per hour and the IV fluids at 125 cc per hour. This rate was selected because the standard rate set by hospital policy was 125 cc per hour if the physician did not specify an infusion rate. Additionally, the nurse elected not to administer both the blood and the IV fluids simultaneously, but to first infuse the blood and then restart the IV fluids. In fact, the physician, given the amount of bleeding and the decreasing blood pressure of the patient, wanted the blood infused as quickly as possible and the IV fluids given with the blood. Though the case has been remanded back to the lower court for additional facts, the nurse was faulted for not clarifying the initial orders, for failure to assess and notify the physician that the patient's blood pressure was dangerously low, and for failure to follow orders in that the ordered telemetry was never initiated. Had the telemetry been used, the nurse would have noted that the patient was in dire distress and he might have survived.

An additional responsibility in the area of assessment and notification is the duty to report suspected child abuse. Instances where such abuse is suspected most often occurs in acute care settings, primarily in the emergency center when these children are evaluated for falls and or other "accidents." *Cooper Clinic v. Barnes* (2006) illustrates the importance for health care providers to report such suspected abuse and protect the child. In that case, a 3-year-old was treated for a bump on his head, which the father told the admitting staff had been done by another child who hit him with a golf club. In examining the boy, the physician and nurses noted multiple bruises on his body and that his teeth were clipped and decaying. The father told staff members that his ex-wife had abused the child and that he was going to alert the authorities in the state where she lived about the abuse. The child was brought back to the emergency center a week later for stomach pains, nausea, and vomiting, and was treated and released.

Ten months after his first visit, the child died from blunt force trauma to his abdomen for which his father and stepmother were convicted of negligent homicide. A civil lawsuit was brought against the health care providers for their failure to report the suspected child abuse. In holding the physician and nursing staff liable, the court noted that there is a mandatory duty to report suspected child abuse so that it can be appropriately investigated. Had the first incident been properly reported, the authorities should have been able to show that it was the father and not the child's mother who was responsible for the abuse, and the child would have been removed from the abusive household.

Courts have also been supportive of staff members who do assess and notify appropriate health care providers of changes in a patient's condition. In *Fiqueredo v. St. Alphonsus Regional Medical Center* (2007), the nurse was commended by the court for her observation that the patient's potassium level was dangerously high (8.9) and for promptly notifying the physician. The physician ordered Kayexalate to be given immediately. However, the nurse neglected to transcribe the order and thus the medication was never administered. The patient died 3 days later in the intensive care unit.

Failure to Communicate with Interdisciplinary Health Care Members

Nurses have a responsibility to communicate with interdisciplinary health care members, particularly if there is a change in patient status. In *Rademacher v. Katuna* (2007), a patient who had a comatose event at home was taken to the emergency center. The emergency center physician called a neurologist, who was unable to rule out a cerebrovascular event versus a seizure, and the patient was admitted to a general medical-surgical unit. X-rays were taken and the nurse was unable to rouse the patient, even though she used a deep sternal rub to attempt arousal. She made a notation in the patient record, but did not notify the physician about this finding. Over the next 10 hours, there was no record of any communication between the nurses and the physicians regarding the patient's changing neurological status, including the fact that the patient was having difficulty moving his limbs, complained of right-sided numbness, could not lift his right arm, and was not able to squeeze his right hand. The physician was notified, some 12 hours after the patient's admission, that the patient was experiencing difficulty swallowing, and a diagnosis of a cerebrovascular accident was made. The patient was awarded a $1,000,000 award for the failure to timely diagnose and treat his medical condition.

A $600,000 award was made to a 46-year-old patient who suffered compression damage to her femoral nerve following a surgical repair of an incisional hernia that resulted from an earlier hysterectomy (*Confidential v. Confidential*, 2007c). After the surgical procedure, the patient told the nurses that she was experiencing severe pain at the surgical site. Later she reported the pain spreading down her left leg. When she was assisted to stand, the patient's left leg gave way and she fell. The nurses communicated the severe pain at the surgical site to the surgeon, but did not mention that the pain radiated down the left leg or that the patient had fallen when her leg did not support her.

During the night, the nurses continued to document the increased level of pain and radiation, but did not call the surgeon. He was apprised of the continuing pain, radiation of the pain, and fall the next morning as he was making his rounds. A neurologist was consulted and an MRI done, which confirmed the compression damage to the femoral nerve. The patient subsequently underwent a second operation for revision at the incisional hernia site. After the second operation, the patient continued to experience problems with the femoral nerve damage.

The patient in *Renz v. Northside Hospital* (2007) had undergone a C-2 nerve block treatment for migraine headaches. Ninety minutes after the treatment, the patient was discharged by the recovery room nurse without consulting the physician, even though the patient was complaining of nausea, a continuing headache, and was crying. A few hours later, the patient called and spoke with another nurse, who advised her to have her prescription for an anti-inflammatory medication filled, take the medication, and lie down in a quiet and darkened room. This nurse also failed to communicate with the physician about the patient's call and continuing pain. In the lawsuit that ensued, the nurses were found liable for not communicating with the physician. Subsequent follow-up showed that the physician had negligently injected the nerve block into an artery.

The failure to communicate medically significant changes to the patient's physician also caused patient injuries in *Confidential v. Confidential* (2008b). In that case, an 18-year-old obstetrical patient who had been diagnosed at age 9 with systemic lupus erythematosus entered the hospital for treatment of her lupus erythematosus. She was treated and discharged, then returned 4 days later because she was in active labor. At 1:00 A.M., she was dilated 8 cm, 90% effaced, and at a minus 2 station. An epidural was initiated, the fetal heart monitoring showed normal tracings, and a Pitocin drip was begun at 1:30 A.M. An hour later, her membranes ruptured, and at 4:45 she was seen by a perinatologist who instructed her to begin pushing. There were some late decelerations on the fetal heart monitor, but the perinatologist was not concerned.

Shortly after the perinatologist left, the Pitocin was stopped, as the nurse was concerned about continuing late decelerations on the monitor. An hour later, the nurse restarted the Pitocin, let it run for about 45 minutes, then again stopped the medication. She did not convey these happenings to the perinatologist, as she thought he was aware of the situation. When the nurses changed shifts at 7:00 A.M., the day nurse was immediately concerned about the monitor tracings, but the night nurse informed the day nurse that the perinatologist knew about the monitor tracings and was in the process of deciding what to do. At 8:00 A.M., the day nurse contacted the perinatologist, who immediately saw the need for a cesarean section, and the infant was delivered at 9:01 A.M. In its conclusions, the court faulted the nurses for not communicating with the primary physician and the perinatologist for the hour delay in performing the cesarean section.

A case vividly illustrating the need to assess, monitor, and communicate and then to document that these were performed is *O'Donnell v. Holy Family Hospital* (1997). In that case, the labor and delivery nurses noted carefully the specific time that the monitoring strips began to show fetal distress and that the physician was informed of these tracings. He arrived to view the monitor tracings for himself and to assess the patient within a 6-minute time frame. The nurses noted the exact time the cesarean section was decided upon, when the anesthetist and neonatologist were called, when the mother was prepped for surgery, and the exact time the initial incision was made. All of these events occurred within an acceptable 30-minute time frame.

Based on the notes at delivery, the court, through expert testimony, was able to conclude that the fetus was essentially born dead, with the airways so hopelessly obstructed in utero that the child could not be brought back to life. Although this was a tragedy, it did not result from failure to assess or to monitor the mother and the unborn child.

Perhaps *Gabaldoni v. Board of Physician Quality Assurance* (2001) best illustrates the role of the nurse in assessing and communicating with members of the health care team. The court in this case upheld a reprimand imposed on an obstetrician by the State Board of Medicine for a patient's avoidable death. In contrast to this negligence, the court praised the nurses' competence. The court record is full of reference to the nurses' notes, exact times when tests were ordered by the physician, exact times when results were returned or when someone was sent to get the reports, and exact times of when and how the physician was notified of the patient's test results.

EXERCISE 17.6

The patient had been admitted to the hospital for the birth of her first child. She was 2 weeks past her due date, her membranes had ruptured at home, and she was in active labor. She and her husband had twice declined the midwife's recommendation that a Pitocin drip be initiated, based on the negative information about Pitocin that they had been given at their natural childbirth class. The nurse midwife informed the couple that the mother's physician had ordered the Pitocin and that she was going to initiate the drip, despite their refusal. At this point, the mother was several hours into her labor, with 60- to 90-second contractions at 5- to 7-minute intervals.

The Pitocin was started and both the nurse directly caring for the mother and the nurse midwife continued to increase the amount of Pitocin that the patient was receiving. This increase in Pitocin dosage continued even though the hospital's policy stated that Pitocin was to be discontinued if contractions became more frequent than every 2 minutes or became tetonic. The Pitocin was still infusing 3 hours after the mother's uterine contractions had become hyperstimulated. At this point, the fetus' heart rate became bradycardic and the severely retarded infant was delivered by cesarean section.

How should the court find in this particular case? Were either of the nurses meeting the standards of care for this patient? If you were able to see a failure to communicate in this case, with whom was the failure to communicate identified? How could better assessment and communications have made a difference in the outcomes?

Failure to Communicate with Patients

Obstetrical nurses must also be attentive to communication of relevant patient data. In *Bryant v. John Doe Hospital and John Doe, M.D.* (1992), the patient had 2 hours of late decelerations, but the nurse failed to communicate these late decelerations to anyone. Sometimes, though, the physician fails to listen to the nurse. In a separate case that same year, the nurses did notify the physician of fetal distress on the monitor, and one nurse even begged him to do an immediate cesarean section to no avail. The physician continued to order drugs to further induce labor and was absent when the woman finally delivered a profoundly retarded neonate (*Herron v. Northwest Community Hospital*, 1992).

The importance of nursing communications cannot be overemphasized because treatment decisions may be made based on those communications or lack of communications. In *Lopez v. Southwest Community Health Service* (1992), a woman who was 28 weeks pregnant experienced pain at home and called the physician's office. She was instructed to go to the hospital, and the physician's nurse called the hospital to inform employees there of the impending admission and that the patient was in labor. Two nurses worked with her in the hospital. The first nurse failed to examine her, and the second nurse, after doing a pelvic examination, determined that she was 10 cm dilated and that the membranes were bulging. When the physician was notified of these results, he ruptured the membranes and delivered the baby, who is now a quadriplegic, deaf, blind, and brain damaged.

Neither of the nurses questioned the patient or her mother when they arrived at the hospital. Neither did a history of the patient, and they must have not talked with her. If they had, they would have known that neither the patient nor her mother believed that she was in labor but were concerned about her persistent pains. And the physician would not have delivered the child had he not listened to the nurses.

Other cases reflect this failure to listen to patients and what they are trying to tell the staff. In *Parker v. Bullock County Hospital Authority* (1990), the patient fell while taking a shower in the hospital. The patient had had surgery, and she told the nurse when the nurse helped her to the shower that she was dizzy and lightheaded, but the nurse left her unattended to take her shower, obviously ignoring her statement.

What nurses fail to communicate is equally important. Several cases have held nurses directly liable for the failure to communicate pertinent patient data or for not informing the primary health care provider in a timely manner. In one case, a 6-year-old boy lost the use of his hand because the nurse had written an accurate assessment in the nursing notes but failed to bring that same data to the attention of the attending physician before permanent injury occurred (Mandell, 1993).

The duty to communicate is not directed exclusively to nurses. In *Riley v. West Paces Ferry Hospital, Inc.* (1990), the court held that physicians have a duty to alert nurses to the fact that they should anticipate a significant change in the patient's condition and a possible medical emergency. In this case, a 24-year-old patient was admitted for shortness of breath and chest tightness. The x-ray indicated air in the subcutaneous neck tissues and mediastinum, and the patient was intubated and placed on a ventilator. The physician, however, failed to tell the staff about the air seen on the x-ray and the possibility of a tension pneumothorax developing. The physician left the facility, and the patient subsequently arrested and could not be successfully resuscitated.

A case that extends the duty of health care providers to warn patients of danger of contact with persons at risk is *Troxel v. A. I. Dupont Institute* (1996). A mother and her newborn infant were diagnosed with cytomegalovirus (CMV). Despite their diagnosis, the mother and child were visited at home by a friend who assisted with feeding and bathing the infant and with changing diapers. The friend herself had just become pregnant. Six months after she began visiting the mother and baby, the friend discovered that CMV is highly contagious and poses a special threat to pregnant women. She also learned that she herself was probably infected with CMV. Her infant was born 3 months later. The friend's infant died from CMV, having been affected in utero. The friend filed suit against the medical facility that diagnosed and treated her friend and her friend's infant, claiming damages for her infant's death and for her own infection.

The court held that health care professionals have the legal duty to warn their patients who have highly contagious diseases, such as CMV, hepatitis C, and human immunodeficiency virus (HIV), of the possibility of spreading their diseases to others in certain specific circumstances and to point out to their patients examples of persons they might encounter who are particularly at risk of contracting their diseases from them.

Communicating with the Culturally and Ethnically Diverse

Some of the issues concerned with communication involve working with culturally and ethnically diverse patients and health care workers. English is not the primary language for approximately 47 million U.S. residents over the age of 5, and this may result in communication difficulties (U.S. Census Bureau, 2002). Health literacy (discussed earlier in Chapter 8) may also compound the health care providers' ability to communicate effectively. Limited case law supports not hiring personnel because of their inability to communicate effectively with the public, an essential requirement of jobs in which the individual interfaces with people daily. Review Chapter 13 for additional information regarding this topic.

Though an important aspect of health care delivery, limited case law exists showing the harm that can occur when English is not the primary language for the patient. For example, in *Nevarez v. New York City Health and Hospitals Corporation* (1997), a patient who did not speak English was brought into the hospital by her brother. She was having labor contractions and was bleeding. The brother brought her to the information desk rather than to the emergency center. The information desk staff phoned the physician, who told them to have her wait for his arrival, which occurred some 3 hours later.

She was in labor with a difficult breech presentation, requiring transfer by ambulance to a second facility for a cesarean section. The baby was born with severe hypoxic brain damage, and the mother was awarded $10 million in damages.

The court found that the patient should have been sent to the emergency center, even though the physician requested that she wait there. Additionally, if the patient had been able to better describe her distress or if the facility had provided a translator, the patient would have been able to make herself understood and she would have been timely seen in the emergency center.

GUIDELINES

Communicating with Non-English-Speaking Patients

1. Use a hospital-provided translator if at all possible. These individuals are more accustomed to medical phrases and conditions and are less likely to be affected by "false fluency," the incorrect use of a word or phrase or the use of a term for which there is no direct translation.
2. Even when using a hospital-provided translator, avoid medical jargon and use words or phrases that are more easily understood by people outside of health care.
3. If this is the first time you have worked with this translator, take a few minutes to speak with the translator. Inform the translator in advance of the subjects to be covered and the potential questions. Ensure that he or she will translate the words as literally as possible or inform you when there is no literal translation.

4. Ensure in advance that the translator understands the need for confidentiality and that anything said during the session is confidential. Make sure that the patient also understands that anything he or she says is confidential.

5. When questioning the patient, speak directly to the patient as if the translator was not present. Do not speak through the translator. This allows your words to be translated exactly as you have spoken them.

6. Look at the patient while the translator speaks to the patient and when the patient replies. Pay attention to the patient's nonverbal body language as well as the spoken words.

7. Speak slowly and pause frequently, so that the translator can complete each question and the patient can respond. Avoid compound sentences as much as possible, as the translator or the patient or both may become confused and you will not get the information you need.

8. When completing the session, ask if there are any questions and allow sufficient time for the patient to answer. If instructions have been given, it is a good idea to have the patient repeat the instructions so that you can validate patient understanding.

Because of this diversity, state laws, JC standards, and the American Hospital Association Bill of Rights for Patients have included provisions for ensuring that patient rights means being able to meet their communication needs, particularly if patients do not speak English or speak it so brokenly that they are unable to express themselves or understand what is said to them. To prevent such a happening, most institutions now provide interpreters for non-English-speaking patients, and nurses must make reasonable efforts to ensure that patients understand care issues and discharge education and instructions. Remember, though, that when family members or patients' friends serve as interpreters, issues concerning patient sensitivity and completeness of information as well as the interpretation to the patient may be compromised. Some patients will not share confidential information with their family members, nor will family members necessarily tell patients the whole truth about their condition/prognosis. Thus, it is advisable to use hospital-provided interpreters whenever possible.

Nurses should document who was used as the interpreter, family member or hospital-provided interpreter, the instructions given, and means of ensuring that the patient understood the instructions or conversations. Means that may be employed to ensure comprehension include having the patient repeat the material back to the nurse or asking questions and requiring that the patient respond. As more non-English-speaking patients enter the health care delivery system, the profession may see additional causes of action based on their noncomprehension and failure to follow instructions because they did not understand the instructions.

EXERCISE 17.7

Jimmie Cho, admitted for minor surgery, tells you he is having some chest discomfort and shortness of breath. The patient, a known cardiac patient, had nitroglycerin prescribed for chest pain, and you give him the ordered medication, then go back to the task you were doing when he called for assistance. You do not notify the physician of the chest discomfort, nor do you check back with the patient to see if the medication eased the pain or had any effect at all. Later in the day, during a preoperative visit by the nurse anesthetist, the nurse anesthetist asks about the patient's status and recent cardiac history and again you say nothing. If the patient suffers a massive heart attack during surgery the next morning, could liability for failure to assess, monitor, and communicate be found against you? What would you plead as your best defense in such a case?

FAILURE TO ACT AS A PATIENT ADVOCATE

As the profession develops, it has become apparent that nurses owe a higher duty to patients than merely following physician's orders. Professional nurses serve in the role of patient advocate, developing and implementing nursing diagnoses and exercising good patient judgment as they monitor the care given to patients by physicians as well as peers. The failure to function in this independent role has long been recognized by the courts as a failure to act as a patient advocate, and court decisions continue to emphasize this vital function of nursing. Review Chapter 2 for an in-depth discussion of this topic.

PATIENT EDUCATION

The issue of early discharge also addresses the crucial need for early and ongoing discharge planning and education of patients. In a home health care case, *Ready v. Personal Care Health Services* (1991), a child was discharged from home health care services, developed pneumonia, and died. The parents brought suit, in part, for the failure of the nurses to adequately address potential complications and to educate the parents about the possibility of such life-threatening conditions.

A more recent case supports the need for proper patient teaching. The court in *Wiley v. Henry Ford Cottage Hospital* (2003) concluded that nurses must first assess the patient, then teach the patient to perform the needed tasks, and finally determine how well the patient understood the patient teaching done in conjunction with the tasks to be performed. The key is that unless and until the nurse is satisfied that the patient teaching has been understood and the patient can perform the task, the nurse has not met the standard for patient teaching.

Nurses have a duty to protect patients, to question orders that are inappropriate or likely to cause harm to the patient, and to provide adequate, early discharge education. If directly speaking with the attending physician does not result in the desired outcome, then nurses have a duty to inform their supervisors and mid-management personnel so that other means of providing safe and competent health care may be obtained. Communication is vital and interventions taken on behalf of patients should be promptly and adequately charted in the patient record.

ETHICAL ISSUES IN ACUTE CARE SETTINGS

Perhaps the most obvious ethical issue concerns the right of the person to be free from restraint and allowed his or her freedom. With confused and demented patients, there are few options available except to restrain the person in the least restrictive manner possible to prevent self-harm or harm to others in the area. With the elder patient, the one sometimes confused but generally fairly aware of his or her circumstances and surroundings, physical or chemical restraints may be seen as demeaning to the person. Thus health care providers are challenged to find ways to prevent injury to the person while enhancing his or her quality of life. Though some of the more obvious measures are employed currently in health care settings, health care providers are ever challenged to discover additional means of assisting persons who might need some degree of restriction.

A second ethical issue concerns the respect due the patient with a psychiatric diagnosis when he or she presents to the health care delivery system as a possible suicide or because of self-harm. Nurses are generally the first health care providers that these patients encounter, and a recent study noted that unfavorable attitudes toward these patients may prevent seeking care and/or cause substandard care to be delivered (McCann, Clark, McConnachie, & Harvey, 2007). Though the study concluded that overall the nurses in the emergency center had sympathetic attitudes toward this population of patients, additional study is needed, as attitudes can affect care decisions and the client's request for needed health care. An earlier study (Austin, Bergum, & Goldberg, 2003) had found that mental health nurses experienced moral distress because of the inability to adequately provide quality care for mental health patients. Though that study noted that this moral distress stemmed from lack of resources, including time and numbers of staff, lack of respect was also noted as being an important factor in treating these patients. Both studies concluded that continuing professional education was needed to begin to assist staff members to better understand their distress and attitudes in relation to respect for this population of patients and their care needs.

Nurses often face ethically difficult situations when trying to find the most appropriate actions to implement in patient care settings. Differences of opinion among health care providers regarding the most appropriate course of treatment and care for patients and conflict between the nurses' value systems and those of the organization may be described as sources of ethical difficulties. Open and honest discussions between health care providers about these issues is one way to begin to address these ethical concerns, especially if the discussions are based on the ethical principles of beneficence, veracity, and respect for others.

Medication errors, particularly the nonreporting of such errors, may present ethical concerns. A recent study noted that nurses may fail to report such errors if they perceive that the error was relatively insignificant, the time taken to report the error and complete required paperwork prevents them from readily reporting the error, or fear that reports, once filed, will be used in an adverse way against them at future evaluations (Wood, 2009). But the nonreporting of such errors may also prevent adequate treatment for the patient, especially if the patient received a medication that was not ordered. Essentially, the nonreporting of such an incident may result in the health care providers scrambling to further treat the patient because they are clueless about the cause of the patient's presenting signs and symptoms.

A final ethical issue concerns standards of care and the possible injury that often results from substandard care. Patients place their trust in their health care providers, with the expectation that the care provided is the most competent and complete care available. The principle of beneficence, the duty to do good, underlies the actions of these health care providers, assuring that actions will continue to meet or exceed standards of care, whether in preventing patient falls, promoting patient safety, preventing medication errors, or ensuring that members of the health care team are informed regarding changes in a patient's condition or response to therapy.

EXERCISE 17.8

Juan Ramirez, a newly diagnosed insulin-dependent diabetic, is to receive discharge planning about his condition. You are the diabetic coordinator for the hospital and have developed a wonderful diabetic teaching protocol. Dr. Nygen, one of the "good old boys," tells you not to teach his patient anything. "He's my patient and I'll teach him what he needs to know. I do not want you interfering in my patient's care, not now or ever." How would you proceed in this instance? Does Dr. Nygen have the final say about his patients in all aspects of their care? What if Mr. Ramirez later suffers significant harm and files a lawsuit because of your failure to teach?

What are the ethical principles involved in working with this physician? With the patient? Can the nurse ethically not teach the patient about his diabetes, merely because the physician does not want the patient taught by the discharge nurse? If Mr. Ramirez should later develop complications from his lack of patient education, what ethical implications would that have for the nurse?

SUMMARY

- Ensuring patient safety remains one of the most important aspects of nurses' responsibilities, with prevention of violence one of the greatest needs.
- Prevention of suicide and self-harm in psychiatric patients often occurs because of nurses' appropriate observations and timely interventions.
- Nurses have an obligation to ensure that potential known victims targeted by patients capable of such violence are appropriately notified.
- Involuntary commitment of mental health patients is allowable only for patients who are a danger to themselves or others.
- Restrains, either physical or chemical, are allowable to prevent patient self-harm or harm to others, with the least restrictive method of restraint used.
- Medication errors may be prevented if one remembers the five rights of medication

administration: right patient, right medication, right dose, right route, and right time.
- Patient falls are among the top incidents that cause or create the potential for serious patient injury or death.
- Advances in technology and equipment have created special problems of liability for nurses.
- Nurses have accountability for adequately assessing and monitoring patients and for communicating these observations to all members of the health care delivery team.
- Nurses also have a responsibility to communicate with patients so that appropriate and timely interventions may be initiated.
- Patient advocacy and patient education are additional responsibilities of the professional nurse.
- Ethical concerns include the patient's right to be free from restraint, right of respect regardless of the medical diagnosis, and upholding standards of care.

APPLY YOUR LEGAL KNOWLEDGE

1. If a patient falls and suffers injury, is the nurse always liable? What defenses could the nurse argue in his or her own support?
2. What can nurses do to prevent medication errors? How can technology assist in improving correct medication delivery?
3. Are there areas of the hospital in which potential liability as a staff nurse is greater? What actions can staff nurses take to prevent potential lawsuits?

4. How do communications prevent lawsuits? What must be communicated and to whom?
5. Are there ever times when the nurse cannot be the patient's advocate? Give examples to support your answer.

YOU BE THE JUDGE

Judy, age 20, was admitted to an inpatient psychiatric facility for acute depression and suicidal ideation. She had gone to the local police station the previous afternoon, stating that she was suicidal. The police transported her to the emergency center, and Judy was admitted on a 24-hour emergency mental health hold.

On admission, Judy was obviously depressed and stated that she was still tormented with thoughts

about killing herself. Later that evening, the nurses heard a crash from Judy's room and, upon investigation, found her sitting on the bed with an overturned chair next to the bed. She had torn her robe, tied the pieces together as a rope, and fell from the chair as she was attempting to tie the homemade rope to the ceiling. Judy was immediately placed on a 15-minute observation protocol.

The following morning, the patient was still on observation every 15 minutes. The nurse at that point determined that Judy was more coherent and noted that Judy was disturbed by her appearance as she had not bathed in some days. The nurse unlocked the bathroom door so that Judy could shower.

Soon after the bathroom door was unlocked, Judy's psychiatrist came to speak with her. She remained with Judy for about 45 minutes, left the room, and entered a charting area that was next to the nurses' station. The nurse caring for Judy did not see the psychiatrist leave Judy's room, nor did the psychiatrist inform the nurse that Judy was now alone in her room.

The nurse checked on Judy approximately 15 minutes later. She found Judy hanging by the belt of her bathrobe from the shower rod. Judy was in full cardiac and respiratory arrest, a code was called, and Judy now has severe and permanent anoxic brain injury. Her parents have brought this lawsuit alleging breach of the standard of nursing care.

QUESTIONS

1. Was the nurse negligent for unlocking the bathroom door and allowing Judy to shower by herself?
2. Was it below the standard of care for the nurse to leave the bathroom door unlocked when the psychiatrist came to see Judy?
3. How significant are the hospital policy and procedures in this instance?
4. How would you decide this case?

REFERENCES

American Transitional Care Centers of Texas, Inc. v. Palacios, 46 S.W.3d 873 (Texas, 2001).

Angell v. State, 719 N.Y.S.2d 158 (N.Y. App., 2000)

Application of Anthony M. v. Sanchez, 645 N.Y.S.2d 23 (N.Y. App., 1996).

Austin, W., Bergum, V., & Goldberg, L. (2003). Unable to answer the call of our patients: Mental health nurses' experience of moral distress. *Nursing Inquiry,* 10(3), 177–183.

Ball v. Charter Behavioral Health, 2006 WL 2422866 (La., App., August 23, 2006).

Bartlett, E. E., & Rehmar, M. I. (1997). *The difficult patient: How to reduce your liability risk.* Rockville, MD: EBA Publications.

Bazel v. Mabee, 576 N.W.2d 385 (Iowa App., 1998).

Biggs v. United States, 655 F. Supp. 1093 (W.D. La., 1987).

Blas v. University of California, 2007 WL 2872325 (Super. Ct. Sacramento Co. Cal., August 30, 2007).

Blevins v. Hamilton Medical Center, 2007 WL 1866744 (Louisiana, June 29, 2007).

Brown v. Tift Health Care, Inc., 2006 WL 1194752 (GA. App., May 3, 2006).

Bryant v. John Doe Hospital and John Doe, M.D. (1992). *Medical Malpractice Verdicts, Settlements, and Experts,* 8(1), 35.

Bullock v. The Rapides Foundation, 2006 WL 2873217 (La. App., October 11, 2006).

Cedars Healthcare Group, Ltd. v. Freeman, 2002 WL 31466407 (Fla. App. November 6, 2002).

Christus Health v. Lanham, 2007 WL 473301 (Tex. App., February 15, 2007).

Cockerham v. LaSalle Nursing Home, Inc., 2006 WL 1155871 (La. App., May 3, 2006).

Colombini v. Westchester County Healthcare Corporation, 2005 WL 3543186 (N.Y. App., December 27, 2005).

Confidential v. Confidential, 2007a WL 2983130 (Super. Ct. Orange Co., Cal, August 10, 2007).

Confidential v. Confidential, 2007b WL 2363269 (Super. Ct. Riverside Co., Cal., July 19, 2007).

Confidential v. Confidential, 2007c WL 4208529 (Super. Ct. Los Angeles, Cal., August 29, 2007).

Confidential v. Confidential, 2008a WL 2020374 (Super. Ct. Riverside Co., Cal., January 17, 2008).

Confidential v. Confidential, 2008b WL 2020372 (Super. Ct. Los Angeles, Cal., May 1, 2008).

Cooper Clinic v. Barnes, 2006 WL 1644635 (Arkansas, June 15, 2006).

Copeland v. Northwestern Memorial Hospital, 964 F. Supp. 1225 (N.D. Ill., 1997).

Cox v. (Name Withheld-Confidential) Nursing Facility, 2007 WL 686055 (Cal. Super., January 2, 2007).

Craig v. Sina, 2007 WL 4643854 (Cir. Ct. Pinellas Co., Fla., April 12, 2007).

Cruzbinsky v. Doctors' Hospital, 188 Cal. Rptr. 685 (Cal. App., 1983).

Czarney v. Porter, 2006 WL 1360593 (Ohio App., May 18, 2006).

Danesh, V. C., Malvey, D., & Fottler, M. D. (2008). Hidden workplace violence: What your nurses may not be telling you. *The Health Care Manager, 27*(4), 357–363.

DeJesus v. United States Department of Veterans Affairs, 2007 WL 454726 (3rd Cir., March 14, 2007).

Demers v. United States. (1990). *Medical Malpractice: Verdicts, Settlements, and Experts, 6*(3), 34.

Department of Mental Health v. Hall, 2006 WL 2437830 (Miss., August 24, 2006).

De Stasio v. Kocsis, 2007 WL 1542607 (N. J. App., May 30, 2007).

Dutton v. Scott and White Memorial Hospital, 2007 WL 866411 (Tex. Dist., February 28, 2007).

Eden Park Management, Inc. v. Schrull, 2007 706583 (Conn. Super., February 14, 2007).

Espinosa v. Baptist Health System, 2006 WL 2871262 (Tex. App., October 11, 2006).

Estate of Gehrich v. St. Frances Hospital, 2008 WL 1051810 (Super. Ct. Marion Co, Ind., February 4, 2008).

Estate of Hollan v. Brookwood Medical Center, 2007 WL 912202 (Ala. Cir. Ct., February 15, 2007).

Estate of Seenandan v. Dependable Ambulette Service, 2007 WL 1287730 (Super. Ct. Queens Co., N.Y., February 2, 2007).

Evans v. Benson, 2007 WL 1299261 (Iowa, May 4, 2007).

Farrow v. Health Services et al., 604 P.2d 474 (Utah, 1979).

Fiqueredo v. St. Alphonsus Regional Medical Center, 2007 WL 2749158 (Dist. Ct., Ada Co., Idaho, July 16, 2007).

Frias v. King, 2008 WL 1959944 (Super. Ct. Queens Co., N.Y., March 6, 2008).

Gabaldoni v. Board of Physician Quality Assurance, 785 A.2d 771 (Md. App., 2001).

Groves v. State, 2007 WL 4898281 (Cir. Ct., Dane Co., Wisc., July 1, 2007).

Hall v. Arthur, 141 F.3d 844 (8th Cir., 1998).

Hanson v. Hospital of Saint Raphael, 2007 WL 2317825 (Conn. Super., July 20, 2007).

Harris v. Sumpter Regional Hospital, 2008 WL 1808397 (Super. Ct. Dougherty Co., Georgia, March 10, 2008).

Heater v. Southwood Psychiatric Center, 49 Cal. Rptr.2d 880 (Cal. App., 1996).

Herron v. Northwest Community Hospital. (1992). *Malpractice Verdicts, Settlements, and Experts, 8*(10), 33.

Hill v. Sacred Heart Medical Center, 2008 WL 500055 (Wash. App., February 26, 2008).

Hofflander v. St. Catherine's Hospital, 635 N.W.2d 13 (Wis. App., 2001); confirmed 2001 WL 21499928 (Wisconsin, July 1, 2001).

Hogan v. Washington Nursing Facility, 2007 WL 922250 (D. C., March 29, 2007).

Hooper v. County of Cook, 2006 WL 1319458 (Ill. App., May 15, 2006).

Hughes v. Boyd, 2008 WL 1733644 (Dist. Ct., Dallas Co., Tex., January 9, 2008).

In re Adam S., 729 N.Y.S.2d 734 (N.Y. App., 2001).

In re Baptist Hospitals of Southeast Texas, 2006 WL 2506412 (Tex. App., August 31, 2006).

In re Dorothy W., 692 N.E.2d 388 (Ill. App., 1998).

In re J. S., 621 N.W.2d 582 (North Dakota, 2001).

In re Mental Health of S.C., 15 P.3d 861 (Montana, 2000).

In re S. B., 763 A.2d 930 (Pa. Super., 2000).

In re Turnbough, 34 S.W.3d 225 (Mo. App., 2000).

In the Interest of "J. P.," 574 N.W.2d 340 (Iowa, 1998).

Institute of Medicine of the National Academies. (2000). *To err is human: Building a safer health system.* Washington, DC: Author.

Involuntary psychiatric commitment: Court reviews legal criteria for holding patient. (1998). *Legal Eagle Eye Newsletter for the Nursing Profession, 6*(5), 4.

Jensen v. Longwood Management Corporation, 2007 WL 1765191 (Super. Ct. Orange Co., Cal., March 12, 2007).

Joint Commission for the Accreditation of Healthcare Organizations. (2003). *Hospital accreditation standards.* Oakbrook Terrace, IL: Author.

John Doe v. Confidential Hospital, 2007 WL 4788549 (Super. Ct., Riverside Co., Cal., December 7, 2007).

Johnson v. Methodist Hospital of Dallas, 2007 WL 143888547 (Dist. Ct. Dallas Co., Tex., March 16, 2007).

Kinchen v. Gateway Community Service Board, 2006 WL 3803014 (11th Cir., December 28, 2006).

Kunz v. Little County of Mary Hospital, 2007 WL 1309558 (Ill. App., May 4, 2007).

Lake Cumberland v. Dishman, 2007 WL 1229432 (Ky. App., April 6, 2007).

Lakos v. Kaiser Permanente, 2008 WL 382331 (Medical Malpractice Arbitration, Los Angeles, Cal., February 5, 2008).

Lance v. Moores, 2007 WL 1977077 (Super. Ct. Albany Co., N.Y., May 29, 2007).

Lawson v. United States, 2006 WL 2819833 (D. Md., October 2, 2006).

Lewandowski v. Mercy Memorial Hospital Corporation, 2003 WL 22850024 (Mich. App., December 2, 2003).

Lopez v. Southwest Community Health Service, 833 P.2d 1183 (New Mexico, 1992).

Mandell, M. (1993). What you don't say can hurt you. *American Journal of Nursing, 93*(8), 15–16.

Maris, R. W., Berman, A. L., & Silverman, M. M. (2000). *Comprehensive textbook of suicidology.* New York: The Guilford Press.

Marvel v. County of Erie, 2003 N.Y. Slip Op. 15822, 2003 WL 21513056 (N.Y. App., July 3, 2003).

McAllen Hospital v. Muniz, 2007 WL 4340867 (Tex. App., December 13, 2007).

McCann, T. V., Clark, E., McConnachie, S. M., & Harvey, I. (2007). Deliberate self-harm: Emergency department nurses' attitudes, triage, and care intentions. *Journal of Clinical Nursing, 16*, 1704–1711.

McKenna Memorial Hospital v. Quinney, 2006 WL 3246524 (Tex. App., November 10, 2006).

McLaughlin v. Firelands Community Hospital, 2006 WL 1047499 (Ohio App., April 21, 2006).

Michael v. Medical Staffing Network, Inc., 2007 WL (57604 (Fla. App., January 10, 2007).

Moc v. Children's Hospital, 2007 WL 4624414 (Super. Ct. Los Angeles, Cal., March 23, 2007).

Moeltner v. Rubio, 2007 WL 224684 (Super. Co. Essex Co., N.J., March 6, 2007).

Morrison v. Mann, 2007 WL 656578 (N.D. Ga., February 27, 2007).

Morton v. Brookhaven Memorial Hospital, 2007 WL 2850371 (Super. Ct. Suffolk Co., N.Y., January 31, 2007).

Nevarez v. New York City Health and Hospitals Corporation, 663 N.Y.S.2d 190 (N.Y. App., 1997).

O'Donnell v. Holy Family Hospital, 682 N.E.2d 386 (Ill. App., 1997).

Ohlen v. Piskacek, 717 N.Y.S.2d 221 (N.Y. App., 2000).

Page v. Daybreak Venture, 2007 WL 18398324 (Dist. Ct. Dallas Co., Tex., April 3, 2007).

Parker v. Bullock County Hospital Authority, A9OAO 762 (1990).

Paullin v. Oconomowoc Memorial Hospital, 2007 WL 2728281 (Wisc. App., September 20, 2007).

Pedraza v. Wyckoff Heights Medical Center, 2002 N.Y. Slip Op. 22094, 2002 WL 1364153 (N.Y. Sup., June 4, 2002).

People v. Gutierrez, 2006 WL 2875504 (Cal. App., October 11, 2006).

People v. Simon, 2007 WL 1966120 (Cal. App., July 9, 2007).

Perby v. East Rockaway Progressive Care, 2008 WL 612034 (Super. Ct. Queens Co., N.Y., February 22, 2008).

Rademacher v. Katuna, 2007 WL 4925066 (Dist. Ct. Boulder Co., Colo., May 24, 2007).

Ready v. Personal Care Health Services, #842472 (California, 1991).

Reid v. Altieri, 2007 WL 750596 (Fla. App., March 14, 2007).

Reinhardt v. Sunrise, 2008 WL 611997 (Super. Ct. Kings Co., N.Y., January 29, 2008).

Renz v. Northside Hospital, 2007 WL 1732805 (Ga. App., June 18, 2007).

Riley v. West Paces Ferry Hospital, Inc., 916 F.2d 608 (Georgia, 1990).

Rodriquez v. Palm Springs General Hospital, 2007 WL 4247300 (Cir. Ct. Dade Co., Fla., November 21, 2007).

Romaro v. Marks, 647 N.Y.S.2d 272 (N.Y. September 25, 1996).

Rose v. Hakim, 335 F. Supp. 1121 (D.C.C. 1971).

Safe Medical Devices Act of 1990, Public Law 101-629, 21 *United States Code*, Section 306i et seq, (November 28, 1990).

Safe Medical Devices Amended Act of 1992, 21 *United States Code*, section 201 et. seq. (1992).

Salcido v. Woodbury County, 119 F. Supp.2d 900 (N.D. Iowa, 2000).

Schroeder v. Northwest Community Hospital, 2006 WL 3615559 (Ill. App., December 12, 2006).

Sheliga v. Cumberland River Comprehensive Care, 2007 WL 4632231 (Cir. Ct. Laurel Co. Ken., October 18, 2007).

Simon v. Sierra Madre Skilled Nursing, 2007 WL 685830 (Cal. Super., February 9, 2007).

Sobti v. Prince William Hospital, 2008 WL 942629 (Cir. Ct. Prince William Co., Va., January 16, 2008).

Soderman v. Smith, 2007 WL 2389564 (Super. Ct. Sacramento Co. Cal., July 13, 2007).

Spohn Hospital v. Mayer, 46 Tex. Sup. Ct. J. 604, 2003 WL 1923002 (Texas, 2003).

S. P. v. City of Takoma Park, 134 F.3d 260 (4th Cir., 1998).

State v. Nguyen, 43 P.3d 1218 (Or. App., 2002).

Stewart v. North Coast Center, 2006 WL 1313098 (Ohio App., May 12, 2006).

Sturgill v. Ashe Memorial Hospital, 2007 WL 3254411 (N.C. App., November 6, 2007).

Tarasoff v. The Regents of the University of California, 554 P.2d 347 (California, 1976).

Tarzian, A. J., & Marco, C. A. (2008). Responding to abusive patients: A primer for ethics committee members. *HEC Forum, 20*(2), 127–136.

Thomas v. Greenview Hospital, Inc., 2004 WL 221198 (Ky. App., February 6, 2004).

Troxel v. A. I. Dupont Institute, 675 A.2d 314 (Pa. Super., 1996).

United States Census Bureau. (2002). *Title 1: Language use, English ability, and linguistic isolation for the population 5 years and over by state: 2000.* Washington, DC: Author.

Umbarber v. Hayes Green Beach Memorial Hospital, 2007 WL 624996 (Mich. App., March 1, 2007).

Unnamed Patient v. Unnamed Private Psychiatric Hospital, 2007 WL 1765189 (Sup. Ct. Los Angeles Co. Cal., May 30, 2007).

Vela v. Bay Area Healthcare Group, 2007 WL 1412614 (Dist. Ct. Nueces Co., Tex., April 2, 2007).

Villarreal v. Rio Grande Regional Hospital, 2008 WL 859667 (Dist. Ct. Hidalgo Co., Tex., March 5, 2008).

Waters v. Andalusia Regional Hospital, 2007 WL 4983148 (Cir. Ct. Covington Co., Ala., October 29, 2007.).

Weeks v. Byrd Medical Clinic, Inc., 2006 WL 862966 (La. App., April 5, 2006).

Weeks v. Eastern Idaho Health Services, 2007 WL 600830 (Idaho, February 28, 2007).

Wert v. (Name Withheld-Confidential) Hospital, 2007 WL 901630 (Cal. Super., February 9, 2007).

Wilcox v. Gamble Guest Care Corporation, 2006 WL 932027 (La. App., April 12, 2006).

Wiley v. Henry Ford Cottage Hospital, 2003 WL 21568688 (Mich. App., July 10, 2003).

Wood, D. (2009). Nurses hesitate to report errors. *AMN Healthcare.* Available online at http://www.nursezone.com/Nursing-News-Events/more-news.aspx?ID=18857

World Health Organization, Department of Mental Health and Substance Abuse. (2006). *Preventing suicide: A resource for counselors.* Geneva, Switzerland: Author.

CHAPTER 18

Nursing in Ambulatory and Managed Care Settings

PREVIEW

The health care delivery trend toward more careful management of scarce health care resources has placed new emphasis on primary prevention and has led to increased opportunities for professionals in traditional ambulatory care settings. These ambulatory settings include traditional clinics, freestanding surgicenters, nurse-managed and nurse-run clinics, and telenursing, among other innovative settings for advanced quality health care. Additionally, the continued growth of managed care as a system for health care financing and delivery creates nursing challenges and opportunities. The restructuring of the health care system has resulted in many cost-containment measures, including the silent replacement of the registered nurse (RN) with unlicensed assistive personnel and other ancillary personnel. Within many managed care organizations, nurses have identified opportunities to achieve original managed care goals, ensuring safe, quality health care for patients. They have also learned to avoid many of the potential legal challenges in managed care. This chapter explores legal issues involved in both settings, considerations for nurses who donate their services, either through disaster nursing or volunteer services, and the potential legal aspects of nursing in managed care organizations.

LEARNING OUTCOMES
After completing this chapter, you should be able to

18.1 Describe the area of ambulatory nursing, including its emergence, the role of risk management, and the focus on patient education in ambulatory nursing.

18.2 Discuss the field of telehealth and telenursing, including potential for growth as well as legal issues involved in delivery of health care via telehealth.

18.3 Analyze the nurse's role in caring for victims of violence.

18.4 Describe the nurse's legal liabilities when volunteering nursing services, including donating health-related advice to consumers.

18.5 Define managed care, including health maintenance organizations, preferred provider organizations, point-of-service plans, and indemnity plans.

18.6 Describe four types of health maintenance organizations.

18.7 Discuss the Employment Retirement Income Security Act and its application in managed care settings.

18.8 Discuss the Emergency Medical Treatment and Labor Act and its application in managed care.

18.9 Define antitrust laws and explain their importance to registered nurses in all practice settings.

18.10 Enumerate patient rights that arise as part of managed care.

18.11 Describe some of the ethical concerns that arise in ambulatory and managed care nursing.

KEY TERMS

ambulatory care nursing
antitrust laws
disaster nursing
donating health-related
    advice
Emergency Medical
    Treatment and Labor Act
    (EMTALA)
Employment Retirement
    Income Security Act of
    1974 (ERISA)

end-of-year profit sharing
gag rules
health maintenance
    organizations (HMOs)
indemnity (fee-for-service
    [FFE]) plans
managed care
National Committee for
    Quality Assurance
    (NCQA)
patient rights

point-of-service (POS) plans
preferred provider
    organization (PPO)
telehealth
telemedicine
telenursing
utilization review
verbal abuse or workplace
    bullying
violence in the workplace
volunteer services

AMBULATORY CARE NURSING

Ambulatory care nursing describes nursing care that is delivered in practice settings outside the traditional acute care and long-term care settings, including physicians' offices, nurse-based practices, wellness programs, freestanding clinics, and health maintenance organizations, evolving into a specialty whose practice setting emphasizes health promotion and disease prevention and nursing care with extensive patient and family involvement (Norwicki & Haas, 2003). The growth of ambulatory nursing practice sites is even more apparent since the onset of managed care has resulted in increasingly greater needs for outpatient care services. As more clients are cared for in ambulatory settings, the role of professional nurses, skilled in the role necessary for this practice arena, continues to expand.

The American Academy of Ambulatory Care Nursing (AAACN) and the American Nurses Association (ANA) have jointly defined professional ambulatory care nursing as:

those clinical, management, educational, and research activities provided by registered nurses for and with individuals who seek care for health-related problems or concerns or seek assistance with health maintenance and/or health promotion. These individuals engage predominately in self-care and self-managed health activities and receive care from family and significant others outside an institutional setting. (Norwicki & Haas, 2003, p. 14)

The AAACN (2004) notes that its mission is to advance and influence the art and science of ambulatory care nursing through excellence in health care delivery, collaborative leadership, partnerships and alliances among providers and other health care organizations, proactive innovation and risk taking, customer-focused services, and continued advancement of the profession.

A case that illustrates the need for partnerships and alliances among providers and health care organizations is *McGill v. Newark Surgery Center* (2001). A surgery center opened in a geographic area that was served by a full-service acute care hospital that also had an outpatient surgical center and housed the only blood bank in the community. A highly competitive climate arose between the top-level executives at both facilities, and the acute care facility refused to enter into an agreement to supply blood to the outpatient facility.

A patient at the outpatient facility was scheduled for a laporoscopic tubal ligation. During the operation, the patient developed serious bleeding and the surgeon requested four units of O-negative blood from the acute care hospital's blood bank. The supervisor at the blood bank refused to release the blood, as she stated she was under strict orders not to supply blood to the outpatient center under any circumstance. After approximately 2 hours and multiple phone calls, the supervisor released two units of blood to the outpatient center. The blood was immediately transfused, but the patient died in transport to the acute care facility. Her family sued both facilities.

The court, in noting that this was the first case in this area of the law, disregarded the long-held legal rule that a hospital's duty of care extends only to the hospital's patients. In emergencies, said the court, hospitals must take reasonable steps to aid a nonpatient. Specifically, a community blood bank cannot refuse to supply blood to a patient in need merely because the person is not a patient of the blood bank's parent facility.

Aspects of the ambulatory care nurses' roles, such as adherence to standards of care, risk management principles, and the duty to assess, notify, and communicate, are as important in ambulatory care nursing as these aspects are in the acute care nurse's role. Patient education, important in all health care settings, takes on additional importance in the ambulatory and managed care nursing roles.

Patient Education

While important in all health care settings, the emphasis on prevention of disease and the promotion of health stresses the need for patient education in all ambulatory settings. This is particularly true as most patients continue to seek care at ambulatory settings over long periods of time and are involved with a variety of interdisciplinary health care members. The major emphasis thus is on quality patient education and patient compliance with the prescribed course of therapy. Included in the concept of patient education is the entire issue of discharge planning.

To be effective educators, nurses must remain current in their knowledge of disease processes, therapies and medications to manage these processes, complications that could occur during the course of treatment, and innovative educational models. It is not sufficient, though, that nurses are knowledgeable about the latest medical treatments or interactions of medications. Nurses must be effective educators, blending teaching styles to fit learner needs and objectives, incorporating educational models into their presentations and discussions, and using culturally competent models with a diversity of clients and family members. Staff in-service education programs in the ambulatory setting should include programs on educational models, learning styles and preferences, assessment of cultural components of learning, assessment of learner readiness, and evaluation of learner objectives. Merely understanding the medical concepts and newer technologies does not make one an effective teacher. The teacher role also requires intense study, adaptation, and motivation to continuous master teaching strategies and content.

DISTANCE DELIVERY OF HEALTH CARE

Telehealth is the use of telecommunications technologies for the provision of long-distance clinical health care, patient and professional education, and health administration. Because telehealth services are widely varied, constantly changing, and technologically complex, the concept is difficult to grasp without some basic definitions.

Telecommunications encompasses the transmission of information from one site to another, using a variety of equipment to transmit information in the form of signals, signs, words, or pictures by cable, radio, telephone systems, cable television programming, facsimile transmissions, satellite paging systems, and electronic mail. *Telehealth* is the use of telecommunications equipment and communications networks for transferring medical health information between participants at different locations. Telehealth can be found in nearly every area of health care, from emergency medical response systems to hospitals and home care. It can be used for direct patient care, patient and health practitioner education, and health services administration. Equipment used in telehealth includes computers, telephones, monitors, and telecommunications networks connecting two or more sites.

Telehealth systems permit the provision of care in situations in which a face-to-face meeting between health care provider and patient is not possible or would be accomplished only with great difficulty and at great cost. **Telenursing,** a subset of telehealth, refers to the use of telecommunications and information technology for providing nursing services in health care whenever a large physical distance exists between the patient and the nurse or between nurses. Telenursing thus allows a nurse to deliver care through a telecommunications system. Most nurses already use simple forms of telenursing by telephoning a patient status report to another nurse or by making a phone call to an ambulatory surgical patient to assess discharge status. Other examples of telenursing include home health visits via telecommunications for monitoring and educating patients.

Telemedicine, another subset of telehealth, allows medical clinicians to provide care via telecommunications. Many telemedicine subspecialties are already recognized, including teleradiology, telepathology, and teleoncology. *Telepresence* combines robotics and virtual reality to allow a surgeon equipped with special gloves and proper video and audio equipment to manipulate surgical instruments at remote sites. Research in telepresence is vital to both military and civilian health centers, especially for the care of individuals in remote areas of the world.

Video *teleconferencing* transmits sounds and images between two or more sites, allowing participants to interact. Health care providers at various sites can discuss a patient's status, a health care provider at a remote site can consult with a patient and family members, and educators at multiple sites can discuss new innovations and interventions as well as provide pertinent and continuous patient education.

The concept of telehealth is not new; it dates back to the 1950s when closed circuit audio and video transmission at larger medical conventions allowed participants in several rooms to simultaneously participate in a presentation. By 1965, surgery to replace a defective aortic valve was performed in Texas and transmitted via the Communications Satellite Corporation's "Early Bird" satellite to the Geneva University Medical School in Switzerland.

Since the early 1990s, there has been renewed interest in telehealth for two primary reasons. First, the quality of computers and telecommunications technology has greatly improved. Second, problems that have persistently plagued the health care delivery system in the country—such as inadequate access to health care, uneven distribution of health care providers in large, metropolitan areas as opposed to smaller, rural communities, quality management, and escalating costs—can be alleviated through the effective use of telehealth, telemedicine, and telenursing.

Today, a variety of innovative uses of telehealth continue to facilitate consultations among professionals, diagnosis and assessment of disease states, interviews with patients, patient histories, and prescriptions of medications and therapies. Some of the innovative uses include:

1. Mobile telehealth applications ensure that patients' real-time vital signs and data and video images of patients are transmitted during ambulance travel.
2. Educational and emotional support programs for families with high-risk newborns are being done through a hospital monitoring system that allows parents to watch their babies' care from home on a television monitor and receive guidance from hospital staff after discharge.
3. Systems for monitoring child abuse establish an around-the-clock monitoring system between the hospital emergency center and child protective team clinicians.

Legal issues with telehealth and telenursing are varied and have the potential to escalate as the entire field continues to expand. Security and confidentiality issues abound because telehealth allows the transmission of patient information electronically. The federal government, recognizing the potential for lack of privacy in transmitted telecommunications, charged the Computer Sciences and Telecommunications Board (CSTB) with studying the privacy and security of electronic health data. The CSTB, which was established in 1986 to provide independent advice to the federal government in technical and public policy issues related to computing and communications, has declared that the protection of patient data requires both organizational and technical measures. The CSTB continues to work on more effective means of ensuring the confidentiality of transmitted patient data. The issue of patient confidentiality with telecommunications is also a part of the Health Insurance Portability and Accountability Act of 1996 (HIPAA). Review Chapter 9 for a discussion of this content.

A second issue with telenursing is licensure, either within single states or with a single license that allows nurses to be licensed in one jurisdiction and practice in several jurisdictions. A major impetus for multistate licensure was the implementation of telenursing, since nurses are in one location and the patients they treat, counsel, and/or educate may be located in any of the 50 states or U.S. territories. Review Chapter 11 for additional information regarding multistate licensure.

A third legal issue involves practice standards, especially as nurses from multiple states are involved in patient care through telenursing. Among the basic concepts included in these practice standards are quality, scope of practice issues, patient safety issues, documentation, and the need for further research in this area of nursing practice.

To date, case law involving telenursing has centered on consultation and information given by nurses to patients who telephone requesting health care advice. For example, in *McCrystal v. Trumbull Memorial Hospital* (1996), the nurse who took the patient's phone call and her nursing supervisor both failed to assess the patient's situation correctly and failed to give the patient appropriate health care advice. The patient was pregnant with her fourth child. She had carried three other pregnancies to full term, but each of them had been delivered by cesarean section. She came to the emergency room believing she was in labor but was reassured that she was not. Six days later, she came back in the morning to the same hospital emergency room believing that she was in labor and again was sent home. She returned that same afternoon, was examined, and was again reassured that she was not in labor.

When the patient returned home, she began to experience vaginal bleeding. She phoned the women's care clinic at another hospital and spoke with the nurse. The nurse, before giving any specific advice, spoke with her nursing supervisor. The nurse and her supervisor both agreed that it was not necessary for the woman to return to the emergency room. They both assured her that she should stay home and wait for the bleeding to stop.

The woman then telephoned her physician and received the same advice from him. Later that day, the woman went to the emergency center anyway. During the cesarean delivery of the child, it was discovered that her uterus had ruptured along the old incision line from a previous cesarean operation. The fetus had already experienced serious brain damage from lack of oxygen.

The court held that both nurses were negligent for failing to make a correct assessment. They believed that the bleeding was some minor spotting from the previous vaginal examination and failed to listen to her description of her complaints or explore the full history of the situation. The physician was also negligent, said the court. A similar conclusion was reached in *Starkey v. St. Rita's Medical Center* (1997), when the nurse correctly assessed that the patient was having a myocardial infarction, but failed to advise the patient and his wife of the gravity of a myocardial infarction and said he could wait until later to seek treatment.

In *Havard v. Children's Clinic of Southwestern Louisiana, Inc.* (1998), a 13-year-old's grandmother withheld the girl's morning insulin injection because the granddaughter was sick, had stayed home from school, and was vomiting. As a child, the 13-year-old had once become hypoglycemic after getting insulin while nauseated and vomiting. The grandmother called the clinic and asked to speak with the child's physician, but he was unavailable. The grandmother told the nurse the girl was diabetic and had not had her morning insulin. She asked for a prescription for Phenergan suppositories to stop the vomiting.

The nurse said she would check the chart and see if she could send the suppositories. The nurse had the suppositories delivered, apparently without checking the chart or consulting the physician. The girl was taken to the emergency room that night and died in the intensive care unit early the following morning from diabetic ketoacidosis. The family sued the clinic and was awarded an $183,000 verdict, which was reduced by 20% for the grandmother's negligence in withholding the morning insulin and ignoring two elevated blood sugar levels later in the afternoon.

The Court of Appeals upheld the jury's verdict, awarding an additional $10,000. The court ruled that the nurse was negligent in her assessment of the child and her treatment of the child's condition.

An additional area of concern with telenursing concerns the individual who dispenses the health care advice. Nursing organizations, primarily the National Council of State Boards of Nursing and the American Nurses Association, have articulately debated licensure issues for the individuals dispensing health care advice and patient education. In *Snider v. Basilio* (2005), a case that involved a 6-month-old infant with a high fever and repeated episodes of vomiting, the individual dispensing health care advice had graduated from a foreign nursing school and had three times failed the NCLEX examination. She told the mother to mix a soft drink, such as Sprite or 7-Up, with Pedialyte and feed the child bananas, rice, applesauce, and toast. When the parents took the infant to the hospital 2 days later, it was discovered that he had bacterial meningitis. The Georgia court held that, among other areas of negligence in this particular case, it was negligent to allow a nonlicensed person to dispense medical advice over a telephone.

GUIDELINES

Telenursing

1. Because privacy and confidentiality are to be afforded all patients, previously established confidentiality and privacy protections for health information must be used with telenursing and reviewed often to ensure that these protections are adequate and used by all personnel. Review HIPAA laws in this regard; request that the agency conduct nursing education classes in this area of the law.

2. Obtain informed consent from all patients before using telenursing, including expanded information about risks and benefits that are unique to telecommunications. Risks include images that may not be as clear as what one would be able to detect were the patient in a more traditional health care setting, and the limitations on some of the finer aspects of physical assessment, such as the use of smell and touch. Benefits include availability of services to patients in distant and hard-to-reach places as well as not having to travel far distances to receive quality health care.

3. Remember to ask patients and secure their written approval before information concerning them is shared with others, such as by telecommunicating data and images of the patient to other health care providers. Patients should also be informed if others outside the health care team will be involved in the telecommunications, such as observers and technical staff.

4. Telenursing should augment health care delivery, not be a substitute for established, competent nursing care. Standards of care must be maintained at all times.

5. Adhere to agency policies and protocols regarding telenursing, especially in the use of telephone triage or counseling via telecommunications. Remember, too, that assessment of patients via telephone is dependent on information as relayed by family members and patients. If you are uncertain about the patient's symptoms or have any doubts that the patient should be seen, err on the side of caution and advise the patient or family member to call 911 or go to an emergency center immediately.

6. Document all data used to decide on the care recommended, as well as care or education given to patients.

EXERCISE 18.1

Mr. Johnson, age 42, began experiencing symptoms "including feeling agitated and upset, nausea, and an urgent need, but inability, to vomit," during the early evening hours. According to the terms of his health care policy, he was required to contact the company at a specific phone number and consult with the nurse prior to seeking medical attention. Mrs. Johnson testified that at approximately 11 P.M. she contacted the advisory nurse on her husband's behalf and informed the nurse of his symptoms and the history of heart trouble in his family. Mrs. Johnson told the nurse she wanted to be sure her husband was not having a heart attack. The nurse told Mrs. Johnson that the symptoms were probably due to excess stomach acid and that he would be fine. Mrs. Johnson again telephoned at 11:30 P.M. She informed the nurse that the symptoms were intensifying and that her husband was experiencing pain in the middle of his chest.

The nurse instructed the patient to sit at a 40-degree angle, drink some milk, which would allow the stomach acids to recede, and to call back in the morning. When his symptoms failed to lessen,

Mrs. Johnson drove her husband to the local emergency department. He became unresponsive during the drive, and cardiopulmonary resuscitation performed at the hospital was unsuccessful. The cause of death, according to the medical examiner, was an acute myocardial infarction.

Did the nurse violate the standard of care due this patient? What would you have done in such a case? How does this type of scenario illustrate the types of potential liability incurred in telenursing? What ethical issues are involved in such a scenario? Do these ethical concerns influence what you would have done if you were the nurse involved in this patient's care?

VIOLENCE

Because of the prevalence of physical and psychological violence in society, nurses frequently care for the victims, perpetrators, and witnesses of physical and psychological violence. Additionally, nurses are also at risk for experiencing **violence in the workplace.** Such workplace violence greatly affects the ability of nurses to be productive members of their facility; sick leave, absenteeism, and general nonproductivity increase the costs to businesses when workers are hurt by violence in the workplace. A recent federal agency noted that approximately 1.7 million workers are victimized annually in the United States, with more than 800 deaths attributable to workplace violence (Bureau of Labor Statistics, 2006). Many of these assaults occur in service settings such as hospitals, nursing homes, and social service agencies. **Verbal abuse or workplace bullying,** defined as the deliberate repeated, hurtful mistreatment of a person by a cruel perpetrator, was encountered by approximately one in five workers in 2002, involving supervisory personnel, co-workers, patients, and/or patients' family members (Bureau of Labor Statistics, 2006).

No one knows the full extent of the problem, because many employers do not maintain such files and may actively discourage staff from reporting incidents. Similarly, many cases of violence and abuse outside formal health care settings are also not reported, because the victims fear greater violence if they come forward, and because of shame and guilt.

Nursing organizations are now beginning to recognize all types of violence, especially domestic violence, as a major public health threat, one with high incidence and prevalence that requires significant health care interventions. The reduction of violence is targeted as one of the major goals of the U.S. National Health Plan in *Healthy People 2010.* (U. S. Department of Health and Human Services, 2000) Often, domestic violence is noted first by nurses in ambulatory settings.

Domestic violence affects a significant proportion of the U.S. population, either as direct victims or as witnesses of abuse directed toward spouses or partners, children, and elders. In addition to immediate physical, emotional, and psychological injury, the sequelae of such abuse are often serious and lifelong. Long-term effects include permanent disabilities, sexually transmitted diseases, and complications of pregnancy and birth, including low-birth-weight babies. Mental health effects include depression, post-traumatic stress disorder, alcohol and drug abuse, and suicide. Health-related costs of domestic violence exceeded $5.8 billion in 2007, with $4.1 billion directly related to cost for medical and mental health care (American Institute on Domestic Violence, 2008).

To begin to address this issue, the American Association of Colleges of Nursing (AACN) (2005) recommends that nursing educational programs at the undergraduate and graduate level address this important health care need. Curriculum content spans understanding the scope of the issue, needed assessment skills, possible interventions, cultural issues to be considered, and public educational needs.

To meet the legal and ethical issues involved in domestic violence, nurses must be aware of state and national legal mandates regarding domestic violence, including mandatory reporting laws. Such mandatory laws include reporting of child abuse and elder abuse in all states. Nurses must also become more cognizant about the appropriate methods for collection and documentation of data so that both the patient and the provider are equally protected. The field of forensic nursing is a testament to the importance of this collection and documentation of data. Nurses must respect confidentiality issues and the individual's right to remain silent. Unfortunately, the abused adult woman or man is not protected as are children and the elderly, presumably because they can "speak for themselves." Thus, they are not considered vulnerable under the law.

Nurses are also becoming better informed about how to approach the issue of abuse with potential victims, asking questions in a way that promotes honest answers rather than mere silence. Nurses, especially those in ambulatory care settings, are also becoming more comfortable addressing the issues, rather than avoiding the hard questions as was so often done in the past. Educational offerings are increasingly becoming available to all nurses about addressing potential victims of violence. As assessment tools are refined, it is hoped that all nurses, in all clinical settings, will address this critical issue.

Finally, patient education concerning victims' rights, possible safe harbors, and better career opportunities for adult victims is slowly beginning to make changes in the lives of these individuals. As nurses become better educated about violence and more comfortable speaking with potential victims about violence, the educational opportunities for these victims are also increasing.

GUIDELINES

Nursing Victims of Violence

1. Understand the immense prevalence of violence in the United States today, especially the silence of its victims. Merely because victims do not report attacks of violence does not mean they are not occurring.
2. Enroll in formal and informal courses to better understand the vast impact of violence in the community. An alternative approach to taking such courses is to review the numerous articles, many with continuing education credit, that are now appearing in many of the nursing journals. Learn as much as you can about the issue and how to assess patients for incidents of violence.
3. When you work with patients from other countries and cultures, remember that assessment techniques must be reflective of cultural norms and practices (American Nurses Association, 1998).
4. Include questions about the possibility of violence in all assessments of patients, even if they do not appear to be victims of violence. Remember, psychological violence leaves no physical scars, and patients may be able to hide their emotional scars during the short time of assessment. Additionally, the more you include such gentle questions in assessment, the more comfortable you will be with them and the less likely you will be to fail to assess the incidence of violence.
5. Learn all you can about community resources for the victims of violence so that you can fully assist patients when they ask for help. You can also include such community resources in your discussions with patients who request no assistance, so that they will know their options should they need them.
6. Educate all patients about the subtleties of violence, as many patients do not know that violent behavior affects much more than merely physical behaviors. Help individuals to

understand how they can help better their situation, including formal educational opportunities, programs to enhance self-image and self-worth, support groups for victims of violence, and preparing in advance an escape plan, as applicable.

EXERCISE 18.2

Research the statistics concerning domestic violence in your geographic area. How do these statistics differ from the national statistics? How are local health agencies attempting to reduce such incidents of violence? How can you affect the staggering statistics in your everyday clinical practice?

VOLUNTEER SERVICES

Many health care providers routinely provide **volunteer services,** usually as a vital part of community services. Volunteer status may also arise when one agrees to care for a sick neighbor or a family member. Examples of volunteer services generally encompass the nursing skills one uses when helping to conduct a hypertension screening program or presenting a lecture on juvenile diabetes for the local parent-teacher association.

Keep several points in mind about volunteer status:

1. The legal statutes are not well defined because donated services do not fall within the auspices of the state nurse practice act. Most nurse practice acts apply only to compensated services, so the strict rules and regulations generated by the state board of nurse examiners do not apply to donated services.
2. Responsibilities and professional actions are not lessened when donating professional services. The nurse is still a professional and is responsible for ensuring that at least a standard of care is delivered to patients or clients.
3. The fact that services are donated does not exempt the nurse from a possible lawsuit or from the standard of the reasonably prudent nurse. The state nurse practice act still guides one's professional responsibilities.
4. The state board of nursing may subject the nurse to disciplinary action should the care delivered fall below minimum standards. This is true even if no civil suit is filed against the nurse in conjunction with legal action that a board of nursing may take in response to the filing of an official complaint naming the nurse.
5. The nurse–patient relationship is initiated when care is first given to the patient. Once established, the duty of care owed this patient is equal to the duty owed patients in formal health care settings (*Lunsford v. Board of Nurse Examiners,* 1983).

To protect oneself legally, follow this basic advice:

1. Never administer any treatment or medication without first obtaining a doctor's order or, in the majority of jurisdictions, without a valid standing order. This is true even if the medication is an over-the-counter drug. Professional nurses are responsible for knowing indications, mechanisms of action, contraindications, dosages, adverse reactions, and drug interactions for all medications they give to patients.
2. Reread carefully one's professional liability insurance policy. Does it cover gratuitous services? Depending on the type of services volunteered (e.g., to a large group as opposed to volunteering

to care for a sick relative) and the number of lawsuits filed against nurses in the given geographic area, the nurse may want to increase the dollar amount of the policy. Nurses might also want to increase the coverage limits if they frequently volunteer professional services and/or if they come in contact with large numbers of persons as they donate their services.

3. A system of record keeping should be initiated and accurate records maintained. Even though there is no formal chart, the records may prove to be invaluable should a lawsuit be filed later. The notes will help to refresh the defendant's memory and may make him or her a more reliable witness.

4. Know the state's Good Samaritan laws. Many states fail to cover nurses for voluntary work done outside of an emergency or away from an accident scene.

5. Above all, one should know the provisions of the applicable nurse practice act. Understand standards of care, and perform to that minimal level or better at all times. If the purpose of the donated services is the better education of the public, as with a mass hypertension screening program, carefully review with the sponsoring agency what the questionnaire should say and the types of questions normally asked. Such review will allow the professional nurse to answer the questions and to conduct a mass-learning program at an optimal standard-of-care level.

GUIDELINES

Volunteering Professional Services

Before donating professional services:

1. Reread your nurse practice act to see if such donated services are covered by the nurse practice act.
2. Check your professional liability insurance policy to ensure that you are covered financially should such services result in a malpractice suit being filed against you.
3. Consider carefully the impact of your decision on public relations and the nursing community should you refuse.

If you decide to volunteer your professional services:

1. Stay within the confines of the nursing scope of practice.
2. Refrain from crossing into a medical scope of practice; do not make medical diagnoses or distribute medical therapies and treatments.
3. Maintain the same standard of care you would maintain if you were a paid employee.
4. Keep accurate notes for your personal files.
5. Use this opportunity wisely to expand the positive image of nursing to the public at large.

DONATING HEALTH-RELATED ADVICE

Most health care practitioners have been asked at some time for health-related advice. It may have been at a fashionable party, at the grocery store, or over the telephone. Although unlikely, a lawsuit could be filed if the advice given falls below the accepted nursing and community standard or actually endangers the person's life and future health.

As with volunteer services, nurses must make a decision about **donating health-related advice.** There is no mandatory duty to do so, but once started, the nurse has a duty to give competent and safe advice. No duty is incurred under the state nurse practice act, because most nurse practice acts exclude gratuitous actions.

The advice given must reflect accepted nursing and community standards and be as current as possible. The nurse should be as open and honest as possible. If the nurse is not sure of the best advice to give or if the person seeking advice asks about an area of nursing practice in which the nurse has no expertise, it is advisable to avoid giving advice. It is perfectly acceptable to have a specialty area (e.g., cancer or pediatric nursing) and to be unfamiliar with other areas of nursing practice (e.g., neurological or rehabilitative nursing). No liability is incurred if the nurse honestly refrains from giving advice, but there may be liability if the nurse guesses and gives incorrect information.

The advice given should be within the scope of nursing practice. Even though freely given, the nurse may not make a medical diagnosis or interfere with the physician–patient relationship. Instead, the nurse should make general statements such as "From what you have described, it could be a mild stroke or a prestroke condition. You should make an appointment and see your doctor as soon as possible," or "I'm not sure. It's been a long time since I had any experience with sick children." Such statements prevent problems with scope of practice issues. Likewise, a statement such as "I don't know the doctor you mentioned. I always see Bob Smith" prevents charges that the nurse recommended changing physicians or that the nurse advised ignoring the primary physician's advice.

Another factor to consider concerns a possible nurse–patient relationship and the reliance of the other person in adhering to the health-related advice given. For example, a neighbor calls and asks a nurse about the neighbor's son who cut his elbow. The teenager had attempted to catch a ride on the hood of a moving car and fell into the street. The nurse examines the obvious wound and applies a sterile dressing, telling the mother that an antibiotic cream should help prevent an infection and that a doctor's visit at this time is unwarranted. The nurse also questions the teenager about the fall, asking exactly how he hit the pavement, and he reassures the nurse that he took the full brunt of the fall on his arm and elbow. The next day the mother calls to say that the injured arm looks better, but she is concerned with her son's erratic gait. He is bumping into doors and furniture. Now the nurse's professional advice is to have the son immediately see his physician. The mother's reliance on the nurse for advice demands that the advice is current and specific as the situation changes.

This reliance type of relationship seldom follows a casual party conversation or a one-time encounter. There are two points to remember. First, if health care questions are asked in an informal manner, the answers given must meet the standard of any reasonably prudent nurse, and second, there is no duty to recontact the person to see how or if the advice was implemented.

It is always acceptable to suggest that the person seeking advice consult with his or her own physician. For example, "If it were me, I would see my doctor immediately" is an appropriate response. The law does not require that nurses make such a suggestion if, in their professional judgment, such a suggestion is not necessary or if a reasonably prudent nurse would likewise not make the suggestion. Similarly, the law does not place liability if the person seeking advice fails to follow the advice. The person asking advice can choose to ignore advice given.

GUIDELINES

Health-Related Advice

1. Before the situation ever arises, reread both the state nurse practice act and your professional liability insurance policy to see if you are covered financially and if the nurse practice act covers such free advice.

2. If you decide to give advice:
   a. Give only current, up-to-date advice.
   b. Stay within the nursing scope of practice and refrain from medical diagnoses and treatments.
   c. Refrain from suggesting that the physician currently being seen is wrong in his or her advice.
   d. Refrain from false reassurance.
   e. Keep a personal written account of your advice.
3. If you are unsure of what to say or how the advice will be taken, suggest that the person seeking advice see his or her own physician, or state that you are unqualified to answer. You will not be sued for advice not given, but you can be sued for incorrect or potentially harmful advice.

One final word of caution: Always refrain from reassuring the person who has asked about a particular disease or symptom that there is nothing to worry about or that "everything will be fine." Reassurance is appropriate only if the condition is indeed minor. As a general rule, ask yourself the following question: If you were at your regular employment and a patient asked the same question, how would you answer it? That very same answer should be given to the person asking for free health care advice.

EXERCISE 18.3

Your next-door neighbor knocks on your door late one night, stating that his wife has fallen and hit her head, and asking that you come to see her. When you arrive, you find her conscious, inebriated, and bleeding from a 4-cm gash over her left eyebrow. You help her bandage the cut and recommend that she seek medical advice, particularly since she hit her head on a sharp object and was dazed and unconscious for about 5 minutes. She also tells you she does not know when she had her last tetanus booster.

The next day you discover that the neighbor has not sought medical advice and is lightheaded and somewhat unsure on her feet. She still refuses to see a doctor or to go to the local emergency center. What are your potential legal liabilities if further harm comes to the neighbor? Are you liable? If yes, what would the neighbor's cause of action be against you? Does the husband also have any reason to name you in a lawsuit?

What are the ethical implications of this scenario? Do you have an ethical obligation to see that the patient seeks additional assistance, such as assistance regarding her alcohol intake?

MANAGED HEALTH CARE ORGANIZATIONS

Managed care is loosely defined as a health care system that integrates the financing and delivery of health care services to covered individuals, most often by arrangements with selected providers. Managed care organizations, sometimes abbreviated MCOs, represent a major shift away from the domination of the fee-for-service system toward networks of providers supplying a full range of services. Managed care is the process of structuring or restructuring the health system in terms of financing, purchasing, delivering, measuring, and documenting a broad range of health care services and products. Though often seen as a concept of the late 1980s and 1990s in the United States, managed care has existed in some form for several decades.

Managed care organizations offer a package of health care benefits, standards for the selection of health care providers, formal programs for ongoing quality assurance and utilization review, and significant financial incentives for its members to use providers and procedures associated with the given plan. Major objections to these organizations tend to be twofold: limitations on the choice of providers by the consumer and requirements for prior authorization to obtain services.

Managed care is generally a prepaid or capitated payment mechanism, which means that a stipulated dollar amount is established to cover the cost of the health care delivered for a person and is paid periodically, usually as monthly or quarterly payments, to a health care provider or a health care plan. The provider or plan is responsible for arranging the delivery of all health care services required by the person under the terms of the contract.

A variety of managed care organizations are operating in the United States today. **Health maintenance organizations (HMOs)** are comprehensive health care financing and delivery organizations that provide or arrange for provision of covered health care services to a specified group of enrollees at a fixed periodic payment through a panel of providers. HMOs are the most highly regulated of the managed care options, and all 50 states have laws regulating these organizations. Most of these organizations are accredited nationally.

These entities act as both an insurer and a provider of services. They charge employers a fixed premium for each subscriber, and individuals who subscribe to an HMO are generally limited to the group of physicians who have contracted with the HMO to provide services to the subscribers.

HMOs may be sponsored by the federal government, medical schools, hospitals, employers, labor unions, consumer groups, insurance companies, and hospital medical plans. To be federally qualified as an HMO, the organization must have the following three aspects:

1. An organized system for providing health care in a geographic area
2. An agreed-upon set of basic and supplemental health maintenance and treatment services
3. A voluntarily enrolled group of persons

Four types of HMOs are common:

1. Staff model: A health care model in which providers practice as employees and are usually paid a set salary.
2. Independent practice association model: A separate legal entity contracts with an HMO for a negotiated fee. The health care providers continue in their existing individual or group practices, seeing HMO patients as a part of the practice.
3. Group model: A health plan contracts with a multispecialty group to provide care to plan members. The providers are not employees of the HMO, but are employed by the group practice and are paid a negotiated salary.
4. Network model: A model that contracts with two or more independent group practices and/or independent practice associations to provide services. Enrolled members pay a fixed monthly fee.

A second type of managed care organization is the **preferred provider organization (PPO),** seen by many in the industry as the model with the most current growth. This type of managed care plan involves contracts with independent providers for negotiated, discounted fees for services to members. Usually, the contract provides significantly better benefits for services received from preferred providers, thus encouraging enrollees to use those providers. Enrollees are often allowed benefits for nonparticipating providers' services, usually on an indemnity basis with significant co-payments. Thirty-five states have some regulation requirements, and most of the organizations are accredited by the Joint Commission (JC) or other federal accrediting body.

Point-of-service (POS) plans, sometimes referred to as an HMO–PPO hybrid or open-ended HMO, provide a set of health care benefits and offer a range of health services, and subscribers are given the option of using either the managed care program or out-of-plan services. This option is given each time the enrollee seeks care. Subscribers usually pay substantially higher premiums, increased deductibles, and coinsurance if they select a provider outside the panel of participating providers. Many plans have this option for the convenience of enrollees who travel and need medical assistance when away from their usual provider. There is little state regulation of these organizations, and they are infrequently accredited.

   Indemnity plans, also known as **fee-for-service (FFS)** plans, allow patients to access their provider of choice and the provider files a claim to the insurance company, which then reimburses the provider for the service. This type of managed care is managed only by the individual patient, and typically the patient pays a portion of the costs through coinsurance plans and deductibles. Regulation of this model is high, as all 50 states have regulating laws, and the plans generally are not accredited through the JC or other federal agencies.

EXERCISE 18.4

Review your own health policy. Does your individual health policy fit into one of the various managed care models? What are the advantages of your plan? Would other plans better fit your health care needs? What health care needs are not covered in your individual plan? How would you go about discovering other plans and/or deciding among various plans if you had such an option?

   Utilization review has become a part of the managed care operations. **Utilization review** is the process whereby a third-party payer evaluates the medical necessity of a course of treatment. The review may be conducted prospectively, concurrently, or retrospectively. Most insurance companies rely on prospective and concurrent review to determine whether care is necessary, as well as the level of care that is appropriate. Utilization review has become a necessary part of cost containment and may also involve some degree of case management. Case management involves identifying at an early point which patients can be treated more cost effectively in an alternative setting or at a lower level of care without negatively affecting the overall care of the patient. Case management is frequently employed with patients whose care is catastrophic.

   Utilization review must be done ethically and with caution. The following case illustrates the dangers of this type of review. In *McEvoy v. Group Health Cooperative of Eau Claire* (1997), the court held that an HMO may be liable under the same standards as an insurance company for bad-faith refusal for out-of-network treatment. This is especially true of the company making such a bad-faith use of out-of-network providers when driven by unreasonable and economically motivated judgments.

   McEvoy involved a 13-year-old girl covered under a group health cooperative (GHC) plan providing 70 days of coverage for inpatient psychological care. Her GHC physician diagnosed anorexia nervosa and recommended treatment in a non-GHC residential treatment center for patients with eating disorders. GHC approved the plan, but discontinued treatment coverage after 6 weeks despite strong opposition from the girl's treating physician and an out-of-network psychiatrist, who protested that she was not ready for release. Instead, the HMO approved a weekly outpatient therapy group for compulsive overeaters. The girl immediately relapsed and lost 21 pounds by the time GHC readmitted her to an out-of-plan center less than 2 months after her initial discharge. The period of coverage ended a week later, and she remained in treatment at her own expense. She filed suit against GHC for breach of contact and bad faith in failing to authorize care.

The Supreme Court of Wisconsin upheld the allegations against the HMO, stating that the purpose of a bad-faith tort is to help redress the bargaining inequality between insurance companies and patients, who frequently have little or no ability to influence the terms of their medical coverage. The HMO, said the court, is "under a contractual duty to provide or pay for reasonable services to remedy the subscriber's condition . . . up to policy limits" (at 404). The court further held that this was not a malpractice issue, because the cooperative made its decision based on administrative, not medical, considerations.

As the network of managed care organizations continued to evolve, the Health Care Quality Improvement Act of 1986 (HCQIA) was enacted as a response to the multiple antitrust suits against participants in peer-review and credentialing activities. The purpose of this act was to provide persons giving information to professional review bodies and those assisting in review activities limited immunity from damage that might arise as a result of adverse decisions affecting staff privileges. Institutions had created quality review committees, sometimes referred to as *quality assessment committees,* to evaluate patient care and patient outcomes within the new framework of managed care. At issue was the potential liability of members of this quality review committee when they reported their findings. Under the HCQIA, to be immune from liability, anyone involved with an internal peer-review body must act with a reasonable belief that his or her actions are in furtherance of quality health care and there must be a reasonable effort to obtain the facts (*Berg v. Shapiro,* 2001).

In the *Berg* case, two physicians reported a third physician to the internal review committee based upon an incident report written by the attending nurse in the obstetrics department. The case centered on whether it was "in bad faith" that these two physicians reported their colleague or whether they were acting "in good faith" and furthering quality care within this institution. The court, in dismissing the lawsuit, noted that it was not bad faith for the physicians to rely on an incident report written by someone who was an eye witness to the care delivered.

Similar to other internal reports, courts have ruled that internal quality review documents are not discoverable in subsequent lawsuits (*Nalder v. West Park Hospital,* 2001; *Subpoena Duces Tecum to Jane Doe, Esq.,* 2003; *Welsh v. Galen of Virginia, Inc.,* 2001). "Gathering information to report as candidly as possible whether improvement is indicated cannot be hampered by fear that the notes will be used against the hospital in a lawsuit" was the conclusion reached in *Nalder v. West Park Hospital* (2001, at 1173). Nor may a patient's lawyer take the deposition of the hospital's quality review officer (*Van Bergen v. Long Beach Medical Center,* 2000).

In 2003, the Centers for Medicare and Medicaid Services (CMS) announced that as a new condition for participation, hospitals must develop and maintain a quality assessment and performance improvement program that meets the CMS guidelines. The focus of this new condition is not on new standards for hospitals, but on the process by which institutions systematically examine themselves (CMS, 2003).

The Ethics in Patient Referral Act (1989) became law as part of the Omnibus Budget Reconciliation Act of 1989. Effective January 1, 1992, the act prohibits physicians who have ownership interest or compensation arrangements with a clinical laboratory from referring Medicare patients to that laboratory. The law also required all Medicare providers to report the names and provider numbers of all physicians or their immediate relatives with ownership interests in the provider entity prior to October 1, 1991.

A system of accreditation for managed care organizations has also emerged. The **National Committee for Quality Assurance (NCQA)** is the independent, nonprofit health maintenance organization accrediting agency. The NCQA is composed of independent health quality experts, employers, labor union officials, and consumer representatives. The NCQA focuses on quality improvement, credentialing, members' rights and responsibilities, utilization management, preventive health services, and medical records. Though none of these standards currently focuses on nursing-specific measures of patient care outcomes, nurses may find themselves equally involved in causes of action against a managed care corporation.

An example of this concept is *Nold v. Binyon* (2001). In that case, the jury awarded $800,000 for a young child who was not given gamma globulin or a hepatitis vaccination in the hospital's newborn nursery despite her mother's positive hepatitis B antigen status. The primary verdict had been against the physicians and residents who cared for the mother and newborn infant; the court of appeals remanded the case for a new trial based on the conclusion that the nurses, and thus the hospital, were equally liable in this case.

In a managed care environment, concluded the court, nurses have a heightened responsibility to see that critical patient assessment data are documented in the nurses' notes so that nurses caring for a patient at a later time will initiate appropriate interventions or ensure that appropriate interventions have already been implemented. In this case, the nurses failed to read the patient's prenatal records. If the nurses had read these records, they would have known of the mother's positive hepatitis B antigen status. This information could then have been relayed to the nurses caring for the newborn infant. The court also faulted the nurses in the newborn nursery for not assessing that the mother's prenatal history was incomplete.

Many health care experts agree that, at least in theory, managed health care is an effective manner in which to deliver quality health care. Patients receive care through a single, seamless system as they move from wellness to illness and back to wellness. Continuity of care, prevention, promotion of wellness, and early intervention are stressed. In reality, though, managed care organizations have become a means of financing health care and not a system of organizing patient care. Many of the measures currently adopted by managed care companies illustrate this financial concern, including early discharge, gag rules, incentives for cost-saving measures that fail to take into consideration the overall health status of the patient, and staff shortages. Such issues, exclusively aimed at cost cutting, have raised several legal issues surrounding managed care.

LEGAL ISSUES SURROUNDING MANAGED CARE

Several sources of legal concern arise under the concept of managed care, including Employment Retirement Income Security Act issues, gag rules and end-of-year profit sharing, standards of care, Emergency Treatment and Active Labor Act issues, and antitrust issues.

Employment Retirement Income Security Act

One of the earliest issues to emerge with managed care concerned potential legal liability under the federal **Employment Retirement Income Security Act of 1974 (ERISA).** The ERISA amendment was designed to ensure that employee welfare benefit plans conform to a uniform body of benefits law. The federal ERISA laws preempt state laws in the area of employee benefit plans. The laws, though, do not regulate the content of the benefit plans, merely that the plans are uniform. Because of their role as both insurer and health care provider, ERISA has shielded HMOs from liability for questionable health care. ERISA requires that every plan describe procedures for the allocation of responsibilities for its operation and administration and specify the basis on which payments are to be made to and from the plan.

Countless stories of poor medical decisions, untoward patient outcomes, and premature patient demise have been told by patients and families, with the HMOs protected under ERISA laws. Congress passed the original ERISA amendments to reserve for the federal government the power to enact any laws or regulations that relate to employer-sponsored benefit plans. These benefits have been broadly interpreted by the courts to include pensions, health plans, and other benefits. ERISA also was created to prevent unfounded actions from eroding benefits and to prevent conflicts among state laws. The act leaves to the states the right to regulate commercial health insurance plans. Since states have been active in this area of the law and the federal government has not, many large employers have established "self-insured" health plans that are not subject to state regulations on health plan rates, benefits, and other protections.

Congress never intended, however, for ERISA to bar lawsuits against HMOs, health insurers, or health plans regarding patient management decisions. There is now acknowledgment that patients' and beneficiaries' lawsuits against health plans may go forward regarding these patient management decisions. Courts still adhere, though, to the rule that patients and beneficiaries do not have the right to file lawsuits in state or federal courts to challenge benefit schedules, internal management decisions, and financial priorities. These areas remain protected under ERISA.

What is occurring is the allowance for patients and beneficiaries to sue health plans, insurance companies, and HMOs for acts that can be characterized as medical care decisions rather than administrative matters. A health care professional who prepares a beneficiary's health plan while working for a health insurer, health plan, or HMO and following its rules can commit malpractice and can be sued along with the health insurer, health plan, or HMO, if the health plan falls below acceptable professional standards, said the court in *Moreno v. Health Partners Health Plan* (1998).

States have been active in promoting greater accountability on the part of HMOs to their patients. For example, legislation in selected states has made managed care providers legally responsible for adverse medical decisions that cause damages to patients. For example, some state legislation has held that managed care providers may be considered medical practitioners and may be liable for treatment decisions and reimbursement denials that result in patient harm. Other state laws impose a duty of ordinary care on managed care providers when making treatment decisions. States continue to pass into laws protections for patients who have been severely harmed by the medical decisions made by managed health care organizations.

Legal examples of this application of the law can be seen in the following cases. In *Land v. CIGNA Healthcare of Florida* (2003), a patient's hand had become infected and he was diagnosed with osteomyelitis. The patient was admitted to the hospital for aggressive intravenous antibiotic therapy. Shortly after admission, the approval nurse employed by the patient's HMO decided that the patient did not require hospitalization. The patient was subsequently discharged; he was to continue with intravenous antibiotic therapy at home. The patient was treated on an outpatient basis for continuing complications and ultimately had the middle finger of his hand amputated.

The patient sued the HMO for negligence. The court, reiterating the original purpose of ERISA laws, made the distinction that this lawsuit was for a patient care decision, rather than for employee benefits. The patient can sue, in a state court, for pain and suffering, loss of earning capacity, and permanent disfigurement causes of actions for the nurse's negligent patient care decision. Similar results were reached in *CIGNA Healthcare of Texas, Inc. v. Pybas* (2004), *Krasny v. Waser* (2001), and *Lazorko v. Pennsylvania Hospital* (2000).

Gag Rules and End-of-Year Profit Sharing

Managed care plans, in order to be financially successful, may restrict patients' choices and redirect health care away from high-cost options and providers. To encourage providers within the HMO to keep costs as minimal as possible, many HMOs initiated **gag rules** that prevent health

EXERCISE 18.5

Explore the managed care options in your geographic setting. Are the plans traditional HMOs or some other type of managed care, such as PPO or POS plans? How many enrollees does the plan cover? What are the advantages to the community of offering an HMO rather than more traditional insurance coverage to people in the area? What are the disadvantages? How has the quality of health care delivery changed in your area with the advent of HMOs?

care providers from offering certain more expensive therapies as options and restricting service to the complaint about which the patient presented to the HMO. Under the gag rule, health care providers are prevented from informing patients about concomitant illnesses or diseases.

End-of-year profit sharing, sometimes called a *performance bonus,* is an incentive given to reward health care providers for keeping costs at a minimum. A certain percentage of profits are distributed at the end of the calendar year to health care providers who did not order expensive tests or who did not prescribe extensive therapy. The more the health care provider assisted the HMO in making a profit, the more profit that is given back to the health care provider.

Both means of keeping costs low have the potential for substandard treatment of patients and would seem to directly conflict with the purpose of HMOs in ensuring preventative care and promoting health at the primary level. In 1998, the federal government prohibited gag clauses in the Federal Employees Health Benefits Program (Office of Personnel Management, 1998). Following this lead, the majority of states now also outlaw both gag rules and end-of-year profit sharing.

A case that illustrates the HMO's potential liability for end-of-year profit sharing through bonuses is *Fox v. Health Net* (1994). In that case, a jury rendered a $90 million verdict against an HMO for its decision to refuse to cover a needed bone marrow transplant. The patient claimed that the decision was based on a decision made by the HMO medical director, who received a performance bonus that encouraged him to deny payment for expensive procedures and treatments. The court concluded that such end-of-year bonuses totaling significant amounts of money can alter the decision-making ability of a medical director.

Standards of Care

Health care providers have a duty to render quality, competent care. This is true whether or not the ERISA laws apply. For example, in *Hand v. Tavera* (1993), a patient presented to an emergency center in considerable distress. The court preempted the case against the HMO based on the ERISA laws, but the patient was still able to prevail against the health care physician. The physician whom the patient initially saw did not have admitting privileges with the hospital. He called the health care plan's on-call primary physician. This second physician, who was the patient's assigned physician, had never met the patient and failed to order an admission to the hospital. The patient subsequently suffered a stroke in the hospital's parking lot. The court held that when a patient who is fully enrolled in a prepaid plan goes to the emergency center and the plan's designated physician is consulted, the physician–patient relationship exists and the physician owes the patient a reasonable duty of care in compliance with established medical standards of care.

Two cases illustrate potential HMO liability, *Shannon v. McNulty* (1998) and *Alejandre v. Kaiser Foundation Hospitals* (2007). In the first case, the patient belonged to an HMO when she became pregnant with her first child. She was given a choice of six different physicians as her primary prenatal care provider, and she chose one of the six. Her HMO membership card instructed her to contact either her chosen primary care provider or the HMO itself if she had questions about her health care. If the subscriber phoned the HMO directly, the subscriber would speak with a telephone triage line staffed by registered nurses employed by the HMO.

The patient saw her primary physician frequently during the pregnancy for abdominal pain and back pain. She was seen in his office on three consecutive days for these complaints. On the third of these three consecutive visits, the physician informed her that she had a fibroid uterus. He did not perform any tests and did not instruct her about the symptoms of preterm labor. The patient called the physician's office several more times in the ensuing days, and he insisted that she was not in labor. The next time the patient called, she could not reach her primary physician and she then called the HMO. A nurse listened only very briefly, then simply told the patient to call her primary physician. On the next 2 days, the same scenario happened. None of the nurses working on the triage telephone line knew her history or listened long enough to find out that she was in the fifth month of a very difficult pregnancy.

When the patient called the HMO the fourth time, still complaining of back pain, she was put in contact with an in-house orthopedic physician-consultant. He instructed her to drive to the emergency center at West Penn Hospital, a facility 1 hour away, further from her home than three other hospitals. At the hospital, the patient was treated as an orthopedic patient, since her referral had been through an orthopedic physician-consultant. The patient was allowed to go to the labor and delivery unit for a check-up.

In the labor and delivery unit, it was decided that the patient was in premature labor and, a few hours later, a small preterm infant was delivered. The infant survived for 2 days before he died due to his extreme prematurity. The patient sued the HMO and her primary physician under a corporate or vicarious liability theory, and the trial court dismissed her suit.

The appeals court, however, upheld her lawsuit and ruled that corporate liability duties are applicable to HMOs. Though providers do not practice medicine, they do involve themselves in decisions affecting their subscribers' medical care. When decisions are made to limit the subscriber's access to treatment, the decision must pass the test of medical reasonableness. There is no reason, said the court, why the duties applicable to hospitals should not equally apply to an HMO when the HMO is performing the same or similar functions as the hospital. When an HMO is providing health care services rather than merely paying for services, the HMO should be judged the same as a hospital or other health care provider.

Similarly, the court reasoned, the patient had established a cause of action for vicarious liability. An HMO has a nondelegable duty to select and train competent primary care providers. Likewise, the HMO provided a medical service in the form of telephone advice nurses. The adequacy of that service and the reasonableness of the patient's use of that service under the circumstances are questions for a jury.

In *Alejandre*, a 22-year-old diabetic patient, 40 weeks pregnant with her first child, called the HMO to report that the fetus did not seem to be moving and requested to be admitted for fetal monitoring. Three days earlier, she had a regularly scheduled appointment, during which a non-stress test was done, indicating that the fetus was healthy. At that time, she had been instructed to call the hospital in 3 days, as that was the end of her 40th week of pregnancy, for instructions regarding admission for the delivery of the baby. When the mother called the hospital, the hospital staff, failing to appreciate that this could be an emergency, waited over 5 hours to call the mother back, stating that there was a bed on the labor and delivery unit and that she should come immediately to the hospital. When she was finally admitted, the fetal heart tracings showed late decelerations without variability, a cesarean section was done, and the infant died shortly after birth.

Two medical experts testified that labor for this high-risk maternity patient with insulin-dependent diabetes should have been induced no later than the 39th week of pregnancy. Thus, liability was found against the HMO for the mismanagement of the patient and wrongful death of her infant.

Emergency Medical Treatment and Labor Act

In 1986 Congress passed the **Emergency Medical Treatment and Labor Act (EMTALA)**, establishing a right of access to medical care regardless of one's ability to pay for that care. The need for the law had become paramount because patients were being turned away from hospitals or "dumped" on other hospitals, primarily through the emergency departments, based solely on their inability to pay for health care. To prevent untoward outcomes, Congress passed the EMTALA.

Essentially, the law applies to every health care institution that has a Medicare provider agreement in effect and requires the following:

1. Examination and treatment for emergency medical conditions and women in labor must be provided.
2. Medical screening is required whenever a patient comes to the emergency department and requests examination or treatment for a medical condition. The hospital must provide for an appropriate medical screening examination within the capability of the hospital's emergency department, including ancillary services routinely available to the emergency department, to determine whether or not an emergency condition exists.
3. Necessary stabilizing treatment for emergency medical conditions and labor is required. When the individual comes to the emergency department requesting treatment and the hospital determines that the individual has an emergency medical condition, the hospital must provide either available treatment within the hospital or transfer the individual to another medical facility for treatment.
4. Transfers are restricted until the individual is stable, unless (1) the individual or legally responsible person acting on the individual's behalf, after being informed of the hospital's obligation to treat and the risk of transfer, in writing requests transfer to another facility; (2) a physician may sign a certificate based on the time of transfer that the medical benefits reasonably expected from the provision of appropriate medical care at another institution outweigh the increased risk to the individual or the unborn child; or (3) a qualified medical person may sign a medical certificate after consultation with the physician and the physician subsequently countersigns the certificate of transfer.
5. An *appropriate transfer* is defined as a transfer in which the transferring hospital provides the medical treatment within its capability that minimizes risks to the individual's health or the health of the unborn infant, and in which the receiving facility has available space and qualified personnel for the treatment of the individual and has agreed to accept the transfer of the individual and to provide appropriate medical treatment.
6. *Emergency medical condition* refers to a medical condition manifesting itself by acute symptoms of sufficient severity, including severe pain, such that the absence of immediate medical attention could reasonably be expected to result in placing the health of the individual or unborn child in serious jeopardy, serious impairment of bodily functions, or serious dysfunction of any bodily organ or part.
7. *Stabilize* means, with respect to the medical condition, to provide such treatment of the condition as may be necessary to assure, with reasonable medical probability, that no material deterioration of the condition is likely to result from or occur during the transfer of the individual from the facility or during the delivery of the unborn infant. (42 U.S.C., Section 1359dd)

New regulations for hospital emergency department policies and procedures were enacted in 2003 ("EMTALA: New Regulations," 2003). The new rules expand the definition of *emergency patient* to include persons that a reasonably prudent layperson would interpret as having an emergency medical condition, whether or not they are in an emergency center per se. If a patient (or a person acting on the patient's behalf) refuses examination or treatment, after fully comprehending the risks and benefits, the medical record must contain a description of the examination, treatment, or both, if applicable, that was refused by or on behalf of the individual. Reasonable steps must be taken to secure this refusal in writing. As before, medical treatment must not be delayed based on insurance status, but may be delayed while contacting the patient's previous physician, if the consultation does not inappropriately delay required services. Similarly, reasonable registration processes may not duly delay screening or treatment or discourage individuals from remaining for further treatment.

Two additional EMTALA amendments were enacted in 2008. Effective October 1, 2008, the amendments further ensure the care for all patients. The first amendment created a community call plan, which directly addressed the increasing problems with availability of specialty physicians. Though the original EMTALA act mandated the establishment of a complete roster of physicians in the facility, the community call plan allows for the names of physicians who work at other area hospitals and who participate in the community call plan to also be listed on such rosters. The second amendment concerns the "good-faith" requirement of the original act. Once a patient is admitted to a treating health care facility, EMTALA no longer applies. But facilities may still encounter challenges with managing the unstable patient. This provision would extend the good-faith requirement of EMTALA to specialty facilities to accept the transfer of these unstable patients if they have the capacity to treat them.

Despite the fact that the law has been in force for more than 10 years, cases still arise under the EMTALA. This area of the law continues to be highly litigious across the United States. The advent of HMOs, with their cost-cutting measures, has seemed to intensify such cases.

Perhaps the earliest challenges to the law concerned patient "dumping" by hospitals. For example, in *Johnson v. University of Chicago* (1990), city fire department paramedics had been called for emergency care of an infant in cardiac arrest. The paramedics contacted the University of Chicago Hospitals telemetry system and were instructed to take the infant to a hospital other than the one five blocks from the infant's home. The telemetry nurse recommended the alternative hospital because the University of Chicago Hospital's pediatric intensive care unit was full and had no place to admit the child for treatment. The child later died.

The child's parents brought suit, claiming that the hospital had violated the EMTALA requirements. In the court's holding for the hospital that no EMTALA violation had occurred, the court noted that it would reconsider the evidence if it could be shown that the hospital used the telemetry system as part of a "scheme to dump patients" (at 236).

In 1995, the U.S. Court of Appeals in *Eberhardt v. City of Los Angeles* further defined the role of a hospital in treating medical conditions. In this case, the paramedics had responded to a call that a man was experiencing a heroin overdose. The paramedics administered Narcan and transported him to a hospital emergency center. At the hospital, the man reported to the triage nurse that he had used cocaine and smoked heroin immediately before the paramedics arrived. He initially refused treatment, but was persuaded to let a physician see him. The physician administered additional Narcan, and his examination of the patient revealed that the man's vital signs had returned to normal levels and that the patient was alert and oriented. He advised the man to seek long-term help through a methadone program at another facility.

The patient then removed his own intravenous line and left the hospital. As he was leaving, he stated that he had a feeling of doom and was upset because the hospital had saved his life. The next day he was shot and killed by police as he attacked them with a machete in a disturbed mental state, and his family brought this lawsuit, alleging an EMTALA violation.

The court ruled that the hospital had met its obligations by attending to the patient's acute medical condition with appropriate care to meet his immediate medical needs. The hospital was not responsible for his death 1 day later at the hands of the police.

Parker v. Salina Regional Health Center, Inc. (2006) clarified regulations regarding the timing of triage and insurance status inquiries. A hospital may adhere to its patient registration policies so long as they do not conflict with the goals of EMTALA. Hospital registration procedures, including insurance inquiries, for persons presenting in the emergency center for needed health care, are allowable so long as these inquiries do not discourage individuals from remaining for evaluation or do not delay triage, initial screening, or necessary stabilizing medical treatment. Hospital staff must appreciate the gravity of a patient's presenting signs and symptoms and the need for immediate medical assessment and intervention. *Henderson v. Medical Center Enterprise* (2006) held that the patient registration resulted in a significant delay that served to discourage the patient from remaining for treatment, and that this is a direct EMTALA violation.

A 1996 case, *Rios v. Baptist Memorial Hospital System*, reiterated the need for the patient to request care to qualify under the EMTALA laws. In *Rios,* a patient with his arm in a sling from a recent industrial accident walked through the emergency department with a family member, stopping only to ask for directions to the admitting department. Unable to find the admitting department, they left and went to another hospital. There was no treatment until 4 days later, when the injury was significantly worse.

The patient sued the first hospital, alleging an EMTALA violation. The court ruled, however, that a patient must first come to the emergency department and present for care before the hospital's obligations under the EMTALA come into play. This patient and family member requested no treatment, but merely asked for directions. Thus, the patient had no basis for a lawsuit.

Similarly, the court in *Johnson v. Nacogdoches County Hospital* (2003) ruled that there was no violation under EMTALA for a patient who voluntarily left the emergency center before receiving care. In *Johnson,* the patient was triaged in the emergency center, classified as nonurgent, and reassessed 25 and 40 minutes after her initial assessment. Her family then took her by wheelchair to the hospital parking lot and placed her in their car, insisting that they were taking her elsewhere for care. The patient died later that evening at another facility. The court of appeals found no violation of EMTALA.

Courts have also defined when patient screening is appropriate (*Trivette v. North Carolina Baptist Hospital,* 1998). The key, said the court, is uniform treatment of emergency patients with similar signs and symptoms, regardless of the ability to pay. In this case, the patient received a battery of tests, including x-rays, and was admitted to the hospital. The next day, he was seen by his primary medical provider and released. The court said in its conclusion that EMTALA does not concern itself with possible misdiagnosis, but whether the patient has had a proper screening examination and has been offered appropriate treatment to stabilize the emergency condition that brought him to the emergency center.

The court, in *Scott v. Dauterive Hospital Corporation* (2003), specifically noted that "in EMTALA cases, the courts do not second guess the professional judgment of nurses and doctors who screen and treat patients. . . . The question is whether the patient was given the same care and attention a patient would get with the same history, signs, and symptoms" (at 3). This case involved an intoxicated patient who presented with a small laceration; he was alert and oriented, pupils were equal and reactive, and he was released without having undergone a CT scan. He was subsequently treated at a second facility for right frontal and temporal lobe hematomas. These holdings were also upheld by courts in *Brenord v. Catholic Medical Center* (2001), *Bryant v. Archbold Memorial Hospital* (2006), *Godwin v. Memorial Medical Center* (2001), and *Kilroy v. Star Valley Medical Center* (2002).

Other cases have discussed the appropriateness of screening examinations. In *Marshall v. East Carroll Parish Hospital Service District* (1998), a hospital was sued for sending a teenager home with what seemed like only an upper respiratory infection. In fact, the young woman had suffered a cerebrovascular accident consistent with a left middle cerebral artery infarction. The teenager's parents sued only the institution, not the nurses or physicians at the facility.

The court noted that EMTALA applies to nursing assessment in the emergency center as well as to the physician's examination and treatment under the general term *appropriate medical screening examination.* The court further noted that when patients sue over a substandard emergency center medical screening examination, the court looks only at whether the patient was given the same screening examination as other patients presenting with similar signs and symptoms. In dismissing this case, the problem for the court was that staff could not show that this patient was treated any differently than other patients coming into the emergency center with the same signs and symptoms.

In dismissing this case, the court expressly discounted the testimony of a nurse who had overheard a heated discussion between the emergency center physician and a second nurse. The second nurse was vehemently arguing with the physician that the teenager should either be admitted or transferred to another facility rather than being sent home.

In *Spillman v. Southwest Louisiana Hospital Association* (2007), a young patient was evaluated for complaints of lower right quadrant abdominal pain. The nurse practitioner evaluated the patient and allowed him to be discharged after the CT scan was noted to be "normal." The next day another radiologist and a pediatrician read the scan, noting that it indicated acute appendicitis. The patient, later on the same day he was discharged, had been taken to a second acute care facility, where he was admitted and his appendix surgically removed. His mother brought suit against the nurse practitioner and the hospital for negligence and violation of EMTALA. The court found no liability against the nurse practitioner and the hospital, but left open a possible negligent lawsuit against the radiologist who had determined that the CT scan was within normal limits.

Morrison v. Colorado Permanente Medical Group (1997) illustrates that nurses and physicians may be liable for their actions as well as extending liability to their institution for EMTALA violations. In *Morrison,* the patient had presented to the emergency center with elevated vital signs and flank and buttock lesions that the nurse thought were uninfected bedsores. The patient was seen and released, even though he had necrotizing fasciitis/myositis, for which he should have been immediately treated.

This court examined the language regarding stabilizing treatment in deciding that the physician and nurses were in violation of the EMTALA. The patient was not adequately screened and was thus sent home despite the fact that his medical condition was, within reasonable medical probability, likely to deteriorate. The court also reiterated that all patients, whether or not they have insurance or the ability to pay privately for care, have the right to sue for an EMTALA violation.

Brodersen v. Sioux Valley Memorial Hospital (1995) illustrates the requirement that a nurse's assessment may trigger the hospital's duty to provide stabilizing care. In this case, the hospital's policy was for the emergency center charge nurse to oversee initial screening in the emergency center. For patients presenting with chest pain, an electrocardiogram was to be obtained simultaneously with the physician's being notified of the patient's arrival. According to the testimony of two emergency department staff nurses, it was the hospital practice for the nurse to move acutely ill patients to cardiac or intensive care before the emergency center physician saw the patients, if that was warranted by the patient's initial screening and nursing physical assessment.

When this patient, who was on public assistance, was not given an electrocardiogram and was left to be seen by the emergency center physician, with chest pains for which his physician had instructed him to go to the emergency center and with signs of acute myocardial infarction, the court read a discriminatory motive into the nurse's conduct and ruled that the hospital had indeed violated the EMTALA.

Note that the opposite conclusion can also be triggered by the nurse's actions. In *Fischer v. New York Health and Hospitals Corporation* (1998), a 6-year-old patient was brought in by ambulance with a fever and headache 18 hours after he was hit in the head with a snowball. The emergency triage nurse saw him at 12:30 A.M. His vital signs were taken, revealing a temperature of 104.6°F. The mother told the nurse of his injury with the snowball and that he had complained of a headache, loss of appetite, and generalized body pain ever since the incident. At 1:00 A.M., he was given 180 mg of Tylenol to reduce his fever.

The nurse was required by the institution policy to categorize each patient as "routine," "high priority," or "emergent." She classified this patient as "high priority." The patient was seen by the emergency center physician at 1:15 A.M. for a pediatric examination. By 2:20 A.M., the fever was 102.0°F and the patient was sent home.

He returned 2 days later and was admitted, and a brain scan showed a serious brain abscess. The family sued for an EMTALA violation, which was dismissed by the court. The court reiterated that the key to avoiding EMTALA violations is equal treatment of emergency center patients. Emergency center physicians and nurses must follow the hospital's same standard screening procedures that they would follow for any other patient in the emergency center with the same medical condition. Here, the emergency center had met its obligations to this patient.

Johnson v. Health Central Hospital (2006) reached a similar conclusion, noting that the patient received the same medical screening and stabilizing care any similar patient would have received. The patient had also alleged that he was transferred in direct violation of the EMTALA act. This case held that a patient who leaves against medical advice (AMA) does not meet the issue of "transferred" as defined in the act.

Departure from the emergency center's standard screening procedures can trigger liability, as "*C. M.*" v. *Tomball Regional Hospital* (1997) illustrates. In this case, the nurse conducted an entire screening for a 15-year-old rape victim in the emergency department waiting room, crowded with 10 to 15 other persons, rather than providing for the emotional support and medical detection screening that was part of the institution's policy manual.

The nurse was told that the teenager had been raped by a 27-year-old man and was in severe pain. The nurse assessed no vital signs, nor did she ask any questions about the teenager's medical history. There was no physical examination of the teenager. The nurse did ask questions concerning how the rape had occurred, asking only if the patient had bathed since the alleged attack. Learning that the girl had taken a bath, the nurse said there was nothing further the hospital could do for her, and she instructed the girl and her mother to see their private physician. No other instructions were given by the nurse.

The court reported that the mother had repeatedly asked for a physical examination to see if the girl was all right, but that the nurse repeatedly said there was nothing the hospital could do for her. One of the persons in the waiting room knew the victim and quickly spread the news of the alleged rape to those in the neighborhood, causing the mother and child to relocate to a new home and new school district due to emotional trauma. The mother also testified that her daughter became physically ill when discussions arose about seeking medical care, was afraid of any type of medical activity, and would not trust anyone with private information about herself.

The court ruled that the hospital, emergency center physician, and nurse had violated the EMTALA. The court pointed out that the nurse herself had testified that she followed none of the hospital's own rape crisis procedures.

EXERCISE 18.6

Juanita, a 22-year-old woman, is admitted to the emergency center complaining of lower abdominal pain and a sudden "passage of water." She is fairly fluent in English and tells you that her last menstrual cycle was approximately 19 weeks ago. She states the pain only recently began and that she is afraid she may be losing her baby, if she is indeed pregnant.

You proceed to take her vital signs, noting that they are within normal limits, that she has no allergies, and that she is not taking any medications. You calculate that she is approximately 17 weeks pregnant and assign her to a treatment area rather than sending her to the labor and delivery unit. Juanita, while waiting for the physician to examine her, passes a large clot, and she subsequently brings a lawsuit, alleging EMTALA violations.

The hospital policy for pregnant patients notes that the triage nurse will:

1. Document the patient's expected date of confinement (EDC) and last menstrual period (LMP) on the triage form.
2. Assess the patient for signs and symptoms of active labor.
3. Assign pregnant patients estimated to be less than 20 weeks' gestation to a treatment area appropriate to her needs.

Was the care provided this patient appropriate and competent? Did the nurse follow the prevailing standard of care for pregnant patients within this institution? Was there a violation of EMTALA in the care given this patient? How might the nurse have avoided this lawsuit?

Note, though, that the mere fact that a hospital standard is not followed will not automatically translate to liability against the institution. In *Torres Otero v. Hospital General Menonita* (2000), a patient presenting with chest pains was assessed in the emergency center. No electrocardiogram (EKG) was performed as part of the assessment data, he was not given aspirin, and a cardiologist was not consulted, even though the hospital policy mandated these measures. The patient was subsequently diagnosed as experiencing a myocardial infarction, transferred to the intensive care unit, placed on anticoagulant therapy, and transferred to a second hospital 7 days later for open-heart surgery. He later sued for failure to adequately assess him while in the emergency center.

The court agreed that the provisions of EMTALA were not met. The care required was administered belatedly in the intensive care unit rather than the emergency center. But the burden of proof remains with the patient to show that this delay adversely affected his care or caused aggravated harm to the patient, and he could not show this at trial. Thus, even though EMTALA was violated, there was no liability on the part of the hospital or its staff.

Court cases have also given guidance with patient stabilization prior to transfer. In *Cherukuri v. Shalala, Secretary of the Department of Health and Human Services* (1999), the court determined that medical and nursing personnel at the first hospital were genuinely concerned about the patients' well-being and were trying to respond to an overwhelmingly difficult situation. Several bad automobile accident trauma victims were brought into a rural hospital. The hospital had an emergency department but no trauma center and no equipment for monitoring anesthesia during neurosurgery; it had in place a longstanding policy against attempting such surgery.

Two patients required brain surgery, but were also bleeding into their abdomens. The physicians wanted to operate for the internal bleeding, then send the patients to a teaching-trauma center 85 miles away. The on-call anesthesiologist, however, refused to come to the hospital, insisting that the procedure was too risky, and that the patients should be immediately transferred.

The nurses assisted in the initial triage. Then they cared for three less seriously injured patients while the physicians concentrated on the two more serious victims. They monitored the patients' blood pressures, phoned the anesthesiologist repeatedly to try to get him to come in, and tried to get a helicopter. They were forced to use ambulances for the transport. The physicians and nurses communicated with the trauma center during the transport, and the patients suffered no harm during the transport.

Technically speaking, a patient does not have to be stabilized to be transferred from the hospital that first accepted the patient as an emergency case. However, the physician must make a written certification based on the information available at the time of transport that the provision of appropriate medical care at another medical facility outweighs the increased risk to the patient from making the transfer, and only if the receiving institution has agreed to accept transfer of the patient and to provide the patient with appropriate medical treatment. A patient who has been stabilized can be transferred to another hospital without a physician's certification and without an agreement from the other hospital to accept the patient. When a transfer is being contemplated, the patient's immediate situation is paramount; long-term goals are not the primary focus. Here, the court held that these patients were stabilized within the first hospital, so that no EMTALA violation occurred.

The patient does not need to be stabilized if the hospital initially treating the patient lacks the full ability to treat the patient's condition and transfer would be more beneficial to the patient in question (*Prickett v. HSC Medical Center*, 2007; *Williamson v. Roth*, 2000). Nor does EMTALA require that an institution admit a patient when the institution does not have the needed services at the facility. In *Bowden v. Walmart Stores, Inc.* (2000), an 8-year-old child suffered a serious eye injury when a helium balloon, which the child punctured with a toy from the store's shelf, exploded. The grandparents rushed the child to the nearest hospital emergency center. The physician patched the eye and told the grandparents to take the child to a specific hospital, because that hospital was the only one that had an ophthalmologist on staff. The child's grandparents instead took the child to an alternate hospital.

The child was eventually treated, but not in time to save the eyesight in the eye that was injured. The parents brought this lawsuit against the retail store and both hospitals. The court dismissed the first hospital from the case, noting that there was no evidence of "patient dumping" when a hospital performs an emergency medical screening that determines the patient requires immediate medical care the hospital cannot provide.

A similar outcome was reached in *Baker v. Adventist Health, Inc.* (2001), involving a patient who committed suicide 2 days after he was seen in the emergency center of a 40-bed rural community hospital. The patient was seen, determined to be physically stable, though suffering from depression and apathy, but not suicidal, and the county mental health professional was called to see the patient. The court later determined that this was the hospital's policy with patients presenting with psychiatric emergencies and that it had been followed. The hospital was under no legal obligation to provide in-depth psychiatric care merely because a patient might present with such an emergency. The key was that the hospital had a policy for screening and stabilizing such cases and followed that policy with each patient who presented with a psychiatric emergency.

Torres Nieves v. Hospital Metropolitano (1998) also held that transfer of a patient was appropriate. In this case, the patient was transferred to a public hospital for surgery after being stabilized at a private institution. The court ruled that the private institution did not have to perform surgery on a charity basis, since the patient was stable and could be transferred to a public hospital without deterioration of her condition during or as a result of the transfer. The opposite finding occurred in *Roberts v. Galen of Virginia, Inc.* (1999) when a patient was transferred prematurely to a skilled nursing home. Here, there was a violation of the EMTALA as the patient still needed care at an acute facility, and her medical condition was compromised as a result of the transfer. The court further noted that for a successful lawsuit, the patient did not need to show that the transfer was motivated by financial considerations, only that the transfer was inappropriate.

Each hospital, said the court in *Ingram v. Muskogee Regional Medical Center* (2000), has the right to set its own policy concerning its capabilities and the care it can reasonably provide to patients. As long as the institution then follows its own policies with each patient, there is no EMTALA violation.

GUIDELINES

Working in Managed Care Settings

1. Understand the impact of ERISA within health care settings; courts will evaluate whether the issues of a case concern employee welfare benefit plans or the quality of the medical and nursing care delivered to the patient. There is no protection under ERISA for less-than-quality, competent health care.

2. If you are involved in end-of-year profit sharing or any type of gag rules, remember that these incentives are means of limiting quality care and have been greatly discouraged by the court system and by selected state legislatures. Involvement in either incentive greatly increases your potential liability.

3. Know and maintain standards of care in all interactions with patients and their family members.

4. Understand that the main aspect of EMTALA is to ensure the same quality health care to all individuals, regardless of their ability to pay for that care. Patients must be seen and evaluated by appropriate staff and afforded all medical interventions and tests that another individual with the same diagnosis (or potential diagnosis) would receive in the medical facility. EMTALA does not mandate that institutions must have all medical services; it does mandate that if the service exists, all patients with like diagnoses must receive the same care.

5. Follow the established policies and procedures of the institution when treating patients. If a policy or procedure needs to be modified or updated, speak with the nursing supervisor or nurse-manager about the issue.

6. Ensure that the rights of patients are honored within the institution, including the right to informed consent and confidentiality. Report to the appropriate persons individuals who do not afford these rights to patients within your institution.

EXERCISE 18.7

Fred, a 21-year-old with severe chest pain and pneumonia-like symptoms, is brought to the urgent care clinic at your hospital. You are the nurse triaging patients in urgent care this evening. How would you proceed with Fred's care? What would you do if the urgent care clinic had no policies for care of this type of patient? Whom would you consult and what types of questions would you ask of the person you chose for consultation?

Assume that Fred was seen and stabilized at the hospital, then released to the care of his parents. Two days later, he is seen at the local health clinic for similar signs and symptoms. Five days later he is admitted with acute bacterial endocarditis at a regional medical center, where he subsequently dies. Does Fred's death change how you would have cared for Fred the first time he was seen in the urgent care clinic? How might the courts view such a case?

Aside from EMTALA rights, what ethical issues does Fred's case present? Which ethical principles did you decide were the most important to apply in this fact scenario?

Antitrust Issues in Managed Care

Health care delivery systems are becoming dominated by large, for-profit centers in most American cities today. Mergers and acquisitions, coupled with the integration of services and insurance, give greater market power to competitors and an opportunity to provide more competent care of patients.

With these mergers and large, for-profit centers come the questions about antitrust and monopolies in the health care industry. **Antitrust laws** contain specific restrictions for exclusive contracts, resisting utilization reviews, and collusion. Antitrust laws do not merely monitor the anti-competitive services of large corporations; they also regulate the practice of health care providers.

Historically, the move toward health care reform has been anchored by three broad promises:

1. Enhanced coordination of clinical services for all eligible enrollees
2. Reduced medical costs and wastes
3. Improved quality of care

The overall goal of America's antitrust laws is to promote competition while creating efficient markets. These antitrust laws apply to all settings and scenarios that limit competition. The laws are based on the premise that larger numbers of individuals and corporations will bring more efficient allocation of resources, improve quality of care, and increase innovation and technology, access, and services to all.

Until the landmark case of *Goldfarb v. Virginia State Bar* in 1975, health professionals were exempt from the antitrust laws due to their "learned profession" status. Since that lawsuit, extensive antitrust litigation has spurred significant changes in the health care delivery system. The Federal Trade Commission (FTC) vigorously challenged the merger of Hospital Corporation of America (HCA) with Hospital Affiliates International (HAI) and Health Care Corporation (HCC) as the possibility existed that such a merger would eliminate healthy sources of competition and make an already concentrated market more conducive to collusion (Furrow et al., 1997). Some of the more likely forms of collusion that could result from such a merger involve:

1. Collective resistance to emerging cost-containment pressures from third-party payers
2. Conspiracies to boycott certain insurance companies that offer competitive prices
3. Refusal to undergo utilization review programs or provide information needed by third-party payers

The court found that the merger violated specific sections of the Clayton Act and the FTC Act and ordered HCA to divest two of the hospitals it had acquired. Without such FTC action, the marketplace would have had fewer providers, and the reduced supply may have resulted in increased prices and a decreased quality of services (Furrow et al., 1997).

Lessons for nurses to be learned from antitrust laws and mergers in managed health care include the fact that such factors force nurses to become more valuable in the health care delivery system. For example, nurses must continue to closely examine the new organization's cost-containment measures to prevent the devaluation and compromise of the nursing profession. Reduction in licensed professionals and the silent replacement of registered nurses with unlicensed assistive personnel has forced nursing to examine continually the delivery of competent patient care and has emphasized the role of the professional nurse as patient advocate and patient educator. It has also emphasized the concept of delegation in health care settings, with the result that more efficient and effective nursing care is now being delivered to patients across the United States.

The inclusion of antitrust laws within the entire health care delivery system has also strengthened the use of mid-level practitioners in a variety of clinical settings, both acute care and community settings. This increased utilization of mid-level practitioners has primarily occurred among advanced practice nurses. When one considers the issues that will shape nursing in the future, including cost containment, improved patient outcomes, empowerment of consumers, and a realignment of the private-sector health care industry, it is not surprising that the use of all advanced practice nurses continues to rise in health care settings.

PATIENT RIGHTS

As managed care has continued its measures of cost containment, many health care providers have become increasingly concerned with issues of **patient rights.** Though some of the factors that caused such concerns are now eroding, such as the strict interpretation that consumers were barred from filing suits against HMOs under the ERISA laws, gag rules, end-of-year profit sharing, and patient "dumping" violations, many still fear that individuals have no true rights in managed care settings. Patients frequently cannot select their own practitioner, but must use the options available under the health care plan. They have no means of questioning who or what status of person will be caring for them. Morbidity rates, infection rates, and rates of complications are not published about individual health care practitioners or settings, and preapproval must be obtained for most health care treatments.

As a response to these issues, the president, the Congress, and individual state legislatures have been working on a variety of patient rights bills over the past several years. In 1997, President Clinton appointed the Advisory Commission on Consumer Protection and Quality in the Health Care Industry, charging it to "advise the President on changes occurring in the health care system and recommend measures as necessary to promote and assure health care quality and value, and protect consumers and workers in the health care system" (Advisory Commission on Consumer Protection, 1997, p. 1). Part of its charge was to draft a consumer bill of rights.

The commission adopted eight areas of consumer rights:

1. *Information disclosure.*   Consumers have the right to receive accurate, easily understood information, and some require assistance in making informed health care decisions about their health plans, professionals, and facilities.
2. *Choice of providers and plans.*   Consumers have the right to a choice of health care providers that is sufficient to ensure access to appropriate high-quality health care. Public and private group purchasers should, whenever feasible, offer consumers a choice of high-quality

health insurance products. Small employers should be provided with greater assistance in offering their workers and their families a choice of health plans and products.

3. *Access to emergency services.*   Consumers have the right to access emergency health care services when and where the need arises. Health plans should provide payment when a consumer presents to an emergency department with acute symptoms of sufficient severity, including severe pain, such that a "prudent layperson" could reasonably expect the absence of medical attention to result in placing that consumer's health in serious jeopardy, serious impairment to bodily function, or serious dysfunction of any bodily organ or part.

4. *Participation in treatment decisions.*   Consumers have the right and the responsibility to fully participate in all decisions related to their health care. Consumers who are unable to fully participate in treatment decisions have the right to be represented by parents, guardians, family members, or other conservators.

5. *Respect and nondiscrimination.*   Consumers have the right to considerate, respectful care from all members of the health care system at all times and under all circumstances. An environment of mutual respect is essential to maintain a quality health care system. Consumers must not be discriminated against in the delivery of health care services consistent with the benefits covered in their policy or as required by law based on race, ethnicity, national origin, religion, gender, age, mental or physical disability, sexual orientation, genetic information, or source of payment. Consumers who are eligible for coverage under the terms and conditions of a health plan or program or as required by law must not be discriminated against in marketing and enrollment practices based on the preceding discrimination factors.

6. *Confidentiality of health information.*   Consumers have the right to communicate with health care providers in confidence and to have the confidentiality of their individually identifiable health care information protected. Consumers also have the right to review and copy their own medical records and request amendments to their records.

7. *Complaints and appeals.*   All consumers have the right to a fair and efficient process for resolving differences with their health plans, health care providers, and the institutions that serve them, including a rigorous system of internal review and an independent system of external review.

8. *Consumer responsibilities.*   In a heath care system that protects consumers' rights, it is reasonable to expect and encourage consumers to assume reasonable responsibilities. Greater individual involvement by consumers in their care increases the likelihood of achieving the best outcomes and helps support a quality improvement, cost-conscious environment. Such responsibilities include taking responsibility for maximizing healthy habits, such as exercising, not smoking, and eating a healthy diet, becoming involved in specific health care decisions, and working collaboratively with health care providers in developing and carrying out agreed-upon treatment plans. (Advisory Committee on Consumer Protection, 1997, pp. 1–8)

These recommendations continue to be enforced, primarily through EMTALA and the enacted provisions of the Health Insurance Portability and Accountability Act of 1996 (HIPAA). The Health Care Financing Administration (HCFA) also enacted new standards for hospitals that participate in Medicare and Medicaid funding to ensure minimum protection of patients' rights. These standards, which took effect in 1999, include:

1. Notification of rights. This section includes informing patients about their rights in advance of furnishing or discontinuing patient care and the establishment of a grievance procedure for prompt resolution of patient grievances.

2. Exercise of rights in regard to care. This section allows the patient to participate in the development and implementation of the plan of care, and to make informed decisions about care issues. It also includes the right to formulate advanced directives.

3. Privacy and safety rights. Rights under this section include personal privacy, care in a safe setting, and freedom from all forms of abuse or harassment.

4. Confidentiality of records. This section includes the right to access the medical record.

5. Freedom from restraints that are not clinically necessary. Restraints are both chemical and physical, and the restraint can be used only if needed to improve the patient's well-being and less restrictive interventions have been determined to be ineffective. Restraint orders may not be written as a standing or "PRN" order.

6. Freedom from seclusion and restraints used in behavior management unless clinically necessary. This section allows the patient to be free from restraints imposed as a means of coercion, discipline, convenience, or retaliation by staff members. Hospitals must report to HCFA any death that occurs while a patient is restrained or in seclusion, or where it is reasonable to assume that a patient's death is the result of restraint or seclusion. (HCFA, 1999, pp. 36069–36089).

Congress continues to work on legislation that would more fully address patients' rights to information about health care providers, staff-to-patient ratios, staffing mix, and other factors that would potentially influence the consumer's choice of health care plans and health care providers. Although some states have already passed such legislation, there is currently no federal legislation that gives these rights to all persons in the United States. Several states have enacted legislation that supports some type of patient rights, though the protections provided by these enactments vary considerably.

EXERCISE 18.8

Draft a patients' bill of rights that would address all the issues you feel are ethically important in today's health care environment. If your state already has such a law, read it carefully for its completeness. What more should the bill contain? Review the voting records of major legislators in your state. Would they support such a bill? What would you need to do to assure the bill's passage? Is it ethical not to support a bill that is primarily designed to afford rights to all patients?

ETHICAL ISSUES IN AMBULATORY AND MANAGED HEALTH CARE

Telenursing and the ability of the nurse to reside in one area and serve patients in countless other areas present ethical issues in a variety of ways. One of the more obvious concerns involves the inability to assess the patient who uses the telephone for health care advice. The nurse responding to the patient is restrained by what the person communicates and is unable to better assess the person's actual health status because there is no visual contact. In the instance where there is visual contact via electronic media, the assessment is only as accurate as the transmission. If the nurse fails to appreciate the gravity of the situation or does not ask more probing questions, it is possible that vital symptoms and presenting signs can be missed and the patient can come to harm.

An additional question that arises with telenursing is the need for certification or additional credentialing for nurses practicing in this arena. Because the technologies used in telenursing are complex and ever evolving and the possibility that incorrect information may severely harm a patient or, in the case of obstetrical patients, more than one patient, the concern that nurses working in this arena must evidence additional knowledge will most likely continue. Telenursing holds tremendous possibilities for advancing the health of individuals, especially in remote areas, and the discipline should continue to work for its advancement, whether through additional education and credentialing or by promoting standards of care.

The issue of beneficence may also arise in instances where there are conflicting values, especially seen in the early days of the managed care models. Remembering that a major impetus in the creation of such models involved financial considerations, conflicts often arose between all levels of nursing, from the staff nurse to mid- and higher-level nursing management, and administration concerning the appropriate care of patients. These conflicts and what nurses often perceived as inadequate care management frequently lead to the moral distress that causes many nurses to question remaining in the profession. Though gag rules and end-of-year profit sharing have been outlawed in most states, these practices still exist in a minority of institutions.

Violence, whether it occurs in the workplace or involves nursing care of persons who have been victims or are perpetrators of the violent actions, triggers a variety of ethical concerns. Nurses may be faced with dilemmas when requested not to report violence, as the victim may be afraid that the reporting of the violence will cause further threats of violent actions in the future. The victim may also deny the violence, causing the nurse to question if it is better to report the obvious violent action or attempt to help the victim see that it is in his or her best interest to report the violence. Finally, nurses may be required to care for the perpetrator, respecting the person but not the actions of the person. For many nurses, caring for this person creates additional ethical issues.

SUMMARY

- Ambulatory nursing describes nursing care that is delivered in practice settings outside the traditional acute care and long-term care settings.
- Ambulatory nursing practice sites have steadily grown with the advent of managed care, which greatly increased the need for outpatient care services.
- Telenursing refers to the use of telecommunications and information technology for providing nursing services in health care.
- Violence in the workplace continues to escalate, and nurses frequently care for the victims, perpetrators, and witnesses of physical and psychological violence.
- Volunteer services arise when one agrees to care for a sick neighbor or a family member, and also includes donating health care advice.
- Managed care is a health care system that integrates the financing and delivery of health care services to covered individuals.
- Managed care includes four models: health maintenance organizations, preferred provider

organizations, point-of-service plans, and indemnity or fee-for-service plans.
- The Employment Retirement Income Security Act of 1974 (ERISA) has previously shielded health maintenance organizations from liability for questionable health care, but that has changed over the past several years, allowing successful lawsuits for poor medical decisions that have caused significant patient harm.
- Gag rules and end-of-year profit sharing have been outlawed in the majority of states.
- The Emergency Medical Treatment and Labor Act of 1986 (EMTALA) established a right of access to medical care regardless of one' ability to pay for that care.
- Patient rights under managed care have been carefully scrutinized because of the cost-containment measures underlying the delivery of health care in the managed care system.
- A variety of ethical issues arise in this area of nursing.

APPLY YOUR LEGAL KNOWLEDGE

1. How will the legal issues involved in telehealth continue to expand, and what can nursing as a profession do to address these potential issues?

2. Give three reasons why ambulatory nursing will expand as a practice arena in the next century, and what nursing must do to prepare for its expansion.

3. How can nursing as a profession affect the issue of domestic violence?

4. Why is accreditation an important concept for HMOs? How does accreditation protect consumers?

5. What additional provisions might be included in ERISA that will begin to address the concept that health maintenance organizations must be accountable for actions and decisions that cause significant harm to health care consumers?

6. How do you think patient rights will continue to expand in the next century?

YOU BE THE JUDGE

Mr. Gonzales was admitted to a surgical center for a routine colonoscopy during which three polyps were removed. The procedure began at 11:00 A.M. and he was released at 12:30 P.M. The patient began experiencing abdominal pain the following day. He tried to phone the attending physician at 2:00 P.M. and later called the physician's nurse at 5:00 P.M. Mr. Gonzales told the nurse he was experiencing severe abdominal pain and that he was flushed and felt he had a fever. The nurse told Mr. Gonzales that everyone had gone home for the day, and she advised him to take aspirin for the fever and call back in the morning.

Mrs. Gonzales drove her husband to the hospital the following morning at 10:00 A.M. He was placed on antibiotics, which did not resolve the problem, and he had surgery on the fifth day following the original colonoscopy. At that time, it was determined that the patient's intestine was perforated at the time of the polyp removal, and Mr. Gonzales now has a permanent colostomy. The patient has now filed a lawsuit against the nurse and physician for malpractice.

QUESTIONS

1. Was the nurse negligent in the advice she gave Mr. Gonzales concerning his condition?

2. Did the nurse exceed her scope of practice in the advice she gave the patient?

3. Should the nurse have instructed Mr. Gonzales to go immediately to the local emergency center?

4. How would you decide this case? Who, if anyone, is liable in this case?

REFERENCES

Advisory Commission on Consumer Protection and Quality in the Health Care Industry. (1997). *Consumer bill of rights and responsibilities: Report to the president of the United States.* Washington, DC: U.S. Government Printing Office.

Alejandre v. Kaiser Foundation Hospitals, 2007 WL 816773 (Medical Malpractice Arbitration, Cal., January 27, 2007).

American Academy of Ambulatory Care Nurses. (2004). About AAACN. Retrieved from http://aaacn .org/cgi.bin

American Association of Colleges of Nursing. (2005). *Position statement: Violence as a public health problem:*

Suggested leveling for selected competencies. Washington, DC: Author.

American Institute on Domestic Violence. (2008). *Domestic violence statistics.* Ruidoso, NM: Author.

American Nurses Association. (1998). *Culturally competent assessment for family violence.* Washington, DC: Author.

Baker v. Adventist Health, Inc., 260 F.3d 987 (9th Cir., 2001).

Berg v. Shapiro, 36 P.3d 109 (Colo. App., 2001).

Bowden v. Walmart Stores, Inc., 124 F. Supp.2d 1228 (M.D. Ala., 2000).

Brenord v. Catholic Medical Center, 133 F. Supp.2d 179 (E.D. N.Y., 2001).

Brodersen v. Sioux Valley Memorial Hospital, 902 F. Supp. 931 (N.D. Iowa, 1995).

Bryant v. Archbold Memorial Hospital, 2006 WL 1517074 (M. D. Ga., May 23, 2006).

Bureau of Labor Statistics. (2006). *National census of fatal occupational injuries.* Washington, DC: United States Department of Labor.

Centers for Medicare and Medicaid Services. (2003, January 24). Quality assessment: New CMS regulations for hospitals. *Federal Register,* 3435–3455.

Cherukuri v. Shalala, Secretary of the Department of Health and Human Services, 175 F.3d 446 (6th Cir., 1999).

CIGNA Healthcare of Texas, Inc. v. Pybas, 2004 WL 253941 (Tex. App., February 12, 2004).

"C. M." v. Tomball Regional Hospital, 961 S.W.2d 236 (Tex. App., 1997).

Eberhardt v. City of Los Angeles, 62 F.3d 1253 (9th Cir., 1995).

Emergency Medical Treatment and Labor Act of 1986. Public Law 99-272, 42 *United States Code.* Section 1359dd (April 7, 1986).

Emergency Medical Treatment and Labor Act: 2008 Amendments. (2008, October 1). *Federal Register,* 48657–48658.

Employment Retirement Income Security Act of 1974. Public Law 93-406, 88 *Statutes* 829 (September 2, 1974).

EMTALA: New Regulations for Hospital Emergency Department Policies and Procedures. (2003, September 9). *Federal Register,* 53221–53264.

Ethics in Patient Referral Act. Public Law 101-239, 103 *Statutes* 2106 (December 19, 1989).

Fischer v. New York Health and Hospitals Corporation, 989 F. Supp. 444 (E.D. N.Y., 1998).

Fox v. Health Net, No. 216992 (Riverside County Superior Court 1994).

Furrow, B., et al. (1997). *Health law: Cases, materials, and problems* (3rd ed.). St. Paul, MN: West Publishing.

Godwin v. Memorial Medical Center, 25 P.3d 273 (N.M. App. 2001).

Goldfarb v. Virginia State Bar, 421 U.S. 773, 95 S. Ct. 2004, 44 L. Ed.2d 572 (1975).

Hand v. Tavera, No. 04–92–00618CV (4th Cir., September 22, 1993).

Havard v. Children's Clinic of Southwestern Louisiana, Inc., 722 So.2d 1178 (La. App., 1998).

Health Care Financing Administration. (1999, July 2). Patient rights: Major new conditions for participation in Medicare and Medicaid. *Federal Register,* 36069–36089.

Health Care Quality Improvement Act of 1986. Public Law 99-660, 100 *Statutes* 3743. (November 14, 1986).

Health Insurance Portability and Accountability Act of 1996. Public Law 104-191, 110 *Statutes* 1936 (1996).

Henderson v. Medical Center Enterprise, 2006 WL 2355467 (M. D. Ala., August 14, 2006).

Ingram v. Muskogee Regional Medical Center, 235 F.3d 550 (10th Cir., 2000).

Johnson v. Health Central Hospital, 2006 WL 709320 (M. D. Fla., March 20, 2006); 2006 WL 3473741 (11th Cir., November 20, 2006).

Johnson v. Nacogdoches County Hospital, 2003 WL 21999408 (Tex. App., August 20, 2003).

Johnson v. University of Chicago, 982 F.2d 230 (7th Cir., 1990).

Kilroy v. Star Valley Medical Center, 2002 WL 31845956 (D. Wyo., December 18, 2002).

Krasny v. Waser, 147 F. Supp.2d 1300 (M.D. Fla., 2001).

Land v. CIGNA Healthcare of Florida, 2003 WL 21751247 (11th Cir., July 30, 2003).

Lazorko v. Pennsylvania Hospital, 237 F. 242 (3rd Cir., 2000).

Lunsford v. Board of Nurse Examiners, 648 S.W.2d 391 (Tex. Civ. App., Austin 1983).

Marshall v. East Carroll Parish Hospital Service District, 134 F.3d 319 (5th Cir., 1998).

McCrystal v. Trumbull Memorial Hospital, 684 N.E.2d 721 (Ohio App., 1996).

McEvoy v. Group Health Cooperative of Eau Claire, 570 N.W.2d 397 (Wisconsin, 1997).

McGill v. Newark Surgery Center, 756 N.E.2d 762 (Ohio Com. Pl., 2001).

Moreno v. Health Partners Health Plan, 4 F. Supp.2d 888 (D. Ariz., 1998).

Morrison v. Colorado Permanente Medical Group, 983 F. Supp. 937 (D. Colo., 1997).

Nalder v. West Park Hospital, 254 F.3d 1168 (10th Cir., 2001).

Nold v. Binyon, 31 P.3d 274 (Kansas, 2001).

Norwicki, C., & Haas, S. (2003). Ambulatory care nursing conceptual framework. *Viewpoint, 25*(3), 14.

Office of Personnel Management. Prohibition of "gag clauses" in Federal Employee Health Benefit Program. 48 *Code of Federal Regulations,* Part 1609 (1998).

Parker v. Salina Regional Health Center, Inc., 2006 WL 3488765 (D. Kan., December 1, 2006).

Prickett v. HSC Medical Center, 2997 WL 2928662 (W. D. Ark., October 5, 2007).

Rios v. Baptist Memorial Hospital System, 935 S.W.2d 799 (Tex. App., 1996).

Roberts v. Galen of Virginia, Inc., 119 S. Ct. 685, 142 L. Ed. 648 (1999).

Scott v. Dauterive Hospital Corporation, 2003 WL 1916273 (La. App., April 23, 2003).

Shannon v. McNulty, 718 A.2d 828 (Pa. Super., 1998).

Snider v. Basilio, 2005 WL 2715854 (Ga. App., October 24, 2005).

Spillman v. Southwest Louisiana Hospital Association, 2007 WL 1068489 (W. D. La., April 4, 2007).

Starkey v. St. Rita's Medical Center, 690 N.E.2d 57 (Ohio App., 1997).

Subpoena Duces Tecum to Jane Doe, Esq., 2003 N.Y. Slip Op. 11299, 2003 WL 4419990 (N.Y. App., February 25, 2003).

Torres Nieves v. Hospital Metropolitano, 998 F. Supp. 127 (D. Puerto Rico, 1998).

Torres Otero v. Hospital General Menonita, 115 F. Supp.2d 253 (D. Puerto Rico, 2000).

Trivette v. North Carolina Baptist Hospital, 507 S.E.2d 48 (N.C. App., 1998).

U.S. Department of Health and Human Services. (2000). *Healthy people 2010: Understanding and improving health.* Washington, DC: Author.

Van Burgen v. Long Beach Medical Center, 717 N. Y. S.2d 191 (N. Y. App., 2000).

Welsh v. Galen of Virginia, Inc., 71 S.W.3d 105 (Ky. App., 2001).

Williamson v. Roth, 120 F. Supp.2d 1327 (M.D. Fla., 2000).

CHAPTER 19

Public and Community Health Care

PREVIEW

As nursing emerged beyond the more traditional acute care setting, new and innovative opportunities opened for professional nursing in a variety of public and community health settings, including parish nursing, school health nursing, occupational nursing, home health nursing, and nursing in correctional settings. Although hospice care nursing may be covered within the auspices of community health nursing, nursing in this health care setting is incorporated into the last chapter of this text. All public and community health care settings offer new and exciting roles for nurses, including more autonomous roles, and all have potential liability for the nurses practicing in the roles. This chapter presents potential legal liability for nurses who are employed in public and community health settings.

LEARNING OUTCOMES
After completing this chapter, you should be able to:

19.1 Briefly describe the historical beginnings of public and community health nursing.

19.2 Describe the various settings in which public and community health nurse are employed, including:

Home health care nurses

Parish nurses
School health nurses
Occupational health nurses
Correctional nurses
Disaster nursing

19.3 Describe ethical issues that are involved in public and community health nursing.

KEY TERMS

abandonment
agency policies
community and public health nurses
correctional nursing

disaster nursing
home health care nursing
occupational health nursing
parish nursing

Public Health Service Act of 1944
refusal of care
school health nursing
Social Security Act of 1935

OVERVIEW OF PUBLIC AND COMMUNITY HEALTH NURSING

Confusion over the title for nurses who focus primarily on the prevention of illness and the promotion of health in nonacute populations has led to the debate regarding public and community health nursing (Lundy & Janes, 2009). *Community health nursing* had been the preferred title for some years, though *public health nursing* has reemerged as the preferred title for nurses who work with the entire public population to improve its health. The primary purpose of either public or community health nursing is to promote and maintain the health of communities, families, and individuals in nonacute care settings. Actions undertaken to promote and maintain the health of the public at large has a basis in law and is subject to legal sanctions of one type or another. Perhaps the best starting point for understanding these legal concepts in community health nursing is to have an appreciation for the federal and state laws affecting community health nursing.

FEDERAL STATUTES

Few pieces of legislation have affected the country's health and welfare systems as have the Social Security Act of 1935 and the Public Health Service Act of 1944, with their respective amendments.

Social Security Act of 1935

The **Social Security Act of 1935** was signed into legislation by President Franklin D. Roosevelt, as a direct result of the Great Depression of 1929. The act was based on European health and welfare practices, and many of its roots can be traced back to early European poverty laws.

The Social Security Act of 1935 provided for the general welfare by establishing a system of federal benefits for the aged population and by enabling states to make provisions for aged persons, blind persons, dependent and crippled children, maternal and child welfare, public health, and administration of state unemployment compensation laws. Programs were defined as *contributory,* financed through taxation and individual contributions, and *assistance* or *noncontributory,* financed only through taxation. Historically, contributory programs have offered more comprehensive benefits than assistive programs.

The act has been amended numerous times since its enactment, with the addition of Medicare and Medicaid in 1965 being one of the most important additions. The act affects the services that nursing provides to its clients. Through Medicare-reimbursable services, regulations specify which clients nurses see, what type of care is provided, how the care is provided, and how long the care is provided. Medicare benefits have changed greatly since their enactment; some of the more recent provisions include the addition of alcohol detoxification facility benefits in 1980, hospice reimbursements in 1983, and a 1990 amendment allowing Medicare Part B premiums to be paid for eligible beneficiaries.

Public Health Service Act of 1944

The **Public Health Service Act of 1944** consolidated all existing public health legislation under one law and became the major piece of health legislation for the country. This piece of legislation, through the original act and its amendments, provides a variety of resources and services, including the National Institutes of Health; nursing training acts; traineeships for graduate students in a variety of nursing specializations; health services for migratory workers; family planning services; health research facilities; and programs and services for the prevention and control of heart disease, cancer, stroke, kidney disease, sudden infant death syndrome, sickle cell anemia, and diabetes. These services are administered by several federal and state agencies.

Implications of this broad and comprehensive act are extensive with regard to nursing. It provides funding for services to at-risk aggregates in the community, such as migratory workers; persons with acquired immune deficiency syndrome (AIDS), tuberculosis, and other communicable diseases; and programs for persons with chronic problems, such as heart disease, stroke, kidney disease, and diabetes. This act financially covers at least some aspects of nursing in all acute care, home health care, and institutional settings. It provides funding for nursing education and funding for all levels of disease prevention: primary, secondary, and tertiary.

The amendments to this act have brought about numerous changes over the years since its enactment. There are now block grants to states, allowing the individual states to decide which programs are most needed in their territories, and monies remain available for specific programs such as immunizations, family planning, and venereal disease programs.

LEGAL RESPONSIBILITIES

Serving in a variety of settings, **community and public health nurses** care for persons in need of their services in clinics, schools, individual homes, and the workplace. Many of the legal responsibilities of these nurses are slightly different, depending on the setting. For ease of understanding, the various nurses working in these multiple settings are discussed separately.

Public and Community Health Nursing

Public and commuity health nursing dates back to the turn of the last century in the United States, though historians date the beginnings of these specialties in nursing to the Egyptians and Greeks. Early leaders of public health in the United States were such women as Lillian Wald, who is credited with creating the title "public health nurse," Dorothea Dix, who led the fight for competent nursing in prisons and mental health institutions, and Mary Breckenridge, who founded the Frontier Nursing Service, the first organized midwifery service in the United States (Lundy & Janes, 2009).

Public or community health nursing is a systematic process by which the health care needs of a population are assessed in order to identify subpopulations, families and individuals who would benefit from health promotion or are at risk of illness, injury, disability, or premature death. A plan for intervention is then developed with the community to meet identified needs. The plan takes into account available resources and the range of activities that contribute to health and the prevention of illness injury, disability, or premature death. The plan is then implemented effectively, efficiently, and equitably. Evaluations are conducted after the plan has been implemented to determine the extent to which the interventions have had an impact on the health status of individuals and the community. The results of the entire process are used to influence and direct the delivery of care, deployment of health resources, and development of local, regional, state, and national health policy and research to promote health and prevent disease.

Services provided by public and community health nurses include the monitoring of health status, disease case identification, community education, community organization, policy development, health regulation enforcement, participation in organized education sessions, evaluation of the effectiveness of programs as implemented, and participation in research. These services are provided to accomplish the goal of public health nursing, which is to improve the health of the public as a whole by systematically providing appropriate nursing interventions to communities, families, and individuals. These services are provided through the multiple roles of public and community health nurses. Some of these roles are depicted in the sections that follow.

Home Health Care

One of the fastest growing fields of nursing today, **home health care nursing** refers to the delivery of health services for the purposes of restoring or maintaining the health of individuals and families in the home. These services cover a broad range, including skilled professional and paraprofessional services, custodial care, pharmacy services, and delivery and use of durable medical equipment, such as ventilators, enteral feeding pumps, and oxygen concentrators. To be covered by either private insurance or public assistance, the services must be medically indicated, ordered by a qualified health care provider, and necessary to maintain or improve the health care of the recipient. Traditionally, home health care services are provided on a visit basis rather than on an hourly basis. A variety of personnel may be involved in delivering these services, including all levels of nurses. The most commonly seen diagnoses for patients cared for in the home include diabetes, essential hypertension, heart failure, chronic ulcers, and osteoarthritis (National Association for Home Care and Hospice [NAHCH], 2008). In 2008 there were more than 9,000 Medicare-certified home health care agencies in the United States, serving more than 3,000,000 beneficiaries (Centers for Medicare and Medicaid Services, 2009).

Home health care nursing emerged as a key component of health care delivery in the 1990s, serving as a facilitator by providing support, treatment, and education so that patients may be successfully managed in their homes. These nurses provide care that ranges from assistance with activities of daily living to complex, highly technical nursing skills. Examples of activities provided by these nurses include acute, continuing, preventative, and palliative care, which reduces admission or readmission to acute care settings or long-term care settings and allows the person to remain in his or her home.

Federal legislation sets requirements for all home health care nurses. The 1987 provisions to the Omnibus Budget Reconciliation Act of 1986 substantially changed the federal law relating to participation of home health care agencies in the Medicare program. Clients must be screened for eligibility, and the signatures of clients must be witnessed after client rights and legal contracts for service have been explained to them. Important provisions of the statute include an extensive listing of consumer rights, including the right to be fully informed in advance about the care and treatment to be provided by the agency, to be fully informed in advance of any changes in the care or treatment to be provided by the agency that may affect the individual's well-being, and to participate in planning care and treatment or changes in care or treatment. The act also enumerates the right of individuals to confidentiality of clinical records, the right to have one's property treated with respect, and the establishment of a grievance hotline to be established by each state.

A separate provision under this act sets strict criteria of qualifications for home health care aides who have a predominant role in direct, hands-on contact with clients. Under this provision, the agency may not use any individual who is not a licensed health care professional, unless the individual has successfully completed a training and competency evaluation program that meets minimum federal standards and the individual is actually competent to provide the services assigned.

Amendments were also made to the Older Americans Act (1987) that directly affects home health care agencies. These amendments were intended to develop demonstration projects to strengthen home care consumer protection mechanisms, such as rights of people with developmental disabilities. Many of these demonstration projects were successful, and regulations concerning home health care consumer protection and corresponding provider obligations have been incorporated into more recent amendments to the original act, with the most current amendment in 2008.

Other federal legislation affecting home health care delivery of services includes the Patient Self-Determination Act of 1990. Under this regulation, agencies that receive federal funds, including home health agencies, must inquire whether patients being admitted for their services have executed a living will and/or special directive such as a durable power of attorney for health care. If the patient has such a document, then the agency is obligated to abide by its provisions. If there is no such directive and the patient so desires to complete a directive, the agency must provide guidance on completing such directives.

Additional legislation that took effect in 1999 applies to home health care agencies that participate in the Medicare program. Specifically, this rule requires that each patient receive from the home health agency a patient-specific, comprehensive assessment that identifies the patient's need for home health care and meets the patient's medical, nursing, rehabilitative, social, and discharge planning needs. In addition, the final rule requires that as part of the comprehensive assessment, home health agencies use a standard core assessment data set, the Outcome and Assessment Information Set (OASIS), when evaluating adult, nonmaternity patients (*Federal Register,* 1999). These changes are an integral part of efforts to achieve broad-based quality improvements through federal programs and in the measurement of that care.

The data required to be collected on the OASIS include:

1. Clinical record items
2. Demographics and patient history
3. Living arrangements
4. Supportive assistance
5. Sensory status
6. Integumentary status
7. Activities of daily living
8. Medications
9. Equipment management
10. Emergent care
11. Data items collected at inpatient facility admission or discharge only (Section 484.55)

These data sets were again updated in 2005 to include the provision that encoding and transmission of these data sets must be done electronically to the state agency or other appropriate Center for Medicare and Medicaid Services OASIS contractor in accordance with the federal reporting mandates (Electronic Submission of OASIS, 2005).

Under these standards, the home health agency must continue to comply with physicians' orders. Verbal orders must be transferred into a written format, signed, and dated with the receipt of the registered nurse or qualified therapist responsible for furnishing or supervising the ordered services. Verbal orders are accepted only by personnel authorized to do so by applicable state and federal laws and regulations as well as by the home health agency's internal policies (Section 484.18).

The initial assessment visit must be conducted by a registered nurse to determine the immediate care and support needs of the patient and to determine eligibility for Medicare home health benefits, including homebound status, if the patient qualifies for Medicare. The initial assessment visit must be within 48 hours of referral, within 48 hours of the patient's return home, or on the physician-ordered start-of-care date. If the only ordered service is rehabilitative therapy service (speech/language pathology, physical therapy, or occupational therapy), the initial assessment service may be performed by the appropriate skilled rehabilitation professional (Section 484.55).

The comprehensive assessment must be completed within 5 days after the start of care. The comprehensive assessment must include a review of all medications the patient is currently using to identify any potential adverse effects and drug reactions, including ineffective drug therapy, significant side effects, significant drug interactions, duplicate drug therapy, and noncompliance with drug therapy (Section 484.55).

The comprehensive assessment must be updated and revised as frequently as the patient's condition warrants due to a major decline or improvement of the patient's health status, but not less frequently than:

1. Every second calendar month beginning with the start-of-care date
2. Within 48 hours of a patient's return to home from a hospital admission of 24 hours or more for any reason other than diagnostic tests
3. At discharge (Section 484.55)

A second part of this rule requires electronic reporting of data from the OASIS as a condition of participation for home health agencies. Specifically, this rule provides guidelines for the electronic transmission of the OASIS data set as well as responsibilities of the state agency or Health Care Financing Administration (HCFA) OASIS contractor in collecting and transmitting this information to HCFA. The final rules set forth mandates concerning the privacy of patient-identifiable information generated by the OASIS (Sections 484.11 and 484.20).

Finally, federal law also requires that all individuals receiving home care services be informed of their rights. Table 19.1 enumerates a model patient bill of rights based on the patient rights currently enforced by law.

State Legislation

State laws encompass a variety of issues that may arise within home health care settings. Nurses working in these settings are advised to explore individual state law in such areas as protection of uninsured persons, abused persons, or homeless persons; rights of renters or tenants; and laws that protect individuals from eviction under certain circumstances. All caregivers should be aware of the state abuse laws, knowing how and when to report suspected abuse. (Elder abuse is covered in more detail in Chapter 20.) Family law issues, such as the right to decide for another, rights of guardians, and consent to perform procedures on minors or incompetent persons, also vary from state to state.

Standing Orders

Because of the relative isolation of home health care, nurses should have written standing orders in case of emergencies or unexpected needs of clients. Such standing orders complement verbal orders, and both types of orders should be clarified when used by the home health care nurse. Standing orders should be reviewed and updated on a regular basis and must be signed by the attending physician(s) before being implemented. Some agencies prefer protocols that are jointly written by nursing and medicine. Both standing orders and protocols must be specific about their implementation and approval by agency physicians.

If verbal orders are used, the home health care nurse should document the orders and have the physician co-sign them as soon as practical. If a patient was injured when the nurse relied on a verbal order and no written documentation of the order is evident, the nurse may have difficulty in demonstrating that the physician's order was accurately followed. The agency should develop a plan by which verbal orders are to be co-signed, such as a system to mail the order to the

TABLE 19.1   Model Patient Bill of Rights

Home health care patients have the right to:

- Be fully informed by the home care agency of all rights and responsibilities.
- Choose care providers.
- Receive appropriate and professional care in accordance with physician orders.
- Receive a timely response from the agency to requests for service.
- Be admitted for service only if the agency has the ability to provide safe, professional care at the level of intensity needed.
- Receive reasonable continuity of care.
- Receive information necessary to give informed consent prior to the start of any treatment or procedure.
- Be advised of any change in the plan of care, before the change is made.
- Refuse treatment within the confines of the law and be informed of the consequences of that action.
- Be informed of rights under state law to formulate advance directives.
- Have health care providers comply with advance directives in accordance with state law requirements.
- Be informed within a reasonable time of anticipated termination of service or plans for transfer to another agency.
- Be fully informed of agency policies and charges for services, including eligibility for third-party reimbursements.
- Be referred elsewhere, if denied service solely on inability to pay.
- Voice grievances and suggest changes in service or staff without fear of restraint or discrimination.
- Receive a fair hearing for any individual to whom any service has been denied, reduced, or terminated, or who is otherwise aggrieved by agency action. The fair hearing procedure shall be set forth by each agency as appropriate to the unique patient situation (i.e., funding source, level of care, diagnosis).
- Be informed of what to do in the event of an emergency.
- Be advised of the telephone number and hours of operation of the state's home health hotline that receives questions and complaints about Medicare-certified and state-licensed home care agencies.

physician and have the physician mail the signed order back to the agency for inclusion in the client record.

Contract Law

Home health nurses must honor contracts made with clients. Contracts include both written and oral agreements of understanding between the agency and the receiver of health care services. Contracts made with clients include the advertised services included in agency brochures and advertisements as well as formal contracts signed by clients and agency staff. Provisions that should be included in all contracts include:

1. Provider's and client's respective roles and responsibilities
2. Length, type, frequency, and limitations of services
3. Cost and payment schedules
4. Provisions for informed client or surrogate consent for specific interventions on an initial and continuing basis

EXERCISE 19.1

You are a home health care nurse and have been assigned to assess a family's potential health care needs. A school health nurse recently referred the family to your agency. Mrs. A. is a 68-year-old grandmother caring for the three children of her youngest daughter: a 5-year-old boy and twin girls who are 6. The family lives in a one-story, one-bedroom home. The twins attend an elementary school about six blocks away; their brother also attends this school during the morning hours. The children's mother and father have both deserted their children; Mrs. A. has not heard from her daughter for about 2 years and the son-in-law has been gone for more than 4 years. Mrs. A. has not formally adopted the children.

Mrs. A. has insulin-dependent diabetes and is currently being treated for severe hypertension. She receives Social Security benefits and has applied for additional benefits for the care of her grandchildren. The school health nurse recently screened the 5-year-old child, and Mrs. A. was notified that he has a hearing loss and will need glasses for his impaired vision. The school nurse also notified the agency that she is concerned about the health and care of all three children because they have been coming to school hungry and in soiled clothing.

What state and federal laws provide guidance for the health care worker in assessing this family? Where would you find out about applicable laws? Speak with a home health nurse about applicable laws once you have decided which laws fit this case scenario. Were you surprised at the number of laws applicable to this one family group?

Be careful of promises that one may not be able to meet, such as a provision in a brochure ensuring that clients will be evaluated within 12 hours of contacting the agency.

All of the agency's legal duties to the client stem from the legal relationship formed between the two parties. Thus, the referral as well as the initial evaluation periods are crucial. Medicare and Joint Commission (JC) standards require that a home health care agency accept clients based on a reasonable expectation that the patient's medical, nursing, and social needs can be adequately met by the agency in the client's residence. New referrals must be carefully evaluated from a referring physician aspect and a nursing aspect to ensure that:

1. The client is medically stable or that a medically unstable condition, as with the dying client, can be managed.
2. There is a desire for home care.
3. The needs of the client can be safely and effectively met by the home care agency.
4. Satisfactory financial arrangements can be made.

Any deficiencies or inability to provide adequate care should be discussed with both the physician and potential client before entering a contract. Client education and informed consent issues as well as client options and other available resources and services should be discussed and agreed upon before entering the contract.

At the initiation of the contract, clients should be instructed about the availability of 24-hour staffing, how to contact staff at other-than-routine office hours, and reasons when such 24-hour staff may be needed. Agencies are advised to have written guidelines on the appropriate use of 24-hour staffing and financial responsibilities of the client if such 24-hour staffing is used.

Clients may be transferred or their care terminated by the agency after a formal contract is entered. Before transferring the care of the client, a discussion about the advantages and disadvantages should be conducted between the client and agency. Issues such as adverse physical and mental reactions to the transfer must be considered as well as better or more acceptable levels of care by the transferring agency.

Contracts may also help protect the home health care agency. *Rovaldi v. Courtemanche* (2005) illustrates this statement. After she was discharged from the hospital in frail health due to a fractured hip, the patient signed a contract to receive in-home care from a visiting nurse association. The contract gave express permission to the association "for authorized personnel of the association to perform all necessary procedures and treatments as prescribed by [her] physician for the delivery of home health care."

The visiting nurse who was assigned to care for this patient needed to visit the patient on a weekend. On Friday, the patient's medication had been changed. Also, the nurse understood that the patient's son who normally lived with her would be out of town that weekend, leaving the patient alone at home. When the nurse phoned the patient, there was no answer. The next day the nurse again phoned and again there was no answer. She then went to the patient's home, knocked several times on the front and back doors and received no response. At the time of the court case, the nurse noted that she thought she had heard someone moaning inside the house when she knocked on the back door.

The nurse phoned her supervisor, then called the police. The police had the fire department come and remove the back door so that they could enter the house. The nurse, police, and fire department personnel entered the house and found the patient in a satisfactory condition, albeit very upset at the way they had entered the house. The patient's son sued the visiting nurse association for civil trespass. The case was dismissed by the court.

The law defines civil trespass as entry into the property of another without authorization or consent. The court found that the admission contract that the patient had signed gave the visiting nurse authorization and consent to take all reasonable and necessary steps to protect the patient's safety and health. Under the circumstances, the police and fire department also acted properly in what appeared to be an emergency, based on what the nurse had told them about the situation. The court also pondered what legal repercussions might have occurred if the nurse has ignored the signs of danger and the patient was lying injured inside her home.

Health care providers need to understand and avoid **abandonment** of the client, defined as the unilateral termination of the professional relationship without affording the client reasonable notice and health care services. Two cases illustrate a home health agency's commitment to clients.

In *Winkler v. Interim Services, Inc.* (1999), a lawsuit was filed against the home health agency by several elderly and disabled Medicare beneficiaries who had been receiving home health services. The lawsuit alleged that the clients were essentially "dumped" and abandoned as a result of recent changes to Medicare reimbursement rules. They alleged that the agency's refusal to continue to provide medically necessary home health care services was based on the simple fact that the clients were all heavy service users and thus economically undesirable to the agency.

The court found that these clients were terminated when the new reimbursement rules went into effect without any evaluation, assessment, or documentation that they no longer needed home health services. A home health agency cannot discriminate against Medicare patients who are heavy users of services and are thus economically less desirable. A federal law, the Rehabilitation Act of 1973, gives handicapped persons the right to sue if they are excluded from participation, denied benefits, or subjected to discrimination with respect to any program that receives assistance from the federal government. A federally funded program that serves the less handicapped while failing to accommodate more severely handicapped persons is operating in an illegal discriminatory manner.

The court also noted in its finding that the home health agency had a contract with the patients to provide services. Thus, the court said, the agency had no legal right arbitrarily and unilaterally to suspend its own obligations under the contract simply because it was no longer profitable.

Morris v. North Hawaii Community Hospital (1999) involved a patient who was notified by his home health agency that his services were being terminated. He, too, claimed that his service termination was motivated by financial considerations. Caps per patient Medicare home health benefits were part of the Balanced Budget Act of 1997. The ostensible reason given to the patient in this case for his discharge was that he was no longer "homebound" and thus not eligible for Medicare home health benefits.

The court noted that an individual is considered to be confined to the home if the individual has a condition due to illness or injury that restricts ability to leave his or her home without the assistance of another individual or the aid of a supportive device, such as crutches, a cane, a wheelchair, or a walker, or if the individual has a condition that makes leaving home medically contraindicated. Although an individual does not have to be bedridden to be considered confined to his or her home, the person's condition should be such that there exists a normal inability to leave home, that leaving home requires considerable and taxing effort, and that absences from home are infrequent or of relatively short duration or are attributable to the need to receive medical treatment.

The court then redefined *homebound,* based on the condition and care of this patient. He was a 40-year-old quadriplegic who used a motorized wheelchair as the result of an automobile accident. Though he was occasionally seen out of the home, he still qualified as a homebound patient given the following facts:

1. He could not leave his bed or home without the aid of at least one other individual, and it required considerable and taxing effort to transfer him from his bed to the wheelchair.
2. He could not leave his home without the use of a wheelchair. Leaving home required at least 1 1/2 hours of preparation, even for a visit to his physician.
3. His absences from home were infrequent and of relatively short duration, usually for the purpose of physician visits at the clinic or office.

A final case illustrates the vital need for home health care providers to ensure that they comply with the contracted services. In *Villarin v. Onobanjo* (2000), a home health care aide left the patient's home during the last hour of the home health care aide's shift. The patient was severely disabled and bedridden; he lived in a rented house with his extended family. A home health care aide was to stay with him at all times when family members were not present.

After the home health care aide left and before the client's 17-year-old stepdaughter arrived at the home, a fire started in the home. When the stepdaughter arrived at the residence, she rushed in the house in an attempt to save her stepfather. Both she and the patient perished in the fire.

The court concluded that the home health care aide was at fault for abandoning the patient during the final hour of the aide's shift. The court further concluded that, because the aide was liable for abandonment, the agency was likewise liable to the patient's family for the two deaths. Though the court conceded that the patient might still have perished in the fire, the aide could have "prevented or detected the fire, called the fire department, and/or saved the patient" (*Villarin v. Onobanjo,* 2000, at 94).

Remember, though, that a contract involves at least two parties and that both parties have roles and responsibilities. Agencies do not have perpetual, ongoing responsibilities to provide services in the absence of compensation, nor do agencies need to continue to provide care if the safety of the agency staff is threatened. To avoid liability for client abandonment or dumping, the agency must develop and implement a satisfactory discharge program. Discharge planning should be started with the initial evaluation of the client, and clients should be involved in the plan throughout their care. Potential clients should be made aware of this discharge program before a formal contract is signed.

GUIDELINES

Home Health Care Nursing

1. Know areas of the law that pertain to home health care nursing, including federal and state laws, and adhere to the mandates of those laws. Request the agency to provide a continuing education program to ensure that all nurses in the agency are knowledgeable about laws affecting home health care nursing.
2. Practice within the scope of nursing practice. If in doubt, request that the agency clarify the issue before proceeding with the treatment or procedure in question.
3. Obtain permission (consent) before caring for clients in the home. This means being able to discuss with patients or their families the risks and benefits of the proposed procedure or intervention before initiation of the intervention.
4. Honor patients' right to refuse care, if that is their wish. If the patient has a living will or other advance directive, honor that document. The patient in the home has the same rights as hospitalized patients to know about such advance directives and to implement such directives. If the patient refuses care, make sure that refusal is communicated to all members of the health care team.
5. Respect the patient's privacy rights, including confidentiality in the nurse–patient relationship. Release forms must be used if patient information is to be given to other health care agencies or health care providers.
6. Follow standing orders and protocols, particularly in times of emergencies or changes in the patient's status. Verbal orders may be secured as needed, and then signed by the physician as per agency protocol.
7. Client education is one of the responsibilities of the home health care nurse. Answer questions as much as possible and tell patients that you will find out needed information and get back to them. Remember, you are most likely the patient's sole reference in health matters and it is vital that you give correct information.
8. Follow agency policies and initiate change in policies as needed.
9. Document all pertinent information, patient condition, and information concerning teaching and referrals you may have made. As with other health care settings, the one way to show and remember what was done is through effective and timely documentation.
10. Delegate wisely, supervise effectively, and train personnel in the delivery of competent patient care and how to respond to emergencies. Much of the case law to date in this area of the law has concerned these three vital concepts, so ensure that all three issues are addressed.

Confidentiality

As a general rule, home care workers and the agency must treat as confidential any information that becomes known as a direct result of the agency–client relationship. Persons and agencies violating this rule may be liable for damages to the client. The Health Insurance Portability and

EXERCISE 19.2

A home health care aide cared for an elderly Alzheimer's patient for about 3 months. Additionally, the patient suffered from Parkinson's disease and was often irritable and disoriented. He had previously been declared mentally incompetent by the court.

As time progressed, the patient became more debilitated and began making crude remarks to the home health care aide, including some that were humiliating, insensitive, and sexually debasing. The home health care agency reported these remarks to her employer and asked to be removed from the care of this patient. The agency then informed the patient's family that it was withdrawing from the case, and the family initiated a lawsuit to prevent the discontinuance of services.

Who would prevail in such a case? Do any ethical principles also prevail in such a case? Should the agency have the right to refuse care to a patient, adjudicated as mentally incompetent, based merely on verbal comments?

Accountability Act of 1996 (HIPAA) laws also protect patients in home care settings. Review Chapter 9 for these laws.

There are some exceptions to this general rule regarding confidentiality. One exception allows the sharing of information among the various health care providers who are responsible for the client's care, including professional staff members, home health care aides, occupational or physical therapists, social workers, and the like. It is advisable to obtain the client's written provision for such sharing of information at the time of the initial contract. If no provision allows this sharing of information, then the client should sign a release form, authorizing such release of information. The release form should include exactly what information is to be released, to whom the information is to be given, and during what time the release is valid. This latter provision may be time-related or event-related.

Other exceptions include the release of information to third-party payers. This will be done by the client or client surrogate because release of this type of information is required before insurance companies and other third-party payers honor requests for payments. The client may also request information from the record, and the agency should have a written policy concerning the release of records to the client or client surrogate. Although the original record is the property of the agency, a copy may be given to clients for their records.

Refusal of Care

An issue of growing concern is clients' right to refuse treatment. Even if clients have previously consented to treatment, they can later withdraw consent. Verbal withdrawal of consent is adequate, and the agency staff should immediately communicate such withdrawal of consent to other members of the health care team and document the refusal or withdrawal of consent in the agency record.

Refusal of care is dependent on informed consent. With informed consent, the client must be given sufficient information on which to base an informed choice. Information needed includes the purpose or expected outcome of the treatment or procedure, risks and complications that accompany the treatment or procedure, who is to perform the treatment or procedure, and alternatives to the treatment or procedure. To refuse treatment, patients need this information as well as the potential and realistic expectations of the refusal or withdrawal of consent. Again, the refusal and the client education must be documented in agency records.

Agency Policies

Home health nurses have a duty to inform themselves about written **agency policies** and procedures, because deviation from these policies may result in substandard care to the client. If the policies are outdated, communicate this to the agency so that there may be changes and more current policies. Additionally, ensure that the policies do not require the nurse to function outside of the scope of nursing practice. The employer's policies and procedures set the standard of care and will be used to show deviation from that standard if a lawsuit develops.

Malpractice and Negligence

Among the major roles of the nurse in community health settings are the responsibilities to assess and instruct patients and their families. The nurse must be able to identify significant changes in the patient's condition and decide if further medical or nursing intervention or hospitalization is required. If changes occur, the home health care nurse must convey clearly any concern and indication for further treatment. While clients have the right to refuse further interventions, nurses must ensure that they or their family members understand the nature and extent of change in their condition. It may be necessary for home health care nurses to contact their supervisor, other family members, and the physician. Because they are working alone in the home setting, it is vital that nurses carefully assess and communicate concerns quickly and appropriately.

In a case that exemplifies negligent training of employees, a home health care aide left a patient unattended in the shower while she did some other work in the patient's home. The patient, disabled and using a shower chair, was unable to control the temperature of the water and was scalded severely. The aide applied ice to the burned areas and attempted to reach her supervisor, who was unavailable at the time. The aide waited before calling an ambulance, and the patient suffered severe third-degree burns over a large portion of her body that required numerous operations and skin grafts (*Loton v. Massachusetts Paramedical, Inc.*, 1987). This case also exemplifies the need to evaluate and call for assistance immediately when needed.

Much of the current case law in this area concerns the duty to train and supervise in the home setting, particularly the training and supervision of home health care aides and nursing staff members. The *Loton* case exemplifies the need to properly train personnel, particularly when the patient is disabled and placed in a position in which harm is likely to occur. In a later case that shows this same need to train and supervise, a home health care aide lost control of a wheelchair on a hill and the 19-year-old quadriplegic was rendered unconscious (*R. W. H. v. W. C. N. S., Inc.*, 1992).

Both of these cases also show the failure to adequately supervise, an issue that is of extreme importance yet difficult to manage, given the isolated nature of home health care nursing. Nursing personnel should institute a system of periodic visits in the home to identify the efficiency and level of care being delivered by the home health care aide as well as other nursing personnel. Patient satisfaction questionnaires may be another means to pinpoint potential trouble areas so that follow-up visits can be made. Issues concerning supervision and proper delegation of care are covered in depth in Chapter 15.

Liability can also ensue for failure to meet standards of care in more traditional nursing interventions. For example, in *Olsten Health Services v. Cody* (2008), the client was discharged from the hospital with an almost-healed lesion near his coccyx. This progressed to a chronic problem that required surgical skin grafting over the course of several months. The client sued the home health care agency for negligence, and the court pointed to several factors in determining that the agency was liable to this particular client.

One of the first factors noted was that the home health care nurse could see that the wound was becoming worse over time, and that there was a smell suggesting that an infection was present. The client's home health aide reported to the home health care nurse that the client was cold and having chills, both indicative of possible systemic septicemia. The home health care nurse visited the client frequently, changing the dressings on the now-open wound, and attempted to inform the client's physician about the worsening wound. She left messages on the physician's answering machine over a period of several days. When she did finally reach the physician, the client was immediately rehospitalized and aggressive therapy begun.

The court faulted the home health care nurse for failure to intercede in a timely manner. When she first was unable to reach the physician, she should have taken the initiative to have the client taken to the physician's office or to the emergency center for immediate treatment.

Home health nurses are also accountable for ensuring that ordered treatments are initiated and completed. In *Wells v. Columbia Valley Community Health* (2006), the care of an elderly patient was compromised when the home health nurses began to focus on end-of-life care rather than continue to treat the patient's pressure ulcers aggressively. They failed to catheterize the patient as had been ordered, instead believing that the patient's son would ensure that his mother's clothing and bedding remained dry when he assured them he would perform these tasks. This failure to follow the order for needed catheterization was a significant factor in the continued ulceration of the patient's sacral area due to the continued presence of urine.

Similar to acute care settings, nurses may also be liable for the failure to deliver intravenous (IV) fluids at appropriate rates. In *McDonough v. Allina Health System* (2004), a home care nurse administered the patient's IV fluids at a rate that exceeded the manufacturer's recommendations; shortly following the rapid infusion of the IV fluids, the patient suffered a nonhemorrhagic infarction of the right middle cerebral artery. The literature that accompanied the IV fluids noted that too-rapid infusion could result in vascular occlusive events. Though the patient was unable to prevail in this lawsuit because the court was not convinced that the rapid IV infusion was the cause of the patient's stroke, the case does serve to reinforce the need for all nurses to maintain standards of care at all times and in all patient settings.

Unlike their hospital counterparts, home health care nurses may be uniquely protected legally when they work in private home settings. In *Tidey v. Holmes* (2007), a home health care aide was bitten by the patient's dog, a Rhodesian Ridgeback, a breed known to have vicious propensities. The law states that the owner of a dog known to have vicious propensities is legally liable if the dog attacks a visitor who has been invited to visit the home. In *Cole v. Hayes* (2007), a home health nurse was successful in her suit for a slip-and-fall injury on a patient's driveway. The court noted that if the patient's home premises are not maintained in a safe condition, a home health nurse has the same right as any other invited visitor to sue for negligence.

Patient Education

The duty to instruct patients is paramount in the home setting, because patients and family members must rely on these instructions when the nurse is not readily available. Education of the patient and family should include both preventative and self-care information, and the nurse must ensure that the patient and/or family member has understood the instructions. Asking for return demonstrations and ensuring that questions are answered appropriately are ways of validating patient understanding. Because references may not be available, nurses should refrain from answering questions or providing information until they are sure the information is correct. Thus, nurses in these settings must remain current in aspects of information they will be responsible for teaching.

EXERCISE 19.3

The assistance of a home health care aide was required by an elderly, home-bound patient who had a diagnosis of a bilateral stroke and decubitus ulcers that were responding slowly to treatment. Though he had difficulty verbalizing his needs and wants, he had been evaluated as being fully cognitive mentally, understanding what was said around him and responding appropriately. In assessing the patient's pre-stroke likes and dislikes, the family reported that the patient had a history of viewing "off-color" and sexually explicit late-night television shows. After his first stroke, he began also watching these types of shows during the day. Frequently, he would become almost combative when a family member turned the station from such shows.

The aide has now come to you, her supervisor, stating that whenever she cares for this particular patient, she is offended by the sexually explicit shows and "off-color" humor that he prefers. She has tried turning the television to other stations or turning it off, but the patient then becomes visibly upset and refuses to cooperate with his nursing care needs.

How do you begin to handle this type of issue? As an invited guest in the patient's home, should the aide be able to change the television station? Can the aide refuse to continue to work while such television shows are playing? Are there laws that protect the health care worker as well as the home health care patient?

PARISH NURSING

One of the newer concepts in the field of home health care nursing is that of **parish nursing,** sometimes referred to as health and faith nursing. Though such nursing has ancient historical roots, the specialization of parish nursing truly emerged in the mid-1980s. Parish nursing is based on the health and healing traditions found in many religions, as seen in the early works of monks, sisters, deacons, church nurses, and traditional healers. The spiritual dimension is central to parish nursing practice. The focus of parish nursing is the faith community and its ministry.

The mission of parish nursing is the intentional integration of the practice of faith with the practice of nursing so that people can achieve wholeness in, with, and through the community of faith in which parish nurses serve. The role of the parish nurse is closest to that of a volunteer nurse, as the majority of parish nurses are not paid workers or are paid by the parish per se as opposed to the recipient of health care. Chapter 18 presents a more complete description of volunteer nursing and the potential legal liabilities for this classification of nurses.

OCCUPATIONAL HEALTH NURSING

The expansion of practice in the area of **occupational health nursing** has greatly increased the potential for liability. This area of practice is greatly influenced by a variety of federal and state laws, particularly workers' compensation laws, mandatory reporting laws, and occupational safety and health laws. Because of the unique interplay between workers' compensation laws and the doctrine of respondeat superior, nurses in this setting face a higher risk of personal liability than do nurses in other settings.

The main law governing occupational nursing practice is the Occupational Safety and Health Act of 1970. Administered through the Department of Labor, it serves the following purposes:

- Encourage employers and employees to reduce workplace hazards and to implement new or improve existing safety and health programs
- Provide for research in occupational safety and health to develop innovative ways of dealing with occupational safety and health problems

- Establish separate but dependent responsibilities and rights for employers and employees for the achievement of better safety and health conditions
- Maintain a reporting and record-keeping system to monitor job-related illnesses and injuries
- Establish training programs to increase the number and competence of occupational safety and health personnel
- Develop mandatory job safety and health standards and enforce them effectively
- Provide for the development, analysis, evaluation, and approval of state occupational safety and health programs

The act does not cover: (1) self-employed persons; (2) farms that employ solely immediate members of the farmer's family; (3) working conditions for which other federal agencies regulate worker safety, such as mining, nuclear energy and nuclear weapons manufacturing, and many aspects of the transportation industries; or (4) employees of state and local governments unless they are on one of the states operating an OSHA-approved state plan. Additional laws that affect the health and safety at the work site include the Americans with Disabilities Act of 1990, the Family and Medical Leave Act, and individual state workers' compensations laws. Review Chapter 13 for a more complete description of these laws.

State workers' compensation laws mandate the compensation of employees who are injured while at work in accordance with specific compensation schedules. These same laws make this the injured employee's sole remedy against the employer and thus deny the employee the legal right to sue the employer for damages even if the employer's negligence was the prime cause of the injury.

In a small minority of states, employees injured on the job may sue any person, including co-workers, but not their employer, for the negligent action that caused the resultant injury. In most states, the immunity extended to the employer is also extended to co-workers of the injured employee. Thus, a nurse employed by a company in these states is protected from civil liability in much the same manner as the employer. However, nurses may work as independent contractors within companies and thus are not protected.

Occupational nurses have responsibilities in a variety of areas, including adequate and rapid assessment of clients, communications with other health care providers who are frequently not at the work site, delivery of nursing interventions using standing orders and protocols, teaching preventative health and safety needs plus the teaching involved with specific diseases and conditions, development of safety programs within the setting, and verification of employees' ability to work. Thus, the job description of the occupational health nurse is of vital importance.

It is also important for these nurses to have specific guidelines, standing orders, and protocols. These written standards give guidance to nurses and serve to prevent greater liability exposure for them. If they were allowed to work under a "do whatever you think is necessary" standard, such a standard would open the nurses to charges of practicing medicine without a license as well as increased malpractice liability. Remember that nurses retain personal accountability for their actions, as well as potentially making other persons liable.

A case that exemplifies some of the nursing responsibilities of this role is *Therrell v. Fonde* (1986). In that case, an employee suffered a crushing hand injury, which was examined by the occupational health nurse. She examined and wrapped the injured hand and gave him an injection of either Vistaril or Demerol. The patient was then directed to wait in the outer waiting room while transportation was being secured. During the patient's hour wait for transportation to arrive, the company-employed physician arrived, was told of the injury, and refused to see the patient.

Eventually, the patient was seen at the health care facility that the company routinely used for its employees, and surgery was performed, resulting in a partial amputation of two fingers and permanent disuse of the index and little finger of his left hand. The suit was brought for negligence, alleging that the company failed to transport promptly and to adequately diagnose and treat his injury and that such conduct was willful, outrageous, and wanton.

Occupational health nurses may also have some accountability for the action of people other than health care providers who render first aid assistance at the work site. If occupational health care nurses have the responsibility to teach first aid or to ensure that needed supplies for first aid intervention are available, they may incur potential liability. Additionally, they will have potential liability if nurses note that first aid assistance is not being delivered correctly and fail to do anything about the lack of quality first aid assistance.

EXERCISE 19.4

Julio Ortis is an occupational health nurse employed in a state that has not granted immunity for co-workers of an employee injured on the job. Dr. Standahl is the plant physician, and a number of written protocols and standing orders guide Julio's practice in Dr. Standahl's absence. A patient who presented to the occupational health clinic during Dr. Standahl's absence was misdiagnosed and negligently treated by Julio; as a result of the negligent nursing care, the patient suffered permanent and extensive injuries.

Who has potential liability in this instance and why? How would the liability change if Dr. Standahl was present at the time of the patient's arrival but was unable to see the patient because of a second worker's injuries? What ethical principles has the nurse violated in giving negligent care to the employee? Which principles did Julio uphold in his care? What ethical advice would you give the nurse?

SCHOOL HEALTH NURSING

According to the National Association of School Health Nurses (1999), **school health nursing** is a:

> specialized practice of nursing that advances the well-being, academic success, and life long achievement of students. . . . School health nurses facilitate positive student responses to normal development; promote health and safety; intervene with actual and potential health problems; provide case management services; and actively collaborate with others to build student and family capacity for adaptation, self-management, self-advocacy, and learning. (p.1)

Laws that affect school health nursing include Section 504 of the Rehabilitation Act of 1973, which mandated specially designed classroom instruction and specialized transportation services for children with disabilities. Two years later, the passage of the Education for All Handicapped Children Act of 1975 broadened the previous law by adding an "inclusion" clause that mandated that children with various disabilities were to be part of the regular classroom instruction. The Office of Comprehensive School Health, which was established in 1979, extended health services to include preschool children; 1979 also saw the advent of the Head Start programs across America. Other laws that indirectly affect student health issues include the Elementary and Secondary Educational Act of 1965 and the No Child Left Behind Legislation of 2001. The first piece of legislation assists funding to educational institutions for children from low-income families, and the No Child Left Behind legislation begins to ensure equality for educational opportunity rather than equalized funding for all schools. The Health Insurance Portability and Accountability Act of 1991 also mandates confidentiality for health information in schools.

School health nurses function is a variety of ways in providing health services, from administration of first aid and prescribed medications to screening for height/weight and visual acuity, counseling for a variety of health conditions, and implementing nursing interventions such as the changing of dressings, suctioning, and catheterizations. These nurses also assist with the formulation and evaluation of individualized educational plans and individualized health plans, depending upon the needs of the children served in the school district.

School health nurses face much of the same type of increased liability issues as occupational health nurses. In most jurisdictions, the school nurse is subject to the same potential liabilities as other governmental workers, because of the relationship of the school district (employer) to the state. This exposes the nurse to greater potential legal liability for injuries.

Because these nurses work in a nonmedical environment, school nurses must exercise considerable independent judgment and must be able to recognize and treat illnesses or injuries or know when to seek immediate assistance. This includes the ability to assess the situation quickly, treat the child if appropriate, or make arrangements for the child to be taken for immediate medical attention.

Two recent lawsuits that illustrate the potential liability for school health nurses are *Garcia v. Northside Independent School District* (2007) and *Gray v. Council Bluffs Community School District* (2006). In the first case, a 14-year old asthmatic high school student had been authorized by his parents to be administered asthma medications on a daily treatment schedule. He was also to have his asthma inhaler with him at all times. The school's physical educational teacher was not apprised of the student's need for immediate access to his asthma inhaler, and the student experienced an asthmatic attack during one of the gym sessions. He did not have his inhaler with him and the student expired before the inhaler could be located and brought to him. The school nurse and the school district were both held liable for the student's untimely demise.

In *Gray*, the young diabetic student had an individualized health plan, and he was to have his blood sugar level checked daily at 10:00 A.M. On the day in question, his blood sugar level was measured at 40 mg/dL and the teacher notified the school nurse of the abnormally low blood sugar level. The nurse administered a glucose gel tube, authorized in advance by his mother, and then the nurse called the mother. Following this phone call, the nurse had the boy eat a snack of milk and crackers, rechecked his blood sugar, and obtained a reading of 56 mg/dL, which rose to 149 mg/dL at 11:00. The remainder of the day was uneventful.

The parents later sued the school district, claiming that their son had experienced a diabetic seizure at school and that the school nurse was responsible for the seizure. The court dismissed the case, noting that it could not find any evidence of negligence on the part of the nurse or other school official in this incidence. The school had followed the individualized health plan and responded appropriately and timely.

Many children visit the school health nurse for traumatic injuries, and the nurse must be competent to provide an emergency standard of care. If injuries occur after school hours, and they frequently do in schools with competitive sports teams, the nurse may be functioning outside the usual scope of her employment, and the standard of the reasonably prudent nurse in an emergency setting will determine potential liability.

One court case that exemplifies this need to follow an emergency standard is *Schlussler v. Independent School District No. 200 et al.*, a 1989 Minnesota case. In that case, a child had come to the nurse's office, suffering from an asthmatic attack. The nurse assessed the situation, gave another child's inhaler to this child, and sent the child back to the classroom. After other children came to the office concerned about this child's breathing pattern, the nurse assessed the child and determined that neither supplemental oxygen nor emergency transportation via an ambulance were needed to transport this child to the physician's office. Within minutes after leaving the school, the child collapsed and died following a brief comatose period.

The court, on hearing evidence from a nursing and an asthma expert witness, concluded that school nurses have a higher duty of care than hospital nurses to make an assessment of the need for emergency medical services. Although they are not expected to provide medical treatment, they are expected to determine the need for those services and for immediate, safe transportation to emergency medical care. The nurse's action also fell below the acceptable standard of care when she used another child's inhaler for this child.

Actions that could have been performed in this case include competent assessment skills, performance to a standard of care and laws governing prescription medications, better monitoring of the student, adherence to school policy concerning the notification of parents (particularly in a case in which the child has no prescription medications for asthmatic attacks), and consultation with other school health nurses and health care providers to develop written criteria for such emergency conditions.

A case that could greatly affect school nurses is *Cedar Rapids Community School District v. Garret F.* (1999). In that case, the U.S. Supreme Court considered the care of a disabled child in light of the Individuals with Disabilities Education Act (IDEA) (20 U.S.C. Section 1400[c]). The section specifies that to help "assure all children with disabilities have available to them . . . a free appropriate public education which emphasizes special education and related services designed to meet their unique needs," the IDEA authorizes federal financial assistance to states that agree to provide such children with special education and related services as defined by the law (at 993).

Respondent Garret F. was a wheelchair-bound and ventilator-dependent schoolchild who required, in part, a responsible individual nearby to attend to his physical needs during the school day. The Community School District refused to accept financial responsibility for the services that Garret required, believing it was not legally obligated to provide continuous one-on-one nursing care. The requested services in this case were supporting services because Garret could not attend school without them, and the requested services were not medical services, but rather those that could be provided by registered nurses educated in the care of ventilator-dependent patients.

The Supreme Court held in this case that the school district was obligated to provide these services for Garret F. during school hours. The related services are those needed by Garret F. to be assisted to "meaningfully access public schools" as a disabled child. The holding has great implications for school districts, beyond financial implications. Public school nurses will become responsible either as the direct provider of care or indirectly as the coordinator of care to students with respirators, feeding tubes, and other chronic health needs that require services that are not medical services.

Correctional Nursing

A newer role is that of **correctional nursing,** and the health care needs of this population present unique challenges for nurses. Nurses in this setting provide care for persons from the time of arrest and entry into the correctional system, through transfers to other facilities, to the person's final release from custody back into the community setting. The American Correctional Health Service Association (2009) describes the functions of health professionals working in this setting. Correctional nurses assess the need for and implement medical treatment as needed, based on the informed consent of the confined person and recognizing that the confined person has the right to refuse such treatment. Emergency treatment may be undertaken in situations in which there is the potential for grave disability and immediate threat of danger to the inmate or others in the area. The privacy rights of the inmate are continually respected, and health care is provided to all inmates regardless of their custody status. Specimens are collected and analyzed only for diagnostic testing based on sound medical principles. Body-cavity searches are only conducted after proper training and not by health care providers in a provider–patient relationship with the inmate. All medical information is confidential and health care records are maintained and transported, as appropriate, in a confidential manner. Biomedical research may only be conducted when the research methods meet all federal requirements and the individual inmate or prison population is expected to derive benefits from the results of the research.

The majority of the health care delivered in these settings involves primary health care and is often preventative, including prenatal care, immunizations, violence prevention, and screening for suicide risk. Nurses also treat a variety of illnesses and disease conditions, including infections, minor injuries, asthma, diabetic care needs, injury rehabilitation, and monitoring for conditions such as coronary artery disease, congestive heart failure, chronic lung diseases, and other long-term chronic conditions. Persons in this setting are also at an increased risk for communicable diseases, violence-associated risks, and substance abuse.

An inmate's right to the provision of appropriate health care is based on the Eighth Amendment of the U.S. Constitution, under the "cruel and unusual punishment" clause. Inmates can and do sue prison medical and nursing personnel who are indifferent to their serious health needs. The court noted in *Spann v. Roper* (2006) that these types of lawsuits have become far more numerous than lawsuits for professional malpractice in instances where inmates receive inadequate health care based on their medical needs. The vast majority of these lawsuits alleging violation of the right to be free from cruel and unusual punishment in the form of indifference to the inmate's serious medical needs are dismissed by the courts. For example, in *Rix v. Strafford County Department of Corrections* (2006), the nurse mixed Lantus insulin with another brand of insulin, then gave the injection to the diabetic inmate, causing a serious reaction. The court found the nurse liable for the drug reaction, but not for deliberate indifference to the inmate's medical needs. Thus, there was no Eighth Amendment violation in this case.

In *Carter v. Benevides* (2007), a prison inmate woke in a pool of blood and requested medical treatment. He was seen in the prison infirmary and then transported to the emergency center of a hospital. The prison contracted with this private hospital for medical care of the inmates requiring medical care that the prison infirmary was unequipped to provide. While at the emergency center, the inmate received supplemental oxygen and an IV was started. He was forced to stand and move to another bed, then left alone for an extended period of time. When the nurse returned, she discontinued the IV and supplemental oxygen, informed the inmate that there was nothing wrong with him, and had him transported back to the prison. No physician ever saw the inmate and, at trial, testimony revealed that no physician was ever informed of the inmate's presence in the emergency center. The inmate was subsequently transferred to another acute care facility where he underwent surgery for a bleeding ulcer.

The nurse and hospital in this case were both liable to the inmate for the deliberate indifference to the inmate's serious medical needs. The court noted that the Eighth Amendment rights of the inmate attached to this private hospital and its personnel because of their contract with the prison for the provision of medical care.

Graham v. Secure Care, Inc. (2007) illustrates some of the unique legal challenges of working in this setting. Unknown to the arresting officers, the suspect had swallowed an ounce of cocaine at the time of his arrest. He was booked into the county jail, where he became violently ill.

The nurse who had completed his routine jail admission assessment tried to find out what might have caused this sudden illness. The suspect denied that he had any immediate medical needs as well as denying that he had taken any medications or narcotics. When his condition changed for the worse, he was taken to the jail medical clinic and then to the hospital, where he expired from the cocaine ingestion. His sister brought a wrongful death cause of action, naming the nurse, her employer, and the company under contract to provide inmate medical services as defendants.

The Court of Appeals of Michigan dismissed the lawsuit. The basic rule is that no one is allowed to sue for damages for the consequences of his or her own actions. Thus, it was legally irrelevant in weighing civil liability for substandard health care whether the patient's medical condition stemmed from inadequate self-care or was actually self-inflicted. The patient's active concealment of the true nature and cause of his medical condition caused the health care team to be unable to intervene in time to save him from the end-effects of his own wrongful conduct.

EXERCISE 19.5

The nurse in a correctional facility gave an inmate three tablets, which he protested were not his usual medications. When he asked what the medications were and why they were ordered for him, the nurse told him that they were a new order and "just take them." After additional resistance, the inmate finally took the medications. Returning to the jail infirmary, the nurse realized that the medications, three potent antipsychotics, were meant for another inmate.

The nurse waited 3 hours before re-checking on the inmate who had taken the medications. During that time interval, the mediations caused the inmate to collapse in his cell and to hit his head as he fell. He was promptly taken to an acute care facility, and he fully recovered from his head injuries. After being transported back to the prison, he filed a lawsuit naming the nurse and the prison as defendants. His cause of action was for violation of his Eighth Amendment rights and for negligence in giving him the mediations.

How should the court respond in this issue? Did the nurse meet the criteria for a valid Eighth Amendment lawsuit? Was there negligence in how this patient was treated?

Disaster Nursing

Some broad guidelines may be applied to **disaster nursing,** in which a nurse either volunteers or is compensated for aid given during a disaster. The standard of care in a time of a disaster usually becomes similar to the standard of care given in emergency situations. Once having decided to render aid, the level of skill and competency is that which a reasonably prudent nurse would do under the same or similar conditions. If the practitioner meets or exceeds these standards, there is no negligence.

A second consideration concerns assuming duties that one ordinarily does not assume. In a true disaster, the professional nurse may be asked to perform actions usually reserved for physicians and medical residents or for nurses with advanced education and skills. Provided the nurse has the knowledge and skills required to perform the actions competently, he or she is permitted to give such substituted care. An emergency exception to either the nurse practice act or other statutory or common laws allows the expanded scope of practice in emergency settings.

Health care providers, once committed to aiding those injured in a disaster, have a duty to give safe, competent care. Remember, though, that no one can meet the standards of safe and competent care when physically or emotionally exhausted. Allow time for needed rest. The quality of the health care provider's work will greatly increase if the individual is able to reach sound decisions, and the probability of a negligent action will be diminished.

GUIDELINES

Disaster Situations

1. Be prepared. Know in advance your capabilities and what to do should a disaster occur. Know the limits of your professional liability policy and the provisions of your nurse practice act. Ensure that certifications such as advanced cardiac life support and pediatric advanced life support are current.
2. Maintain at least an emergency standard of care. Perform functions that you are qualified and skilled to do, even if they are outside your normal nursing actions, when instructed to do so by those in authority.
3. Allow for needed rest periods. If you are so exhausted you cannot make valid judgments, no one benefits from your care or presence.
4. Make notes and record happenings as quickly as possible after rendering nursing care. These notes and records will help to refresh your memory as needed.
5. Volunteer to be a part of community disaster planning committees. Such committees function to ensure that the needed planning and coordination are done before a disaster happens, effecting a more unified and prepared response to the disaster situation.

Nurses, especially those working in community and public health arenas, and other health care providers may also be involved in disaster response. The National Disaster Medical System is a federally coordinated system that was primarily established to integrate national response capability for assisting state and local authorities in dealing with the medial impact of natural disasters. Nurses are involved in every level of this coordinated system, serving to prepare guidelines and policies for implementation in the event of a natural or national disaster; planning for disasters with state and local agencies; collaborating with other disaster team members on plans, procedures, and tasks; coordinating the disaster team at various locations within the community; triaging at community area health care facilities; and treating victims.

SELECTED ETHICAL ISSUES

Ethical issues in public health nursing may arise from a variety of aspects. Relationships may pose ethical concerns, especially with physicians who devalue the unique knowledge of patients that so many home health care nurses develop over time. This may be especially seen when one considers that home health care nurses and aides generally see the patient on a daily basis or several times a week, as opposed to the primary health care physician who sees the patient on a very infrequent basis.

The allocation of resources and the maintenance of quality in the face of diminishing resources pose ethical issues for many public health nurses. As health care agencies, particularly public health agencies, are forced to minimize operating costs and decrease their workforce, multiple concerns about the adequacy and appropriateness of allocation of the remaining resources are emerging. If the goal of public health nursing is the prevention of illness and the promotion of the healthiest state possible for individuals and communities, then how does one justify the suspension of home health care programs that serve diabetic clients or supply milk and other essential nutrients to women and infants? Can one justify the potential outcomes if reduction of school health nurses force schools merely to set medications in a safe place for the child to come and take the medication on his or her own? This could be the result if schools are not able to afford school health nurses or to train other staff members to safely administer the medications needed for school-age children.

Empowerment of persons through educational programs and the importance to support autonomy in clients may also emerge as ethical issues for public and community health nurses. Both of these concerns involve the need for nurses to advocate for the clients they serve and not to allow the clients to become overly dependent on the nurse, but to become more reliant on themselves for meeting their own health care goals. But what if the person refuses to become more reliant on himself or herself? Can the public health nurse merely become a bystander and allow the person to adopt an unhealthy lifestyle? Can the school health nurse stand aside and watch a child not receive the care he or she needs merely because the parent has not provided the necessary permission form?

Nurses must recognize their own personal values and attitudes in relation to the programs under the Social Security Act of 1935 and realize that these attitudes and values may cause conflicts for them. For example, if the nurse believes that single mothers should not receive monetary support from the government, the nurse may have difficulty working with mothers receiving Aid to Families with Dependent Children (AFDC) assistance or even letting clients know that they are eligible for the services. Personal values and conflicts can also affect the standard of care with which one provides care, resulting in substandard care and potential harm to the patient or client.

Multiple unique ethical issues arise with caring for inmates and detainees. Issues may arise with the collection of evidence for forensic purposes, such as collecting blood or urine samples for evidence of alcohol usage, presence of illegal drugs, or for DNA samples. X-rays may be requested and taken solely as a means of searching for contraband so that the person can be charged with additional crimes. Body-cavity searches, done to discover the existence of illegal drugs and contraband, is a procedure reserved for the correctional system and may be requested of the nurse or other health care provider. Most health care professionals have only experienced the acquiring of blood or urine samples for solely medical purposes, including the diagnosing of disease states or to ensure the effectiveness of selected medical treatments, and the American Correctional Health Service Association principles mandate that health care providers collect and/or analyze specimens only for diagnostic testing based on sound medical principles.

SUMMARY

- Though the term *community health nursing* has been used for a number of years, the preferred title today is *public health nursing*.
- Multiple federal laws, predominately the Social Security Act of 1935 and the Public Health Service Act of 1944, are the driving forces that affect the U.S. health and welfare systems.
- Serving in a variety of settings, public and community health nurses care for persons

in need of their services in clinics, schools, individual homes, and the workplace.
- Community and public health nurses fulfill multiple roles, including home health care nursing, parish nursing, occupational nursing, school health nursing, correctional nursing, and disaster nursing.
- The legal responsibilities for each of these roles vary greatly, depending upon applicable state and federal laws or the absence of

such regulatory laws, practice site, and whether a paid or volunteer service.

- Perhaps the role with the greatest potential legal liabilities is that of the home health care nurse, with case law supporting this statement.
- Correctional nursing is one of the newest roles, presenting some of the more unique legal challenges for nursing.

- The standard of care for disaster nursing is similar to an emergency standard of care and allows individual nurses to use the full potential of their nursing and critical thinking skills.
- Multiple ethical issues may be evidenced with public and community health nursing.

APPLY YOUR LEGAL KNOWLEDGE

1. How have the Social Security Act of 1935 and the Public Health Service Act of 1944, with their respective amendments, changed the health care delivery system in the past 10 years?
2. What advice should be given to nurses seeking employment as occupational health nurses or school health nurses about their potential legal liability?
3. What is the applicable standard of care for community health nursing? How does this standard differ from that in acute care settings? Why are there different standards of care between the two arenas of nursing?
4. How could your assistance be best utilized in the event of a natural or national disaster? Name three things you can begin to do today to ensure your competency should a disaster affect your community.

YOU BE THE JUDGE

Mrs. McGrady was a home health care aide. She worked exclusively with an elderly woman who had limited mobility and who lived alone. Mrs. McGrady worked a regular 6:00 A.M. to 3:30 P.M. shift. She assisted the patient with bathing, dressing, personal care, housekeeping, and meal preparation. She drove the client to various places in town, and did the client's grocery shopping, including getting her fresh fruit from the local farmer's market.

One day after breakfast, the client asked Mrs. McGrady to take the dog out to the yard. Mrs. McGrady did this on a fairly regular basis, sometimes two to three times per day. While in the yard, the aide saw a pear growing on a tree in the client's yard, and Mrs. McGrady decided to climb the tree to pick the pear. Mrs. McGrady had done this type of activity on previous occasions without incident. While climbing the tree on this occasion, Mrs. McGrady fell, sustained a severe compression fracture, and filed for workers' compensation.

QUESTIONS

1. Was Mrs. McGrady within the course and scope of her employment when she fell from the tree?
2. Was Mrs. McGrady negligent in her actions?
3. Was this aide entitled to workers' compensation for this specific injury?
4. How would you decide this case?

REFERENCES

American Correctional Health Service Association. (2009). *Principles of correctional health services.* Alpharetta, GA: Author.

American with Disabilities Act of 1990. Public Law 110-325, 104 *Statutes* 327 (July 26, 1990).

Carter v. Benevides, 2007 WL 676686 (S. D. Tex., March 1, 2007).

Cedar Rapids Community School District v. Garret F., 119 S.Ct. 992 (1999).

Centers for Medicare and Medicaid Services. (2009). *Home health quality initiatives: An overview.* Baltimore, MD: Author.

Cole v. Hayes, 2007 WL 1228053 (Dist. Ct. Tulsa Co., Okla., February 14, 2007).

Education for All Handicapped Children Act of 1975. Public Law 94-142 (December 2, 1975).

Electronic Submission of OASIS, Part 484. (2005, December 23). *Federal Register* (pp. 76199–76208). Washington, DC: Government Printing Office.

Elementary and Secondary Educational Act of 1965. Public Law 89-10, 79 *Statutes* 27 (April 11, 1965).

Family Medical Leave Act of 1993. Public Law 103-3 (February 5, 1993).

Federal Register. (January 25, 1999). *Home health: HCFA now requires OASIS, electronic reporting for Medicare patients.* Sections 484.11, 484.20, 484.18, 484.55, 3747–3785. Washington, DC: Government Printing Office.

Garcia v. Northside Independent School District, 2007 WL 26803 (W. D. Tex., January 3, 2007).

Gray v. Council Bluffs Community School, 2006 WL 33313947 (Iowa App., November 16, 2006).

Graham v. Secure Care Inc., 2007 WL 122127 (Mich. App., January 18, 2007).

Health Insurance Portability and Accountability Act of 1996. Public Law 104-191, 110 *Statutes* 1936 (1996).

Loton v. Massachusetts Paramedical, Inc. (Mass. Sup. Ct., 1987). *National Jury Verdict Review and Analysis* (1989).

Lundy, K. S., & Janes, S. (2009). *Community health nursing: Caring for the public's health.* (2nd ed.). Boston: Jones and Bartlett Publishers.

McDonough v. Allina Health System (Minnesota App., August 17, 2004).

Morris v. North Hawaii Community Hospital, 37 F. Supp.2d 1181 (D. Hawaii, 1999).

National Association for Home Care and Hospice. (2008). *Basic statistics about home care.* Washington, DC: Author.

National Association of School Health Nurses. (1999). *Definition of school nursing.* North Branch, MN: Sunrise River Press.

No Child Left Behind Act of 2001, Public Law 107-110, 115 *Statutes* 1425 (January 8, 2002).

Occupational Safety and Health Act of 1970. Public Law 91-596, 84 *Statutes* 1590 (December 29, 1970).

Older Americans Act of 1987. Public Law 100-175 (November 29, 1987).

Olsten Health Services v. Cody, 2008 WL 583687 (Fla. App., March 5, 2008).

Omnibus Budget Reconciliation Act of 1987. Public Law 100–203, 101 Statutes 1330 (December 22, 1987).

Patient Self-Determination Act, Sections 4206 and 4751 of the Omnibus Reconciliation Act of 1990. Public Law 101-508 (November 5, 1990).

Public Health Service Act of 1944. Public Law 410, 58 Statutes 682 (July 1, 1944).

Rix v. Strafford County Department of Corrections, 2006 WL 2873623 (D. N. H, October 5, 2006).

Rehabilitation Act of 1973. Public Law 93-112. (September 26, 1973).

Rovaldi v. Courtemanche, 2005 WL 3455131 (D. Conn., December 16, 2005).

R. W. H. v. W. C. N. S., Inc. (1992). No. 88-CV-18315, *Medical Malpractice Verdicts, Settlements and Experts, 6,* 34.

Schlussler v. Independent School District No. 200 et al. Case No. MM89–14V, Minnesota Case Reports (Minnesota, 1989).

Social Security Act of 1935. Public Law 271. (August 14, 1935).

Spann v. Roper, 2006 WL 1912983 (8th Cir., July 13, 2006).

Therrell v. Fonde, 495 So.2d 1046 (Alabama, 1986).

Tidey v. Holmes, 2007 WL 2640658 (Super. Ct. St. Joseph Co., Ind., June 13, 2007).

Villarin v. Onobanjo, 714 N.Y.S.2d 90 (N.Y. App. 2000).

Wells v. Columbia Valley Community Health, 2006 WL 38131705 (E. D. Wash., December 27, 2006).

Winkler v. Interim Services, Inc., 36 F. Supp.2d 1026 (M.D. Tenn. 1999).

CHAPTER 20

Nursing in Long-Term Care Settings

PREVIEW

Though nurses have been employed in long-term care settings, primarily in nursing homes, for most of the last century, newer models for long-term care continue to evolve. Some of these newer models include rehabilitation centers, retirement homes, assisted living centers, and elder day care centers. Many of these newer models offer new and exciting opportunities for nurses, including more autonomous roles; all have some potential liability for the nurses practicing in these roles. This chapter presents an overview of these long-term care settings and the potential legal liability for nurses who are employed in these settings.

LEARNING OUTCOMES

After completing this chapter, you should be able to:

20.1 Define the various long-term care settings, including nursing homes, assisted living centers, hospice care centers, and elder day care centers.

20.2 Discuss aspects of providing quality care in long-term care settings, including:
- **a.** Falls and restraints
- **b.** Skin and wound care
- **c.** Nutrition and hydration
- **d.** Patient safety issues
- **e.** Patient transfer
- **f.** Duty to assess, monitor, and communicate

20.3 Describe the provisions and purposes of the Nursing Home Reform Act of 1987.

20.4 Discuss the nurse's potential liability issues for international and quasi-intentional torts in long-term care nursing.

20.5 Describe the purpose and potential liability involved in involuntary discharge.

20.6 Discuss the concept of elder abuse in the United States.

20.7 Describe ethical issues that can arise in long-term care settings.

KEY TERMS

assisted living
elder abuse
elder day care
hospice care

involuntary discharge
Nursing Home Reform Act
    of 1987

nursing homes
Residents' Bill of Rights

LONG-TERM CARE SETTINGS

As managed care continues to affect the size, structure, and length of stay in acute care facilities, more nurses are employed by long-term health care facilities, including nursing homes, assisted living centers, extended care facilities, day care facilities for adults, hospice centers, and skilled nursing homes. Though these types of settings have many similarities, there are also some differences that affect nursing care issues. A brief overview of the various settings examines these differences.

Nursing Homes

Nursing homes, residential living centers offering nursing care primarily for elders on a 24-hour basis, were the first model of long-term care to evolve and remain the type of facility that houses the majority of individuals receiving long-term care. Today, there are about 15,000 certified nursing homes in the United States, serving approximately 1.8 million residents. Approximately half of all residents are 85 years of age or older; virtually all residents are 65 or older. The median age of all residents is 83.2 years. The majority (69.2%) of residents are women, 97.3% have a least one disability, and approximately 83% of all residents require assistance with three or more activities of daily living (El Nasser, 2007; Harrington, Carillo, & Blank, 2007).

Nursing homes offer a variety of care services, including assistance with activities of daily living. Typical services in nursing homes include assistance with bathing, dressing, toileting, feeding, skin care, range of motion exercises, and ambulation, though other services such as dressing changes, medication administration, supplemental oxygen administration, and frequent repositioning are also provided in most nursing home settings.

Employees in nursing homes include administrators, social workers, registered nurses (RNs), licensed practical/vocational nurses (LPN/LVNs), certified nursing assistants (CNAs), and selected ancillary staff. Many of the nursing employees of these agencies are unlicensed assistive personnel (UAPs) and LPN/LVNs working with minimal supervision. Contract personnel include physicians and dentists.

Assisted Living Centers

Assisted living is a long-term care alternative for seniors who need more assistance than is available in a retirement center, but who do not need the more intensive nursing and medical care that is provided in nursing homes. Assisted living centers bridge the gap between independent living and nursing homes. Residents live in a congregate residential setting that generally provides personal services, 24-hour supervision and assistance, and planned activities and health-related services. These planned activities and services accommodate residents' changing preferences; maximize their dignity, autonomy, independence, and safety; and encourage family and community involvement. Assisted living services can be provided in freestanding facilities, in sites that are adjacent to nursing homes and hospitals, as components of continuing care retirement centers, or at independent housing complexes.

Approximately 900,000 individuals live in assisted living centers. The typical resident of an assisted living center is an 86-year-old woman who is mobile, but requires assistance with approximately two activities of daily living. Current data indicate that 76% of residents in assisted living centers are female and 24% are male. Most frequently, the two activities of daily living that these individuals need assistance with are bathing and dressing. Most of the residents also need assistance with instrumental activities of daily living, including telephoning, shopping, preparing meals, completing housework, taking medications, and managing money. Generally, the assisted living center employees supervise, assist, or administer medications as dictated by state rules and regulations. The average length of stay in an assisted living center is 27 months; 34% of the residents move to nursing homes from the assisted living centers and 30% die while living in assisted living centers (National Center for Assisted Living, 2006).

Employees in assisted living centers generally include registered nurses, certified nursing assistants, personal care attendants, health/wellness directors, activity directors, and administrative staff. Contract services include physicians, dieticians, and physical therapists.

Hospice Nursing Centers

Hospice care is a concept rooted in the centuries-old idea of offering a place of shelter and rest to weary and sick travelers. In 1967, this concept was expanded to describe the specialized care that may be given to terminal patients when they no longer benefit from curative care. Hospice treats the person rather than the disease, offering comfort care to individuals who are within the last 6 months of life. Care may be provided in home settings, and care may be provided in specialized care units, such as those attached to nursing homes, skilled care facilities, and hospitals, or provided in freestanding hospice centers. Provided by an extensive interdisciplinary team, hospice care entails spiritual, home, respite, and bereavement care. Because of the multiple facilities that provide hospice care, there is no current estimate of the numbers of patients currently cared for by hospice staff members or the number of these facilities in North America today.

Elder Day Care Centers

Elder day care is a concept that parallels the numerous child care centers provided in the United States. Initiated in the 1970s, there were approximately 300 centers nationwide in 1978, and today the number of adult day care centers exceeds 4,000. These elder care facilities provide care to adults who are unable to stay at home by themselves, allowing caregivers to continue to work outside the home. There are three types of day care centers:

- Adult day social care provides social activities, meals, recreation, and some limited health-related services.
- Adult day health care offers more intensive health, therapeutic, and social services for individuals with severe medical programs and for those at risk of requiring nursing home care.
- Alzheimer-specific adult day care provides social and health services only to persons with Alzheimer disease or related dementia.

Hours of operation generally are from early morning until 6:00 or 7:00 P.M.; individuals may access the care facilities on a daily basis or as needed. Most programs do not offer care on weekends, though some have a half-day service on Saturdays ("Adult Day Care," 2008).

LONG-TERM CARE NURSING: PROVIDING QUALITY CARE

Given the variety of facilities that provide long-term care and the extent of care that is delivered by these facilities, the nurse's potential for liability differs greatly. Generally, the potential liability for these nurses is similar to the potential liabilities of nurses working in home health care/ community agencies.

The majority of cases filed against nurses and long-term care facilities involve malpractice issues, and the standards of care differ somewhat from the applicable standards in acute care settings. Though the definition and elements remain constant, the application is unique to the circumstances and settings in which the care is provided.

Falls and Restraints

Similar to acute care settings, falls are one of the primary reasons that lawsuits are filed against long-term care facilities. Current statistics report that 3 out of 4 residents in nursing homes fall each year, averaging 2.6 falls per person per year. These falls result in serious injuries to between 10% and 20% of residents, and cause increasing disability, functional decline, and reduced quality of life (Centers for Disease Control, 2008). In this setting, unlike the acute care setting, falls are frequently more preventable and are thus less able to be defended (*Dubin v. United Nursing Services,* 2007; *Harrison v. Meriter Health Services,* 2007; *Shapiro v. Nyack Manor Nursing Home,* 2007).

For example, in *Gray v. Grenada Health and Rehabilitation* (2007), a nursing home resident fell repeatedly while attempting to ambulate to a bathroom, ultimately injuring herself to the extent that she incurred fatal injuries. The nursing home staff members were aware that the resident was continually getting up and going to the bathroom unattended, despite her cognitive deficits and ambulation problems. The court found that a fall-risk assessment should have been completed on admission, which would have shown that the resident was a high risk for falls and that a toileting schedule would have prevented the repeated falls. The expert nurse witness in this case noted that a toileting schedule is mandated when a cognitively impaired patient falls repeatedly to minimize the need for the patient to try to attempt to get up on her own. A toileting schedule also assures that there will be someone to assist the resident in ambulating to and from the bathroom, thus decreasing the possibility of falls.

Similarly, in *Estate of Myers v. NHC Healthcare* (2007), an elderly male resident fell eight times, each time while trying to ambulate from his bed to the bathroom. The final fall resulted in complete immobility due to his injuries, which then led to open bed sores for which he received substandard skin care. These outcomes, ruled the court, could have been prevented if the facility had implemented a toileting plan for the individual, ensuring that he used the bathroom on a regular basis rather than calling for assistance and waiting until someone could assist him.

Two cases (*Labarge v. Wisconsin Veterans Home,* 2007 and *Riverside Hospital, Inc. v. Johnson,* 2006) also held that bed alarms would have assisted in preventing patient falls. Both patients, one a 68-year-old Alzheimer patient and the other a 78-year-old patient with confusion and disorientation, among other diagnoses, fell when there were no bed alarm devices in use. Both courts concluded that such devices, if used properly, could have prevented the patients' falls.

The need to order restraints has been addressed by the courts. In *Danna v. Marina Manor, Inc.* (2003), the court determined that the nursing home where an 81-year-old resident resided had the legal duty to use a Posey restraint to keep the patient in bed and an additional duty to observe this resident more closely than she had been observed. The patient required, and the nurses should have sought a medical order for, restraints, as such mechanisms were needed to assure the resident's safety. A similar decision was reached in *Estate of Birdwell v. Texarkana*

Memorial Hospital, Inc. (2003). In this case, the patient's documented confusion and her inability to be taught safety measures indicated a need for further protection of the patient.

Courts, though, have also found that restraints are not always appropriate. For example, in a case cited earlier (*Gray v. Grenada Health and Rehabilitation,* 2007), the court deliberated on the appropriateness of restraints in preventing the resident's falls. An expert witness in the case testified that restraints would have increased the resident's confusion and decreased her quality of life. Interventions that were seen as appropriate included additional padding on the floor and/or additional padding on the resident herself to minimize the effect of a potential fall. The facility had already lowered the bed so that it was in its lowest position.

In *Yamin v. Baghel* (2001), an 89-year-old resident fell and broke her right hip while attempting to go from her bed to the bathroom without assistance. Though the resident was a high risk for falls, the resident was assessed as alert, oriented, and cooperative, with her short-term and long-term memory intact and with good safety awareness. She was instructed to use her call bell to summon assistance and not to attempt independent ambulation. The resident had demonstrated that she could and would call for assistance rather than attempt to ambulate on her own. In fact, she had called for assistance to use the bathroom a few hours before she attempted the ambulation that resulted in her fall.

In its finding, the court noted that restraints may not be routinely applied to patients whose individualized assessments do not point to a need for restraints to protect their safety. A facility will not be penalized merely because, in hindsight, the patient would not have fallen if restrained.

If restraints are used, then they must be used correctly and the resident properly supervised. *Lakeridge Villa Health Care Center v. Leavitt* (2006) concerned an inspection by the state health agency that occurred in response to a resident's complaints. Noting that federal regulations require nursing facilities to provide adequate supervision and assistance devices to prevent accidents, the inspection revealed three instances creating immediate jeopardy to the health and safety of actual residents. One resident, who had an impaired cognitive status and a history of falling out of bed, was restrained, with the bed rails in their lower position, and unsupervised. The inspectors in this instance noted that there had been no documentation of supervision for several hours. A second resident was also restrained and unsupervised; similar to the first resident, there was no documentation of supervision for this resident. The third resident was placed in an improperly sized vest restraint and became suspended while the inspectors were in the facility. He, too, was unsupervised. Finally, the inspectors reported that the restraints in use were found attached to immovable objects in a manner warned against by the manufacturer of the restraint devices.

The inspection also revealed that the facility failed to provide ongoing assessment and reassessment of the impact and appropriateness of patients' restraints. One resident was ordered to be restrained pending the healing of a hip fracture. Though the fracture had fully healed 3 months earlier, the patient was still in a restraint device. Two other residents were to be released from their restraints at least every 2 hours, but both were kept in their restraints for the 4-hour interval while the survey inspectors were on the premises. Based on the assessments of the survey inspectors, the facility incurred a significant monetary penalty. A second case where state inspectors' investigations resulted in significant monetary penalties for the nursing home concluded that actual harm to the residents does not need to occur. All that is necessary to justify imposing a penalty is a threat of more than minimal harm to a resident due to substandard compliance with Medicare participation requirements (*Harmony Court v. Leavitt,* 2006).

Residents must also be adequately restrained during transport. In *Health Facilities Management Corporation v. Hughes* (2006), a wheelchair-bound resident was transported in the nursing home's van to a dental appointment. When the nurse driving the van suddenly applied the brakes to avoid a collision with another vehicle, the resident, who was not strapped into the wheelchair, was thrown forward, striking her head and face on the seat in front of her. The injuries from this accident started a downward spiral in her overall condition. As her mood, mobility, and appetite decreased, she became more contractured, and developed both open bed sores and a urinary tract infection. She eventually died from sepsis, and the jury awarded her estate almost $2,000,000 compensation.

In some cases, patient falls and the use of restraints are both pled. In *Abrahams v. King Street Nursing Home, Inc.* (1997), the resident's family had filed a lawsuit alleging a preventable fall. The court found for the defense for the following reasons. There was no meaningful evidence presented showing how the defendant nursing home was negligent in its supervision of the care of the resident. The resident's physician had not ordered restraints during the day, and the nursing home's policy was that residents were not to be restrained without a physician's order. Additionally, there was no evidence presented that the resident's condition warranted the application of restraints.

In long-term care settings, the adverse effects of therapies must be evaluated when the best course of therapy for patients is considered. Restricting a patient's mobility can prevent falls, but can also force the elderly to live far more restricted lives than their limitations actually require them to live. Since the late 1980s, the federal government has discouraged the use of restraints, both physical and chemical, in the elderly, especially in long-term care facilities (Omnibus Budget Reconciliation Act of 1987). In settings in which restraints are seldom used, rates of falls increase, but the incidence of long-term injuries has not changed, supporting interventions that avoid the use of restraints, if possible.

EXERCISE 20.1

A patient weighing 450 pounds had surgery for a partial knee replacement on his left leg. The patient's right leg had been surgically fused at the knee 9 years earlier. Following acute care in the hospital setting, he was transferred to a combined nursing home–rehabilitation center for long-term convalescence.

At the rehabilitation center, the patient was being transferred from his wheelchair to a commode. Two nurse's aides assisted with the transfer, standing by his side in case they were needed to assist and allowing the patient to put his weight on his nonoperative leg. When the patient placed his weight on the nonoperative leg, he suddenly lost his balance and fell forward. Neither nurse was able to assist him as he fell, further injuring both knees.

Was this a type of incident in which the patient's fall was preventable and thus actionable? Were the nurses justified in their assessment of the patient as requiring only minimal assistance in the transfer to the commode? What additional facts would help in determining the extent of liability in this instance?

Skin and Wound Care

Due to the length of time residents remain in long-term care facilities, some types of cases become more prominent. Most lawsuits regarding decubitus ulcers arise in long-term care settings or in home care settings. For example, in *Convalescent Services, Inc. v. Schultz* (1996), a 77-year-old resident suffered from end-stage Alzheimer's dementia. The patient was bedridden and incontinent, and his extremities were contracted. On admission to the facility, the nursing staff noted a large, reddened area on his coccyx and buttock, classified as a stage I or stage II pressure ulcer. The ulcer worsened as the skin became broken 11 days after admission to the long-term care facility.

After a month, the patient was transferred to an acute care hospital for aggressive treatment of the ulcer, which now extended to the bone. He had several surgical procedures and was hospitalized for 3 months.

The family alleged that the long-term care facility was negligent in the care of the resident, specifically by the failure to:

1. Turn the patient every 2 hours.
2. Notify the physician when the ulcer worsened.
3. Follow the physician's orders for daily whirlpool therapy.
4. Ensure adequate nutrition.
5. Provide the appropriate mattress to relieve pressure on the ulcer.

The facility alleged that these were merely deficiencies in documentation. The court noted the rapid deterioration of the resident in upholding the verdict that substandard care had been given this resident. Additionally, he had developed new decubitus ulcers during his stay in the facility.

The court awarded punitive damages to the resident, based on a finding of gross negligence by the nursing home staff and administration. In doing so, the court used the following definition of gross negligence:

1. The act or omission, viewed objectively from the standpoint of the actor, involved an extreme degree of risk, considering the probability and magnitude of the potential harm to others.
2. The actor had actual, subjective awareness of the risk involved, but nevertheless proceeded in conscious indifference to the rights, safety, or welfare of others. (*Convalescent Services, Inc. v. Schultz*, 1996, at 736)

The court cited the extreme degree of dependency and vulnerability of this resident in determining the seriousness of the risks. Additionally, the facility continued to violate its own policies and procedures in caring for this resident. The facility also allowed the resident to rapidly deteriorate without informing the family of his status. The court held that these actions offended a public sense of justice and properly warranted the imposition of damages both as punishment and as a deterrent to such practices in an effort to ensure quality care for elderly persons in nursing homes.

The opposite finding was concluded in *Pack v. Crossroads, Inc.* (2001). The patient was discharged from an acute care setting to the nursing home following hip surgery. Six weeks after his admission to the nursing home, the patient was rehospitalized and died a week after his admission to the acute care setting. The attending physician at the acute care setting contended that the patient had suffered abuse and neglect in the nursing home, as evidenced by the patient's signs of dehydration and decubiti on both heels and his right hip. In the subsequent lawsuit, the court found for the nursing home and against the patient's family.

The most important factor in finding for the nursing home setting was the nursing documentation created at the nursing home. The admitting nurses had carefully assessed the patient when he was first admitted to the nursing home, noting that the patient already had pressure sores on both heels and redness and excoriation on his buttocks and perineal area on admission. The nursing notes also documented that the patient had been turned every 2 hours and that the patient received closer monitoring to ensure that he remain repositioned and off his back. Additionally, there was a flow chart that indicated how much fluid the patient was receiving with his meals and during the day. Output was not monitored as the patient was incontinent. Additional IV fluids were not administered, as the nursing home did not have the capability to administer IV fluids.

Finally, the nurse's notes documented the progression of the patient's skin lesions, noting that the physician was notified of this fact and that new orders, including an antibiotic and debriding agent, had been initiated during the patient's stay at the nursing home. The nurses also documented that the family had been approached about a transfer back to the hospital because of the increasing skin lesions, but the family refused such a transfer. Finally, while the patient was diagnosed with sepsis, there was no proof that this had developed in the nursing home rather than in the acute care hospital. Additional court cases, *Alexander v. Amelia Manor Nursing Home, Inc.* (2006), *Beverly Healthcare Kissimmee v. Agency for Health Care Administration* (2004), *Crestview Parke Care Center v. Thompson* (2004), and *Renfro v. E. P. I. Corporation* (2004), all supported the conclusion that pressure ulcers/decubiti do not in themselves result in a finding of negligence on the part of the nursing home.

An interesting twist to these cases occurred in *Emerald Oaks v. Agency for Health Care Administration* (2000). The court noted that quality of care may be met and residents who enter nursing homes without any evidence of skin breakdown may develop such pressure sores as their individual clinical conditions allow the development of such pressure sores. When this happens, the responsibility and weight of evidence is on the long-term care facility to show that the developing pressure sore was unavoidable, with all necessary treatment having been provided in a timely manner.

EXERCISE 20.2

The patient was ambulatory when she entered the nursing home and was assessed as being capable of turning herself in bed. She had a diagnosis of renal failure, hypertension, and peripheral vascular disease, all conditions that can predispose a person to skin breakdown. The resident's medical record showed that wound care nurses were seeing the resident on a regular basis and also indicated that a sacral skin lesion that began while the resident was in the facility had fully healed. At the time of her death, there was an open wound on her leg.

Her family brought a negligence lawsuit, alleging that the substandard care for the resident's skin integrity issues led to bed sores that progressed to serious lesions, eventually causing the need for amputation of her leg. Following this amputation, the resident became despondent, refused to eat, had difficulty sleeping, and finally refused to comply with her care interventions.

How should the court react to this case? Was the long-term care facility negligent in the resident's care? Did the staff have a further duty to ensure that this resident was turned in bed, despite the fact that the patient was capable of turning herself?

Nutrition and Hydration

Providing quality care includes the responsibility to feed residents who cannot safely feed themselves, the court ruled in *Thrasher v. Houston Northwest Medical Investors d/b/a Vila Northwest Convalescent Center* (1997). In that case, a 79-year-old resident with Alzheimer's dementia could not feed herself. Her family brought suit, alleging that the nursing assistants fed her improperly, causing her to choke and aspirate food into her lungs. Additionally, the family alleged that the facility failed to call emergency medical assistance quickly and to adequately oxygenate the resident while waiting for medical assistance to arrive. The resident was ultimately admitted to an acute care hospital, where she died 11 days after the aspiration from complications caused by the aspiration and hypoxia.

The defense was able to show that the patient choked because of her difficulty swallowing and not because of improper feeding techniques. They also showed through documentation that the resident was promptly assessed and treated and that she was oxygenated while awaiting the 911 ambulance. The court found for the defense.

The court may also find against the nursing home, however, as it did in *Beverly Enterprises Inc.-Virginia v. Nichols* (1994). The allegation was that the resident, an elderly patient with Alzheimer's dementia, died because employees failed to assist her with feeding. The resident's mental capacity was greatly diminished, and she was restrained and unable to eat unassisted. The resident had difficulty with choking prior to admission to the home, and the administrator and nursing staff had been informed by the family of the resident's need for assistance with feeding. During one visit, a relative of the resident noted that no one assisted the resident with eating, but merely left the tray at her bedside.

The following day, an employee placed the dinner tray by the resident, and a nursing assistant who was feeding the resident in the adjacent bed noted that the resident was having difficulty. The aide ran for assistance and returned with the nurse, but the resident had expired. Testimony from the nurse indicated that the resident did need to be spoon-fed, and that if a tray of food was left at the bedside, it would have been a mistake. The medical examiner testified that the autopsy revealed that the resident had died of asphyxia. No expert witness was required because the act of negligence clearly fell within the range of the jury's common knowledge and experience. The jury awarded the family $100,000.

Sometimes, the failure to provide quality care is termed *negligence of the elderly* by the court. The failure of a designated caregiver to meet the patient's basic care needs is generally accepted as a form of neglect. For example, in *Musgrove v. Medical Facilities of America* (2007), an elderly patient suffering from heart disease, diabetes, and peripheral vascular disease was admitted to the nursing home. Twice he was sent from the nursing home to an acute care facility. Both times the hospital found pressure sores and evidence of dehydration. He died in the hospital the second time he was admitted, and the attending physician listed dehydration as the cause of death on his death certificate.

In their case for negligence, the family's attorney was able to show that fluid output greatly exceeded fluid intake during the 10 days prior to this second admission and that the care facility had a fundamental responsibility to provide adequate hydration to a basically vulnerable adult such as this resident. If he was receiving adequate hydration, then that fact should have been properly recorded in the medical record. Additionally, the infrequent charting in the resident's medical record created the general impression that this resident was not adequately assessed or monitored.

Scampone v. Grane Healthcare Company (2007) reached a similar conclusion. In that case, the resident was transported by paramedics to the hospital after her son found her in bed lethargic and unresponsive. At the hospital, she was diagnosed as severely dehydrated and septic. Shortly after her admission, she had a major myocardial infarction and died. The nursing expert witness, using the resident's record for evidence, testified to the substandard and negligent nursing care that this resident had received. On only 4 days during the month prior to her admission to the hospital was there a notation in the medical record. There was no follow-up to the physician's order for lab cultures to see about a possible urinary tract infection, and thus there was no treatment for the infection that led to her sepsis and ultimate demise.

Patient Safety Issues

Failure to provide for the patient's safety has been addressed in court cases (*Miller v. Terrace at Grove Park*, 2007; *Ostrom v. Manorcare Health Services, Inc.*, 2007; *Pelletier v. Manor at Woodside*, 2007). In *Miller*, an elderly Alzheimer resident was fitted with an ankle bracelet meant to trigger an alarm if he tried to leave the facility. The bracelet system did not work and the resident eloped.

While wandering the neighborhood, he fell and cut his leg, which was not properly treated, leading to sepsis and his ultimate death. The facility was found liable for not preventing the resident's elopement and for failure to adequately treat his injury, once it occurred. Additionally, the assisted living care facility was also cited for accepting an Alzheimer resident when it did not have the capacity to adequately care for such a resident. In *Pelletier*, a 90-year-old-resident eloped from an assisted living facility and died due to hypothermia. This case also directly questioned the adequacy of care for a deteriorating Alzheimer resident to be in an assisted living center, even though the center had locked doors and an alarm on the door.

The final case also concerned the elopement by a resident with an Alzheimer diagnosis. Here the resident exited the facility into an enclosed courtyard, where he fell and sustained a serious head injury as he was attempting to run from the facility staff member who was chasing after him. The court noted that facilities that serve Alzheimer residents must be aware of their propensity for elopement.

Nursing homes also have a responsibility to protect patients from assaults by other residents. In *Dupree v. Plantation Pointe* (2003), a resident was known to wander into the rooms of other residents. He was abusive, both with physical violence and crude sexual displays and comments. Although the nursing staff knew of this behavior and appreciated the danger this patient presented, the only action taken to prevent such behaviors was an attempt to have the resident transferred to another nursing home. When a female resident was assaulted by this individual, the nursing home was found liable. The nursing home's defense was that Alzheimer patients often verbalize sexually inappropriate content. The court, though, held that verbal comments are very different from a resident who acts out in a frightening manner and one whom even the nursing staff is afraid to be left alone with in the same room.

The court in *Pollock v. CCC Investments* (2006) held an assisted living facility responsible when one resident of the facility murdered another resident. In finding liability, the court noted that the resident, diagnosed with major depressive disorder, dementia, and psychosis, had expressed to staff members that he could hurt himself or others. His psychiatrist ordered antipsychotic medications, and that his medication compliance and mental status were to be monitored by a psychiatric nurse. Since the facility had no psychiatric nurse, the resident should have been immediately transferred to an institution that could treat him.

Providing appropriately for a resident's safety entails the timely transfer of a resident to more appropriate care facilities should the resident's condition warrant such a transfer. In *Franklin v. Britthaven, Inc.* (2006), an 85-year-old resident was admitted to a nursing home with diagnoses of new-onset diabetes, urinary tract infection, agitation, confusion, angina, congestive heart failure, coronary artery disease, hypertension, and a history of transient ischemic attacks.

At about 7:00 one morning, he became pale. His oxygen saturation was noted to be low, so he was started on supplemental oxygen. He was seen by his physician at about 8:30, and it was decided that he needed to be transferred to an acute care hospital. The transport van arrived at 9:30 and he was moved to the hospital. At 7:00 that evening he died, and the causes of death were listed as an acute myocardial infarction, cardiopulmonary arrest, and probable sepsis.

His family sued the physician and the nursing home for wrongful death, noting that he should have been immediately transferred when he first became pale and his oxygen saturation fell. The court agreed that there is a legal responsibility to timely transfer a nursing home resident when his or her condition dramatically changes. If there is a delay and harm ensures, the nursing home and staff can be held liable. However, in this case there was lack of evidence to support that a 2-hour delay significantly caused this patient's demise.

As with acute care nursing, facilities have a responsibility to ensure that the equipment used in long-term care facilities is safe and is used appropriately. Liability was assessed against a nursing home when the back of a shower chair used for a resident's bath broke when he sat on the chair and leaned back. Visual inspection of the shower chair showed that one or more of the screws holding the back of the shower chair had rusted or were missing (*Wilson v. Invacare Corporation*, 2006). In *Quigley v. Tacoma Home* (2007), an aide used a shower chair to transport a resident. When she lowered the back of the chair to roll the resident over a raised doorway threshold, the resident struck his head, resulting in a subdural hematoma that caused his death 2 days later.

A final example of failure to safeguard a resident occurred in *Liberty Commons Nursing and Rehabilitation Center v. Leavitt* (2007). A nursing assistant wore latex gloves while caring for a resident with a known allergy to latex, causing the resident to suffer an allergic reaction that required hospitalization. This event triggered a state inspection of the facility, in relationship to federal regulations requiring long-term care facilities to develop and implement written policies and procedures that prohibit mistreatment, neglect, or abuse of residents (Nursing Home Reform Act, 1987). The facility was cited for a series of four staff errors, including:

1. the nursing assistant was unfamiliar with the resident and his allergies;
2. warning signs about the latex allergy were missing from the resident's room;
3. the nursing assistant did not receive a verbal warning in the report at the beginning of her shift about the allergy; and
4. the nursing assistant herself failed to consult the resident's chart until the end of the shift.

In upholding the assessed penalty for failure to follow federal regulations, the court noted that this was not an isolated error but instead showed a wider pattern of failure to implement protective measures for the safety of dependent patients. Thus this particular violation of federal regulations did pose immediate jeopardy to the health and safety of the other residents.

Patient Transfer

Patient transfer and the provision of sufficient numbers of staff to ensure that such transfer is performed competently serves as the basis for cases among this population. For example, in *Pock v. Georgian Rehabilitation House* (2007), a 65-year-old resident was unable to stand and could not bear weight on her left leg. She was assessed as needing two persons to transfer her, and a sign over her bed alerted staff that a two-person transfer was mandatory. One nurse alone attempted to move her and the resident fell, fracturing her ankle. The resident required surgery and the facility was assessed $200,000 as a settlement to the resident's family for the facility's substandard care of the resident. A similar result occurred in *Ingarra v. Rosewood Care Center* (2007).

Providing quality care during patient transfers may result from understaffing to the point that staff members have little time to read care plans. In *Penalver v. Living Centers of Texas, Inc.* (2004), the resident's care plan called for two attendants to work with her at any time she was transferred from her wheelchair to her bed, as she was considered a "dependent" transfer. Additionally, a transfer belt was to be used. On the day before her death, one certified nursing assistant attempted to transfer the resident by herself. The resident fell during the transfer, and trauma was ruled as the cause of the resident's death.

The aide testified that she had not read the nursing care plan as she did not have time to read the plan and that, had she read the plan, she would have known that this patient was a two-person transfer. On the day in question, the nursing home was critically understaffed. Two aides had called in sick and the administrator did not call in off-duty personnel nor did she telephone the facility's four sister facilities to locate available staff. She also had not called a staffing agency for additional help. The court laid the blame for this incident completely on the administrator and director of nursing, noting that they had deliberately allowed the facility to be understaffed. The family was awarded damages of $856,000.

EXERCISE 20.3

The resident was transferred to the hospital after she complained of leg pain and the nurses began to notice swelling of her leg. At the hospital, an orthopedic surgeon found a hip fracture he believed had to be at least 2 weeks old. He also said that the fracture most likely had to have been caused by a fall of some sort. The family sued the nursing home, alleging that an aide must have dropped the 79-year-old woman during a dependent transfer.

    The nursing home convinced the court to dismiss the case at trial level, basing its request on the fact that there was nothing in the nursing documentation about the resident being mishandled or falling. The case was then remanded to the appellate level for further determination. How should the appellate court rule in this case? Can you envision at least two possible bases for the family's lawsuit? What would the family be required to show to prevail in this case? Who should prevail in the end?

Duty to Assess, Monitor, and Communicate

Quality of care ensures that information about a resident's condition is conveyed in a timely manner, as illustrated by *McMackin v. Johnson County Healthcare Center* (2003). In that case, the resident had frequent transient ischemic attacks (TIA) during which she would become confused and unable to verbalize. These TIAs occurred fairly regularly and were well documented in the nursing progress notes. Nothing was said to the resident's physician about these episodes, nor were steps taken to refer this resident for a neurological work-up. Shortly before she died, the resident had another episode early one afternoon during which she had difficulty verbalizing and was crying; the aides reported this finding to the professional nursing staff. The night nurse finally decided to notify the physician at about 4:30 A.M the next morning. The resident was transferred to an acute care facility, where she died the next week. In finding for the resident's family, the court ruled it was not necessary to prove conclusively that timely and aggressive follow-up would have prevented her terminal stroke. It was only necessary to prove that the nurses failed to take appropriate measures, including notifying the physician of a change in the resident's condition, in a timely manner.

    Liability issues in long-term care facilities differ from liability issues in acute care settings because of the lack of direct physician contact with residents. The need for nursing staff to adequately assess changes and potential problems and notify the resident's physician or the medical director of the facility is critical. In *State v. Peoples* (1998), the court held that negligent actions by a director of a nursing home were not criminal negligence, but would support a finding of civil negligence. In *Peoples,* aides in the nursing home repeatedly told the director that a certain resident was vomiting. The resident vomited 17 times in a 42-hour interval, and the director was notified at home on the first night he had problems, was told throughout the day that he was still vomiting, and was called the second night at home because of the continued vomiting. She neither notified the resident's physician nor instructed the aides to notify the resident's physician. Even though the resident died of heart failure related to a lower gastrointestinal bleed, unrelated to his vomiting, the court held that the nurse would be liable for malpractice in a civil lawsuit.

    To further protect these patients, the **Nursing Home Reform Act of 1987,** part of the Omnibus Budget Reconciliation Act of 1987, was passed. This specific piece of legislation came as a direct result of a 1986 study that showed residents of nursing homes were being abused, neglected, and given inadequate care. The basic objective of the Nursing Home Reform Act of 1987 was to ensure that residents of nursing homes receive quality care that will result in their achieving or maintaining their "highest predictable" physical, mental, and psychological well-being. To secure quality care, the act requires the provision of specific services to each resident and establishes a **Residents' Bill of Rights.** Enumerated in the Residents' Bill of Rights are the following provisions:

- The right to freedom from abuse, mistreatment, and neglect
- The right to freedom from physical restraints
- The right to privacy
- The right to accommodation of medical, physical, psychological, and social needs
- The right to participate in resident and family groups
- The right to be treated with dignity
- The right to exercise self-determination
- The right to communicate freely
- The right to participate in the review of one's care plan, and to be fully informed in advance about any changes in care, treatment, or change in status in the facility
- The right to voice grievances without discrimination or reprisal (Nursing Home Reform Act of 1987, section 483.10)

In addition to this federal statute, states and selected nursing homes have instituted individual Residents' Bills of Rights. These bills outline the rights of persons in the nursing homes, and courts have uniformly upheld the rights of residents when such rights have been violated. Case examples include *St. Angelo v. Healthcare and Retirement Corporation of America* (2002) and *Terry v. Red River Center Corporation* (2003).

Intentional and Quasi-Intentional Torts

Nursing homes and other long-term care facilities also have a responsibility to protect residents from intentional and quasi-intentional torts. Case examples of such decisions include those in the area of confidentiality and privacy rights, freedom from harm, and freedom from assault and battery. *State v. Larson* (2003) held that all areas of a nursing home, including the dining areas, are not public areas but private areas and essentially the equivalent to a resident's home setting. Thus, it is proper for a nursing home to have a policy that prohibits residents from being photographed without their consent and to prohibit residents not able to give their consent from being photographed altogether.

In *Starkey v. Covenant Care, Inc.* (2004), the court ruled that a health care provider could not release medical records to a third party without the proper written permission from the patient. In this case, the patient's daughter presented a document that stated the patient had appointed the daughter as her power of attorney. Pages were missing from the document, the daughter presented only a photocopy of the document, and the facility referred the matter to its legal department, at which time the facility refused to release the patient's medical record. The court upheld this refusal, ruling that the facility could not release such records without proper and legal authorization.

In *Healthcare Centers of Texas, Inc. v. Rigby* (2002), a resident was acting out sexually at a nursing home. The extent and nature of his behavior were well documented in the nursing record. He had attempted to sexually assault an elderly male resident who was blind, disoriented, and suffering from Alzheimer disease. When a resident's daughter was threatened, the nursing director wrote in the nurse's note that "This resident is at risk for harming others" (*Healthcare Centers of Texas, Inc. v. Rigby,* 2002, at 31769624). He was discharged from the nursing home, temporarily admitted to a state psychiatric facility, and subsequently admitted to a second nursing home. The staff nurses and aides at this second nursing home immediately began to see that there were problems with having this patient in their facility. However, they did not take any steps to prevent him from assaulting a helpless female resident in her room some 10 days after his admission. In its decision, the court noted that when it is foreseeable that a patient can and will harm another person, it is imperative for the health care facility to take steps to prevent such harm.

Finally, in *Marchbanks v. Borum* (2001), the question of assault and battery arose when a patient was sedated with Haldol and transferred to a nursing home setting. In this particular case, the patient had established a pattern of allowing her niece to give valid informed consent on her behalf. At the time of the incident, the patient had become extremely combative, aggressive, and agitated. The treating physician determined that the best course of action to care for this patient was to transfer her to a nursing home setting where she could be adequately supervised during her recovery from gallbladder surgery. The court noted that this was a judgment call, but given the facts of the case and the patient's previous actions, this was not a case of assault and battery, and placement in the nursing home was reasonable.

Involuntary Discharge

Involuntary discharge from the nursing home, similar to discharge from home health agencies, may be permitted under the law. For example, in *Robbins v. Iowa Department of Inspections* (1997), a nursing home discharged a patient for violent conduct and verbal abuse of others, specifically running his wheelchair into other residents and restraining their freedom of movement, and for directing abusive language at both residents and staff members. The facility attempted several times to stop the resident's acting out to no avail, and the court held that, with proper notice, the home could discharge this resident. In fact, the court noted that an extended care facility risks liability for keeping a resident who poses a threat of harm to other residents.

In *Board of Health Facilities Administrators v. Werner* (2006), an elderly gentleman was admitted to a long-term care facility with a diagnosis of organic brain syndrome. For almost 3 years, he had numerous incidents of aggression toward staff members and other residents. Some of the incidents involved physical assaults on other residents, while other incidents were merely verbal.

The resident was seen numerous times by psychiatric professionals. Recommendations were made that he needed a structured behavior program, something the facility did not have. With organic brain syndrome, he was not a candidate for hospitalization in an acute psychiatric hospital. At times his acting out would subside and at other times his acting out was quite alarming to the facility staff.

The administrator began the process of involuntary removal from the facility to a facility that had a structured behavior program. The state long-term care ombudsman told him that she would block any such transfer, and the administrator halted the involuntary process proceedings. The resident then attacked a vulnerable female resident, who used a walker, pushing her against a wall. The injured resident died from her injuries and the episode prompted a state inspection.

During the inspection, the department found a violation of federal regulations, specifically the requirement that long-term care facilities attend to their residents' psychosocial needs. In addition, the administrator was cited for not proceeding with the involuntary transfer of this resident, as he should have known that the ombudsman had no legal authority to block an involuntary transfer.

To discharge a resident involuntarily, written notice must be given to the resident, a responsible party, a state agency, or an ombudsman. The resident has the right to social work counseling and a written plan of care. Residents can also ask the court to oversee that their rights are being honored or to negate the whole process if they are not honored.

Emergency transfers may be done without the required 30-day federally mandated notice, dependent upon the circumstances warranting the transfer. In *Florida Department of Veterans*

Affairs v. Cleary (2008), inappropriate sexual acting out toward other residents and staff was becoming more of a behavior pattern. The family was approached about a possible transfer of the resident to a facility that could better handle the resident, but the family refused. The nursing home went forward with the transfer, which occurred 23 days later, 7 days short of the federal regulations mandating 30 days' notice prior to such an involuntary transfer. The court supported this early transfer, noting that the transfer should occur as soon as practical, as the health and safety of other residents in the facility were at stake.

The Nursing Home Reform Act of 1987 also applies to nursing home admission practices, stating that a nursing home must not require a third party to guarantee payment to a facility as a condition of admission or continued stay in the facility. This act applies whether the nursing home accepts Medicare and Medicaid applicants or is a private-pay extended facility. A family member who voluntarily agrees to co-sign as a financially responsible party is entitled to advance written notice before a nursing home can legally discharge the patient. The court in *Podolsky v. First Healthcare Corporation* (1996) held that it is unfair and a deceptive trade practice to allow a family member to sign as a third-party guarantor without advising that a co-signer is not required for admission, but only gives the co-signer the right to notice if the resident is to be discharged. A later case (*Guardianship of Skrzyniecki,* 1997) held that a nursing home does have the right to take legal action if a resident's guardian exhausts the resident's assets to pay for nursing home care but then neglects to apply for Medicaid or Medicare benefits for the resident.

As with admission to acute care facilities and home health care, patients or their surrogate decision makers sign contracts that outline the patient's rights and obligations and the facility's rights and obligations. Three cases, *Howell v. NHC Healthcare-Fort Saunders, Inc.* (2003), *Raiteri v. NHC Healthcare/Fort Sanders, Inc.* (2003), and *Romano v. Manor Care, Inc.* (2003), have all concerned the right of the patient/surrogate decision maker when arbitration is involved. All of the cited cases have upheld the use of arbitration when disagreements arise.

End-of-Life Care and Patient Education

Residents who are admitted to long-term care facilities have the same rights as all inpatients under the Right to Self-Determination Act of 1990. A research study investigating patients' understanding of the benefits and burdens of cardiopulmonary resuscitation, artificial hydration, and nutrition in the elderly concluded that, in general, the elderly actually perceive more benefit from these interventions than was previously thought (Corpolla et al., 1998). This underscores the need for continued patient education about the resident's right to self-determination as well as the benefits of the variety of therapies and treatments available to the elderly. Nurses should continue to teach patients about their options, empowering the patient and family members so that they remain competent decision makers.

EXERCISE 20.4

Julia works in the independent living section of a retirement community. Mrs. Chu is a patient who is terminally ill with cancer but is still able to care for herself and performs her own activities of daily living. Mrs. Chu executed a living will just prior to her admission, and her physician has signed a do-not-resuscitate order in the event of her demise. The retirement community has just enacted a new policy stating that all residents will be resuscitated in the event of a cardiopulmonary arrest, regardless of the resident's wishes. Should Mrs. Chu suddenly experience a cardiopulmonary arrest, what should Julia do? Whose rights prevail in such a situation? What types of ethical issues are involved with such a policy? Do patients retain their right of autonomy when they enter retirement communities?

Elder Abuse

The mistreatment of the elderly has prompted a legislative response to the issue, much as was done with child abuse some years ago. All states now have elder abuse laws, designed to protect the older, vulnerable adult from abuse, neglect, and financial exploitation. Though the laws differ from state to state, they generally define vulnerable adults as persons with a mental or physical condition that significantly impairs their ability to care for themselves. Some states also use a specific age, generally 60, though some states do not specify when the person is chronologically considered an elder adult for purposes of the law.

Although definitions vary, the term **elder abuse** overtly refers to the maltreatment of older people. Such abuse usually includes physical and psychological abuse and can be either intentional or unintentional, resulting from the actions or inactions of other people, usually caregivers. Physical abuse means intentional infliction, or allowing someone else to intentionally inflict, bodily injury or pain. Examples of such injury or pain include slapping, kicking, biting, pinching, burning, and sexual abuse. Examples may also include the inappropriate use of medications and physical restraints. Unintentional abuse is the failure of the caregiver to provide the goods, services, or care necessary to maintain the health and safety of the vulnerable adult. Neglect may be repeated conduct or a single incident that endangers the elder's physical or psychological well-being. Psychological abuse includes verbal harassment, intimidation, denigration, and isolation, as well as repeated threats of abandonment or physical harm.

Financial exploitation occurs when family members, friends, or paid caregivers take financial advantage of the person, stealing from bank accounts, selling possessions, and taking the elder person's Social Security checks for their own benefit. Financial exploitation includes the improper or unauthorized use of funds, property, powers of attorney, and guardianships. Exploitation may also include making elderly persons work against their wishes.

A case example of such exploitation is *Miller v. Dunn* (2006). An aide caring for an elderly resident in a nursing home wrote one of the resident's personal checks to herself in the amount of $15,000. Though the aide's name and the amount of the check were in the aide's handwriting, the signature on the check was genuinely that of the resident. The aide endorsed the check and deposited it into her bank account. The resident's niece, who had legal power of attorney for the resident, discovered the check about a month later and reported it to the nursing home administrator. The administrator contacted the state Department of Health and Senior Services along with the local police.

In her defense, the aide claimed that the patient had voluntarily given her the money as a down payment on a home purchase. Gifts and bequests from vulnerable persons to caregivers come under scrutiny for undue influence, defined by the court as meaning when a person uses dishonest motives to substitute his or her will for the will of another. Undue influence amounts to over-persuasion, force, or coercion. Coercion, in this case, was further defined as occurring when one person exploits another person's special vulnerability. In this case, the resident's extreme age and impaired mental and physical state easily led to the conclusion that undue influence was involved in this transfer of money to the aide. The court also noted that a vulnerable person's mental capacity does not have to amount to full-blown incompetence to find undue influence has occurred. Finally, the court noted the fact that there was no independent advice before this transaction in finding that undue influence had occurred.

United States v. Ashworth (2006) upheld the finding that identity theft is a form of financial exploitation and abuse if the victim of the identity theft is a vulnerable, elderly individual. In this case, an aide in a nursing home had stolen the identity of an elderly resident, and the aide subsequently emptied the resident's personal bank account. *Iroabuchi v. Commissioner of Human Services* (2007) upheld the disqualification of a licensed practical nurse from working with vulnerable nursing home patients when it was revealed that she had been previously convicted of shoplifting. In its finding, the court specifically noted that although the shoplifting conviction was a relatively minor criminal offense, it was a major drawback to being allowed to work in a position of trust with persons who are extremely vulnerable to thefts of their property.

Elder abuse is not an isolated problem in the United States today. Rather, all indicators suggest that the maltreatment of the elderly is widespread and occurs within all subgroups of the aged population. Estimates range from a 2% to 10% incidence of such abuse, based on various sampling, survey, and case definitions, although it is widely agreed that the accuracy of this estimate is difficult to ascertain due to underreporting of cases and the multiple definitions used by individual states (National Center on Elder Abuse, 2005). The profile of the person most likely to be abused is an elderly woman, unable or minimally able to care for herself, with limited periods of competency, and often depressed, with the oldest elders the most frequently abused. In over 67% of the reported cases, the abuser is an adult child or spouse who abuses by neglect, psychological abuse, exploitation, and physical abuse. Geroff and Olshaker (2006) reported that 48.7% of abuse cases involved neglect, 35.4% were psychological in nature, 30.2% concerned final exploitation, 25.6% involved physical abuse, 3.6% were caused by abandonment of the elderly person, 0.3% involved sexual abuse, and the remaining 1.4% were classified as other.

The overwhelming majority of states mandate the reporting of elder abuse, with the minority of states continuing to encourage the reporting of abuse. The standard for reporting is a reasonable belief that a vulnerable person has been, or is likely to be, abused, neglected, or exploited. Note that one does not need to be certain that abuse has occurred, but must have a legitimate basis for suspecting that abuse has or will occur. Reporting is thus done in "good faith." Most states grant immunity from civil and criminal action for reporting, and some prevent employment retaliation for reporting. Since the procedure for reporting and the agency to which the report is made varies from state to state, nurses are advised to explore their individual state laws regarding elder abuse.

Court cases that have resulted because of elder abuse involve physical, verbal, and sexual abuse of the elderly. For example, *Wyatt v. Department of Human Services* (2007) held that using a pillow to muffle a resident's cries constitutes physical abuse of a vulnerable person. It was immaterial, said the court, that the nurse's intent was to prevent other vulnerable residents from becoming alarmed by the resident's cries for help. In *Livingston v. Department of Employment Security* (2007), an aide was fired for slapping the face of an elderly resident, and the court noted that any touching of a resident is considered abusive if it is not directly related to the provision of nursing care. In this case, the aide had attempted to use the fact that she merely touched the resident's face to get her attention and had not truly "slapped" the resident.

Some courts distinguish whether the action of the caregiver is intentional or a reflex behavior. In *Wiley v. Department of Health and Human Services* (2002), a resident spit at an aide, who responded by slapping the resident. The resident was highly combative and frequently acted out toward staff members. The court in this case stated that the staff member's action was a reflex behavior and that the action was not willful, but merely a reaction to the resident's behavior. Abuse, said this court, is the willful infliction of injury, unreasonable confinement, intimidation, or punishment with resulting physical harm, pain, or mental anguish.

Abuse can also be a finding for what is often considered part of ordinary nursing care. *Taylor v. Department of Veterans Affairs* (2006) concerned a resident who was undergoing inpatient treatment for paranoid schizophrenia. Though the facility had a barber shop where residents could get a haircut and a shave, this particular resident did not like having his hair cut or his face shaved. Two nurses decided to provide these services when the resident was in his wheelchair by locking the wheels and holding his hands so that one of the nurses could cut his hair and shave his face. The court found that abuse of a vulnerable person includes mental, physical, sexual, or verbal abuse, such as actions or behaviors that conflict with a person's rights, willful violation of a person's privacy, or willful physical injury. The court upheld the nurses' termination for abuse of this vulnerable resident.

Note, though, that there must be some solitary evidence that abuse did occur for courts to hold a health care provider liable for that abuse. In *In re Abuse Finding* (2008), the court was unable to conclude that any abuse had occurred because the investigation into an alleged abuse situation was not fully conducted and the resident who alleged the abuse and who suffered from confusion could not distinguish which of two similar-looking aides was the abuser. Additionally, the resident was receiving Trental, an anticoagulant that made her more prone to bruising, thus the bruises on her wrists did not necessarily prove that anyone had handled her roughly.

Abuse can occur in home care settings, and *In the Interest of E. Z., Dependent Adult* (1998) is an example of the need for nurses to report such abuse. In this case, the court applauded the nurse who reported a case of elder abuse by her caretaker. E. Z. was 96 years old, suffering from organic brain syndrome and multiple medical conditions, and was living with her grandson. They both subsisted on her Social Security checks. On two occasions, a visiting nurse found the woman alone, helpless, and in serious need of attention. The nurse reported the situation to the human services department, so that an emergency court order could be obtained to take the woman to a hospital and then to a nursing home. A guardian ad litem was appointed by the court to represent the woman's interests. The court ruled that she was a victim of dependent adult abuse by her grandson-caretaker, who had apparently abandoned her.

Staff members may also be terminated for their failure to report abuse in nursing home settings. In *Brewington v. Sunrise Regency* (2007), an aide was terminated when he failed to report sexual abuse of a resident by another resident. The court noted that consenting adults who happen to live in nursing homes have the same privacy rights as everyone else to have consensual sexual relationships, and when such sexual acts involve a resident who is not mentally competent to give consent, the sexual contact is not consensual and thus there is an affirmative duty on the part of the witnessing employee to report the abuse.

Abuse can be based on the verbal comments made to a resident. In *Allen v. Department of Health and Human Services* (2002), the court held that a verbal threat may be considered abuse, even if there is no proof that the threats result in physical harm or pain to the resident. In that case, the resident kicked one of the nursing aides as she was being transferred from her wheelchair to a shower chair. The aide threatened to either beat or pinch the resident if she ever kicked her again. Though the court conceded that it was possible that the resident was not cognizant of the threat, the law presumes that instances of abuse of any sort cause physical harm, pain, or mental anguish. In *Mason v. Department of Public Health* (2001), the court concluded that even one incident of such verbal abuse is sufficient to discipline a staff member for elder abuse.

The court in *Appeal of Staley* (2007) held that the use of obscene and demeaning language was sufficient for verbal abuse of a resident. In this case, an aide was overheard using demeaning language while assisting a resident to use the bedside commode. Following this verbal abuse, the resident was noted to be visibly upset and reluctant to request assistance from other staff members when he again needed to use the bedside commode. This court noted that mistreatment of a vulnerable elder includes disparaging, derogatory, humiliating, harassing, or threatening language or gestures, and not just abusive physical contact. *Swift v. Evangelical Lutheran Good Samaritan Society* (2007) reached a similar conclusion when an aide, with a history of verbal abuse of vulnerable adults, responded in a harsh tone to a resident's call bell over the intercom that she was turning off the resident's call bell and that the resident had better not turn it on again.

Sexual abuse can also occur in long-term care settings. In *Dixon Oaks v. Long* (1996), an elderly resident could not walk or get out of bed on her own. The 79-year-old resident had a medical diagnosis of Alzheimer's dementia. Her daughter discovered a large bruise on her mother's buttocks and inner thigh. She was told by the nurse that her mother had fallen a few days earlier, and this was the possible source of the bruise. Two days later, while changing her mother's clothes, the daughter saw severe bruising and swelling in her mother's anal and genital area.

The following day, the daughter was contacted by the nursing home and told that a male resident had been caught fondling her mother's genitals. The same male resident had been found kissing and fondling her on more than one occasion. The male resident admitted having sex with the woman, and was arrested and charged with deviant sexual assault.

In *Regions Bank v. Stone County Skilled Nursing* (2001), the court held that health care facilities must observe the work performance of nurse's aides and must see them demonstrate competency in specific care tasks. Newly hired or newly certified male aides who are to work with vulnerable female patients must be observed by supervising nurses before they are allowed to work independently with these female patients.

Abuse can result in criminal charges being brought against the abusers. In *State v. Easton* (1998), two nonlicensed personnel working in a residential care facility were convicted of a felony offense and sentenced to 2 to 10 years in prison. Their crimes were committed when they tried to restrain a resident residing in the facility where they were employed. The two defendants refused to take directions from an experienced worker who knew how to take down and safely restrain a combative patient. Instead, they taunted and cursed the resident, tore his clothing, and struck him for 2 1/2 hours while the resident's agitation escalated, apparently trying to intimidate him into behaving and following the rules. Also, the defendants had created the emergency situation because their actions showed they had the willful intent to abuse this resident. Their convictions and sentences were appropriate, the court ruled. In *Goodlett v. Adventist Health Systems* (2007), the court upheld the criminal conviction of an aide who sexually abused a partially paralyzed 62-year-old stroke resident.

EXERCISE 20.5

An 83-year-old resident of a nursing home was physically in good health, but had been diagnosed with Alzheimer disease. At times, this resident would become confused and wander toward the doors of the nursing home, looking for her parents and a way to exit the facility. To prevent the resident from leaving the nursing home, she was fitted with a special bracelet that automatically locked an outer door if the resident came within 30 feet of the door. For fire-safety purposes, the door automatically unlocked within a 15-second time frame. Thus, staff members had essentially a 15-second time frame to notice an elopement attempt and redirect the resident.

Early one morning, the resident was trying to get out of the door and a staff member came up behind her, slapped her on the buttocks, grabbed her by the shoulders, turned her around, and shoved her back into an interior hallway. This episode was reported to the director of nurses. The director interviewed the other nursing staff members who were present during this incident; the director also examined the resident, noting that a red mark was present on the resident's buttocks. The director then reported the nursing staff member to the proper state agency, and the staff member was charged with criminal abuse of a nursing home resident.

Without argument, the treatment of this patient was abusive. The question is whether this was mere civil abuse or whether the manner of abusive behavior toward this elderly resident constitutes criminal abuse. State reasons why you believe that the nurse was correctly charged with criminal abuse or reasons why you do not believe that this type of charge was appropriate in these circumstances.

Ethically, how should this resident have been treated? What ethical principles were violated in this case?

GUIDELINES

Warning Signs of Elder Abuse and Neglect

Signs and symptoms frequently associated with abuse of an elder person include the following:

1. Widowed, elder female living on a fixed and limited income
2. Unusual or unexplained injuries such as cuts, bruises, and burns
3. Unkempt appearance and/or dirty and soiled clothing
4. Pressure or bed sores
5. Confinement against the person's will, such as being locked in a room or tied/restrained to a piece of furniture
6. Dehydration and malnutrition without a medical cause for such conditions
7. Fear, apprehension, and/or anxiety
8. Withdrawal or social isolation
9. Inconsistent or "strange" explanations for injuries
10. Helplessness and reluctance to talk with health care providers
11. Visits to multiple physicians and clinics
12. Depression

Signs and symptoms of a potential abuser include the following:

1. Adult, unemployed, and dependent child living with an elderly parent
2. Spouse of an elder person who requires extensive care
3. Verbally assaulting, threatening, or insulting the older person
4. Concerned only with the older person's financial situation, not the older person's health or well-being
5. Problems of the caregiver with alcohol, drug abuse, or gambling
6. Preventing the older person from speaking for himself or herself
7. Continually and constantly blaming the older person
8. An attitude of indifference or anger toward the elder person
9. Socially isolating the older person from outside contacts

All states and the District of Columbia have laws authorizing the Long-Term Care Ombudsman Program, which is responsible for advocating on behalf of long-term care facility residents who experience abuse, violations of their rights, or other issues. This program is mandated as a condition of receiving federal funds under the Older Americans Act of 1987 and the amended act of 1992. In selected states, the program fulfills the role of adult protective services and has the legal authority to investigate and respond to abuse occurring within long-term care settings. Additionally, a bill entitled Elder Justice Act of 2003 was introduced into the U.S. House of Representatives early in 2003 and reintroduced in the 2006 legislative session by both houses of the U.S. Congress. Though it failed to pass in either session, it had some important provisions that many continue to feel are important considerations in this area of the law, such as the following:

1. Establish dual offices of elder justice in the U.S. Department of Health and Human Services and the U.S. Department of Justice to coordinate elder abuse prevention efforts nationally.

2. Require an FBI criminal background check of long-term care nursing aides and better training for workers in the detection of elder abuse.
3. Establish the Office of Adult Protective Services within the U.S. Department of Health and Human Services, Administration for Children and Families.
4. Enhance law enforcement response.

EXERCISE 20.6

Indicate which of the following scenarios are examples of elder abuse and the type of abuse that each scenario depicts:

1. Alice, age 75, lives in a small apartment with her son Frank, 54. Frank moved in with his mother on the condition that he stop drinking and seek counseling for that problem. Frank found a job and began coming home later and later in the evening. Alice thought she smelled alcohol on Frank's breath, and she confronted him with that fact and told him he would need to find alternate living arrangements if he continued to drink. Frank became enraged, ran toward his mother with his fist raised over his head, and Alice fled to the safety of a neighbor's house.

2. Carol, 24, a single mom with two young children, lives in an apartment building where Beatrice, 86, also lives. Because of her arthritis, Beatrice seldom leaves her apartment and Carol frequently visits Beatrice, often helping with the laundry and small household chores in exchange for babysitting services. Carol also does some grocery shopping for Beatrice, frequently keeping the change from the money that Beatrice has given to Carol. Carol thinks this is fair, as she is taking the time and trouble to assist Beatrice.

3. Judy, 82, lives alone and suffers from chronic congestive heart failure and depression. She hates taking her diuretics because it is difficult for her to ambulate to the bathroom and she has had many "accidents." Thus, she has chosen not to take her medications as directed, and now her legs have become so swollen that she is unable to walk at all.

4. John, 72, partially blind and hard of hearing, lives with his son and daughter-in-law. Both the son and daughter-in-law are unemployed and refuse to help John leave the house for relaxation, walks, or doctor's appointments. They also refuse to allow John to use his Social Security money to buy a new hearing aid.

SELECTED ETHICAL ISSUES IN LONG-TERM CARE

One of the main ethical issues in this area of nursing concerns elderly individuals' autonomy, including their capability for decision making. This capability involves understanding what is being considered as well as appreciating the consequences of the decision. The decision should not be made under duress or in times of great stress, and the individual should be able to communicate the decision to others in a way that reflects the understanding of potential consequences and outcomes. Influencing factors, such as pain, depression, psychiatric illness, or effects of mediations, can affect this decision-making capacity. All of these influencing factors are often seen, some to a greater and some to a lesser degree, in the elderly residents of long-term care facilities. Thus, health care providers are ever aware of the need to promote the person's welfare and balance the benefits and burdens of decisions.

A second concern involves doing what is just or fair, especially with the distribution of benefits for all concerned. For example, how many staff resources can be devoted to a single disruptive nursing home resident when other, equally deserving, residents have needs that are not being met? Does partial care, what one can do under the circumstances and with the resources available at the time, meet the ethical principle of justice?

Nurses may be tempted to not report cases of abuse, primarily because of uncertainty concerning how to report such abuse and/or because of fear that they will somehow become involved in the stigma involved with the abuse. This is especially true if the abuse has been particularly shocking, such as occurs in sexual abuse of the elderly or such severe physical abuse that the elderly person is gravely harmed. Failing to report such abuse, though, prevents the person who is abused from obtaining the counseling and care that he or she needs to begin the healing process and prevent future harm. Nurses need to support one another in such instances, reporting the abuse to persons or agencies as appropriate, and assisting in subsequent investigations so that future individuals will not be similarly harmed.

Nurses may also be tempted not to report cases of abuse because the abused person asks that the abuse not be reported. This request is generally made in instances where the abuser is a family member and the person is afraid that reporting the abuse will make future abuse more severe or that he or she will be abandoned if the abuser is jailed. Such a request presents a true dilemma for the nurse or nurses involved. Does one tell the truth and report the abuse, following the principle of beneficence, or do as requested and allow the abuse to continue?

Jogerst, Daly, Brinig, et al. (2003) discovered that cases of abuse were more apt to be reported in states that had mandatory reporting laws than in states where such report was encouraged, but not mandated. Though this is not a surprising outcome, it does suggest that such underreporting may prevent the cessation of such abuse in the future or actually increase the possibility that rates of abuse will accelerate. Should not state legislatures examine these data and enact legislation that mandates the reporting of elder abuse similar to the mandated reporting of child abuse in all states? Though the mandatory reporting of child abuse has not eradicated such abuse, it does begin to assure the safety and care of abuse victims.

SUMMARY

- Long-term and home health care settings include a variety of facilities, including nursing homes, assisted living centers, extended care facilities, day care facilities for adults, hospice centers, and skilled nursing homes.
- Providing quality nursing care in any of these facilities is challenging, and the majority of cases filed by residents and family members concern malpractice and standards of care.
- To protect residents in these facilities, the Nursing Home Reform Act of 1987 was passed, requiring the provision of specific services to each resident and mandating provisions contained in the Residents' Bill of Rights provision of the law.
- In accordance with this federal mandate, states and selected nursing homes have instituted individual Residents' Bills of Rights that generally exceed the provisions of the federal statute.

- Long-term care facilities may also be liable for intentional and quasi-intentional torts and involuntary discharge of residents.
- Elder abuse, an international issue, refers to the maltreatment of older people, including physical, verbal, psychological, sexual, and financial exploitation abuse.
- Nurses, as well as the public at large, have a duty to report cases of elder abuse to the appropriate agency and/or administration of the facility.
- Health care providers can be held both civilly and criminally liable for abuse to elderly, vulnerable individuals.
- The Long-Term Care Ombudsman Program was established to assure advocacy on behalf of long-term care residents who experience abuse, violations of their rights, and other issues.
- Multiple ethical issues may arise when providing nursing care in long-term care settings.

APPLY YOUR LEGAL KNOWLEDGE

1. Why do the potential legal liabilities of nurses in long-term care settings more closely resemble the potential legal liabilities of community health nurses and home health care nurses than the potential legal liabilities of acute care nurses?

2. Should physical restraints be used with the elderly population? Why or why not?

3. How can nurses begin to address the issue of elderly abuse in long-term care settings?

YOU BE THE JUDGE

Mr. Aburu, 81, with a history of a cerebral vascular accident, was hospitalized as an outpatient for a surgical procedure to incise and drain a skin lesion on his chest. After the procedure, he returned to the long-term care facility with sterile packing in the partially sutured incision site. The packing was to remain for 3 days, then be removed, and the wound covered with a dry dressing. The risk of complications for this type of surgery were considered quite low, and both the nursing home administrator and the attending surgeon saw no reason why the patient could not be adequately cared for in the nursing home immediately after surgery.

Approximately 5 hours after Mr. Aburu returned to the nursing home, blood was observed at the incision site. He was transferred back to the acute care hospital, where he died the following day.

Evidence at trial showed that for the 5 hours that Mr. Aburu was at the nursing home, several licensed and unlicensed personnel attended to him. At lunchtime, two aides escorted Mr. Aburu to the dining room; lunch was about 3 hours after his return to the nursing home. None of the personnel examined his dressing until an aide noticed that he was bleeding though his bed sheets. Shortly after discovering the bleeding, the patient was transferred by ambulance to the hospital. His family has filed a lawsuit for the wrongful death of their father, alleging that the care given to the patient after surgery fell below the acceptable standards of care.

QUESTIONS

1. What should the standards of care be for such a patient?

2. Even though the nursing care plan did not specify that the wound should be checked hourly, how should the prudent nurse have acted?

3. Should the lawsuit center primarily on the surgeon for allowing this patient to be sent back to the nursing home for post-operative care rather than insisting he be kept for 24 hours in an acute care facility post-operatively?

4. How would you decide this case?

REFERENCES

Abrahams v. King Street Nursing Home, Inc., 664 N.Y.S.2d 479 (N.Y. App., 1997).

Adult Day Care. (2008). Definition, purpose, and description. Available online at http://www.surgery encyclopedia.com/A-Ce/Adult-Day-Care.html

Alexander v. Amelia Nursing Home Inc., 2006 WL 472289 (La. App., March 1, 2006).

Allen v. Department of Health and Human Services, 2002 WL 31889915 (N.C. App., December 31, 2002).

Appeal of Staley, 2007 730 N. W. 2d 289 (Minn. App., April 24, 2007).

Beverly Enterprises Inc.-Virginia v. Nichols, 441 S.E.2d 1 (Virginia, 1994).

Beverly Healthcare Kissimmee v. Agency for Health Care Administration, 2004 WL 177018 (Fla. App., January 30, 2004).

Board of Health Facilities Administrators v. Werner, 2006 WL 306385 (In. App., February 10, 2006).

Brewington v. Sunbridge Regency, 2007 WL 4522619 (M.D. N.C., December 18, 2007).

Centers for Disease Control and Prevention. (2008). *Falls in nursing homes.* Atlanta, GA: Author.

Convalescent Services, Inc. v. Schultz, 921 S.W.2d 731 (Texas, 1996).

Corpolla, K. et al. (1998). Perceived benefits and burdens of life-sustaining treatment differences among elderly adults, physicians, and young adults. *Journal of Ethics, Law, and Aging, 4*(1), 12–16.

Crestview Parke Care Center v. Thompson, 2004 WL 1432719 (6 Cir., June 28, 2004).

Danna v. Marina Manor, Inc., 2003 WL 22888936 (Mass. App., December 8, 2003).

Dixon Oaks v. Long, 929 S.W.2d 226 (Missouri, 1996).

Dubin v. United Nursing Services, 2007 WL 4954007 (Cir. St. Palm Beach Co., Fla., December 7, 2007).

Dupree v. Plantation Pointe, 2003 WL 22077863 (Miss. App., September 9, 2003).

El Nasser, H. (2007, September 27). Fewer seniors live in nursing homes. *USA Today.* Available at http://www.usatoday.com/news/nation/census/2007-09-27-nursing-homes_N.htm

Emerald Oaks v. Agency for Health Care Administration, 774 So.2d 737 (Fla. App., 2000).

Estate of Birdwell v. Texarkana Memorial Hospital, Inc., 2003 WL 22927420 (Tex. App., December 12, 2003).

Estate of Myers v. NHC Healthcare, 2007 WL 1247215 (Cir. Ct. Warren Co., Tenn., February 22, 2007).

Florida Department of Veterans Affairs v. Cleary, 2008 WL 53644 (Fla. App., January 4, 2008).

Franklin v. Britthaven, Inc., 2006 WL 2947295 (N.C. App., October 17, 2006).

Geroff, A. J., & Olshaker, J. S. (2006). Elder abuse. *Emergency Medicine Clinics of North America, 24,* 491–505.

Goodlett v. Adventist Health Systems, 2007 WL 1976779 (Dist. Ct. Tarrant Co., Tex., May 8, 2007).

Gray v. Grenada Health and Rehabilitation, 2007 WL 4224337 (N.D. Miss., November 27, 2007).

Guardianship of Skrzyniecki, 691 N.E.2d 1105 (Ohio App., 1997).

Harmony Court v. Leavitt, 2006 WL 22188705 (6th Cir., August 1, 2006).

Harrington, C., Carillo, H., & Blank, B. (2007). *Nursing facilities, staffing, residents, and facility deficiencies. Centers for medical services.* Washington, DC: United States Department of Health and Human Services.

Harrison v. Meriter Health Services, 2007 WL 4976341 (Cir. Ct. Dane Co., Wis., July 1, 2007).

Health Facilities Management Corporation v. Hughes, 2006 WL 301084 (Ark., February 9, 2006).

Healthcare Centers of Texas, Inc. v. Rigby, 2002 WL 31769624 (Tex. App., December 12, 2002).

Howell v. NHC Healthcare-Fort Sanders, Inc., 2003 WL 465775 (Tenn. App., February 25, 2003).

In re Abuse Finding, 2008 WL 125238 (Minn. App., January 15, 2008).

In the Interest of E. Z., Dependent Adult, 485 N.W.2d 214 (Iowa, 1998).

Ingarra v. Rosewood Care Center, 2007 WL 5075846 (Cir. Ct. Winnebago Co., Ill., November 29, 2007).

Iroabuchi v. Commissioner of Human Services, 2007 WL 1248177 (Minn. App., May 1, 2007).

Jogerst, G. J., Daly, J. M., Brinig, M. F., et al. (2003). Domestic elder abuse and the law. *American Journal of Public Health, 93,* 2131–2136.

Labarge v. Wisconsin Veterans Home, 2007 WL 2216534 (Cir. Ct. Waupaca Co., Wis., March 17, 2007).

Lakeridge Villa Health Care Center v. Leavitt, 2006 WL 3147250 (6th Cir., November 3, 2006).

Liberty Commons Nursing and Rehabilitation Center v. Leavitt, 2007 WL 2088703 (4th Cir., July 20, 2007).

Livingston v. Department of Employment Security, 2007 WL 2163996 (Ill. App., July 27, 2007).

Marchbanks v. Borum, 806 So.2d 278 (Miss. App., 2001).

Mason v. Department of Public Health, 761 N.E. 794 (Ill. App., 2001).

McMackin v. Johnson County Healthcare Center, 2003 WY 91, 2003 WL 21771691 (Wyoming, August 1, 2003).

Miller v. Dunn, 2006 WL 327850 (Mo. App., February 14, 2006).

Miller v. Terrance at Grove Park, 2007 WL 2216409 (Cir. Ct. Houston Co., Ala., February 9, 2007).

Musgrove v. Medical Facilities of America, 2007 WL 2614655 (Super. Ct., City of Danville, Va., June 18, 2007).

National Center for Assisted Living. (2006). *2006 overview of assisted living.* Washington, DC: Author.

National Center on Elder Abuse. (2005). *Fact sheet: Elder abuse prevalence and incidence.* Washington, DC: Author.

Nursing Home Reform Act of 1987, 42 *Code of Federal Regulations* 483 et seq. (1987).

Older American Act of 1987. Public Law 100–175 (November 29, 1987).

Older Americans Amended Act of 1992. Public Law 102–375 (September 30, 1992).

Omnibus Budget Reconciliation Act of 1987. Public Law 100–203, 101 *Statutes* 1330 (December 22, 1987).

Ostrom v. Manorcare Health Services, Inc., 2007 WL 188132 (E. D., Mich., January 22, 2007).

Pack v. Crossroads, Inc., 53 S.W.3d 492 (Tex. App., 2001).

Pelletier v. Manor at Woodside, 2007 WL 4863935 (Super. Ct. Dutchess Co., N.Y., December 11, 2007).

Penalver v. Living Centers of Texas, Inc., 2004 WL 1392268 (Tex. App., June 23, 2004).

Pock v. Georgian Rehabilitation House, 2007 WL 4616733 (Super. Ct. Pierce Co., WA, July 18, 2007).

Podolsky v. First Healthcare Corporation, 58 Cal. Rptr.2d 89 (Cal. App., 1996).

Pollock v. CCC Investments, 933 So. 2d 572 (Fla. App., May 24, 2006).

Quigley v. Tacoma Home, 2007 WL 4700969 (Super. Ct. Pierce Co., WA., May 23, 2007).

Raiteri v. NHC Healthcare/Knoxville, Inc., 2003 WL 23094413 (Tenn. App., December 30, 2003).

Regions Bank v. Stone County Skilled Nursing, 38 S.W.3d 916 (Ark. App., 2001).

Renfro v. E. P. I. Corporation, 2004 WL 224397 (Ky. App., February 6, 2004).

Riverside Hospital, Inc. v. Johnson, 2006 WL 3106157 (Va., November 3, 2006).

Robbins v. Iowa Department of Inspections, 567 N.W.2d 653 (Iowa, 1997).

Romano v. Manor Care, Inc., 2003 WL 22240322 (Fla. App., October 1, 2003).

Salmon v. Department of Public Health, 788 A.2d 1199 (Connecticut, 2002).

Scampone v. Grane Healthcare Corporation, 2007 WL 2728291 (Ct. Cm Pl. Allegheny Co., Penn., June 1, 2007).

Shapiro v. Nyack Manor Nursing Home, 2007 WL 1364523 (Super. Ct. Rockland Co., N.Y., April 12, 2007).

St. Angelo v. Healthcare and Retirement Corporation of America, 2002 WL 1972320 (Fla. App., August 28, 2002).

Starkey v. Covenant Care, Inc., 2004 WL 206209 (Cal. App., February 4, 2004).

State v. Easton, 510 S.E.2d 465 (West Virginia, 1998).

State v. Larson, 2003 WL 22766043 (Wash. App., November 24, 2003).

State v. Peoples, 962 S.W.2d 921 (Mo. App., 1998).

Swift v. Evangelical Lutheran Good Samaritan Society, 2007 WL 2472347 (Minn. App., September 4, 2007).

Taylor v. Department of Veterans Affairs, 2006 WL 678926 (Fed. Cir., March 17, 2006).

Terry v. Red River Center Corporation, 2003 WL 22901004 (La. App., December 10, 2003).

Thrasher v. Houston Northwest Medical Investors d/b/a Vila Northwest Convalescent Center (1997). No. 94-15038, *Medical Malpractice Verdicts, Settlements, and Experts, 13*(9), 27.

United States v. Ashworth, 2006 WL 2591933 (4th Cir., September 7, 2006).

Wiley v. Department of Health and Human Services, 2002 WL 31895023 (N.C. App., December 31, 2002).

Wilson v. Invacare Corporation, 2006 WL 167675 (La. App., January 25, 2006).

Wyatt v. Department of Human Services, 2007 WL 911892 (Iowa App., March 28, 2007).

Yamin v. Baghel, 728 N.Y.S.2d 520 (N.Y. App., 2001).

INDEX